Bronchopulmonary Dysplasia

LUNG BIOLOGY IN HEALTH AND DISEASE

Executive Editor

Claude Lenfant
Former Director, National Heart, Lung, and Blood
Institute National Institutes of Health
Bethesda, Maryland

1. Immunologic and Infectious Reactions in the Lung, *edited by C. H. Kirkpatrick and H. Y. Reynolds*
2. The Biochemical Basis of Pulmonary Function, *edited by R. G. Crystal*
3. Bioengineering Aspects of the Lung, *edited by J. B. West*
4. Metabolic Functions of the Lung, *edited by Y. S. Bakhle and J. R. Vane*
5. Respiratory Defense Mechanisms (in two parts), *edited by J. D. Brain, D. F. Proctor, and L. M. Reid*
6. Development of the Lung, *edited by W. A. Hodson*
7. Lung Water and Solute Exchange, *edited by N. C. Staub*
8. Extrapulmonary Manifestations of Respiratory Disease, *edited by E. D. Robin*
9. Chronic Obstructive Pulmonary Disease, *edited by T. L. Petty*
10. Pathogenesis and Therapy of Lung Cancer, *edited by C. C. Harris*
11. Genetic Determinants of Pulmonary Disease, *edited by S. D. Litwin*
12. The Lung in the Transition Between Health and Disease, *edited by P. T. Macklem and S. Permutt*
13. Evolution of Respiratory Processes: A Comparative Approach, *edited by S. C. Wood and C. Lenfant*
14. Pulmonary Vascular Diseases, *edited by K. M. Moser*
15. Physiology and Pharmacology of the Airways, *edited by J. A. Nadel*
16. Diagnostic Techniques in Pulmonary Disease (in two parts), *edited by M. A. Sackner*
17. Regulation of Breathing (in two parts), *edited by T. F. Hornbein*
18. Occupational Lung Diseases: Research Approaches and Methods, *edited by H. Weill and M. Turner-Warwick*
19. Immunopharmacology of the Lung, *edited by H. H. Newball*
20. Sarcoidosis and Other Granulomatous Diseases of the Lung, *edited by B. L. Fanburg*
21. Sleep and Breathing, *edited by N. A. Saunders and C. E. Sullivan*
22. *Pneumocystis carinii* Pneumonia: Pathogenesis, Diagnosis, and Treatment, *edited by L. S. Young*
23. Pulmonary Nuclear Medicine: Techniques in Diagnosis of Lung Disease, *edited by H. L. Atkins*
24. Acute Respiratory Failure, *edited by W. M. Zapol and K. J. Falke*

For information on volumes 25–186 in the *Lung Biology in Health and Disease* series, please visit www.informahealthcare.com

187. Oxygen/Nitrogen Radicals: Lung Injury and Disease, *edited by V. Vallyathan, V. Castranova, and X. Shi*

188. Therapy for Mucus-Clearance Disorders, *edited by B. K. Rubin and C. P. van der Schans*

189. Interventional Pulmonary Medicine, *edited by J. F. Beamis, Jr., P. N. Mathur, and A. C. Mehta*

190. Lung Development and Regeneration, *edited by D. J. Massaro, G. Massaro, and P. Chambon*

191. Long-Term Intervention in Chronic Obstructive Pulmonary Disease, *edited by R. Pauwels, D. S. Postma, and S. T. Weiss*

192. Sleep Deprivation: Basic Science, Physiology, and Behavior, *edited by Clete A. Kushida*

193. Sleep Deprivation: Clinical Issues, Pharmacology, and Sleep Loss Effects, *edited by Clete A. Kushida*

194. Pneumocystis Pneumonia: Third Edition, Revised and Expanded, *edited by P. D. Walzer and M. Cushion*

195. Asthma Prevention, *edited by William W. Busse and Robert F. Lemanske, Jr.*

196. Lung Injury: Mechanisms, Pathophysiology, and Therapy, *edited by Robert H. Notter, Jacob Finkelstein, and Bruce Holm*

197. Ion Channels in the Pulmonary Vasculature, *edited by Jason X.-J. Yuan*

198. Chronic Obstructive Pulmonary Disease: Cellular and Molecular Mechanisms, *edited by Peter J. Barnes*

199. Pediatric Nasal and Sinus Disorders, *edited by Tania Sih and Peter A. R. Clement*

200. Functional Lung Imaging, *edited by David Lipson and Edwin van Beek*

201. Lung Surfactant Function and Disorder, *edited by Kaushik Nag*

202. Pharmacology and Pathophysiology of the Control of Breathing, *edited by Denham S. Ward, Albert Dahan, and Luc J. Teppema*

203. Molecular Imaging of the Lungs, *edited by Daniel Schuster and Timothy Blackwell*

204. Air Pollutants and the Respiratory Tract: Second Edition, *edited by W. Michael Foster and Daniel L. Costa*

205. Acute and Chronic Cough, *edited by Anthony E. Redington and Alyn H. Morice*

206. Severe Pneumonia, *edited by Michael S. Niederman*

207. Monitoring Asthma, *edited by Peter G. Gibson*

208. Dyspnea: Mechanisms, Measurement, and Management, Second Edition, *edited by Donald A. Mahler and Denis E. O'Donnell*

209. Childhood Asthma, *edited by Stanley J. Szefler and Søren Pedersen*

210. Sarcoidosis, *edited by Robert Baughman*

211. Tropical Lung Disease, Second Edition, *edited by Om Sharma*

212. Pharmacotherapy of Asthma, *edited by James T. Li*

213. Practical Pulmonary and Critical Care Medicine: Respiratory Failure, *edited by Zab Mosenifar and Guy W. Soo Hoo*

214. Practical Pulmonary and Critical Care Medicine: Disease Management, *edited by Zab Mosenifar and Guy W. Soo Hoo*

215. Ventilator-Induced Lung Injury, *edited by Didier Dreyfuss, Georges Saumon, and Rolf D. Hubmayr*

216. Bronchial Vascular Remodeling in Asthma and COPD, *edited by Aili Lazaar*
217. Lung and Heart–Lung Transplantation, *edited by Joseph P. Lynch III and David J. Ross*
218. Genetics of Asthma and Chronic Obstructive Pulmonary Disease, *edited by Dirkje S. Postma and Scott T. Weiss*
219. *Reichman and Hershfield's* Tuberculosis: A Comprehensive, International Approach, Third Edition (in two parts), *edited by Mario C. Raviglione*
220. Narcolepsy and Hypersomnia, *edited by Claudio Bassetti, Michel Billiard, and Emmanuel Mignot*
221. Inhalation Aerosols: Physical and Biological Basis for Therapy, Second Edition, *edited by Anthony J. Hickey*
222. Clinical Management of Chronic Obstructive Pulmonary Disease, Second Edition, *edited by Stephen I. Rennard, Roberto Rodriguez-Roisin, Gérard Huchon, and Nicolas Roche*
223. Sleep in Children, Second Edition: Developmental Changes in Sleep Patterns, *edited by Carole L. Marcus, John L. Carroll, David F. Donnelly, and Gerald M. Loughlin*
224. Sleep and Breathing in Children, Second Edition: Developmental Changes in Breathing During Sleep, *edited by Carole L. Marcus, John L. Carroll, David F. Donnelly, and Gerald M. Loughlin*
225. Ventilatory Support for Chronic Respiratory Failure, *edited by Nicolino Ambrosino and Roger S. Goldstein*
226. Diagnostic Pulmonary Pathology, Second Edition, *edited by Philip T. Cagle, Timothy C. Allen, and Mary Beth Beasley*
227. Interstitial Pulmonary and Bronchiolar Disorders, *edited by Joseph P. Lynch III*
228. Chronic Obstructive Pulmonary Disease Exacerbations, *edited by Jadwiga A. Wedzicha and Fernando J. Martinez*
229. Pleural Disease, Second Edition, *edited by Demosthenes Bouros*
230. Interventional Pulmonary Medicine, Second Edition, *edited by John F. Beamis, Jr., Praveen Mathur, and Atul C. Mehta*
231. Sleep Apnea: Implications in Cardiovascular and Cerebrovascular Disease, Second Edition, *edited by Douglas T. Bradley and John Floras*
232. Respiratory Infections, *edited by Sanjay Sethi*
233. Acute Respiratory Distress Syndrome, *edited by Augustine M. K. Choi*
234. Pharmacology and Therapeutics of Airway Disease, Second Edition, *edited by Kian Fan Chung and Peter J. Barnes*
235. Sleep Apnea: Pathogenesis, Diagnosis, and Treatment, Second Edition, *edited by Allan I. Pack*
236. Pulmonary Hypertension, *edited by Marc Humbert and Joseph P. Lynch III*
237. Tuberculosis, Fourth Edition: The Essentials, *edited by Mario C. Raviglione*
238. Asthma Infections, *edited by Richard Martin and Rand E. Sutherland*
239. Chronic Obstructive Pulmonary Disease: Outcomes and Biomarkers, *edited by Mario Cazzola, Fernando J. Martinez, and Clive P. Page*
240. Bronchopulmonary Dysplasia, *edited by Steven H. Abman*

The opinions expressed in these volumes do not necessarily represent the views of the National Institutes of Health.

Bronchopulmonary Dysplasia

edited by

Steven H. Abman
University of Colorado
The Children's Hopsital
Aurora, Colorado, USA

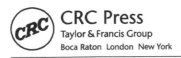

CRC Press
Taylor & Francis Group
Boca Raton London New York

CRC Press is an imprint of the
Taylor & Francis Group, an **informa** business

CRC Press
Taylor & Francis Group
6000 Broken Sound Parkway NW, Suite 300
Boca Raton, FL 33487-2742

First issued in paperback 2017

© 2010 by Taylor & Francis Group, LLC
CRC Press is an imprint of Taylor & Francis Group, an Informa business

No claim to original U.S. Government works

ISBN-13: 978-1-4200-7691-2 (hbk)
ISBN-13: 978-1-138-11504-0 (pbk)

Library of Congress Cataloging-in-Publication Data

Bronchopulmonary dysplasia / edited by Steven H. Abman.
     p. ; cm. — (Lung biology in health and disease ; 240)
   Includes bibliographical references and index.
   ISBN-13: 978-1-4200-7691-2 (hardcover : alk. paper)
   ISBN-10: 1-4200-7691-4 (hardcover : alk. paper) 1. Bronchopulmonary dysplasia. I. Abman, Steven H. II. Series: Lung biology in health and disease ; v. 240.
   [DNLM: 1. Bronchopulmonary Dysplasia—physiopathology. 2. Bronchopulmonary Dysplasia—therapy. 3. Infant, Premature. 4. Lung—embryology. 5. Lung—growth & development. W1 LU62 v.240 2009 / WS 410 B8687 2009]

   RJ320.B75B762 2009
   618.92'23—dc22

                      2009022303

Visit the Taylor & Francis Web site at
http://www.taylorandfrancis.com

and the CRC Press Web site at
http://www.crcpress.com

Introduction

Bronchopulmonary dysplasia (BPD) is a complex and challenging disease. Since its original description by William Northway and his colleagues in 1967, many significant advances have occurred. Yet, it remains a major cause of mortality and morbidity in premature neonates, the rates of which are inversely related to the birth weight.

This new volume, *Bronchopulmonary Dysplasia*, edited by Dr Steven Abman, presents the most recent progress to its readership. The role of genetic determinants and of individual and environmental factors in the occurrence and severity of BPD are extensively addressed throughout the chapters. Of great interest is the discussion of biomarkers in BPD, as eventually they may help predict the occurrence of the disease and thus lead to early application of therapeutic options. This has the potential to reduce mortality and may limit long-term consequences of the disease.

Recent studies underscore the significance of these consequences, that is, residual lung structural changes very similar to those caused by emphysema (1–3). This concept is not new as for years neonatologists and pediatricians have called BPD a "chronic lung disease of early infancy."

Today, chronic bronchitis and emphysema (currently termed chronic obstructive pulmonary disease—COPD) are recognized as major worldwide public health problems. Although smoking is undoubtedly the main risk factor, we are well aware of the occurrence of these diseases in nonsmokers. Thus, emphysema-like lesions and bronchial obstruction that develop in survivors of BPD underscore the need for extended basic and clinical research on BPD. Undoubtedly, as stated in the Preface, this volume will "stimulate the next generation of investigators and clinicians to further improve long-term outcomes of prematurely born infants."

As the executive editor of the series of monographs Lung Biology in Health and Disease, I express my gratitude to Dr Abman for giving us the opportunity to present this volume. Both neonatologists and pulmonologists will benefit from it but, more important, their patients will as well.

Claude Lenfant, MD
Vancouver, Washington, U.S.A.

References

1. Wong PM, Lees AA, Louw J, et al. Emphysema in young adult survivors of moderate-to-severe bronchopulmonary dysplasia. Eur Respir J 2008; 32(2):321–328 [Epub April 2, 2008].
2. Askin DF, Diehl-Jones W. Pathogenesis and prevention of chronic lung disease in the neonate. Crit Care Nurs Clin North Am 2009; 21(1):11–25.
3. Bourbon JR, Boucherat O, Boczkowski J, et al. Bronchopulmonary dysplasia and emphysema: in search of common therapeutic targets. Trends Mol Med 2009; 15(4): 169–179 [Epub March 18, 2009].

Preface

Over 40 years ago, Dr William Northway and his colleagues at Stanford described the clinical, radiologic, and pathologic features of a new disorder—bronchopulmonary dysplasia (BPD). Their comprehensive phenotyping of patients with chronic lung disease following premature birth included numerous insights into the pathogenesis of the disease, including mechanistic links with hyperoxia, ventilator-induced lung injury, inflammation and infection, and its time course. This insightful, landmark study laid a strong foundation and provided the basis for subsequent work in the field, setting the stage for numerous advances in neonatal respiratory care. After all these years, many of these basic observations remain central to our current understanding of BPD.

BPD remains a disease partly defined and altered by its treatments. Despite major differences in the nature of BPD that have followed the introduction of surfactant therapy, prenatal steroids, and changes in neonatal care, BPD remains a major cause of neonatal morbidity and mortality. As survival of the tiniest of premature babies increases, many infants still develop significant impairment of lung function, leading to prolonged ventilator and NICU courses, frequent hospitalizations after NICU discharge, recurrent respiratory exacerbations, and problems with late cardiorespiratory diseases.

Nearly 10 years ago, Drs Richard Bland and Jacqueline Coalson edited an important volume that highlighted the current state of the art in our understanding of BPD (1). This book provided an important resource for basic scientists, clinician-scientists, and practicing clinicians alike. Chapters provided historical perspectives on BPD, highlighted basic mechanisms of lung development, characterized the clinical course and treatment strategies of premature infants at risk for developing BPD or with established BPD, and related topics. Their book especially highlighted the changing epidemiology and clinical course of premature newborns with BPD in the post-surfactant era, providing in-depth reviews of normal lung development, mechanisms of lung injury and repair, and clinical and pathologic features of the disease. In addition to its state-of-the-art reviews, this previous volume was especially useful for helping to define persistent questions and challenges for laboratory investigators and clinicians to better understand and treat premature newborns at risk for BPD.

Over the past decade, much work has been done to address the many challenges of premature birth and to further extend our understanding of BPD. The purpose of this current book is to simply provide an update of recent progress made in this field, and to once again raise new questions worthy of pursuit in the laboratory and clinical settings. The first section presents new advances in lung development, including recent insights into molecular pathways and the integration of growth factors, transcription factors, and cell-cell interactions in this process. The second section highlights mechanisms of lung injury and repair that disrupt normal lung airspace and vascular growth, and lead to the abnormalities of lung structure and function that characterize BPD. The third section highlights novel insights into clinical aspects of BPD, including new information on the genetic basis for BPD, its changing epidemiology, clinical course, and physiology, and updated reviews of its treatment. Finally, the fourth section presents an update on emerging therapies for the prevention of BPD, based on recent preclinical studies and multicenter randomized clinical trials.

Overall, this volume provides new insights into the pathobiology and treatment of BPD. I dedicate this book to our patients and their families, and hope that this work will help stimulate the next generation of investigators and clinicians to further improve long-term outcomes of prematurely born infants.

In addition, I would like to personally thank and acknowledge support in my career as provided by "mentors from afar," including Alan Jobe, Eduardo Bancalari, Richard Bland, and Marlene Rabinovitch, as well as local friends and colleagues who keep me in line, especially David Cornfield, John Kinsella, Vivek Balasubramaniam, Jason Gien, and Peter Mourani. Finally, I thank my family (Carolyn, Ryan, Lauren, Mark, and Megan) for their loving support.

Steven H. Abman, MD

Reference

1. Bland RD, Coalson JJ. Chronic Lung Disease in Early Infancy. New York: Marcel Dekker, 2000.

Contributors

Steven H. Abman Pediatric Heart Lung Center, Sections of Critical Care and Pulmonary Medicine, Department of Pediatrics, University of Colorado Denver, School of Medicine and The Children's Hospital, Aurora, Colorado, U.S.A.

Namasivayam Ambalavanan University of Alabama at Birmingham, Birmingham, Alabama, U.S.A.

Richard L. Auten Duke University Medical Center, Durham, North Carolina, U.S.A.

Phillp L. Ballard University of California at San Francisco, San Francisco, California, U.S.A.

Roberta A. Ballard University of California at San Francisco, San Francisco, California, U.S.A.

Eduardo Bancalari University of Miami Miller School of Medicine, Miami, Florida, U.S.A.

Eugenio Baraldi University of Padua, School of Medicine, Padua, Italy

Vineet Bhandari Yale University School of Medicine, New Haven, Connecticut, U.S.A.

Olivier Boucherat Centre de Recherche en Cancérologie de l'Université Laval, Centre Hospitalier Universitaire de Québec, L'Hôtel-Dieu de Québec, Québec, Canada

Jacques R. Bourbon INSERM, Unité 955-Institut Mondor de Recherche Biomédicale, Faculté de Médecine, Université Paris 12, Créteil, France

Joy V. Browne University of Colorado Denver School of Medicine and The Children's Hospital, Aurora, Colorado, U.S.A.

Waldemar Carlo   University of Alabama at Birmingham, Birmingham, Alabama, U.S.A.

Robert G. Castile   The Ohio State University, Columbus, Ohio, U.S.A.

Nelson Claure   University of Miami Miller School of Medicine, Miami, Florida, U.S.A.

Jonathan M. Davis   Tufts University School of Medicine, Boston, Massachusetts, U.S.A.

Christophe Delacourt   INSERM, Unité 955-Institut Mondor de Recherche Biomédicale, Faculté de Médecine, Université Paris 12, Créteil, France

Marco Filippone   University of Padua, School of Medicine, Padua, Italy

Neil N. Finer   University of California, San Diego, San Diego, California, U.S.A.

Emily Fox   Hospital for Sick Children, Toronto, Ontario, Canada

Anne Greenough   Division of Asthma, Allergy & Lung Biology, MRC-Asthma U.K. Centre in Allergic Mechanisms of Asthma, King's College London, London, U.K.

Henry L. Halliday   Queen's University Belfast and Royal Maternity Hospital, Belfast, Northern Ireland, U.K.

Alison A. Hislop   Institute of Child Health, University College London, London, U.K.

David A. Ingram   Herman B Wells Center for Pediatric Research, Indianapolis, Indiana, U.S.A.

Robert P. Jankov   University of Toronto, Toronto, Ontario, Canada

Alan H. Jobe   University of Cincinnati, Cincinnati, Ohio, U.S.A.

Suhas Kallapur   University of Cincinnati, Cincinnati, Ohio, U.S.A.

John P. Kinsella   The Children's Hospital and University of Colorado School of Medicine, Aurora, Colorado, U.S.A.

Stella Kourembanas Harvard Medical School, Boston, Massachusetts, U.S.A.

Boris W. Kramer Academisch Ziekenhuis Maastricht, Maastricht, The Netherlands

Tina A. Leone University of California, San Diego, San Diego, California, U.S.A.

William M. Maniscalco University of Rochester School of Medicine, Rochester, New York, U.S.A.

Peter M. Mourani Pediatric Heart Lung Center, Sections of Critical Care and Pulmonary Medicine, Department of Pediatrics, University of Colorado Denver, School of Medicine and The Children's Hospital, Aurora, Colorado, U.S.A.

Leif D. Nelin The Ohio State University, Columbus, Ohio, U.S.A.

Sanna Padela University of Toronto, Toronto, Ontario, Canada

Richard Parad Harvard Medical School, Boston, Massachusetts, U.S.A.

Martin Post Hospital for Sick Children, Toronto, Ontario, Canada

Rebecca S. Rose Indiana University, Indianapolis, Indiana, U.S.A.

Ola Didrik Saugstad University of Oslo, Oslo, Norway

Michael D. Schreiber University of Chicago, Chicago, Illinois, U.S.A.

Wei Shi Developmental Biology and Regenerative Medicine Program, Saban Research Institute, Children's Hospital Los Angeles, Keck School of Medicine and School of Dentistry, University of Southern California, Los Angeles, California, U.S.A.

Christian P. Speer University Children's Hospital, Würzburg, Germany

A. Keith Tanswell University of Toronto, Toronto, Ontario, Canada

Bernard Thébaud University of Alberta, Edmonton, Alberta, Canada

Linda J. Van Marter Harvard Medical School, Boston, Massachusetts, U.S.A.

Maximo Vento Hospital Universitario Materno Infantil La Fe, Valencia, Spain

Michele C. Walsh Rainbow Babies and Children's Hospital, Case Western Reserve University School of Medicine, Cleveland, Ohio, U.S.A.

David Warburton Developmental Biology and Regenerative Medicine Program, Saban Research Institute, Children's Hospital Los Angeles, Keck School of Medicine and School of Dentistry, University of Southern California, Los Angeles, California, U.S.A.

Kristi Watterberg University of New Mexico, Albuquerque, New Mexico, U.S.A.

Carl White National Jewish Medical and Research Center, Denver, Colorado, U.S.A.

Mervin C. Yoder Herman B Wells Center for Pediatric Research, Indianapolis, Indiana, U.S.A.

Contents

Introduction   Claude Lenfant   . . . .   *vii*

Preface   . . . .   *ix*

Contributors   . . . .   *xi*

Part I: Mechanisms of Lung Growth and Development

1. **Genetic Mechanisms of Lung Development and Bronchopulmonary Dysplasia: An Integrative View** *1*
   David Warburton and Wei Shi

2. **Growth Factors and Cell-Cell Interactions During Lung Development** *40*
   Emily Fox and Martin Post

3. **Basic Mechanisms of Alveolarization** *56*
   Jacques R. Bourbon, Christophe Delacourt, and Olivier Boucherat

4. **Lung Vascular Development** *89*
   Alison A. Hislop

Part II: Mechanisms of Disrupted Lung Development and Repair in the Pathobiology of BPD

5. **Oxidative and Nitrosative Stress and Bronchopulmonary Dysplasia** *105*
   Richard L. Auten and Carl White

6. **Prenatal Inflammation and Immune Responses of the Preterm Lung** *118*
   Suhas Kallapur, Alan H. Jobe, and Boris W. Kramer

7. **Inflammatory Mechanisms in Bronchopulmonary Dysplasia** *133*
   Christian P. Speer

8. **Disruption of Lung Vascular Development** *146*
   William M. Maniscalco and Vineet Bhandari

9. **Pulmonary Endothelial Progenitor Cells and Bronchopulmonary Dysplasia** *167*
   Rebecca S. Rose, David A. Ingram, and Mervin C. Yoder

10. **Effects of Mesenchymal Stem Cell Therapy in BPD** *178*
    Bernard Thébaud and Stella Kourembanas

11. **Altered Growth Factor Signaling in the Pathogenesis of BPD** *188*
    A. Keith Tanswell, Sanna Padela, and Robert P. Jankov

Part III: Clinical Aspects of BPD and its Management

12. **Evolving Clinical Features of the New Bronchopulmonary Dysplasia** *208*
    Eduardo Bancalari and Nelson Claure

13. **Epidemiology of Bronchopulmonary Dysplasia** *223*
    Linda J. Van Marter

14. **Definitions of Bronchopulmonary Dysplasia and the Use of Benchmarking to Compare Outcomes** *267*
    Michele C. Walsh

15. **Genetics of Bronchopulmonary Dysplasia** *280*
    Vineet Bhandari

16. **Role of Management in the Delivery Room and Beyond in the Evolution of Bronchopulmonary Dysplasia** *292*
    Maximo Vento and Ola Didrik Saugstad

17. **Mechanical Ventilation: Early Strategies to Decrease BPD** *314*
    Tina A. Leone and Neil N. Finer

18. **Lung Function, Structure and the Physiologic Basis for Mechanical Ventilation of Infants with Established BPD** *328*
    Robert G. Castile and Leif D. Nelin

19. **Pulmonary Vascular Disease in Bronchopulmonary Dysplasia: Physiology, Diagnosis, and Treatment** *347*
    Peter M. Mourani and Steven H. Abman

20. **Drug Therapies in the Management of BPD** *364*
    Henry L. Halliday

21. **Lung Function Abnormalities in Infants and Children with Bronchopulmonary Dysplasia** *388*
    Marco Filippone and Eugenio Baraldi

22. **Long-Term Outcomes of Infants with BPD** *405*
    Anne Greenough

23. **Neurodevelopmental Outcomes of Children with Bronchopulmonary Dysplasia** *417*
    Joy V. Browne

Part IV: Emerging Therapies in the Treatment of BPD

24. **Inhaled Nitric Oxide in Premature Infants for the Prevention and Treatment of BPD** *427*
    John P. Kinsella, Philip L. Ballard, Roberta A. Ballard, and Michael D. Schreiber

25. **Vitamin A in the Prevention of Bronchopulmonary Dysplasia** *446*
    Namasivayam Ambalavanan and Waldemar Carlo

26. **The Use of Antioxidants to Prevent or Ameliorate Bronchopulmonary Dysplasia** *458*
    Jonathan M. Davis and Richard Parad

27. **Low-Dose Glucocorticoids for Prevention or Treatment of Bronchopulmonary Dysplasia** *472*
    Kristi Watterberg

Index *485*

1
Genetic Mechanisms of Lung Development and Bronchopulmonary Dysplasia: An Integrative View

DAVID WARBURTON and WEI SHI
Developmental Biology and Regenerative Medicine Program, Saban Research Institute, Children's Hospital Los Angeles, Keck School of Medicine and School of Dentistry, University of Southern California, Los Angeles, California, U.S.A.

I. Lung Development and Bronchopulmonary Dysplasia

The major function of the human neonatal lung is to rapidly clear fluid from the airways and to begin to exchange gas. The gas diffusion surface of the mature human neonatal lung has a honeycomb-like structure, comprising extensively branched, perfectly matched ducts for air and blood. This configuration maximizes the gas exchange surface area between air and blood, and facilitates maximally efficient packing within the chest cavity. In humans, the gas exchange membrane, which is about 1-μm thick, consists of type I alveolar epithelial cells (AECI), basement membrane, and endothelial cells, with a total surface area that increases in the adult to about 70 m^2. This vast and complex structure is developed sequentially by early epithelial tube branching and late septation of terminal air sacs. Perturbation of this developmental process results in abnormal lung structure and, hence, deficiency of the gas exchange function. Thus, premature human delivery interrupts this developmental process, resulting in an injury response phenotype that depends on the stage of lung maturity at the time of delivery. Northway et al. (1) coined the term *bronchopulmonary dysplasia (BPD)* to label the clinical, radiographic, and pathological features of chronic airway obstruction (broncho) and interstitial lung disease (pulmonary) with emphysema-like alveolar destruction and abnormal peripheral lung development (dysplasia). In those now far-off days respiratory distress syndrome (RDS) due to a combination of delayed fluid clearance, structural immaturity, and surfactant deficiency of the premature lung with the radiographic appearance of hyaline membrane disease were recognized as the major etiological factors from about 32 up to 36 weeks' gestation. Supportive treatment (oxygen plus pressure plus time) (2) plus fluid overload and left-to-right shunting through a patent ductus arteriosus (3) were recognized early on as the key postnatal, mostly iatrogenic, factors. With the widespread implementation of prophylactic artificial surfactant therapy, coupled with improvements in neonatal care including control of thermoregulation, judicious fluid therapy, gentler ventilation, and so on, the threshold for survival in human prematurity moved steadily downward toward 24 weeks' gestation. In these extremely premature infants, alveolarization has barely started, and accordingly, the critical feature of the "new BPD" was recognized to be alveolar hypoplasia (4). This chapter provides an overview of the integrated genetic and molecular processes that drive lung development and discusses concisely how lung injury, repair, and regeneration impact them in the context of BPD.

II. Early Lung Development: The Bauplan of the Lung

The lung originates from the ventral surface of the primitive foregut at five weeks' gestation in human. The lung anlage emerges as the laryngotracheal groove, located in the ventral foregut endoderm, which invaginates into the surrounding splanchnic mesenchyme (Fig. 1). Then a pair of primary buds evaginate from the laryngotracheal groove. The respiratory tree then develops by branching morphogenesis, in which reiterated outgrowth, elongation, and subdivision of these epithelial buds occur in a bilaterally asymmetrical pattern. Three lobes on the right side and two lobes on the left side are formed in human lung. There are 23 generations of airway branching in human. The first 16 generations branch stereotypically and are thus highly reproducible, and this is completed by 16 weeks' gestation, whereas the remaining 7 generations are random and are completed by about 20 to 24 weeks' gestation. Alveolarization begins around 20 weeks' gestation in human and continues postnatally at least until 7 years of age.

A. Genes Controlling Induction of the Early Lung

Early lung induction is under control of many gene products that act cooperatively to precisely define the location of laryngotracheal groove formation and specify proximaldistal, dorsal-ventral, and left-right axes of the developing lung. The earliest endodermal signals essential for gut morphogenesis and gut tube closure are the GATA (zinc finger proteins that recognize GATA DNA sequence) and hepatocyte nuclear factor (HNF/Fox) transcription factors. Foxa2 is required for gut tube closure, whereas GATA-6 is required for activation of the lung developmental program in the foregut endoderm. *Hnf-3/Foxa2β* is a survival factor for the endoderm, and its expression is induced by Sonic hedgehog (*Shh*) signaling. Also, *Tbx4* can induce ectopic bud formation in the esophagus by activating the expression of *Fgf10* (5). In addition, left-right asymmetry is controlled by several gene products including *nodal, Lefty-1,2*, and *Pitx-2*. For example, single-lobed lungs are found bilaterally in *Lefty-1$^{-/-}$* mice, and isomerism of lung is found in Pitx2 null mutants. Retinoids and their transcriptional factor receptors also play key roles in induction of the early lung branching process.

B. Complexities of Distal Airway Branching: Some Simplifying Concepts

At first sight, intrapulmonary airway branching in the developing lung distal to the primary bronchi appears to become increasingly complicated as it proceeds distally and the number of individual branches increases into the millions. But, once the laryngotracheal complex and left-right laterality are established, distal airway branching is thought to be driven by a master branch generator routine, with three slave subroutines instructing a periodicity clock that times the appearance of subsequent branches, a rotational orientation subroutine that determines the orientation of the branches around the axis of the airway, and finally, a bifurcation subroutine (6,7). Thus, branching morphogenesis of the bronchi in early mouse embryo lung can be parsed anatomically into three simple geometric forms, termed domain branching, planar, and orthogonal

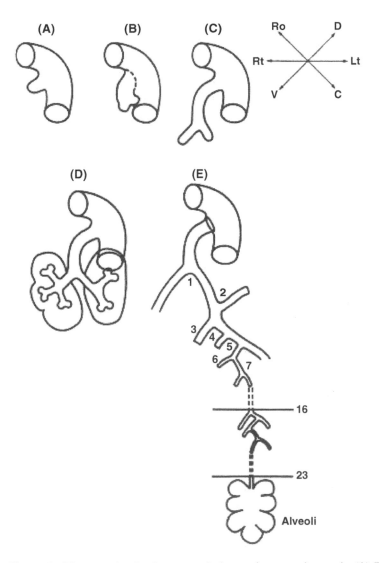

Figure 1 Diagrams showing key events in human lung morphogenesis. (**A**) The primitive lung anlage emerging as the laryngotracheal groove from the ventral surface of the primitive foregut at five weeks' gestation in human. (**B**) The primitive trachea separating dorsoventrally from the primitive esophagus as the two primary bronchial branches arise from the lateral aspects of the laryngotracheal groove at 5 ± 6 weeks' gestation in human. (**C**) The embryonic larynx and trachea with the two primary bronchial branches separated dorsoventrally from the embryonic esophagus at six weeks in human. (**D**) The primitive lobar bronchi branching from the primary bronchi at seven weeks in human. (**E**) A schematic rendering of the term fetal airway in human. The stereotypically reproducible, first 16 airway generations are complete by 16 weeks in human. Between 16 and 23 weeks, the branching pattern is random and is completed by about 24 weeks in human. Alveolarization begins after about 20 weeks in human and is complete by 7 years of age at the earliest.

bifurcation. These basic forms are repeated iteratively to form different arrangements of branches. These arrangements have been termed bottlebrush array, planar array, and rosette array. The bottlebrush array describes the sequential proximal to distal emergence of secondary branches along the airway. The bottlebrush mechanism can be reoriented to form a second row of branches at right angles to the first row. The planar and rosette arrays describe the patterns formed by sequential bifurcation of the tip of secondary, tertiary, and subsequent buds at right angles to each other. Repetition of these simple branching modules together with the hierarchical control and coupling of them may therefore explain how the genome could encode the highly complex yet stereotypic pattern of early bronchial branch formation using a relatively simple toolbox of genetic modules. Genes that drive these specific processes are discussed later on in this chapter.

C. The Impact of Hydraulic Pressure and Airway Peristalsis

The embryonic lung is filled with liquid. Active chloride secretion through the cystic fibrosis transmembrane conductance regulator (CFTR) and other chloride ion channels attracts sodium and thus creates an osmotic gradient, which draws water into the lumen. Lung liquid is produced from the earliest stages of embryonic lung development up to delivery. The hydraulic pressure within the lung lumen is determined by the rate of production of liquid together with the pinch-cock valve function of the primitive larynx. Obstruction of fluid outflow by clipping or cauterization of the embryonic trachea increases the intraluminal pressure by about two- to threefold. This is accompanied by a threefold increase in branching of the airway. Most notably, the rate of bud extension increases by about twofold whereas the interbud distance is halved. These effects of increased intraluminal pressure depend on FGF10-FGFR2b-Sprouty signaling (8). Several clinical trials have been made to determine whether tracheal obstruction to increase intraluminal pressure can accelerate fetal lung maturation in human fetuses with congenital diaphragmatic hernia. However, clinical opinion remains divided on whether there is any therapeutic role for this highly risky intervention. Nevertheless, the connection between physical force, morphogenetic signaling, and lung development is clearly important, and nowhere this is more evident than in BPD where barotrauma clearly plays a major role in the etiology. The discovery that waves of airway peristalsis that are calcium-driven and originate in a rhythm generator in the proximal airways also play a key role in embryonic lung development suggests that airway smooth muscle has an essential function even very early in lung development.

D. Coupling of Endothelial (Blood and Lymphatic Capillaries) with Epithelial Morphogenesis

Tight coupling of endothelial with epithelial development is also clearly important for efficient gas transport and fluid clearance at birth. Capillary plexi surround the primitive airway from the earliest stages of development. Vascular endothelial growth factor (VEGF) signaling from the epithelium to the developing capillary endothelium is essential for the development of the primitive capillary hemangioblasts into mature networks of capillary endothelium. Likewise, the endothelium signals back to the epithelium to coordinate morphogenesis of these tissue compartments. There is a constant stereotypic anatomical relationship between the developing pulmonary capillaries, arteries, and veins (Fig. 2).

The arteries run along the superior surface of the developing lobules, whereas the veins run along the interior surface. The lymphatics also develop under the control of the

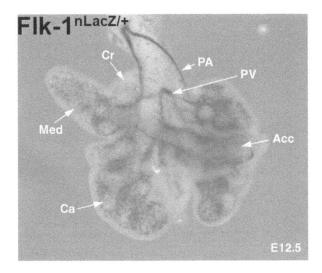

Figure 2 Blood vessels of the developing lung are shown at E12.5 in a special transgenic mouse. The blue signal is generated by staining for LacZ, driven in endothelial cells by the Flk-1 (VEGF receptor) promoter. *Source*: Artwork by Pierre del Moral. *Abbreviations*: PA, pulmonary artery; PV, pulmonary vein; Cr, cranial lobe; Med, median lobe; Ca, caudal lobe; Acc, accessory lobe of right lung.

VEGFR3 isoform of VEGF receptor and play a key role in regulating lung interstitial liquid content. Null mutation of VEGR3 markedly retards mobilization of fetal lung liquid at birth because of lymphatic hypoplasia, leading to failure of lymphatic drainage of interstitial fluid.

III. Histological Stages in Lung Development

Histologically, lung development and maturation has been divided into four stages: the pseudoglandular stage, the canalicular stage, the terminal sac stage, and the alveolar stage (Fig. 3).

A. The Pseudoglandular Stage (5–17 Weeks of Human Pregnancy, Embryonic E9.5–16.6 Days in Mouse Embryo)

This is the earliest lung development stage in which the embryonic lung undergoes branching morphogenesis developing epithelial tubular structures with lining cuboidal epithelial cells that resemble an exocrine gland. However, this fluid-filled respiratory tree structure is too immature to perform efficient gas exchange.

B. The Canalicular Stage (16–25 Weeks of Human Pregnancy, E16.6–E17.4 Days in Mouse Embryo)

The cranial part of the lung develops relatively faster than the caudal part, resulting in partial overlap between this stage and the previous stage. During the canalicular stage,

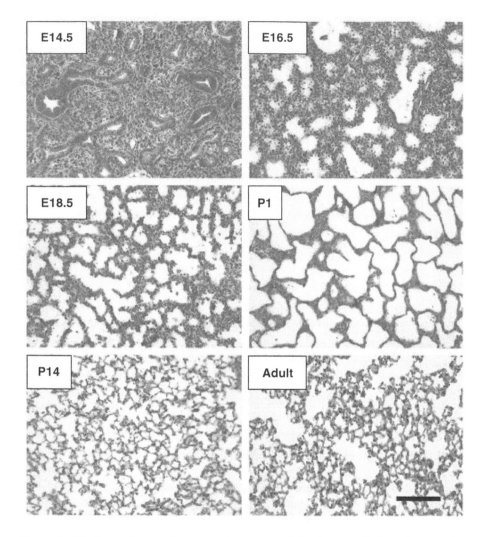

Figure 3 Histology of mouse lungs at various stages of development. Embryonic mouse lung develops from early pseudoglandular stage (E14.5) to canalicular stage (E16.5) and further terminal sac stage (E18.5 and P1). Neonatal lungs undergo further alveolarization, resulting in many septa formation (P14). Finally, a mature honeycomb-like structure with normal respiratory function is formed, as observed in adult. Scale bar: 100 μm.

the respiratory tree is further expanded in diameter and length, accompanied by vascularization and angiogenesis along the airway. A massive increase in the number of capillaries occurs. The terminal bronchioles are then divided into respiratory bronchioles and alveolar ducts, and the airway epithelial cells are differentiated into peripheral squamous cells and proximal cuboidal cells.

C. The Terminal Sac Stage [24 Weeks to Late Fetal Period in Human, E17.4 to Postnatal Day 5 (P5) in Mouse]

There is substantial thinning of the interstitium during the terminal sac stage. This results from apoptosis as well as ongoing differentiation of mesenchymal cells (9,10). Additionally, at this stage, the AEC are more clearly differentiated into mature squamous type I pneumocytes and secretory rounded type II pneumocytes. The capillaries also grow rapidly in the mesenchyme surrounding the saccules to form a complex network. In addition, the lymphatic network in lung tissue becomes well developed. The thick wall of these saccules, also called primary septae, comprises lining epithelial cells on both sides of a connective tissue core, within which there is a double parallel network of capillaries. Toward the end of this stage, the fetal lung can support air exchange in prematurely born human neonates. Although human premature infants can breathe with the lung that has developed to the end of terminal sac stage, the immature lung is nevertheless vulnerable to hyperoxic injury and barotrauma, resulting in the alveolar hypoplasia phenotypes described as new BPD. Maturation of surfactant synthesis and secretion is a key factor in determining whether the newborn lung can sustain gas exchange without collapsing. Another key factor is the rapid switch from chloride ion-driven fluid secretion into the airway to sodium-driven uptake of fluid out of the airway. This latter is driven by the birth response of the adrenergic system to cord cutting at birth.

How lung development is controlled at this stage is still incompletely known. The hydrostatic pressure inside the lumen of the airway, which is due to chloride ion and hence liquid secretion from epithelium in the developing lung (11–13), integrated with chemotactic signals from the mesenchyme such as FGF10 play important roles in forming terminal sacs. Mechanical factors also play an important role. Diaphragm muscle in MyoD$^{-/-}$ mice is significantly thinned and cannot support fetal breathing movements. As a result, lung is hypoplastic, and the number of proliferating lung cells is decreased in MyoD$^{-/-}$ lungs at E18.5. Therefore, mechanical forces generated by contractile activity of the diaphragm muscle play an important role in normal lung growth at this stage (14).

D. The Alveolar Stage (Late Fetal Period to Childhood in Human, P5–P30 in Mouse)

Alveolization is the last stage of lung development. The majority of the gas exchange surface is formed during this stage. Alveolarization can be positively and negatively influenced by many exogenous factors including oxygen concentration, stretch in fetal airway, dexamethasone, and retinoic acid.

Forming new septa within terminal sacs is the key step for differentiation of the saccule into alveoli. This involves a complex interaction between myofibroblasts in the mesenchyme, adjacent airway epithelial cells, and vascular endothelial cells. Controlled multiplication and differentiation as well as migration of the myofibroblast progenitor cells within terminal sac walls are important for new septa formation. Myofibroblasts, smooth muscle precursor cells having the morphology of fibroblasts, migrate to the proper position within nascent alveolar septa, and synthesize and deposit elastin (15,16). This is the first step of new secondary septa development (16). Platelet-derived growth factor-A (PDGF-A) and its receptor PDGF-α play important roles in forming new septa.

Pdgf-a$^{-/-}$ or *Pdgf-α*$^{-/-}$ shows a phenotype comprising loss of alveolar myofibroblasts and elastin, failure of alveolar septation, and this develops into emphysema due to alveolar hypoplasia (15,17). Besides PDGF-A, there are some other key proteins that mediate cell-cell interaction within terminal sac walls. For example, Roundabout (ROBO) is a receptor known to be involved in repellent signaling controlling axonal extension in the developing neuronal system. ROBO and its ligand SLIT are also involved in the regulation of nonneuronal cell migration (18). In E18, one day before birth, *Slit-2* is expressed in the saccular mesenchyme surrounding the airways. At the same time, *Robo* is expressed on the apical aspects of the airway epithelium adjacent to the ligand *Slit-2*, suggesting interactive roles in pulmonary bronchiolar development (19). A *Robo* knockout mouse has been shown to have loss of septation and thickened mesenchyme (20). In addition, transforming growth factor β (TGF-β)-Smad3 signaling in peripheral lung epithelial cells is also essential for secondary alveolar septa formation (21). Abrogation of TGF-β type II receptor in lung epithelial cells results in reduction of AECI and alveolar formation (22).

E. Alveolar Septum Formation

Two additional processes are necessary in septum differentiation to form a septum with final mature morphology and function. One is the thinning out of the septal mesenchyme and the other is the maturation of the double capillary network into a single capillary bed. Thinning of the mesenchymal tissue involves apoptosis of "unwanted" cells in the postnatal lung mesenchyme. There is a substantial reduction in the number of interstitial myofibroblasts resulting from increased apoptosis during this phase of rapid alveolarization (23,24). The immature lung contains at least two morphologically distinct fibroblast populations, lipid-filled interstitial fibroblasts (LFIF) and non-LFIF (NLFIF). After alveolarization, apoptosis occurs preferentially in only one of these fibroblast populations, the LFIF. Apoptosis was correlated with downregulation of insulin-like growth factor I receptor (*Igf-IR*) mRNA and cell surface protein expression (25). This thinning of the previously thickened immature interstitium occurs simultaneously with the ongoing expansion of the epithelial, blood vessel, and airspace compartments in the rapidly developing septa. A mature capillary bed is also vital for the proper function of alveoli, but the mechanism is still incompletely known. In the developing lungs, VEGF isoforms and their receptors have been identified as being important for endothelial survival and proliferation in the alveolar wall. Inhibition of VEGF signaling results in abnormal lung vascular growth and reduced alveolarization (26). Finally, the new septum differentiates into a functional respiratory membrane that consists of AECI, basement membrane, and capillary endothelial cells. The respiratory membrane provides a short distance for gases diffusion and thus facilitates optimal gas exchange. It is estimated that about 50 million alveoli are present in neonatal lung at term. However, by age seven to eight years, when the alveolarization is substantially complete, the number of alveolar units in the lung has grown about six times, to about 300 million alveoli.

Retinoid acid (RA) has been shown to increase the number of alveoli (27) and can partially rescue a block in alveolar formation induced by dexamethasone (28). In adult rats, RA has also been reported to reverse the anatomical features of elastase-induced emphysema, in which there is destruction of septa (27). In the *RAR-γ* gene deletion mouse, there is a developmental defect in alveolar formation most consistent with a defect in elastin deposition. The additional deletion of one retinoid X receptor (*RXRα*) allele results in a decrease in alveolar surface area and alveolar number (29). Retinoids affect multiple cellular functions that are involved in alveolar septal formation such as proliferation, migration, and temporal differentiation of cells (30). Retinoic acid is an active metabolite of vitamin A. Vitamin A deficiency has long been known to injure lungs and impairs function of rat type 2 pneumocytes (29). Taken together, the evidence suggests that RA may play an important role in alveolar development. For more on RA signaling, see following text.

IV. Specific Cell Types in the Lung

More than 40 specific types of cells are differentiated during embryonic lung development. The epithelial cell lineages are arranged in a distinct proximal-distal spatial pattern in the airways.

Cartilage lies outside the submucosa and decreases in amount as the caliber of the bronchi decreases. Cartilage is present in the bronchi, but not in the bronchioles. Two major cell components of the proximal bronchial epithelium are identified: pseudostratified ciliated columnar cells and mucous (goblet) cells. Both of them are derived from basal cells, but ciliated cells predominate in number. Goblet cells release mucus granules into the bronchial lumen to prevent drying of the walls and traps particulate matter. Mucous cells begin to mature around 13 weeks' gestation in humans, when the mature ciliated columnar cells are already present. The molecular markers for mucous cells are mucins (MUC5B, 5A, 5C). The beating of cilia results in a cephalad movement of the mucus blanket, thereby cleaning and protecting the airway. In the case of cystic fibrosis, cilia movement is disabled due to the thick mucous layer that is caused by mutation of the *Cftr* gene, which encodes a transmembrane Na^+ ion transporter protein. This phenotype also makes the airway surface vulnerable to microbial infection. In chronic airway injury, both repair and fully experimental exposure of the epithelium to IL-9 before it becomes fully differentiated result in goblet cell hyperplasia. Exposure to IL-9 resulted in increased lysozyme and mucus production by the epithelia (31). IL-4, IL-13, and allergens enhance the release of TGF-α, which is a ligand for the epidermal growth factor receptor (EGFR) that also stimulates fibroblast proliferation and goblet cell differentiation (32).

There are three different types of cells in bronchial submucosal glands: myoepithelial cells surround the gland, whereas mucous cells (pale cytoplasm) and serous cells (basophilic cytoplasm) produce mucins. These secreted mucins mix with lysozyme and IgA on airway surface.

Kulchitsky cells are also found on the airway surface next to bronchial glands. Their precise function is unclear. It is believed that they are pulmonary neuroendocrine cells that produce a variety of peptide hormones such as serotonin and calcitonin. Their fingerlike cytoplasmic extensions usually reach the airway lumen. Kulchitsky cells expressing the markers gastrin-releasing peptide, calcitonin gene-related peptide, and chromogranin may be related to certain lung neoplasms (i.e., small cell carcinoma and carcinoid tumors). However, pulmonary neuroendocrine cells differentiate earlier by 10 weeks of gestation in humans and are also the first airway epithelial cells to be fully differentiated in mouse.

Clara cells are found in the distal bronchiolar airway epithelium that normally lacks mucous cells. They produce a mucus-poor, watery proteinaceous secretion. They assist with clearance and detoxification, as well as reduction of surface tension in small airways. The most important cellular marker of Clara cell is Clara cell–specific protein (CC10, CCSP, or uteroglobin). Cytochrome P450 reductase and CC10 can also be used as cellular markers for Clara cells. Clara cells begin to mature during the 19th week in humans. In normal mice, only a small number of mucin-positive cells are present in the airway. However, numerous mucous cells that are derived from Clara cells with excessive mucin production or reduced mucin secretion can be detected during mucous metaplasia.

The majority of the alveolar surface is normally covered by type I epithelial cells. These flat cells are believed to be terminal differentiated cells, expressing several specific molecular markers such as T1α and aquaporin 5. T1α is a differentiation marker gene of lung alveolar epithelial type I cells. It is developmentally regulated and encodes an apical membrane protein of unknown function. In the absence of T1α protein, type I cell differentiation is blocked. Homozygous T1α null mice die at birth of respiratory failure, and their lungs cannot be inflated to normal volumes (33). Aquaporin 5 is a water channel in type I epithelial cells.

Type I epithelial cells only account for 40% of the total airway epithelial cells, even though 95% of the surface area of the alveolar wall is covered by this type of cells. The remaining 60% of the epithelial cells are rounded cells that cover only 3% of the alveolar surface, named type II pneumocytes.

Type II pneumocytes are plump or cuboidal and have a finely stippled cytoplasm and surface microvilli. They manufacture surfactant phospholipids and proteins that reduce the surface tension in the lung. This equalizes pressures, stabilizes and maintains alveoli in an open position despite the variation in alveolar size, and prevents atelectasis at end-expiration. Four surfactant proteins, SP-A, -B, -C, and -D, also play critical roles in maintaining lung function. SP-A and -D participate in host defense in the lung, whereas SP-B and -C contribute to the surface tension–lowering properties of the lipoprotein complex termed pulmonary surfactant (34). Type II cells are capable of regeneration and replacement of type I cells after injury. A commonly used cellular marker of type II cell is SP-C (*SftpC*).

Alveolar macrophages constitute a small percentage of the cells in alveoli, but they represent a major cellular sentinel of the host defense mechanism in the alveolar space. They are part of the mononuclear phagocyte system and are derived primarily from blood monocytes. However, once they get into the lung, their turnover rate is extremely slow.

V. Stem and Progenitor Cells in the Respiratory System

Respiratory stem and progenitor cells have important functions in repairing damaged trachea, bronchi, bronchioles, and alveoli. However, the precise identification of lung stem/progenitor cells remains uncertain. The large surface area and highly branched and folded geography of the lung dictates that there must be several kinds of stem or progenitor cells in the respiratory system. In the trachea and bronchi, certain basal cells and mucus-gland duct cells are believed to be stem/progenitor cells. Clara-like cells and type II pneumocytes are also thought to function as stem/progenitor cells in bronchioles and alveoli, respectively. Another population of stem/progenitor cells lies at the bronchoalveolar duct junction (35). They can function as bipotential precursors of both the SP-C and CC10-expressing cell lineages.

It has recently been reported that bone marrow–derived mesenchymal stem cells can differentiate into airway epithelial cells in airway and type I pneumocytes in alveoli, particularly by injury. In contrast, in vitro cell culture indicates that Syrian hamster fetal lung epithelial M3E3/C3 cells can differentiate into Clara cells and type II pneumocytes under different culture conditions. Whether CCSP-expressing cells with pre-Clara cell phenotypes are stem cells for the entire respiratory tract remains to be determined. In addition, the concept of a pluripotent stem cell for the whole lung needs to be further investigated due to the great differences between identified stem cell and progenitor candidates in proximal bronchi and distal alveoli. Recently, we have discovered that lung contains populations of cells with stem or progenitor cell characteristics that can be sorted by FACS from adult rat and also mouse lung. This population is relatively resistant to apoptosis and may possibly be responsible for repopulation of the damaged alveolar surface. Another such population of stem or progenitor cells sorted as "side cells" on FACS has been identified to possibly repopulate in several different tissues, including the bone marrow.

Airway smooth muscle is derived from at least two distinct progenitor cell populations. One population comes from the periphery of the embryonic lung and is derived from the *Fgf10*-expressing progenitor cells that lie in the submesothelial mesenchyme. This population of cells at first plays a key role in mediating branching morphogenesis of the peripheral airway by virtue of expression of FGF10 as a chemotactic and proproliferative growth factor. However, as the airway extends outward into the peripheral mesenchyme, these progenitor cells relocate to lie along the more proximal stalk portion of the distal bud. In this location, they differentiate into smooth muscle cells (SMCs), most probably under the paracrine inductive influence of bone morphogenetic protein 4 (BMP4) and SHH, which are secreted by the underlying airway epithelium (36). On the contrary, another population of smooth muscle progenitor cells arises around the upper airway and proximal bronchi (37). The two populations of smooth muscle progenitor cells appear to meet distal to the major lobar and segmental branches. It is speculated that the size of these smooth muscle progenitor populations that are laid down during airway branching in the embryonic lung may determine the eventual propensity of the airway to undergo obstructive disease processes later in life such as BPD and asthma. Moreover, these progenitor pools may be targets for nicotine derived from maternal smoking.

VI. Molecular Mechanisms of Lung Development

Normal lung development is controlled by many genes as well as physical and chemical factors including intraluminal hydraulic pressure and relative hypoxia. Genetic factors responsible for lung development include (*i*) transcription factors that directly modulate gene expression in the cell nucleus, (*ii*) peptide growth factors and cytokines as well as their related intracellular signaling components that mediate cell-cell interaction, and (*iii*) extracellular matrix (ECM) that provides important environmental cues for developing lung cells to differentiate. The specification of all these integrated regulatory mechanisms are still being explored, but the interaction between epithelium and mesenchyme compartments has long been known to play a critical role during airway branching morphogenesis and lung maturation.

A. Transcription Factors

Lung growth is initiated and developed through changes in specific gene expression. The activity and expression level of relevant transcription factors determine gene expression profiles in the developing lung, and consequently, the morphogenetic process in a particular temporospatial order. Recent advances in mouse genetic technology allow us to evaluate each factor by either overexpressing or knocking out a specific gene. Three major groups of transcription factors such as forkhead box transcription factors, Nkx homeodomain transcription factors, and *Gli* play important roles in lung development.

Forkhead Box Transcription Factor Family

Many members of the forkhead box family transcription factors, such as Foxa1, Foxa2, HFH8, and HFH4, are important regulatory factors involved in lung development. These transcription factors share homology in the winged helix DNA-binding domain and play important roles in pulmonary cellular proliferation and differentiation.

HNF-3α (Foxa1) and HNF-3β (Foxa2) share 93% homology in their amino acid sequences and were first identified as essential factors in hepatocyte differentiation (38). However, *Hnf-3β* is also expressed in developing lung, with higher levels in proximal airway-lining epithelial cells and lower levels in the distal type II epithelial cells (39). Overexpression of *Hnf-3β* under the control of the lung epithelial–specific *SP-C* promoter in vivo inhibits lung branching morphogenesis and vasculogenesis (40). Also, HNF-3α and HNF-3β have important functions in regulating expression of CCSP as well as SPs in both bronchiolar and type II epithelial cells (41–43). *Hnf-3β* is inducible by interferon and, in turn, regulates the expression of the *Nkx* homeodomain transcription factor *Nkx2.1* (also termed *Ttf-1* and *CebpI*), which in turn regulates transcription of the SP genes in lung peripheral epithelium (44,45).

HFH8 is another important member of this family of proteins that contribute to lung development. At E9.5, *Hfh-8* expression is restricted to the splanchnic mesoderm contacting the embryonic gut and presumptive lung bud, suggesting that *Hfh-8* may participate in the mesenchymal-epithelial induction of lung and gut morphogenesis. HFH-8 expression continues in lateral mesoderm-derived tissue during development. By day E18.5, *Hfh-8* expression is restricted to the distal lung mesenchyme and the muscular layer of the bronchi (46). One important regulated target of HFH8 is *Pdgf* receptor that is also expressed in mesenchyme (15,47,48). The level of *Hfh-8* expression is important for normal lung development, as an alveolar hemorrhage phenotype is observed in *Hfh8* (+/−) mice, while *Hfh8* (−/−) mice died in utero. In addition, reduction of *Hfh-8* expression in *Hfh-8⁺/⁻* mutants is accompanied by decreased expression of VEGF and its receptor 2 (Flk-1), BMP4, and the transcription factors of the Brachyury T-Box family (Tbx2–Tbx5) and lung Kruppel-like factor (49). HFH8-binding sites are also found in the promoter region of genes such as *Bmp4*, *Hgf*, and *Hoxa5* that are very important in controlling lung morphogenesis (50,51).

Hfh4 (*Foxj1*) is the key factor in controlling ciliated epithelial cell differentiation. *Hfh4* is expressed in E15.5 airway epithelium just before the appearance of ciliated epithelial cells (52). Defective ciliogenesis in airway epithelial cells and randomized left-right asymmetry are observed in *Hfh4*$^{-/-}$ null mutant mice, mimicking Kartagener syndrome in humans. This congenital syndrome can result in perinatal lethality, but in low penetrance gives rise to situs inversus, sinusitis, bronchoectasis, and sterility, all caused by defects in ciliary beat (53,54). Interestingly, in mesenchyme-free airway epithelial culture, inhibition of endogenous BMP4 signaling by adding exogenous BMP antagonist Noggin results in increased expression of the proximal lung markers CCSP and HFH4 (55).

Foxp1, *Foxp2*, and *Foxp3* are newly discovered members of the forkhead box family of transcription factors that are expressed at a high level in mouse lung and gut tissues. All three proteins are expressed in lung epithelium. *Foxp1* and *Foxp4* are expressed in both proximal and distal airway epithelium, whereas Foxp2 is expressed primarily in distal epithelium. Foxp1 protein expression is also observed in the mesenchyme and vascular endothelial cells of the lung (10).

Nkx and Hox Homeodomain Transcription Factors

One of the most important homeodomain transcription factors in lung development is NKX2.1, also called TTF-1 (thyroid-specific transcription factor) or CEBP-1. *Nkx2.1* is expressed in foregut endoderm-derived epithelial cells including developing lungs, thyroid, and pituitary, as well as in some restricted regions of fetal brain (56,57). *Nkx2.1*$^{-/-}$ mice suffer severe impairment in branching morphogenesis of the lung and tracheoesophageal septum formation. The distal airway branches are totally absent, while only the two main bronchial stems are formed in *Nkx2.1* knockout mice, which indicates that lung development is arrested at a very early stage (58,59). In developing mouse lung, *Nkx2.1* is expressed in the proximal and distal airway epithelia and, at later stages of lung development, in the distal AEC (39). *Nkx2.1* expression is strictly controlled, and increased expression of *Nkx2.1* causes dose-dependent morphological alterations in postnatal lung. Modest overexpression of *Nkx2.1* causes type II pneumocyte hyperplasia and increased levels of SP-B. Higher expression level of *Nkx2.1* disrupts alveolar septation, causing emphysema due to alveolar hypoplasia. The highest overexpression of *Nkx2.1* in transgenic mice causes severe pulmonary inflammation, fibrosis, and respiratory failure, associated with eosinophil infiltration as well as increased expression of eotaxin and IL-6 (60). *Nkx2.1* is critical for SP, *T1α*, and *Ccsp* gene expression (56,61–66). *Nkx2.1*-deficient pulmonary epithelial cells fail to express nonciliated marker genes, including differentiated *Sp-B*, *Sp-C*, and *Ccsp*. *Bmp4* expression in these cells is also reduced. Phosphorylation of NKX2.1 is important. Mice with point mutation of seven serine phosphorylation sites of NKX2.1 died immediately following birth with malformation of acinar tubules and pulmonary hypoplasia. Meanwhile, expression of SPs, secretoglobulin 1A, and *Vegf* was decreased (67). *Nkx2.1* expression can be activated by HNF-3β (44) and GATA-6 (68) transcription factors during lung morphogenesis.

The expression of Hox transcription factors shows a proximal to distal polarity in developing lung. *Hoxa5*, *Hoxb2*, and *Hoxb5* expression are restricted to distal lung mesenchyme. *Hoxb3* and *Hoxb4* genes are expressed in the mesenchyme of both proximal airway and distal lung (69–71). The importance of these genes during lung development is well illustrated in gene-targeting experiments in mice. *Hoxa5*$^{-/-}$ null mutant mice display defects of tracheal formation and impaired lung branching morphogenesis, with tracheal occlusions, diminished SP expression, and thickening of alveolar walls (69).

GLI Family of Zinc Finger Transcription Factors

GLI1, -2, and -3 are very important zinc-finger transcription factors, which are activated by the SHH pathway. All of them are expressed in lung mesoderm rather than endoderm, particularly in the distal portion (72). Null mutation of *Gli2* plus *Gli3* genes results in total absence of lung. Mice with *Gli3* single deficiency are viable, but the size of the lung is smaller and the shape of the lung is also altered (72). In *Gli2*$^{-/-}$ null mutant mice, the right and left lungs are not separated but exist as a single lobe with a reduced size, and the primary branching in right lung is defective. Also, both trachea and esophagus are hypoplastic, though separated from each other. However, proximal-distal differentiation is normal (73). Therefore, *Gli2* plays an important role in the asymmetric patterning of the lung.

B. Peptide Growth Factors That Mediate Lung Morphogenesis

E11 mouse embryo lung can grow and branch spontaneously in serum-free medium in vitro. A variety of growth factors added into the culture medium can influence lung growth in the culture system (74,75). Such experiments indicate that the embryonic lung mesenchymal and epithelial cells can communicate through autocrine or paracrine factors. In this way, different signaling pathways are coordinated to control lung growth at the right time and right place. Many of those factors are peptide growth factors, including FGF, EGF, TGFβ, IGF, PDGF, SHH, etc. The expression and modification of these proteins and their downstream signaling components are strictly controlled during normal lung development. Loss of function of many of these genes perturbs normal lung development and function in mice.

FGF Family

FGF family members can be found in all vertebrate and invertebrate animals. Their regulatory functions during respiratory organogenesis are very well conserved from drosophila (76,77) to mammals. On the basis of their protein sequence homology, FGFs have been divided into several subgroups. Similarly, their cognate transmembrane protein tyrosine kinase receptors are classified into several different types, contributing to the specificity of FGF ligand binding (78). Heparin or heparan sulfate proteoglycan, an ECM protein, has been reported to be essential for FGF ligand–receptor binding and activation (79,80). FGFs play important roles in cell proliferation, migration, and differentiation during embryo development. Inhibition of fibroblast growth factor receptor signaling at different stages of embryo development shows that FGF signaling is required for branching morphogenesis early in lung development. Later inhibition of FGFR signaling in E14.5 lung decreased lung tubule formation before birth and caused severe emphysema at maturity. In E16.5, FGFR inhibition caused mild focal emphysema. Inhibition of FGFR signaling after birth did not alter alveolarization (81).

One of the best-studied FGF family members during embryonic lung development is FGF10. Despite the formation of larynx and trachea, the distal embryonic lung is completely missing in $Fgf10^{-/-}$ null mice (82). $Fgf10$ is expressed in the mesenchyme of E11 to E12 mouse lungs, adjacent to distal epithelial tubules. These sites of expression change dynamically in a pattern that is compatible with the idea that FGF-10 appears in the mesenchyme at prospective sites of bud formation (83). Culture experiments have shown that FGF10 has a chemotactic effect on nearby epithelium, so that the nearby epithelial tips proliferate and migrate toward FGF10-expressing mesenchyme or FGF10 beads (84,85). FGF10 also controls the differentiation of the epithelium by inducing Sp-C expression and by downregulating the expression of $Bmp4$ (55). Several other regulatory molecules such as SHH, BMPs, and TGF-βs may cross talk with FGF10 to coordinate control of embryonic lung morphogenesis. These interactions will be further discussed later in this chapter.

FGF7 (KGF) is found in the developing lung mesenchyme during late stages (86). In early cultured mouse embryonic lung, addition of FGF7 promotes epithelium growth and formation of a cyst-like structure with extensive cell proliferation. FGF7 can also contribute to distal airway epithelial cell differentiation (87,88). Erm and $Pea3$ are ETS domain transcription factors known to be downstream of FGF signaling. FGF7 can induce $Erm/Pea3$ expression more effectively than FGF10. Erm is transcribed exclusively in the epithelium, whereas $Pea3$ is expressed in both epithelium and mesenchyme. When examined at E18.5, transgenic expression of a repressor form of Erm, specifically in the embryonic lung epithelium, shows that the distal epithelium of Sp-C-Erm transgenic lungs is composed predominantly of immature type II cells, while no mature type I cells are observed. In contrast, the differentiation of proximal epithelial cells, including ciliated cells and Clara cells, appears to be unaffected (89,90). FGF7 does not seem to protect against hyperoxic inhibition of normal postnatal alveoli formation and early pulmonary fibrosis, but FGF7 consistently had a significant protective/preventive effect against the development of pulmonary hypertension during hyperoxia (91). However, $Fgf7^{-/-}$ mutant mice have apparently no gross abnormalities in the lung (92), suggesting a redundant function of FGF7 with other factors during lung development.

Another FGF family member FGF9 also regulates branching morphogenesis. In E10.5 lung, $Fgf9$ is expressed in the visceral pleura lining the outside of the lung bud as well as in the epithelium of the developing bronchi. At E12.5 and E14.5, $Fgf9$ expression persists in the mesothelium of the visceral pleura, but is no longer detected in airway epithelium (93). $Fgf9$ null mice exhibit reduced mesenchyme and decreased branching of the airways, but show significant distal airspace formation and pneumocyte differentiation. The reduction in the amount of mesenchyme in $Fgf9^{-/-}$ lungs limits the expression of mesenchymal $Fgf10$ (94). Recombinant FGF9 protein inhibits the differentiation response of the mesenchyme to N-SHH, but does not affect proliferation (95).

The signaling cascade activated by FGF-10 and -9 involves Raf, MAP ERK kinase, and extracellular-regulated kinases (ERK) 1 and 2 as signal transducers. MAP ERK kinase inhibition has been shown to reduce lung branching and epithelium cell proliferation, but increase mesenchyme cell apoptosis in fetal lung explants (13). FGF signaling is regulated at several levels. One of the key negative regulators is the Sprouty family. There are four sprouty (Spry) genes in mouse ($mSpry1$–4) and human ($hSpry1$–4). Murine $Spry2$ is expressed in the distal tip of embryonic lung epithelial branches, but is downregulated between the sites of new bud formation. Murine $Spry4$ is predominantly expressed in the distal mesenchyme of the embryonic lung (96) and may play roles in branching morphogenesis. Sprouties (SPRY1, -2, and -4) act as suppressors of Ras-MAP kinase signaling (97–99). Overexpression of *mSpry2* or *mSpry4* can inhibit lung branching morphogenesis through reducing epithelium cell proliferation (100–102). SPRED-1 and -2 are two sprouty-related proteins, which contain EVH-1 domains. *Spreds* are predominantly expressed in mesenchymal cells. Expression of *Spreds* is especially strong in the peripheral mesenchyme and epithelium of new bud formation. After birth, *Spreds* expression decreases, while the expression of *Sprouties* expression is still high. Both *Sprouties* and *Spreds* play important roles in mesenchyme-epithelium interaction during lung development (9).

TGF-β/BMP Family

The TGF-β superfamily comprises a large number of structurally related polypeptide growth factors including TGF-β, BMP, and activin subfamilies. TGF-β ligands bind to their cognate receptors on cell surface and activate downstream Smad proteins, which translocate into the nucleus and modulate target gene expression (103).

TGF-β Subfamily

TGF-βs are well known for their inhibitory effects on embryonic lung branching morphogenesis. There are distinct expression patterns for the three isoforms of TGF-βs, TGF-β1, -β2, and -β3. In early mouse embryonic lung (E11.5), TGF-β1 is expressed in the mesenchyme, particularly in the mesenchyme underlying distal epithelial branching points, whereas TGF-β2 is localized in distal epithelium. TGF-β3 is mainly expressed in proximal mesenchyme and mesothelium. Each isoform of TGF-βs plays a unique and nonredundant role during embryonic development. Mice lacking TGF-β1 develop normally but die within the first two months of life as a result of aggressive pulmonary inflammation (104). A TGF-β2$^{-/-}$ null mutation results in embryonic lethality around E14.5 in mice, and one of the abnormally developed organs is lung (105). TGF-β3$^{-/-}$ null mutant mice display cleft palate, retarded lung development, and neonatal lethality (106,107). Misexpression of TGF-β1, leading to excessive TGF-β1 activation, always results in an adverse phenotype that depends on the developmental stages at which TGF-β1 is expressed. Overexpression of TGF-β1 in early mouse embryonic lung epithelium inhibits lung branching morphogenesis in vitro (108), while misexpression of *Sp-C* promoter-controlled TGF-β1 in embryonic lung epithelium results in arrest of embryonic lung growth and epithelial cell differentiation as well as inhibition of pulmonary vasculogenesis (109,110). Clinically, the presence of excess TGF-β1 activity in tracheal aspirates of human premature infants who develop more severe BPD suggests a crucial role for TGF-β1 in lung maturation (111,112). On the other hand, misexpression of TGF-β1 in adult rats results in a chronic, progressive interstitial pulmonary fibrosis with increased proliferation and matrix secretion by the mesenchyme (113,114). Misexpression of TGF-β1 in neonatal rat lung using recombinant adenoviral vectors results in neonatal alveolar hypoplasia and interstitial fibrosis that phenocopies BPD (115). In addition, TGF-β1 may be one of the most important factors that are involved in the pulmonary inflammation response to exogenous factors, such as infection, bleomycin, or endotoxin. Blockade of the TGF-β-Smad3 pathway in Smad3$^{-/-}$ null mutant mice strongly attenuates bleomycin-induced pulmonary fibrosis (114). TGF-β-activated kinase-1-binding protein-1 (TAB1) was identified as a molecule that activates TGF-β-activated kinase-1 (TAK1). *Tab1* mutant embryonic fibroblast cells displayed drastically reduced TAK1 kinase activities and decreased sensitivity to TGF-β stimulation. *Tab1* mutant mice died of cardiovascular and lung dysmorphogenesis (116).

The activity of TGF-β signaling is regulated precisely at multiple levels. For example, β6 integrin, LTBPs, and thrombospondin are involved in regulating the release of TGF-β mature peptide, whereas betaglycan, endoglin, or decorin influences the affinity of TGF-β receptor binding. Mutation of the above genes display phenotypes related to malfunction of TGF-βs. For example, loss-of-function mutation both in the human and mouse endoglin gene, whose protein product binds to both TGF-β ligand and its type I receptor (Alk1), causes hereditary hemorrhagic telangiectasia (117). Null mutation of LTBP-3 or -4 causes profound defects in elastin fiber structure and lung alveolarization, which is similar to the phenotypic changes observed in Smad3 knockout mouse lung (118,119). In addition, TGF-β signaling in epithelial cells versus mesenchymal cells of developing mouse lung has distinct regulatory impacts on lung branching morphogenesis and alveolarization in vivo. Selective blockade of endogenous TGF-β signaling in embryonic lung mesenchymal cells results in retarded lung branching after midgestation, while abrogation of epithelial cell–specific TGF-β signaling only causes abnormal postnatal lung alveolarization, but does not have significant impact on prenatal lung development (22).

BMP Subfamily

BMPs, with more than 20 ligand family members, have been shown to regulate many developmental processes, including development of the lung. Expression of *Bmp3, -4, -5,* and *-7* are detected in embryonic lung. BMP4 is an important BMP member that plays a key role in normal lung development. Addition of exogenous BMP4 to intact embryonic lung explant culture stimulates lung branching, as reported by us and other groups (120,121). However, in isolated E11.5 mouse lung endoderm cultured in Matrigel, addition of BMP4 inhibited epithelial growth induced by the morphogen FGF10 (85). On the other hand, transgenic overexpression of BMP4 in the distal endoderm of fetal mouse lung, driven by a 3.7-kb human SP-C promoter, causes abnormal lung morphogenesis with cystic terminal sacs (122). In contrast, SP-C promoter-driven overexpression of either the BMP antagonist *Xnoggin* or the Gremlin to block BMP signaling results in severely reduced distal epithelial cell phenotypes and increased proximal cell phenotypes in the lungs of transgenic mice (51). Interestingly, blockade of endogenous BMP4 in embryonic mouse lung epithelial cells using a conditional gene knockout approach results in abnormal lung development with similar dilated terminal sacs as seen in BMP4 transgenic mouse lung (123), suggesting that appropriate level of BMP4 is essential for normal lung development. As extracellular growth factors, BMPs bind to heteromeric complexes of BMP serine/threonine kinase type I and type II receptors to activate intracellular signal pathway. Three cognate BMP type I receptors (Alk2, Alk3, and Alk6) have been identified. Among them, Alk3 expresses predominantly in distal airway epithelial cells during mouse lung development. Abrogation of Alk3 in mouse lung epithelia either from early lung organogenesis or from late gestation resulted in similar neonatal respiratory distress phenotypes, accompanied with collapsed lungs (124). Early induction of Alk3 knockout in lung epithelial cells causes retardation of early lung branching morphogenesis and reduces cell proliferation and differentiation. But late gestation induction of Alk3 knockout also causes significant epithelial apoptosis accompanied by lack of surfactant secretion (124). Furthermore, canonical Wnt signaling was perturbed, possibly through reduced WIF-1 expression in Alk3 knockout lungs (124). Therefore, deficiency of appropriate BMP signaling in lung epithelial cells results in prenatal lung malformation, neonatal atelectasis, and respiratory failure.

In addition, BMP signaling is also important in lung vasculogenesis and angiogenesis. Mutations of BMP type II receptor (BMPRII) and change in expression level of BMP antagonist Gremlin are associated with primary pulmonary hypertension (125,126). Moreover, upregulation of Gremlin is also associated with pulmonary fibrosis and the severity of the pathology (127,128).

SHH Pathway

Sonic hedgehog is a vertebrate homologue of *hedgehog* (Hh) that patterns the segment, leg, wing, eye, and brain in *Drosophila*. Hh binds to patched (Ptc), a transmembrane protein, and releases its inhibitory effect on downstream smoothened (Smo), which is a G-protein-coupled seven-span transmembrane protein. This leads to the activation of cubitus interruptus (Ci), a 155-kDa transcription factor that is usually cleaved to form a 75-kDa transcription inhibitor in cytosol. Elements of the *Drosophila* Hh signaling pathway and their general functions in the pathway are highly conserved in vertebrates, albeit with increased levels of complexity. Gli1, -2, and -3 are the three vertebrate Ci gene orthologues (129).

The SHH signal transduction pathway plays important roles in mesenchyme-epithelium interaction, which is very important in morphogenesis. In developing mouse lung, *Shh* is detected in the tracheal diverticulum, the esophagus, and later in the trachea and lung endoderm. *Shh* is expressed at low levels throughout the epithelium, whereas at higher level in the growing distal buds (130,131). Null mutation of *Shh* produces profound hypoplasia of the lung and failure of trachea-esophageal septation. Mesenchymal expression of *Ptc*, *Gli1*, and *Gli3* are all downregulated in the *Shh* knockout lung. However, proximal-distal differentiation of epithelial airway is preserved (132,133). Also, *Fgf10* expression is widespread in the epithelium in *Shh* null mutant lung, instead of the precisely location-restricted expression seen in wild-type control. Lung-specific *Shh* overexpression results in severe alveolar hypoplasia and a significant increase in interstitial tissue caused by an increased proliferation of epithelium and mesenchyme (130). Defective hedgehog signaling may lead to esophageal atresia and tracheoesophageal fistula (134). Gli1, -2, and -3 are three zinc-finger transcription factors activated by SHH signaling. Their functions in embryonic lung development have been discussed earlier.

HIP1, a membrane-bound protein, directly binds all mammalian hedgehog (HH) proteins and attenuates HH signaling (135). *Hip1* is transcriptionally activated in response to Hh signaling, overlapping the expression domains of *Ptch1* (135,136). Targeted disruption of *Hip1* results in neonatal lethality with respiratory failure. Although asymmetry in their growth was conserved, the initial stereotyped branching from the two primary buds was absent in *Hip1*$^{-/-}$ lungs. Hedgehog signaling is upregulated in *Hip1* mutants. *Fgf10* expression was slightly downregulated at the distal tips of the primary lung buds in *Hip1*$^{-/-}$ lungs at E10.5, but completely absent from the mesenchyme where secondary branching normally initiates (136). Attenuated PTCH1 activity in a *Hip1*$^{-/-}$ mutant lungs leads to an accelerated lethality. *Hip1* and *Ptch1* have redundant roles in lung branching control (136). Both of them can attenuate SHH signal in lung development and pancreas development (136,137).

Wnt/β-Catenin Pathway

Wnt signals are transduced through seven-transmembrane-type Wnt receptors encoded by *Frizzled* (*Fzd*) genes to activate the β-catenin–TCF pathway, the JNK pathway, or the Ca^{2+}-releasing pathway. The Wnt/β-catenin pathway plays a critical role in many developmental and tumorigenesis processes. Following Wnt binding to the receptor, β-catenin is dephosphorylated and translocates to the nucleus to activate downstream gene expression (138).

Interestingly, all members of the *Fzd* gene family are expressed in embryonic and neonatal lung, albeit at different levels. *Fzd* genes are differentially expressed in the epithelium and mesenchyme. Expression of the *Fzd2*, *Fzd5*, *Fzd6*, and *Fzd8* was observed predominantly in the epithelium, while *Fzd4* and *Fzd10* were expressed in the mesenchyme. Expression of *Fzd1* and *Fzd7* was observed both in the epithelium and the mesenchyme, while *Fzd3* and *Fzd9* were only marginally expressed. This spatial distribution suggests differential roles for different *Fzd* receptor genes in the Wnt signaling pathway during the development of the lung (139).

In mouse lung development, between embryonic days 10.5 and 17.5 (E10.5–E17.5), β-catenin was localized in the cytoplasm, and often also in the nucleus of the undifferentiated primordial epithelium, differentiating alveolar epithelium, and adjacent mesenchyme. Other Wnt/β-catenin pathway members, *Tcf1*, *Lef1*, *Tcf3*, *Tcf4*, *sFrp1*, *sFrp2*, and *sFrp4*, are also expressed in the primordial epithelium, alveolar epithelium, and adjacent mesenchyme in specific spatiotemporal patterns (140). In human fetal lung, nuclear β-catenin is present in pulmonary acinar buds (141). Null mutation of β-catenin in mice results in abnormal cystic structure formation in the lung and prenatal lethality. On the basis of molecular marker detection, the lungs are composed primarily of proximal airways, suggesting that β-catenin is one of the essential components to specify proximal-distal axis of the lung (139).

EGF Family Growth Factors

EGF, TGF-α, and amphiregulin are all EGFR ligands. Loss or gain of function experiments in mice, rat, or other animal models proves that EGF ligands can positively modulate early mouse embryonic lung branching morphogenesis and cytodifferentiation through EGFR (75,142,143). EGF is also expressed in mature AEC and regulates type 2 cell proliferation through an autocrine mechanism both in culture and in vivo (144). However, respiratory epithelial cell overexpression of TGF-α under the control of the *Sp-C* promoter of transgenic mice induces postnatal lung fibrosis (145). Overexpression of TGF-α caused severe pulmonary vascular disease, which was mediated through EGFR signaling in distal epithelial cells. Reductions in VEGF may contribute to the pathogenesis of pulmonary vascular disease in TGF-α mice (146).

EGFR is a tyrosine kinase receptor that transfers EGF signals into the cell. Abnormal branching and poor alveolization are observed in mice deficient in $Egfr^{-/-}$. Mechanical stretch–stimulated EGFR phosphorylation, at least in part, induces differentiation of fetal epithelial cells via EGFR activation of the ERK pathway. Blockade of the EGFR or ERK pathway by specific inhibitors decreased stretch-inducible *Sp-C* mRNA expression. Maybe EGFR is part of a mechanic stimulus signal sensor during fetal lung development (147). Aberrant expression of matrix metaloprotease proteins (MMPs) is also detected in $Egfr^{-/-}$ null mutant mice, which suggests that MMPs may be involved in EGFR-regulated lung growth (148).

TNF-α-converting enzyme (TACE) is a transmembrane metalloprotease-disintegrin that functions as a membrane sheddase to release the ectodomain portions of many transmembrane proteins, including the precursors of TNFα and several other cytokines, as well as the receptors for TNFα, and neuregulin (ErbB4) (149). Neonatal TACE-deficient mice had visible respiratory distress, and their lungs failed to form normal saccular structures, resulting in a reduction of normal air-exchange surface. Mouse embryonic lung explant cultures show that TGF-α and EGF can rescue the inhibition of TACE activity (150).

Platelet-Derived Growth Factors

There are four types of PDGF peptides. The PDGF-A and PDGF-B can form homodimers (AA or BB) or heterodimers (AB). Two types of PDGF receptors, α and β, are present in embryonic mouse lung and are differentially regulated in fetal rat lung epithelial cells and fibroblasts (151). PDGF-A regulates both DNA synthesis and early branching in early mouse embryonic lung epithelium in culture (152). *Pdgf-A* homozygous null mutant mice are perinatally lethal. The pulmonary phenotypes include lack of lung alveolar SMCs, reduced deposition of elastin fibers in the lung parenchyma, and developing lung emphysema due to complete failure of alveogenesis (15,17). Abrogation of PDGF-B chain expression with antisense oligodeoxynucleotides reduces the size of the epithelial component of early embryonic mouse lung explants, but does not reduce the number of branches (153). PDGF-B and its receptor are crucial for vascular growth and integrity during the alveolar phase (16). PDGF-C and -D also dimerize and bind to PDGF-α or -β receptor (154,155). PDGF-C mRNA expression shows a significant increase in lung fibrosis induced by bleomycin (156).

Insulin-like Growth Factors

The IGFs and their receptors are expressed in both rodent and human fetal lung (157–161). Null mutant mice for the cognate type 1 IGF receptor (*Igf1r*) gene always die at birth with respiratory failure and severe growth deficiency (45% of normal birth weight). Dwarfism is further exacerbated (70% of size reduction) in either *Igf1* and *Igf2* double null mutants or *Igf1r* and *Igf2* double null mutants. There does not appear to be a gross defect in primary branching morphogenesis per se; the lungs merely appear hypoplastic (162). IGF signaling may play a role in facilitating other peptide growth factor pathways during lung morphogenesis. IGF1R signaling function is required for both the mitogenic and transforming activities of the EGF receptor (163). The lungs displayed reduced airspace in the *Igf1*-deficient embryos and neonates, and the phenotype was exacerbated in additionally leukemia inhibitory factor (*Lif*) null mutant mice, which showed abnormal epithelial cells and decreased Sp3 expression. In addition, *Nkx2.1* and *Sp-B* expression are reduced in the lung of these double null mutant neonates. Thus, LIF and IGF-I have cooperative and distinct tissue functions during lung development (164). IGF1 is also a potent trophic factor for fetal lung endothelial cells. In human fetal lung explants, inactivation of IGF-IR results in a loss of endothelial cells, attenuates time-dependent increase in budding of distal airway, and increases mesenchymal cell apoptosis (165).

VEGF Isoforms and Cognate Receptors

Lung development must form a fine alignment between the alveolar surface and the surrounding pulmonary capillary system for effective gas exchange. VEGF are potent effectors of vascular development in lung morphogenesis. VEGF signals through the cognate receptors fetal liver kinase-1 (Flk-1, VEGFR2) and fetal liver tyrosinase-1 (Flt-1, VEGFR1) (166). VEGF is regulated by hypoxia-inducible transcription factor-2α (167). During lung organogenesis in mouse, VEGF120, -164, and -188 isoforms are expressed in pulmonary epithelial and mesenchymal cells around E12.5 and play a role in regulating endothelial cell proliferation and maintaining microvascular structure (168,169). Further, as epithelial branching progresses, *Vegf-A* expression becomes restricted to the distal lung (170), which may be partly due to the high affinity of VEGF-A for matrix components that concentrate VEGF-A around the branching tips (171,169). Thus, leading to the speculation that VEGF signaling may play a critical role in lung vascular development and diseases.

Vasculogenesis is initiated as soon as the lung evaginates from the foregut epithelium (172). Development of the vascular system influences branching morphogenesis of the airway as well as alveolarization. In transgenic mice, where the *Vegf* transgene is misexpressed under the control of SP-C promoter, gross abnormalities in lung morphogenesis are associated with a decrease in acinar tubules and mesenchyme (173); thus, suggesting that excessive VEGF signaling may disrupt both vascular and epithelial morphogenesis in the lung. Additionally, VEGF-A signaling through Flk-1 plays a key functional role in mediating cross talk between the epithelial, mesenchymal, and endothelial compartments during epithelial and vascular branching morphogenesis of the early mouse embryonic lung in explant culture (174). VEGF has also been demonstrated to play a role in maintaining alveolar structure (26). Lungs from newborn mice treated with antibodies to Flt-1 were reduced in size and displayed significant immaturity with a less complex alveolar pattern (175) (Fig. 4).

C. ECM and Lung Development

The protein components of extracellular basement membrane, laminins (LNs), entactin/nidogen, type IV collagen, perlecan, SPARC, and Fibromodulin, are important in mediating cell-cell and cell-ECM interaction during fetal lung morphogenesis. Basement membrane components are differentially expressed and have a specific cell distribution during lung morphogenesis. ECM components not only provide the support for tissue architecture but also play an active role in modulation of cell proliferation and differentiation (176). For example, basement membrane components may serve as a barrier

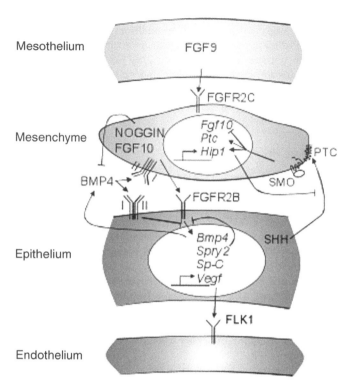

Figure 4 Integrative summary of selected growth factor signaling events during early lung morphogenesis. FGF9 is produced by the mesothelium, which signals through FGFR2c on the underlying mesenchyme. This stimulates *Fgf10, Ptc, and Hip* gene transcription. FGF10 in turn signals from the mesenchyme to FGFR2b on the epithelium. This signaling event is chemotactic for the epithelium, in addition to stimulating *Bmp4, Spry2, Vegf, and Sp-C* transcription. SPROUTY2 is an inducible negative downstream modulator of FGFR signaling. VEGF, produced by the epithelium, signals through FLK1 on the endothelium. BMP4, produced by the epithelium, signals back to the mesenchyme through its cognate receptors to modulate mesenchymal differentiation, particularly into smooth muscle. BMP4 ligand bioavailability is in turn negatively modulated by NOGGIN, which is produced in the mesenchyme. SHH, produced by the epithelium, signals through its cognate receptors Ptc and Smo located on the mesenchyme to both negatively modulate *Fgf10* transcription, but also to positively regulate mesenchyme differentiation into smooth muscle. This network diagram is highly simplified and does not include other key signaling mechanisms including Wnt ligands, Wnt antagonists such as DKK1, and their role in controlling fibronectin deposition at branch points. While all members of the network must interact correctly to control morphogenesis, the ratio of FGF10 to SPROUTY2 is a major factor that determines the periodicity and geometry of branching morphogenesis (7). *Source*: From Stijn de Langhe and Pierre del Moral.

and reservoir of growth factors, which in turn regulate epithelial and mesenchymal cell proliferation. Absence or inhibition of the interaction of epithelial cells with the basement membrane results in failure of normal lung development (177,178).

LNs are glycoproteins involved in cell adhesion, migration, proliferation, and differentiation during tissue development and remodeling. LNs are composed of three chains, one central (α) and two laterals (β and γ), that are linked by disulfide bonds to form a cross-shaped molecule (179). To date, five α, three β, and three γ chain isoforms have been identified, which suggests that their combination can lead to approximately 30 variants of LN (180–189). The α1 chain has been found principally localized in the basement membrane at the epithelial-mesenchymal interface, with a predominant distribution in specific zones. The LN α1 chain has also been identified around some mesenchymal cells. Molecular analysis dissecting the α1 chain isoform has shown that a domain in the cross-region of the α1 chain is involved in the regulation of lung epithelial cell proliferation (190). The α4 chain, found in LN8 and LN9 variants, has been reported to highly express in lung and heart tissues during mouse development (191,183–185). The LN α4 chain, localized principally around vessels in fetal lung, may play a role principally in the organization of lung mesenchyme (188,192). The α5 chain, found in LN10 and LN11, has been indicated abundantly expressed during fetal lung morphogenesis (188,193,194). Mouse embryos bearing mutated LN α5 chain isoform display a poor lobe septation and bronchiolar branching, suggesting that the LN α5 chain isoform might be the most indispensable LN variant for lung branching morphogenesis.

A constant expression of β1 and γ1 is observed during fetal lung development (195). These two chains also have a role in cell adhesion. The globular domains near the N-terminal of β1 and γ1 chains participate in the regulation of cell polarization (196,197). Immunohistochemistry studies have demonstrated that the LN β2 chain isoform is localized in the basement membrane of prealveolar ducts, airways, SMCs of airways, and arterial blood vessels, as well as type II pneumocytes.

Nidogen (150 kDa) is a constituent of the basement membranes. Nidogen binds to the γ1 and γ3 chains of LN and forms a link between LN and collagen IV (187,198,199). Nidogen is actively synthesized by mesenchymal cell during fetal lung development, which suggests that it has a key role in the organization of the basement membrane during lung morphogenesis (200). Blocking the interaction of nidogen with LN affects the progression of lung development (198,200,201). Susceptibility of nidogen to degradation by matrix metalloproteinases may contribute in the remodeling and degradation of the basement membrane (202).

Proteoglycans comprise a core protein with sulfated carbohydrate side chains. They function as flexible structures in the organization of the basement membrane and may also play an important role as a reservoir for growth factors, water, and ions. Perlecan is a predominant proteoglycan in the basement membrane. It is composed of an approximately 450-kDa core protein with three heparan sulfate chains. Perlecan is involved in the control of smooth cell proliferation and differentiation since increased cell proliferation of fetal lung SMCs is accompanied by a highly increased synthesis of perlecan (203). Growth and branching of E13 mouse lung explants can be disrupted by inhibiting PG sulfation. The migration of epithelial cells toward invaded lung mesenchyme as well as toward beads soaked in FGF10 is inhibited when PG sulfation fails; chlorate severely decreased branching morphogenesis in lung mesenchymal and epithelial tissue recombinants (204).

Fibronectin also plays important roles in lung development. In branching morphogenesis, repetitive epithelial cleft and bud formation create the complex three-dimensional branching structures characteristic of many organs. Fibronectin is essential for cleft formation during the initiation of epithelial branching in salivary gland. Immunofluorescence comparisons of fibronectin localization during early branching of lung and kidney also showed an accumulation of fibronectin at sites of epithelial constriction and indentation (205), supporting possible roles for fibronectin in branching morphogenesis of the lung (206). Direct tests for roles of fibronectin, by treatment of developing lung rudiments with antifibronectin antibody or siRNA, inhibited branching morphogenesis, while fibronectin supplementation promoted branching of lung (205). The EIIIA segment of fibronectin is one of the major alternatively spliced segments and modulates the cell proliferative potential of fibronectin in vitro. The EIIIA-containing fibronectin isoform localized in both the epithelial cells and the mesenchyme. Its expression gradually decreased from the pseudoglandular stage to the saccular stage and then slightly increased from the saccular stage to the alveolar stage. This change in expression pattern of EIIIA-containing fibronectin seemed to be in accord with the change in the number of PCNA-positive cells in the distal pulmonary cells throughout lung development (207).

Extracellular matrix is under dynamic control during lung development. The MMPs are a large family of ECM-degrading enzymes. MMPs are inhibited by the family of tissue inhibitors of metalloproteinases, termed TIMPs. Activity of MMPs may be required during development and normal physiology in several ways: (*i*) to degrade ECM molecules and allow cell migration, (*ii*) to alter the ECM microenvironment and result in alteration in cellular behavior, and (*iii*) to modulate the activity of biologically active molecules by direct cleavage, release from bound stores, or modulating of activity of their inhibitors (208). In *Timp3* null mutant mouse, lung airway branching is inhibited. Compared with wild type, the number of bronchioles is reduced and alveologenesis was attenuated in the *Timp3* null (209). The *Timp3* null animals spontaneously develop progressive alveolar air space enlargement similar to that seen in human emphysema (210). Early postnatal exposure to dexamethasone (Dex) influences MMP2 and MMP9, as well as their tissue inhibitors (TIMP1 and TIMP2) in the developing rat lung: the expression of *Timp2* is reduced and that of *Mmp9* increases. These changes may be responsible, in part, for some of the known adverse maturational effects of steroids on lung structure in the newborn (211). MT1-MMP, which acts as a potent activator of MMP2, is a major downstream target of EGFR signaling in lung. $Egfr^{-/-}$ mice had low expression of *MT1-Mmp*. Extracts from lungs of $Egfr^{-/-}$ mice showed a tenfold reduction in active MMP-2. At birth, the abnormal lung alveolization phenotype of $Mmp2^{-/-}$ mice is similar to that of $Egfr^{-/-}$ mice, albeit somewhat less severe (148). The balance between the activity of MMPs and TIMPs is important to normal lung development.

Retinoic Acid and Lung Morphogenesis

Retinoids (all-*trans*, 9-*cis*, and 13-*cis*) are fundamental for normal development and homeostasis of a number of biological systems including the lung. There is a precisely controlled RA synthesis and degradation system in mammals. Retinaldehyde dehydrogenase-2 (RALDH-2) plays a prominent role in generating RA during organogenesis

(212–214). RA signaling is mediated by its nuclear receptors of the steroid hormone receptor superfamily: RAR (α, β, γ) and retinoid RXR (α, β, γ). RAR/RXR heterodimers have also been shown to transduce RA signaling in vivo (215). Within the E13.5 lung, *Rar-β* isoform transcripts are specifically localized to the proximal airway epithelium and immediately adjacent mesenchyme, whereas *Rarα1*, *Rarα2*, and *Rarγ2* isoforms are ubiquitously expressed (216).

RA signaling is required for lung bud initiation. Acute vitamin A deprivation in pregnant rats at the onset of lung development results in blunt-end tracheae and lung agenesis in some embryos, which is similar to $Fgf10^{-/-}$ null mutant mice (217,218). Disruption of RA signaling in *Rarα/β2* knockout mice leads to agenesis of the left lung and hypoplasia of the right lung (219). Interestingly, lung branching morphogenesis is characterized by a dramatic downregulation of RA signaling in the lung. Prevention of downregulating RA signal by treating embryonic lung explants with high concentrations of RA (10^{-6} to 10^{-5} M) results in dramatic disruption of distal budding and formation of proximal-like immature airways (220,221). Continued RA activation by overexpression of constitutively activated *Rarα* chimeric receptors also resulted in lung immaturity. Lungs did not expand to form saccules or morphologically identifiable type I cells. High levels of *Sp-C*, *Nkx2.1*, and *Gata6* but not *Sp-A* or *Sp-B* in the epithelium at birth suggested that in these lungs differentiation was arrested at an early stage. Downregulation of RA signaling, however, is required to allow completion of later steps of this differentiation program that ultimately form mature type I and II cells (222). RA inhibits expression and alters distribution of *Fgf10* and *Bmp4*, which are required for distal lung formation (220,221). Pan-RAR antagonism alters the expression of *Tgf-β3*, *Hnf-3β*, and *Cftr* in proximal tubules and that of *Bmp4*, *Fgf10*, and *Shh* within the distal buds (216).

It is also noteworthy that during early stages of lung branching (day 11–12.5), *Raldh-2* expression is concentrated in trachea (mesenchyme) and proximal lung (mesothelium) at sites of low branching activity. The *Raldh-2* pattern is not overlapping with that of *Fgf-10*, supporting the idea that RA signaling restricts *Fgf-10* expression and helps to define the proximal-distal axis of the developing lung. However, during later postnatal stages of lung development, RA has been shown to increase the number of alveoli, and therefore, partially rescue dexamethasone-induced suppression of alveolarization. In adult rats, RA has also been reported to reverse the anatomical features of elastase-induced emphysema in which there is destruction of septal structures (27,28,223). In *Rarγ* gene deletion mouse, there is a developmental defect in alveolar formation, consistent with a defect in elastin deposition (30). This combined evidence suggests that RA may play an important but rather complex role in alveolar development during late lung development.

Fetal Lung Surfactant Maturation, Lung Liquid Absorption, and the Transition to Air Breathing

Maturation of the fetal lung surfactant system is one of the two key steps to prepare the lung for air breathing. During the last eight weeks of human gestation, fetal lung glycogen is broken down and converted into surfactant phospholipids, the most important of which is disaturated phosphatidylcholine. This maturation is under the control of and can be stimulated by corticosteroids. Null mutation of the glucocorticoid receptors and of corticotrophin-releasing hormone block this maturation in mice. Human mutations in various components of the surfactant system have been found such as SP-B that adversely affect stability of pulmonary surfactant and hence the ability to maintain lung inflation.

The transition to air breathing occurs rapidly in the mature neonatal lung. Immediately following severance of the umbilical circulation, a significant spike in catecholamine levels switches off chloride secretion and stimulates sodium/potassium ATPase (224–226). This reverses the production of tracheal fluid and leads to its rapid absorption into the lung interstitium and thence into the lymphatic and pulmonary capillary circulation. Null mutation of Na/K ATPase in mice leads to failure to absorb fetal lung liquid, which causes significant respiratory distress and even neonatal lethality (227). In human infants, delayed lung liquid absorption can manifest as transient tachypnea of the newborn.

Impact of Lung Injury on the Developmental Program

The lung has a relatively limited genetic repertoire to respond to injury. Initial injury to the epithelium results in an outpouring of cyotokines and chemoattractants including IL1, IL6, IL8, etc. Macrophages are recruited into the lung and enter the airways together with neutrophils and lymphocytes. Physiological levels of TGFβ peptides are actually protective of the airway and prevent inflammation, as revealed by null mutation in mice. Yet excessive amounts of TGFβ1 activity have been detected in the tracheal fluid of human premature infants who go on to get severe forms of BPD and hence have a worse pulmonary prognosis (228). As discussed earlier, transgenic misexpression of TGFβ1 in mice substantially phenocopies BPD (115). Another important feature of the airway cytokine milieu in human prematures who do badly with BPD is deficiency of IL10 (229,230). IL10 is an important anti-inflammatory cytokine, leading to the hypothesis that the airway of the human premature may be particularly prone to acute and eventually chronic inflammation, which in turn leads to production of TGFβ1 by inflammatory cells in the airway. Targets for suppression by excessive TGFβ1 signaling include epithelial and endothelial proliferation, while mesenchymal lineages may be stimulated. Likewise suppressive interactions of TGFβ signaling with morphogenetic pathways such as VEGF, FGF, PDGF, and SHH signaling may also play an important role in mediating the alveolar hypoplasia and airway obstruction phenotype characteristic of BPD.

The Hope of Recovery and Regeneration

Clinical experience in the special care nursery demonstrates that in most cases BPD is apparently at least somewhat reversible, that airway inflammation eventually resolves, and that lung alveolar growth can sometimes resume. This gives hope that with supportive care, even severe cases of BPD may eventually move toward resolution. However, one current view of BPD is that it is a disease in which damage to progenitor cells in the peripheral airway may be compounded by failure to resolve inflammation within a reasonable period. Thus, full recovery may be marred by failure to continue to grow alveoli. Survivors of extreme prematurity are now beginning to appear in adult pulmonary practice with reduced diffusion capacity, airways obstruction, and an "empty chest" on CT radiography as a result of BPD in infancy. Some of this is due to airway epithelial damage and smooth muscle hypertrophy and some due to endothelial vascular damage, while some may be due to subsequent intercurrent infections, particularly RSV. Nevertheless, the neonatal lung is reassuringly relatively resilient. Newer studies in mice show that oxygen-induced BPD models can be ameliorated in terms of alveolarization both by VEGF therapy and by various kinds of exogenous stem cells. Thus, hope springs eternal for improved postnatal lung recovery from the ravages of prematurity, oxygen plus pressure plus time. Translation of this hope into practices that can prevent or improve BPD outcomes may depend on an increasingly thorough integrative understanding of the genetics of lung development, injury, repair, and regeneration in the human premature lung.

References

1. Northway WH Jr., Rosan HC, Porter DY. Pulmonary disease following respirator therapy of hyaline-membrane disease. Bronchopulmonary dysplasia. N Engl J Med 1967; 276:357–368.
2. Philip AG. Oxygen plus pressure plus time: the etiology of bronchopulmonary dysplasia. Pediatrics 1975; 55:44–50.
3. Bell EF, Warburton D, Stonestreet BD, et al. Effect of fluid administration on the development of symptomatic patent ductus arteriosus and congestive heart failure in premature infants. N Engl J Med 1980; 302:589–604.
4. Jobe A H, Bancalari E. Bronchopulmonary dysplasia. Am J Respir Crit Care 2001; 163:1723–1729.
5. Sakiyama J, Yamagishi A, Kuroiwa A. Tbx4-Fgf10 system controls lung bud formation during chicken embryonic development. Development 2003; 130:1225–1234.
6. Metzger RJ, Klein OD, Martin GR, et al. The branching program of mouse lung development. Nature 2008; 453:745–750.
7. Warburton D. Developmental biology: order in the lung. Nature 2008; 453:733–735.
8. Unbekandt M, del Moral PM, Sala FG, et al. Tracheal occlusion increases the rate of epithelial branching of embryonic mouse lung via the FGF10-FGFR2b-Sprouty2 pathway. Mech Dev 2008; 125:314–324.
9. Hashimoto S, Nakano H, Singh G, et al. Expression of Spred and Sprouty in developing rat lung. Mech Dev 2002; 119(suppl 1):S303–S309.
10. Lu MM, Li S, Yang H, et al. Foxp4: a novel member of the Foxp subfamily of winged-helix genes co-expressed with Foxp1 and Foxp2 in pulmonary and gut tissues. Mech Dev 2002; 119(suppl 1):S197–S202.
11. Blewett CJ, Zgleszewski SE, Chinoy MR, et al. Bronchial ligation enhances murine fetal lung development in whole-organ culture. J Pediatr Surg 1996; 31:869–877.
12. Kitano Y, Yang EY, von Allmen D, et al. Tracheal occlusion in the fetal rat: a new experimental model for the study of accelerated lung growth. J Pediatr Surg 1998; 33:1741–1744.
13. Papadakis K, Luks FI, De Paepe ME, et al. Fetal lung growth after tracheal ligation is not solely a pressure phenomenon. J Pediatr Surg 1997; 32:347–351.
14. Inanlou MR, Kablar B. Abnormal development of the diaphragm in mdx:MyoD-/-(9th) embryos leads to pulmonary hypoplasia. Int J Dev Biol 2003; 47:363–371.
15. Bostrom H, Willetts K, Pekny M, et al. PDGF-A signaling is a critical event in lung alveolar myofibroblast development and alveogenesis. Cell 1996; 85:863–873.
16. Lindahl P, Karlsson L, Hellstrom M, et al. Alveogenesis failure in PDGF-A-deficient mice is coupled to lack of distal spreading of alveolar smooth muscle cell progenitors during lung development. Development 1997; 124:3943–3953.
17. Bostrom H, Gritli-Linde A, Betsholtz C. PDGF-A/PDGF alpha-receptor signaling is required for lung growth and the formation of alveoli but not for early lung branching morphogenesis. Dev Dyn 2002; 223:155–162.

18. Wu JY, Feng L, Park HT, et al. The neuronal repellent Slit inhibits leukocyte chemotaxis induced by chemotactic factors. Nature 2001; 410:948–952.

19. Anselmo MA, Dalvin S, Prodhan P, et al. Slit and Robo: expression patterns in lung development. Gene Expr Patterns 2003; 3:13–19.

20. Xian J, Clark KJ, Fordham R, et al. Inadequate lung development and bronchial hyperplasia in mice with a targeted deletion in the Dutt1/Robo1 gene. Proc Natl Acad Sci U S A 2001; 98:15062–15066.

21. Chen C, Chen H, Sun J, et al. Smad1 expression and function during mouse embryonic lung morphogenesis. Am J Physiol Lung Cell Mol Physiol 2005; 288:L1033–L1039.

22. Chen H, Zhuang F, Liu YH, et al. TGF-beta receptor II in epithelia versus mesenchyme plays distinct role in developing lung. Eur Respir J 2008; 32:285–295.

23. Awonusonu F, Srinivasan S, Strange J, et al. Developmental shift in the relative percentages of lung fibroblast subsets: role of apoptosis postseptation. Am J Physiol 1999; 277:L848–L859.

24. Schittny JC, Djonov V, Fine A, et al. Programmed cell death contributes to postnatal lung development. Am J Respir Cell Mol Biol 1998; 18:786–793.

25. Srinivasan S, Strange J, Awonusonu F, et al. Insulin-like growth factor I receptor is downregulated after alveolarization in an apoptotic fibroblast subset. Am J Physiol Lung Cell Mol Physiol 2002; 282:L457–L467.

26. Kasahara Y, Tuder RM, Taraseviciene-Stewart L, et al. Inhibition of VEGF receptors causes lung cell apoptosis and emphysema. J Clin Invest 2000; 106:1311–1319.

27. Massaro GD, Massaro D. Postnatal treatment with retinoic acid increases the number of pulmonary alveoli in rats. Am J Physiol 1996; 270:L305–L310.

28. Massaro GD, Massaro D. Retinoic acid treatment partially rescues failed septation in rats and in mice. Am J Physiol Lung Cell Mol Physiol 2000; 278:L955–L960.

29. McGowan S, Jackson SK, Jenkins-Moore M, et al. Mice bearing deletions of retinoic acid receptors demonstrate reduced lung elastin and alveolar numbers. Am J Respir Cell Mol Biol 2000; 23:162–167.

30. Chytil F. Retinoids in lung development. FASEB J 1996; 10:986–992.

31. Vermeer PD, Harson R, Einwalter LA, et al. Interleukin-9 induces goblet cell hyperplasia during repair of human airway epithelia. Am J Respir Cell Mol Biol 2003; 28:286–295.

32. Lordan JL, Bucchieri F, Richter A, et al. Cooperative effects of Th2 cytokines and allergen on normal and asthmatic bronchial epithelial cells. J Immunol 2002; 169:407–414.

33. Ramirez MI, Millien G, Hinds A, et al. T1alpha, a lung type I cell differentiation gene, is required for normal lung cell proliferation and alveolus formation at birth. Dev Biol 2003; 256:61–72.

34. Whitsett JA, Weaver TE. Hydrophobic surfactant proteins in lung function and disease. N Engl J Med 2002; 347:2141–2148.

35. Kim CF, Jackson EL, Woolfenden AE, et al. Identification of bronchoalveolar stem cells in normal lung and lung cancer. Cell 2005; 121:823–835.

36. DeLanghe S, Carraro G, Warburton D, et al. Levels of mesenchymal FGFR2 signaling modulate smooth muscle progenitor cell commitment in the lung. Dev Biol 2006; 299:52–62.

37. Shan L, Subramanian M, Emanuel RL, et al. Centrifugal migration of mesenchymal cells in embryonic lung. Dev Dyn 2008; 237:750–757.

38. Qian X, Costa RH. Analysis of hepatocyte nuclear factor-3 beta protein domains required for transcriptional activation and nuclear targeting. Nucleic Acids Res 1995; 23:1184–1191.

39. Zhou L, Lim L, Costa RH, et al. Thyroid transcription factor-1, hepatocyte nuclear factor-3beta, surfactant protein B, C, and Clara cell secretory protein in developing mouse lung. J Histochem Cytochem 1996; 44:1183–1193.

40. Zhou L, Dey CR, Wert SE, et al. Hepatocyte nuclear factor-3beta limits cellular diversity in the developing respiratory epithelium and alters lung morphogenesis in vivo. Dev Dyn 1997; 210:305–314.

41. Bingle CD, Hackett BP, Moxley M, et al. Role of hepatocyte nuclear factor-3 alpha and hepatocyte nuclear factor-3 beta in Clara cell secretory protein gene expression in the bronchiolar epithelium. Biochem J 1995; 308(pt 1):197–202.
42. Bohinski RJ, Di Lauro R, Whitsett JA. The lung-specific surfactant protein B gene promoter is a target for thyroid transcription factor 1 and hepatocyte nuclear factor 3, indicating common factors for organ-specific gene expression along the foregut axis. Mol Cell Biol 1994; 14:5671–5681.
43. He Y, Crouch EC, Rust K, et al. Proximal promoter of the surfactant protein D gene: regulatory roles of AP-1, forkhead box, and GT box binding proteins. J Biol Chem 2000; 275:31051–31060.
44. Ikeda K, Shaw-White JR, Wert SE, et al. Hepatocyte nuclear factor 3 activates transcription of thyroid transcription factor 1 in respiratory epithelial cells. Mol Cell Biol 1996; 16:3626–3636.
45. Samadani U, Porcella A, Pani L, et al. Cytokine regulation of the liver transcription factor hepatocyte nuclear factor-3 beta is mediated by the C/EBP family and interferon regulatory factor 1. Cell Growth Differ 1995; 6:879–890.
46. Peterson RS, Lim L, Ye H, et al. The winged helix transcriptional activator HFH-8 is expressed in the mesoderm of the primitive streak stage of mouse embryos and its cellular derivatives. Mech Dev 1997; 69:53–69.
47. Shinbrot E, Peters KG, Williams LT. Expression of the platelet-derived growth factor beta receptor during organogenesis and tissue differentiation in the mouse embryo. Dev Dyn 1994; 199:169–175.
48. Souza P, Tanswell AK, Post M. Different roles for PDGF-alpha and -beta receptors in embryonic lung development. Am J Respir Cell Mol Biol 1996; 15:551–562.
49. Kalinichenko VV, Lim L, Stolz DB, et al. Defects in pulmonary vasculature and perinatal lung hemorrhage in mice heterozygous null for the Forkhead Box f1 transcription factor. Dev Biol 2001; 235:489–506.
50. Ohmichi H, Koshimizu U, Matsumoto K, et al. Hepatocyte growth factor (HGF) acts as a mesenchyme-derived morphogenic factor during fetal lung development. Development 1998; 125:1315–1324.
51. Weaver M, Yingling JM, Dunn NR, et al. Bmp signaling regulates proximal-distal differentiation of endoderm in mouse lung development. Development 1999; 126:4005–4015.
52. Hackett BP, Brody SL, Liang M, et al. Primary structure of hepatocyte nuclear factor/forkhead homologue 4 and characterization of gene expression in the developing respiratory and reproductive epithelium. Proc Natl Acad Sci U S A 1995; 92:4249–4253.
53. Brody SL, Yan XH, Wuerffel MK, et al. Ciliogenesis and left-right axis defects in forkhead factor HFH-4-null mice. Am J Respir Cell Mol Biol 2000; 23:45–51.
54. Chen J, Knowles HJ, Hebert JL, et al. Mutation of the mouse hepatocyte nuclear factor/forkhead homologue 4 gene results in an absence of cilia and random left-right asymmetry. J Clin Invest 1998; 102:1077–1082.
55. Hyatt BA, Shangguan X, Shannon JM. BMP4 modulates fibroblast growth factor-mediated induction of proximal and distal lung differentiation in mouse embryonic tracheal epithelium in mesenchyme-free culture. Dev Dyn 2002; 225:153–165.
56. Guazzi S, Price M, De Felice M, et al. Thyroid nuclear factor 1 (TTF-1) contains a homeodomain and displays a novel DNA binding specificity. EMBO J 1990; 9:3631–3639.
57. Lazzaro D, Price M, De Felice M, et al. The transcription factor TTF-1 is expressed at the onset of thyroid and lung morphogenesis and in restricted regions of the foetal brain. Development 1991; 113:1093–1104.
58. Kimura S, Hara Y, Pineau T, et al. The T/ebp null mouse: thyroid-specific enhancer-binding protein is essential for the organogenesis of the thyroid, lung, ventral forebrain, and pituitary. Genes Dev 1996; 10:60–69.

59. Minoo P, Su G, Drum H, et al. Defects in tracheoesophageal and lung morphogenesis in Nkx2.1(-/-) mouse embryos. Dev Biol 1999; 209:60–71.

60. Wert SE, Dey CR, Blair PA, et al. Increased expression of thyroid transcription factor-1 (TTF-1) in respiratory epithelial cells inhibits alveolarization and causes pulmonary inflammation. Dev Biol 2002; 242:75–87.

61. Boggaram V. Regulation of lung surfactant protein gene expression. Front Biosci 2003; 8:d751–d764.

62. Bruno MD, Bohinski RJ, Huelsman KM, et al. Lung cell-specific expression of the murine surfactant protein A (SP-A) gene is mediated by interactions between the SP-A promoter and thyroid transcription factor-1. J Biol Chem 1995; 270:6531–6536.

63. Ramirez MI, Rishi AK, Cao YX, et al. TGT3, thyroid transcription factor I, and Sp1 elements regulate transcriptional activity of the 1.3-kilobase pair promoter of T1alpha, a lung alveolar type I cell gene. J Biol Chem 1997; 272:26285–26294.

64. Whitsett JA, Glasser SW. Regulation of surfactant protein gene transcription. Biochim Biophys Acta 1998; 1408:303–311.

65. Yan C, Sever Z, Whitsett JA. Upstream enhancer activity in the human surfactant protein B gene is mediated by thyroid transcription factor 1. J Biol Chem 1995; 270:24852–24857.

66. Zhang L, Whitsett JA, Stripp BR. Regulation of Clara cell secretory protein gene transcription by thyroid transcription factor-1. Biochim Biophys Acta 1997; 1350:359–367.

67. DeFelice M, Silberschmidt D, DiLauro R, et al. TTF-1 phosphorylation is required for peripheral lung morphogenesis, perinatal survival, and tissue-specific gene expression. J Biol Chem 2003; 278:35574–35583.

68. Shaw-White JR, Bruno MD, Whitsett JA. GATA-6 activates transcription of thyroid transcription factor-1. J Biol Chem 1999; 274:2658–2664.

69. Aubin J, Lemieux M, Tremblay M, et al. Early postnatal lethality in Hoxa-5 mutant mice is attributable to respiratory tract defects. Dev Biol 1997; 192:432–445.

70. Bogue CW, Lou LJ, Vasavada H, et al. Expression of Hoxb genes in the developing mouse foregut and lung. Am J Respir Cell Mol Biol 1996; 15:163–171.

71. Volpe MV, Martin A, Vosatka RJ, et al. Hoxb-5 expression in the developing mouse lung suggests a role in branching morphogenesis and epithelial cell fate. Histochem Cell Biol 1997; 108:495–504.

72. Grindley JC, Bellusci S, Perkins D, et al. Evidence for the involvement of the Gli gene family in embryonic mouse lung development. Dev Biol 1997; 188:337–348.

73. Motoyama J, Liu J, Mo R, et al. Essential function of Gli2 and Gli3 in the formation of lung, trachea and oesophagus. Nat Genet 1998; 20:54–57.

74. Jaskoll TF, Don-Wheeler G, Johnson R, et al. Embryonic mouse lung morphogenesis and type II cytodifferentiation in serumless, chemically defined medium using prolonged in vitro cultures. Cell Differ 1988; 24:105–117.

75. Warburton D, Seth R, Shum L, et al. Epigenetic role of epidermal growth factor expression and signalling in embryonic mouse lung morphogenesis. Dev Biol 1992; 149:123–133.

76. Glazer L, Shilo BZ. The Drosophila FGF-R homolog is expressed in the embryonic tracheal system and appears to be required for directed tracheal cell extension. Genes Dev 1991; 5:697–705.

77. Sutherland D, Samakovlis C, Krasnow MA. Branchless encodes a Drosophila FGF homolog that controls tracheal cell migration and the pattern of branching. Cell 1996; 87:1091–1101.

78. Ornitz DM, Itoh N. Fibroblast growth factors. Genome Biol 2001; 2:REVIEWS3005.

79. Izvolsky KI, Zhong L, Wei L, et al. Heparan sulfates expressed in the distal lung are required for Fgf10 binding to the epithelium and for airway branching. Am J Physiol Lung Cell Mol Physiol 2003; 285:L838–L846.

80. Izvolsky KI, Shoykhet D, Yang Y, et al. Heparan sulfate-FGF10 interactions during lung morphogenesis. Dev Biol 2003; 258:185–200.

81. Hokuto I, Perl AK, Whitsett JA. Prenatal, but not postnatal, inhibition of fibroblast growth factor receptor signaling causes emphysema. J Biol Chem 2003; 278:415–421.
82. Min H, Danilenko DM, Scully SA, et al. Fgf-10 is required for both limb and lung development and exhibits striking functional similarity to Drosophila branchless. Genes Dev 1998; 12:3156–3161.
83. Bellusci S, Grindley J, Emoto H, et al. Fibroblast growth factor 10 (FGF10) and branching morphogenesis in the embryonic mouse lung. Development 1997; 124:4867–4878.
84. Park WY, Miranda B, Lebeche D, et al. FGF-10 is a chemotactic factor for distal epithelial buds during lung development. Dev Biol 1998; 201:125–134.
85. Weaver M, Dunn NR, Hogan BL. Bmp4 and Fgf10 play opposing roles during lung bud morphogenesis. Development 2000; 127:2695–2704.
86. Post M, Souza P, Liu J, et al. Keratinocyte growth factor and its receptor are involved in regulating early lung branching. Development 1996; 122:3107–3115.
87. Cardoso WV, Itoh A, Nogawa H, et al. FGF-1 and FGF-7 induce distinct patterns of growth and differentiation in embryonic lung epithelium. Dev Dyn 1997; 208:398–405.
88. Deterding RR, Jacoby CR, Shannon JM. Acidic fibroblast growth factor and keratinocyte growth factor stimulate fetal rat pulmonary epithelial growth. Am J Physiol 1996; 271: L495–L505.
89. Liu Y, Jiang H, Crawford HC, et al. Role for ETS domain transcription factors Pea3/Erm in mouse lung development. Dev Biol 2003; 261:10–24.
90. Liu Y, Hogan BL. Differential gene expression in the distal tip endoderm of the embryonic mouse lung. Gene Expr Patterns 2002; 2:229–233.
91. Frank L. Protective effect of keratinocyte growth factor against lung abnormalities associated with hyperoxia in prematurely born Rats. Biol Neonate 2003; 83:263–272.
92. Guo L, Degenstein L, Fuchs E. Keratinocyte growth factor is required for hair development but not for wound healing. Genes Dev 1996; 10:165–175.
93. Colvin JS, Feldman B, Nadeau JH, et al. Genomic organization and embryonic expression of the mouse fibroblast growth factor 9 gene. Dev Dyn 1999; 216:72–88.
94. Colvin JS, White AC, Pratt SJ, et al. Lung hypoplasia and neonatal death in Fgf9-null mice identify this gene as an essential regulator of lung mesenchyme. Development 2001; 128:2095–2106.
95. Weaver M, Batts L, Hogan BL. Tissue interactions pattern the mesenchyme of the embryonic mouse lung. Dev Biol 2003; 258:169–184.
96. Mailleux AA, Tefft D, Ndiaye D, et al. Evidence that SPROUTY2 functions as an inhibitor of mouse embryonic lung growth and morphogenesis. Mech Dev 2001; 102:81–94.
97. Hacohen N, Kramer S, Sutherland D, et al. Sprouty encodes a novel antagonist of FGF signaling that patterns apical branching of the Drosophila airways. Cell 1998; 92:253–263.
98. Kramer S, Okabe M, Hacohen N, et al. Sprouty: a common antagonist of FGF and EGF signaling pathways in Drosophila. Development 1999; 126:2515–2525.
99. Reich A, Sapir A, Shilo B. Sprouty is a general inhibitor of receptor tyrosine kinase signaling. Development 1999; 126:4139–4147.
100. Hadari YR, Kouhara H, Lax I, et al. Binding of Shp2 tyrosine phosphatase to FRS2 is essential for fibroblast growth factor-induced PC12 cell differentiation. Mol Cell Biol 1998; 18:3966–3973.
101. Perl AK, Hokuto I, Impagnatiello MA, et al. Temporal effects of Sprouty on lung morphogenesis. Dev Biol 2003; 258:154–168.
102. Tefft D, Lee M, Smith S, et al. mSprouty2 inhibits FGF10-activated MAP kinase by differentially binding to upstream target proteins. Am J Physiol Lung Cell Mol Physiol 2002; 283:L700–L706.
103. Derynck R, Zhang YE. Smad-dependent and Smad-independent pathways in TGF-beta family signaling. Nature 2003; 425:577–584.

104. McLennan IS, Poussart Y, Koishi K. Development of skeletal muscles in transforming growth factor-beta 1 (TGF-beta1) null-mutant mice. Dev Dyn 2000; 217:250–256.
105. Bartram U, Molin DG, Wisse LJ, et al. Double-outlet right ventricle and overriding tricuspid valve reflect disturbances of looping, myocardialization, endocardial cushion differentiation, and apoptosis in TGF-beta(2)-knockout mice. Circulation 2001; 103:2745–2752.
106. Kaartinen V, Voncken JW, Shuler C, et al. Abnormal lung development and cleft palate in mice lacking TGF-beta 3 indicates defects of epithelial-mesenchymal interaction. Nat Genet 1995; 11:415–421.
107. Shi W, Heisterkamp N, Groffen J, et al. TGF-beta3-null mutation does not abrogate fetal lung maturation in vivo by glucocorticoids. Am J Physiol 1999; 277:L1205–L1213.
108. Zhao J, Sime PJ, Bringas P Jr., et al. Spatial-specific TGF-beta1 adenoviral expression determines morphogenetic phenotypes in embryonic mouse lung. Eur J Cell Biol 1999; 78:715–725.
109. Zeng X, Gray M, Stahlman MT, et al. TGF-beta1 perturbs vascular development and inhibits epithelial differentiation in fetal lung in vivo. Dev Dyn 2001; 221:289–301.
110. Zhou L, Dey CR, Wert SE, et al. Arrested lung morphogenesis in transgenic mice bearing an SP-C-TGF-beta 1 chimeric gene. Dev Biol 1996; 175:227–238.
111. Lecart C, Cayabyab R, Buckley S, et al. Bioactive transforming growth factor-beta in the lungs of extremely low birthweight neonates predicts the need for home oxygen supplementation. Biol Neonate 2000; 77:217–223.
112. Toti P, Buonocore G, Tanganelli P, et al. Bronchopulmonary dysplasia of the premature baby: an immunohistochemical study. Pediatr Pulmonol 1997; 24:22–28.
113. Sime PJ, Xing Z, Graham FL, et al. Adenovector-mediated gene transfer of active transforming growth factor-beta1 induces prolonged severe fibrosis in rat lung. J Clin Invest 1997; 100:768–776.
114. Zhao J, Shi W, Wang YL, et al. Smad3 deficiency attenuates bleomycin-induced pulmonary fibrosis in mice. Am J Physiol Lung Cell Mol Physiol 2002; 282:L585–L593.
115. Gauldie J, Galt T, Warburton D. Transfer of active TGFβ1 gene to newborn rat lung induces changes consistent with Bronchopulmonary dysplasia. Am J Pathol 2003; 163:2575–2584.
116. KomatsuY, Shibuya H, Takeda N, et al. Targeted disruption of the Tab1 gene causes embryonic lethality and defects in cardiovascular and lung morphogenesis. Mech Dev 2002; 119:239–249.
117. Li DY, Sorensen LK, Brooke BS, et al. Defective angiogenesis in mice lacking endoglin. Science 1999; 284:1534–1537.
118. Sterner-Kock A, Thorey IS, Koli K, et al. Disruption of the gene encoding the latent transforming growth factor-beta binding protein 4 (LTBP-4) causes abnormal lung development, cardiomyopathy, and colorectal cancer. Genes Dev 2002; 16:2264–2273.
119. Chen H, Sun J, Buckley S, et al. Abnormal mouse lung alveolarization caused by Smad3 deficiency is a development antecedent of centrilobular emphysema. Am J Physiol Lung Cell Mol Physiol 2005; 288:L683–L691.
120. Shi W, Zhao J, Anderson KD, et al. Gremlin negatively modulates BMP-4 induction of embryonic mouse lung branching morphogenesis. Am J Physiol Lung Cell Mol Physiol 2001; 280:L1030–L1039.
121. Bragg AD, Moses HL, Serra R. Signaling to the epithelium is not sufficient to mediate all of the effects of transforming growth factor beta and bone morphogenetic protein 4 on murine embryonic lung development. Mech Dev 2001; 109:13–26.
122. Bellusci S, Henderson R, Winnier G, et al. Evidence from normal expression and targeted misexpression that bone morphogenetic protein (Bmp-4) plays a role in mouse embryonic lung morphogenesis. Development 1996; 122:1693–1702.
123. Eblaghie MC, Reedy M, Oliver T, et al. Evidence that autocrine signaling through Bmpr1a regulates the proliferation, survival and morphogenetic behavior of distal lung epithelial cells. Dev Biol 2006; 291:67–82.

124. Sun J, Chen H, Chen C, et al. Prenatal lung epithelial cell-specific abrogation of Alk3-bone morphogenetic protein signaling causes neonatal respiratory distress by disrupting distal airway formation. Am J Pathol 2008; 172(3):571–82.
125. Lane KB, Machado RD, Pauciulo MW, et al. Heterozygous germline mutations in BMPR2, encoding a TGF-beta receptor, cause familial primary pulmonary hypertension. The International PPH Consortium. Nat Genet 2000; 26:81–84.
126. Costello CM, Howell K, Cahill E, et al. Lung-selective gene responses to alveolar hypoxia: potential role for the bone morphogenetic antagonist gremlin in pulmonary hypertension. Am J Physiol Lung Cell Mol Physiol 2008; 295:L272–L284.
127. Koli K, Myllarniemi M, Vuorinen K, et al. Bone morphogenetic protein-4 inhibitor gremlin is overexpressed in idiopathic pulmonary fibrosis. Am J Pathol 2006; 169:61–71.
128. Myllarniemi M, Vuorinen K, Pulkkinen V, et al. Gremlin localization and expression levels partially differentiate idiopathic interstitial pneumonia severity and subtype. J Pathol 2008; 214:456–463.
129. van Tuyl M, Post M. From fruitflies to mammals: mechanisms of signalling via the Sonic hedgehog pathway in lung development. Respir Res 2000; 1:30–35.
130. Bellusci S, Furuta Y, Rush MG, et al. Involvement of Sonic hedgehog (Shh) in mouse embryonic lung growth and morphogenesis. Development 1997; 124:53–63.
131. Urase K, Mukasa T, Igarashi H, et al. Spatial expression of Sonic hedgehog in the lung epithelium during branching morphogenesis. Biochem Biophys Res Commun 1996; 225:161–166.
132. Litingtung Y, Lei L, Westphal H, et al. Sonic hedgehog is essential to foregut development. Nat Genet 1998; 20:58–61.
133. Pepicelli CV, Lewis PM, McMahon AP. Sonic hedgehog regulates branching morphogenesis in the mammalian lung. Curr Biol 1998; 8:1083–1086.
134. Spilde TL, Bhatia AM, Mehta S, et al. Defective sonic hedgehog signaling in esophageal atresia with tracheoesophageal fistula. Surgery 2003; 134:345–350.
135. Chuang PT, McMahon AP. Vertebrate Hedgehog signalling modulated by induction of a Hedgehog-binding protein. Nature 1999; 397:617–621.
136. Goodrich LV, Johnson RL, Milenkovic L, et al. Conservation of the hedgehog/patched signaling pathway from flies to mice: induction of a mouse patched gene by Hedgehog. Genes Dev 1996; 10:301–312.
137. Kawahira H, Ma NH, Tzanakakis ES, et al. Combined activities of hedgehog signaling inhibitors regulate pancreas development. Development 2003; 130:4871–4879.
138. Wodarz A, Nusse R. Mechanisms of Wnt signaling in development. Annu Rev Cell Dev Biol 1998; 14:59–88.
139. Mucenski ML, Wert SE, Nation JM, et al. beta -catenin is required for specification of proximal/distal cell fate during lung morphogenesis. J Biol Chem 2003; 278:40231–40238.
140. Tebar M, Destree O, de Vree WJ, et al. Expression of Tcf/Lef and sFrp and localization of beta-catenin in the developing mouse lung. Mech Dev 2001; 109:437–440.
141. Eberhart CG, Argani P. Wnt signaling in human development: beta-catenin nuclear translocation in fetal lung, kidney, placenta, capillaries, adrenal, and cartilage. Pediatr Dev Pathol 2001; 4:351–357.
142. Schuger L, Johnson GR, Gilbride K, et al. Amphiregulin in lung branching morphogenesis: interaction with heparan sulfate proteoglycan modulates cell proliferation. Development 1996; 122:1759–1767.
143. Seth R, Shum L, Wu F, et al. Role of epidermal growth factor expression in early mouse embryo lung branching morphogenesis in culture: antisense oligodeoxynucleotide inhibitory strategy. Dev Biol 1993; 158:555–559.
144. Raaberg L, Nexo E, Buckley S, et al. Epidermal growth factor transcription, translation, and signal transduction by rat type II pneumocytes in culture. Am J Respir Cell Mol Biol 1992; 6:44–49.

145. Korfhagen TR, Swantz RJ, Wert SE, et al. Respiratory epithelial cell expression of human transforming growth factor-alpha induces lung fibrosis in transgenic mice. J Clin Invest 1994; 93:1691–1699.
146. Le Cras TD, Hardie WD, Fagan K, et al. Disrupted Pulmonary Vascular Development And Pulmonary Hypertension in Transgenic Mice Overexpressing Transforming Growth Factor-{alpha}. Am. J. Physiol Lung Cell Mol. Physiol. 2003; 285(5):L1046–L1054.
147. Sanchez-Esteban J, Wang Y, Gruppuso PA, et al. Mechanical stretch induces fetal type II cell differentiation via an EGFR-ERK signaling pathway. Am J Respir Cell Mol Biol 2004; 30(1):76–83.
148. Kheradmand F, Rishi K, Werb Z. Signaling through the EGF receptor controls lung morphogenesis in part by regulating MT1-MMP-mediated activation of gelatinase A/MMP2. J Cell Sci 2002; 115:839–848.
149. Shi W, Chen H, Sun J, et al. TACE is required for fetal murine cardiac development and modeling. Dev Biol 2003; 261:371–380.
150. Zhao J, Chen H, Peschon JJ, et al. Pulmonary hypoplasia in mice lacking tumor necrosis factor-alpha converting enzyme indicates an indispensable role for cell surface protein shedding during embryonic lung branching morphogenesis. Dev Biol 2001; 232:204–218.
151. Buch S, Jassal D, Cannigia I, et al. Ontogeny and regulation of platelet-derived growth factor gene expression in distal fetal rat lung epithelial cells. Am J Respir Cell Mol Biol 1994; 11:251–261.
152. Souza P, Kuliszewski M, Wang J, et al. PDGF-AA and its receptor influence early lung branching via an epithelial-mesenchymal interaction. Development 1995; 121:2559–2567.
153. Souza P, Sedlackova L, Kuliszewski M, et al. Antisense oligodeoxynucleotides targeting PDGF-B mRNA inhibit cell proliferation during embryonic rat lung development. Development 1994; 120:2163–2173.
154. LaRochelle WJ, Jeffers M, McDonald WF, et al. PDGF-D, a new protease-activated growth factor. Nat Cell Biol 2001; 3:517–521.
155. Li X, Ponten A, Aase K, et al. PDGF-C is a new protease-activated ligand for the PDGF alpha-receptor. Nat Cell Biol 2000; 2:302–309.
156. Zhuo Y, Zhang J, Laboy M, et al. Modulation of PDGF-C and PDGF-D expression during bleomycin-induced lung fibrosis. Am J Physiol Lung Cell Mol Physiol 2004; 286(1): L182–188.
157. Batchelor DC, Hutchins AM, Klempt M, et al. Developmental changes in the expression patterns of IGFs, type 1 IGF receptor and IGF-binding proteins-2 and -4 in perinatal rat lung. J Mol Endocrinol 1995; 15:105–115.
158. Lallemand AV, Ruocco SM, Joly PM, et al. In vivo localization of the insulin-like growth factors I and II (IGF I and IGF II) gene expression during human lung development. Int J Dev Biol 1995; 39:529–537.
159. Maitre B, Clement A, Williams MC, et al. Expression of insulin-like growth factor receptors 1 and 2 in the developing lung and their relation to epithelial cell differentiation. Am J Respir Cell Mol Biol 1995; 13:262–270.
160. Retsch-Bogart GZ, Moats-Staats BM, Howard K, et al. Cellular localization of messenger RNAs for insulin-like growth factors (IGFs), their receptors and binding proteins during fetal rat lung development. Am J Respir Cell Mol Biol 1996; 14:61–69.
161. Schuller AG, van Neck JW, Beukenholdt RW, et al. IGF, type I IGF receptor and IGF-binding protein mRNA expression in the developing mouse lung. J Mol Endocrinol 1995; 14:349–355.
162. Liu JP, Baker J, Perkins AS, et al. Mice carrying null mutations of the genes encoding insulin-like growth factor I (Igf-1) and type 1 IGF receptor (Igf1r). Cell 1993; 75:59–72.

163. Coppola D, Ferber A, Miura M, et al. A functional insulin-like growth factor I receptor is required for the mitogenic and transforming activities of the epidermal growth factor receptor. Mol Cell Biol 1994; 14:4588–4595.

164. Pichel JG, Fernandez-Moreno C, Vicario-Abejon C, et al. Developmental cooperation of leukemia inhibitory factor and insulin-like growth factor I in mice is tissue-specific and essential for lung maturation involving the transcription factors Sp3 and TTF-1. Mech Dev 2003; 120:349–361.

165. Han RN, Post M, Tanswell AK, et al. Insulin-like growth factor-I receptor-mediated vasculogenesis/angiogenesis in human lung development. Am J Respir Cell Mol Biol 2003; 28:159–169.

166. Larrivee B, Karsan A. Signaling pathways induced by vascular endothelial growth factor (review). Int J Mol Med 2000; 5:447–456.

167. Compernolle V, Brusselmans K, Acker T, et al. Loss of HIF-2alpha and inhibition of VEGF impair fetal lung maturation, whereas treatment with VEGF prevents fatal respiratory distress in premature mice. Nat Med 2002; 8:702–710.

168. Greenberg JM, Thompson FY, Brooks SK, et al. Mesenchymal expression of vascular endothelial growth factors D and A defines vascular patterning in developing lung. Dev Dyn 2002; 224(2):144–153.

169. Ng YS, Rohan R, Sunday ME, et al. Differential expression of VEGF isoforms in mouse during development and in the adult. Dev Dyn 2001; 220(2):112–121.

170. Healy AM, Morgenthau L, Zhu X, et al. VEGF is deposited in the subepithelial matrix at the leading edge of branching airways and stimulates neovascularization in the murine embryonic lung. Dev Dyn 2000; 219(3):341–352.

171. Acosta JM, Thébaud B, Castillo C, et al. Novel mechanisms in murine nitrofen-induced pulmonary hypoplasia: FGF-10 rescue in culture. Am J Physiol Lung Cell Mol Physiol 2001; 281(1):L250–257.

172. Gebb SA, Shannon JM. Tissue interactions mediate early events in pulmonary vasculogenesis. Dev Dyn 2000; 217:159–169.

173. Zeng X, Wert SE, Federici R, et al. VEGF enhances pulmonary vasculogenesis and disrupts lung morphogenesis in vivo. Dev Dyn 1998; 211:215–227.

174. Del Moral PM, DeLanghe SP, Sala FG, et al. Differential role of FGF9 on epithelium and mesenchyme in embryonic lung. Dev Biol 2006; 293:77–89.

175. Gerber HP, Hillan KJ, Ryan AM, et al. VEGF is required for growth and survival in neonatal mice. Development 1999; 126:1149–1159.

176. Lwebuga-Mukasa JS. Matrix-driven pneumocyte differentiation. Am Rev Respir Dis 1991; 144:452–457.

177. Hilfer SR. Morphogenesis of the lung: control of embryonic and fetal branching. Annu Rev Physiol 1996; 58:93–113.

178. Minoo P, King RJ. Epithelial-mesenchymal interactions in lung development. Annu Rev Physiol 1994; 56:13–45.

179. Burgeson RE, Chiquet M, Deutzmann R, et al. A new nomenclature for the laminins. Matrix Biol 1994; 14:209–211.

180. Bernier SM, Utani A, Sugiyama S, et al. Cloning and expression of laminin alpha 2 chain (M-chain) in the mouse. Matrix Biol 1995; 14:447–455.

181. Ehrig K, Leivo I, Argraves WS, et al. Merosin, a tissue-specific basement membrane protein, is a laminin-like protein. Proc Natl Acad Sci USA 1990; 87:3264–3268.

182. Galliano MF, Aberdam D, Aguzzi A, et al. Cloning and complete primary structure of the mouse laminin alpha 3 chain. Distinct expression pattern of the laminin alpha 3A and alpha 3B chain isoforms. J Biol Chem 1995; 270:21820–21826.

183. Iivanainen A, Sainio K, Sariola H, et al. Primary structure and expression of a novel human laminin alpha 4 chain. FEBS Lett 1995; 365:183–188.

184. Iivanainen A, Vuolteenaho R, Sainio K, et al. The human laminin beta 2 chain (S-laminin): structure, expression in fetal tissues and chromosomal assignment of the LAMB2 gene. Matrix Biol 1995; 14:489–497.
185. Iivanainen A, Kortesmaa J, Sahlberg C, et al. Primary structure, developmental expression, and immunolocalization of the murine laminin alpha4 chain. J Biol Chem 1997; 272:27862–27868.
186. Iivanainen A, Morita T, Tryggvason K. Molecular cloning and tissue-specific expression of a novel murine laminin gamma3 chain. J Biol Chem 1999; 274:14107–14111.
187. Koch M, Olson PF, Albus A, et al. Characterization and expression of the laminin gamma3 chain: a novel, non-basement membrane-associated, laminin chain. J Cell Biol 1999; 145:605–618.
188. Pierce RA, Griffin GL, Mudd MS, et al. Expression of laminin alpha3, alpha4, and alpha5 chains by alveolar epithelial cells and fibroblasts. Am J Respir Cell Mol Biol 1998; 19:237–244.
189. Vuolteenaho R, Nissinen M, Sainio K, et al. Human laminin M chain (merosin): complete primary structure, chromosomal assignment, and expression of the M and A chain in human fetal tissues. J Cell Biol 1994; 124:381–394.
190. Schuger L, Varani J, Killen PD, et al. Laminin expression in the mouse lung increases with development and stimulates spontaneous organotypic rearrangement of mixed lung cells. Dev Dyn 1992; 195:43–54.
191. Frieser M, Nockel H, Pausch F, et al. Cloning of the mouse laminin alpha 4 cDNA. Expression in a subset of endothelium. Eur J Biochem 1997; 246:727–735.
192. Miner JH, Patton BL, Lentz SI, et al. The laminin alpha chains: expression, developmental transitions, and chromosomal locations of alpha1-5, identification of heterotrimeric laminins 8-11, and cloning of a novel alpha3 isoform. J Cell Biol 1997; 137:685–701.
193. Miner JH, Lewis RM, Sanes JR. Molecular cloning of a novel laminin chain, alpha 5, and widespread expression in adult mouse tissues. J Biol Chem 1995; 270:28523–28526.
194. Miner JH, Cunningham J, Sanes JR. Roles for laminin in embryogenesis: exencephaly, syndactyly, and placentopathy in mice lacking the laminin alpha5 chain. J Cell Biol 1998; 143:1713–1723.
195. Durham PL, Snyder JM. Characterization of alpha 1, beta 1, and gamma 1 laminin subunits during rabbit fetal lung development. Dev Dyn 1995; 203:408–421.
196. Schuger L, Skubitz AP, de las MA, et al. Two separate domains of laminin promote lung organogenesis by different mechanisms of action. Dev Biol 1995; 169:520–532.
197. Schuger L, Skubitz AP, Gilbride K, et al. Laminin and heparan sulfate proteoglycan mediate epithelial cell polarization in organotypic cultures of embryonic lung cells: evidence implicating involvement of the inner globular region of laminin beta 1 chain and the heparan sulfate groups of heparan sulfate proteoglycan. Dev Biol 1996; 179:264–273.
198. Dziadek M. Role of laminin-nidogen complexes in basement membrane formation during embryonic development. Experientia 1995; 51:901–913.
199. Reinhardt D, Mann K, Nischt R, et al. Mapping of nidogen binding sites for collagen type IV, heparan sulfate proteoglycan, and zinc. J Biol Chem 1993; 268:10881–10887.
200. Senior RM, Griffin GL, Mudd MS, et al. Entactin expression by rat lung and rat alveolar epithelial cells. Am J Respir Cell Mol Biol 1996; 14:239–247.
201. Ekblom P, Ekblom M, Fecker L, et al. Role of mesenchymal nidogen for epithelial morphogenesis in vitro. Development 1994; 120:2003–2014.
202. Mayer U, Mann K, Timpl R, et al. Sites of nidogen cleavage by proteases involved in tissue homeostasis and remodelling. Eur J Biochem 1993; 217:877–884.
203. Belknap JK, Weiser-Evans MC, Grieshaber SS, et al. Relationship between perlecan and tropoelastin gene expression and cell replication in the developing rat pulmonary vasculature. Am J Respir Cell Mol Biol 1999; 20:24–34.
204. Shannon JM, McCormick-Shannon K, Burhans MS, et al. Chondroitin sulfate proteoglycans are required for lung growth and morphogenesis in vitro. Am J Physiol Lung Cell Mol Physiol 2003; 285(6):L1323–L1336.

205. Sakai T, Larsen M, Yamada KM. Fibronectin requirement in branching morphogenesis. Nature 2003; 423:876–881.
206. Roman J. Fibronectin and fibronectin receptors in lung development. Exp Lung Res 1997; 23:147–159.
207. Kikuchi W, Arai H, Ishida A, et al. Distal pulmonary cell proliferation is associated with the expression of eiiia+ fibronectin in the developing rat lung. Exp Lung Res 2003; 29:135–147.
208. Vu TH, Werb Z. Matrix metalloproteinases: effectors of development and normal physiology. Genes Dev 2000; 14:2123–2133.
209. Gill SE, Pape MC, Khokha R, et al. A null mutation for tissue inhibitor of metalloproteinases-3 (Timp-3) impairs murine bronchiole branching morphogenesis. Dev Biol 2003; 261:313–323.
210. Leco KJ, Waterhouse P, Sanchez OH, et al. Spontaneous air space enlargement in the lungs of mice lacking tissue inhibitor of metalloproteinases-3 (TIMP-3). J Clin Invest 2001; 108:817–829.
211. Valencia AM, Beharry KD, Ang JG, et al. Early postnatal dexamethasone influences matrix metalloproteinase-2 and -9, and their tissue inhibitors in the developing rat lung. Pediatr Pulmonol 2003; 35:456–462.
212. Niederreither K, McCaffery P, Drager UC, et al. Restricted expression and retinoic acid-induced downregulation of the retinaldehyde dehydrogenase type 2 (RALDH-2) gene during mouse development. Mech Dev 1997; 62:67–78.
213. Niederreither K, Subbarayan V, Dolle P, et al. Embryonic retinoic acid synthesis is essential for early mouse post-implantation development. Nat Genet 1999; 21:444–448.
214. Ulven SM, Gundersen TE, Weedon MS, et al. Identification of endogenous retinoids, enzymes, binding proteins, and receptors during early postimplantation development in mouse: important role of retinal dehydrogenase type 2 in synthesis of all-trans-retinoic acid. Dev Biol 2000; 220:379–391.
215. Kastner P, Mark M, Ghyselinck N, et al. Genetic evidence that the retinoid signal is transduced by heterodimeric RXR/RAR functional units during mouse development. Development 1997; 124:313–326.
216. Chazaud C, Dolle P, Rossant J, et al. Retinoic acid signaling regulates murine bronchial tubule formation. Mech Dev 2003; 120:691–700.
217. Dickman ED, Thaller C, Smith SM. Temporally-regulated retinoic acid depletion produces specific neural crest, ocular and nervous system defects. Development 1997; 124:3111–3121.
218. Sekine K, Ohuchi H, Fujiwara M, et al. Fgf10 is essential for limb and lung formation. Nat Genet 1999; 21:138–141.
219. Mendelsohn C, Lohnes D, Decimo D, et al. Function of the retinoic acid receptors (RARs) during development (II). Multiple abnormalities at various stages of organogenesis in RAR double mutants. Development 1994; 120:2749–2771.
220. Cardoso WV, Williams MC, Mitsialis SA, et al. Retinoic acid induces changes in the pattern of airway branching and alters epithelial cell differentiation in the developing lung in vitro. Am J Respir Cell Mol Biol 1995; 12:464–476.
221. Malpel S, Mendelsohn C, Cardoso WV. Regulation of retinoic acid signaling during lung morphogenesis. Development 2000; 127:3057–3067.
222. Wongtrakool C, Malpel S, Gorenstein J, et al. Downregulation of retinoic acid receptor alpha signaling is required for sacculation and type 1 cell formation in the developing lung. J Biol Chem 2003; 278(47):46911–46918.
223. Maden M, Hind M. Retinoic acid, a regeneration-inducing molecule. Dev Dyn 2003; 226:237–244.
224. Olver RE, Strang LB. Ion fluxes across the pulmonary epithelium and the secretion of lung liquid in the foetal lamb. J Physiol 1974; 241:327–357.

225. Brown MJ, Olver RE, Ramsden CA, et al. Effects of adrenaline and of spontaneous labor on the secretion and absorption of lung liquid in the fetal lamb. J Physiol 1983; 344:137–152.
226. Olver RE, Ramsden CA, Starng LB, et al. The role of amiloride-blockable sodium transport in adrernaline-induced lung liquid reabsorption in the fetal lamb. J Physiol 1986; 376:321–340.
227. Hummler E, Barker P, Gatzy J, et al. Early death due to defective neonatal lung liquid clearance in alpha-ENaC-deficient mice. Nat Genet 1996; 12:325–328.
228. Lecart C, Cayabyab R, Buckley S, et al. Bioactive transforming growth factor-beta in the lungs of extremely low birthweight neonates predicts the need for home oxygen supplementation. Biol Neonate 2000; 77(4):217–223.
229. Jones CA, Cayabyab RG, Kwong KY, et al. Undetectable interleukin (IL-10) and persistent IL-8 expression early in hyaline membrane disease: a possible developmental basis for the predisposition to chronic lung inflammation in preterm newborns. Pediatr Res 1996; 39:966–975.
230. Garingo A, Tesoriero L, Cayabyab R, et al. Constitutive IL-10 expression by lung inflammatory cells and risk for bronchopulmonary dysplasia. Pediatr Res 2007; 61:197–202.

Bibliography

Aubin J, Chailler P, Menard D, et al. Loss of Hoxa5 gene function in mice perturbs intestinal maturation. Am J Physiol 1999; 277:C965–C973.

Chiang C, Litingtung Y, Lee E, et al. Cyclopia and defective axial patterning in mice lacking Sonic hedgehog gene function. Nature 1996; 383:407–413.

Costa RH, Kalinichenko VV, Lim L. Transcription factors in mouse lung development and function. Am J Physiol Lung Cell Mol Physiol 2001; 280:L823–L838.

De Moerlooze L, Spencer-Dene B, Revest J, et al. An important role for the IIIb isoform of fibroblast growth factor receptor 2 (FGFR2) in mesenchymal-epithelial signalling during mouse organogenesis. Development 2000; 127:483–492.

Del Moral PM, Sala FG, Tefft D, et al. VEGF-A signaling through Flk-1 is a critical facilitator of early embryonic lung epithelial crosstalk and branching morphogenesis. Dev Biol 2005; 290:177–199.

Jeffery PK. Remodeling in asthma and chronic obstructive lung disease. Am J Respir Crit Care Med 2001; 164:S28–S38.

King JA, Marker PC, Seung KJ, et al. BMP5 and the molecular, skeletal, and soft-tissue alterations in short ear mice. Dev Biol 1994; 166:112–122.

Millarniemi M, Lindholm P, Ryynanen MJ, et al. Gremlin-mediated decrease in bone morphogenetic protein signaling promotes pulmonary fibrosis. Am J Respir Crit Care Med 2008; 177:321–329.

Ohuchi H, Hori Y, Yamasaki M, et al. FGF10 acts as a major ligand for FGF receptor 2 IIIb in mouse multi-organ development. Biochem Biophys Res Commun 2000; 277:643–649.

Shi Y, Massague J. Mechanisms of TGF-beta signaling from cell membrane to the nucleus. Cell 2003; 113:685–700.

Stewart GA, Hoyne GF, Ahmad SA, et al. Expression of the developmental Sonic hedgehog (Shh) signalling pathway is up-regulated in chronic lung fibrosis and the Shh receptor patched 1 is present in circulating T lymphocytes. J Pathol 2003; 199:488–495.

Takahashi H, Ikeda T. Transcripts for two members of the transforming growth factor-beta superfamily BMP-3 and BMP-7 are expressed in developing rat embryos. Dev Dyn 1996; 207:439–449.

Threadgill DW, Dlugosz AA, Hansen LA, et al. Targeted disruption of mouse EGF receptor: effect of genetic background on mutant phenotype. Science 1995; 269:230–234.

Tichelaar JW, Lim L, Costa RH, et al. HNF-3/forkhead homologue-4 influences lung morphogenesis and respiratory epithelial cell differentiation in vivo. Dev Biol 1999; 213:405–417.

Urness LD, Sorensen LK, Li DY. Arteriovenous malformations in mice lacking activin receptor-like kinase-1. Nat Genet 2000; 26:328–331.

Wendel DP, Taylor DG, Albertine KH, et al. Impaired distal airway development in mice lacking elastin. Am J Respir Cell Mol Biol 2000; 23:320–326.

Yoshida M, Korfhagen TR, Whitsett JA. Surfactant protein D regulates NF-kappa B and matrix metalloproteinase production in alveolar macrophages via oxidant-sensitive pathways. J Immunol 2001; 166:7514–7519.

Yuan B, Li C, Kimura S, et al. Inhibition of distal lung morphogenesis in Nkx2.1(-/-) embryos. Dev Dyn 2000; 217:180–190.

2

Growth Factors and Cell-Cell Interactions During Lung Development

EMILY FOX and MARTIN POST
Hospital for Sick Children, Toronto, Ontario, Canada

I. Introduction

The cells comprising the vertebrate lung are derived from the endoderm and mesoderm of the developing embryo. Bidirectional interactions between these two tissue layers have been shown to be essential for the proper development of the lung (1). In the mouse, the lung epithelial cells come from the primitive foregut around embryonic day 9.5 (E9.5) and invade the surrounding splanchnic mesenchyme (2). As development proceeds, these cells proliferate and differentiate into the cells that will form the mature lung. This process requires activation of cell-specific transcription factors and occurs under the influence of a number of growth factors, many of which act in a paracrine or autocrine manner. Epithelial-mesenchymal interactions play an important role in branching morphogenesis and proximal-distal airway differentiation. Epithelial-endothelial interactions assist in vascularization of the lung and development of the blood-air interface, which allows the organ to carry out gas exchange. This chapter focuses on the growth factors involved in early lung development, with emphasis on those factors involved in cell-cell interactions that aid in cell-fate decisions (Fig. 1).

II. Fibroblast Growth Factors

Fibroblast growth factors (FGFs) comprise a family of secreted polypeptide ligands that signal through tyrosine kinase receptors to regulate multiple processes including proliferation, differentiation, and angiogenic activity (3). These molecules are widely expressed from early development and into adulthood, implicating them as key regulators of growth and differentiation throughout life (3). Many FGFs including FGF-7 (4), FGF-9 (5), and FGF-10 (6) have been implicated in various aspects of lung development and play an important role in cell-cell signaling across the various tissue layers.

FGF-7 is an important growth factor in both the developing and postnatal lung, as well as in other organs including the forebrain, breast, and skin (4,7). This factor is sometimes referred to as keratinocyte growth factor (KGF) as it was first discovered to be a potent mitogen for mouse epidermal keratinocytes and later characterized as a member of the FGF family (8). FGF-7 is expressed in the mesenchyme and is unique among the FGF family as it only binds to one specific isoform of the receptor FGFR-2,

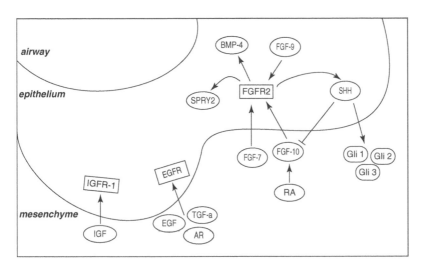

Figure 1 Schematic diagram illustrating the recognized molecular interactions between the epithelium and the mesenchyme of the developing lung. Positive interactions are depicted with arrowheads and negative interactions with a blunt-ended line. Some interactions that may function through intermediate effectors are not shown.

designated FGFR-2-IIIb, which is found exclusively in epithelial cells (3,9). This appositional expression of receptor and growth factor indicate that the FGF-7 is a diffusible mediator of epithelial-mesenchymal interactions (4). In the developing mouse lung, expression of FGF-7 begins at E11 and persists into adulthood, although at much lower levels than is seen at early time points (4). Conditional overexpression of FGF-7 in epithelial cells produced hypoplastic lungs with large interstitial space and an absence of alveolarization, similar to the malformations seen in pulmonary cystadenoma. This overexpressor mouse also had marked epithelial cell hyperplasia in adult lungs (7). These results suggest that FGF-7 plays an important role in lung morphogenesis, a claim that is further supported by inhibition studies in rat lung explants (4). Antisense FGF-7 oligonucleotide treatment of lung explants inhibited branching in a concentration-dependent manner, with addition of rat FGF-7 able to partially rescue these effects (4). Given the results from these studies, and the identification of FGF-7 as an important factor in lung development, it is surprising to note that FGF-7 null mice had a no apparent lung abnormalities (10). The lack of lung defects seen in these mice could be due to a partial compensatory effect of other FGFs. For example, FGF-1 and FGF-10 bind to the same receptor as FGF-7 and are also produced by the lung mesenchyme (6).

    Another role of FGF-7 in the developing lung is to stimulate epithelial differentiation and maturation. Studies using fibroblast-conditioned medium demonstrated that the FGF-7 secreted into the medium was able to stimulate alveolar type II cell proliferation in vitro (11). A similar effect was found in vivo when FGF-7 was injected intratracheally into adult rats and caused hypertrophy of the alveolar epithelium. The hyperplastic airway lining in the FGF-7–stimulated rats was found to produce surfactant protein B (SFPTB) and had an ultrastructure consistent with surfactant-producing type II pneumocytes (12). These results along with other studies (13) suggest that type II cell maturation and the resulting surfactant production is under the control of mesenchymal-epithelial interactions (8).

FGF-9 is expressed in the epithelium of the mouse lung at E10.5 and signals to the adjacent mesenchyme (14), through the FGFR-2B receptor (15). FGF-9 knockout mice show severe lung hypoplasia, reduced mesenchyme, and reduced branching (5). Further evidence for the theory that FGF-9 plays an important role in the regulation of mesenchymal proliferation comes from studies adding recombinant FGF-9 to lung explants. The addition to E12.5 lungs resulted in increased proliferation of the mesenchyme, along with decreased differentiation and reduced epithelial branching (15). This effect was independent of mesenchymal-epithelial interactions, as separate mesenchyme and epithelial layers showed the same response as when the tissue was in contact. Overexpression of FGF-9 using an inducible system showed similar results, with large expansion of the mesenchymal layer and reduced epithelial branching (16).

FGF-10 was initially discovered in E14 rat mesenchymal cells (17), but subsequent in situ analysis in mice demonstrated that it is expressed at the onset of lung development (E9.5) (6). FGF-10 is expressed by the mesenchymal cells of the lung, adjacent from the epithelium of the distal buds, where its receptor FGFR-2-IIIb resides (6). The position of FGF-10 at the distal end of the airway suggests that it is involved in directing the branching morphogenesis. Studies using FGF-10–soaked heparin beads have shown that mouse lung bud epithelium will grow toward this stimuli within 24 hours of culture. This effect was not seen in the proximal lung epithelium, suggesting that FGF-10 is a powerful chemotactic agent for the distal, but not the proximal lung (18). FGF-10 has also been found to be the only lung-associated FGF that is essential for lung development. This was demonstrated in FGF-10 null mice which completely lacks lung buds below the trachea as well as a number of other abnormalities including absence of limb buds, thyroid, and kidney malformations (19). Overexpression of FGF-10, driven by promoter elements from SFPTC or Clara cell secretory protein, resulted in disrupted branching and pulmonary adenomas, indicating that FGF-10 expression is critical for directing branching at the distal bud of the growing lung (20). The ability of FGF-10 signaling to adjust expression levels as lung growth progresses suggests that the endoderm is signaling back to the mesenchyme to regulate its expression. This is most likely occurring through interactions with Sonic hedgehog (SHH), bone morphogenetic protein 4 (BMP-4), and Sprouty 2 (Spry2), all of which are expressed in the epithelium of the distal tips of the developing lung (21). More recent studies ectopically expressing FGF-10 from the pancreatic and duodenal homeobox 1 promoter suggests that this factor is also involved in regulating differentiation of distal lung cells (22).

III. Sprouty

The Spry family of genes were initially discovered in *Drosophila*, where they were discovered to be antagonists to Breathless, the homologue of the FGF receptor in vertebrates (23). In these studies, mutations in Spry leading to loss of function caused excessive lung branching due to overactive FGF signaling. Forced expression of Spry blocked branching in the more distal airways (23). Similar results occurred when the mouse homologue Spry2 was overexpressed (24). Spry2 mRNA is detectable in the epithelium of the primary bronchial buds at E10.5. While low message levels of Spry2 are found in the adjacent mesenchyme at this stage, its expression quickly becomes restricted to the epithelium of the growing bud tips (24). Given the positions of Spry2 and FGF-10 in the developing lung, they have been implicated in epithelium-mesenchyme interactions. Further evidence to support this claim comes from studies using FGF-10–coated beads placed at the caudal lobes of E12 lungs. Spry2 expression was found to be significantly upregulated in the adjacent epithelium at the tips of the buds. FGF-10 antisense oligonucleotides resulted in reduced branching and levels of Spry2, signifying that FGF-10 plays a role in activating this factor (24). Overexpression studies demonstrate that an increase in Spry2 also results in reduced branching morphogenesis and an inhibition of epithelial cell proliferation (24). This phenotype was also noted when FGF-10 was blocked, although the authors were unable to conclusively show that Spry2 was a negative regulator of FGF-10 (24). While the details of their interactions remain to be characterized, it is clear that interplay between Spry2 and FGF-10 is needed to finely regulate branching morphogenesis in the embryonic lung.

IV. Bone Morphogenetic Protein

BMPs are part of a conserved family of secreted growth factors that are related to the transforming growth factor β (TGF-β) superfamily. BMP-5 and BMP-7 are expressed in both the mesenchyme and the epithelium of the developing lung, whereas BMP-4 is expressed in the epithelium of the distal lung buds, suggesting a role for it in epithelium-mesenchymal interactions (25). Despite their expression in early lung development, BMP-5 null mice do not show any obvious lung phenotype, although they do possess bone and external ear abnormalities (26). In contrast to the viable BMP-5 null mice lacking BMP-7 die within one month of birth and have global developmental defects (27). However, lung development was not found to be affected. BMP-4 null mice die early in gestation, between E6.5 and E9.5, before the initiation of lung development, indicating the pivotal role it plays in development (28). BMP-4 signaling can be detected in the embryonic lung from E11.5 at the distal tips of developing buds (29). FGF-10 has been shown to regulate BMP-4 expression in mice and can induce ectopic expression of the factor (30). These studies also indicate that FGF-10 signaling is required for maintenance of BMP-4 expression, as BMP-4 signaling decreased when FGF-10–soaked beads were moved to another area (30). The same study also found that adding exogenous BMP-4 inhibited outgrowth of lung endoderm toward FGF-10 beads, implying that there is antagonistic cross talk between these molecules (30). BMP-4 has also been shown to help establish proximal-distal cell fate in embryonic lungs. Overexpressor studies using *Xenopus* noggin (Xnoggin), an inhibitor of BMP-4, from an SFPTC promoter showed a severe reduction in cell types characteristic of the distal epithelium (25). On the basis of the results from these experiments, the authors hypothesize that cells exposed to high levels of BMP-4 assume a distal airway phenotype, whereas cells that receive negligible amounts adopt a proximal airway phenotype (25).

V. Sonic Hedgehog

SHH is expressed early in lung development at the tracheal diverticulum and is later restricted to the trachea and lung endoderm (31). SHH transcripts can be found in the entire epithelium of the mouse lung, with the highest expression levels present at the distal buds. SHH signals through its receptor patched (Ptc), a membrane protein found in the lung mesenchyme (32). Ptc is found at high levels adjacent to SHH expression at the distal lung mesenchyme, and is also detectable in low levels in the epithelium. Around E16.5, at the end of the pseudoglandular period, the levels of both SHH and Ptc begin to decline, especially in the distal epithelium (32). By postnatal day 24, SHH was undetectable in the bronchial and alveolar epithelium, indicating its major role in lung development is complete around birth (33). The primary role of Ptc is to regulate transcription of SHH target genes. In the absence of SHH, Ptc represses genes that are induced by SHH. SHH signaling causes Ptc to release the repression of the target genes and ultimately results in an upregulation in their activity (34). Overexpression of SHH in the distal epithelium using the SFPTC promoter resulted in an increase in the amount of mesenchyme and an absence of functional alveoli, indicating the SHH is acting as a regulator of mesenchymal cell proliferation. Ptc was also found to be upregulated in the lungs of these mice (32). SHH null mice have foregut defects such as trachea-esophageal fistulas and esophageal stenosis. In addition, the lung is hypoplastic and each lung bud has only one lobe with sac-like morphology instead of a system of alveoli. This model also demonstrated a lack of mesenchymal proliferation and epithelial branching, although proximal-distal differentiation seemed to be intact (35). This result indicates that SHH plays an important role in branching in the developing lung. The SHH null model shows a downregulation of Ptc, and when taken with the results of the overexpressor model, suggests a positive feedback between SHH and Ptc expression (36). There is evidence that the Gli family of zinc-finger transcription factors, namely Gli1, Gli2, and Gli3, play a role in the transduction of SHH signaling in the lung. Similar to Ptc, these Gli genes are expressed in the mesenchyme and at higher levels in the distal airway, across from SHH expression and act primarily as mediators of SHH signaling (37).

VI. Retinoic Acid

Retinoic acid (RA) is the oxidized form of vitamin A and plays a major role in regulating cell homeostasis, proliferation, migration, and differentiation. RA is stored in fibroblasts of the mesenchyme of the alveolar walls and its expression peaks around the time of alveolar septation (38). RA signals through two families of receptors: RA receptors (RARs) and retinoid X receptors (RXRs), each composed of three subtypes α, β, and γ. RAR can bind *trans*-RA and 9-*cis*-RA, whereas the RXR can only bind 9-*cis*-RA. These two receptors are capable of forming a heterodimer that binds to the RA DNA response elements upstream from promoters on target genes (39). While expression of RAR-α and RXR are found throughout the epithelium of the developing lung, RAR-β and RAR-γ expression is regulated temporally and spatially (40). Expression profile studies of RAR in rats have demonstrated that RAR-α expression peaks in the transition period between the pseudoglandular and canalicular stage of development

(E17–E18). This is consistent with its roll in promoting epithelial cell differentiation (40). RAR-β induces differentiation of type I and type II cells in the distal epithelium in the terminal saccular stage (E22), and RAR-γ is restricted to the mesenchyme (40). Double null mutations in RAR-α and RAR-β lead to severe lung abnormalities, including agenesis, and tracheal cartilage abnormalities (41). A deletion in RAR-γ results in a decrease in the elastic tissue of the lung, as well as a reduction of alveoli (42). These defects demonstrate that alveolarization and septation are dependent on proper signaling between RA from the mesenchyme to the RAR located in the epithelium. This cross talk has also been shown to play a role early in lung development. Knocking out an enzyme required for early embryonic RA synthesis, retinaldehyde dehydrogenase 2 (RALDH2), results in death at E10.5 due to heart abnormalities (43,44). The lungs of these knockout animals are very immature, with the primary lung buds failing to grow. Studies using this model have found that FGF-10 signaling is disrupted in the lung and is not restored after exogenous RA treatment. This led the authors to hypothesize that endogenous RA signaling plays a role in generating the local gradients of FGF-10 expression in the foregut derivatives (44). This disruption in FGF-10 leads to downstream effects on many other factors regulated by this gene, including BMP-4 and Spry. This combination of inappropriate gene expression leads to the phenotype seen (44), and suggests a role for RA in regulating early lung development.

VII. Vascular Endothelial Growth Factor

Vascular endothelial growth factor (VEGF) is known to play a central role in the initiation of vasculogenesis and angiogenesis in the developing lung (45). VEGF-A, the main isoform involved in vascular development, is found in both the mesenchyme and the epithelium as early as E12.5, and then becomes restricted primarily to the epithelium of the developing lung bud by E14.5 (16). This factor has been shown to induce migration and proliferation of endothelial cells (46). The actions of VEGF are mediated through two tyrosine kinase receptors Flk-1 (aka VEGFR-2) and Flt-1 (aka VEGFR-1) (47). Flk-1 is one of the earliest markers of endothelial cells and is expressed in mesodermal cells before any differentiation to endothelial cells is apparent. Endothelial cell differentiation fails to occur in embryos lacking Flk-1, which results in an absence of blood vessels and embryonic lethality, as in the VEGF knockout animals (48). Conversely, targeted disruption of Flt-1 results in excessive endothelial cell recruitment with little structural organization, indicating that it may play a role in downregulating VEGF-A activity (49). These studies illustrate the great importance of VEGF signaling in the development of the vasculature in concert with the lung (34). VEGF protein is localized to the basement membrane beneath the epithelial cells of the distal airway (50). The position suggests that VEGF is important in directing the location of capillaries by signaling the underlying endothelial cells in a paracrine fashion. These epithelial-endothelial interactions are essential in the formation of a proper blood-air interface. Once the blood vessels are formed, VEGF continues to interact with the endothelial cells and is thought to regulate the expression of endothelial nitric oxide synthase (eNOS). Nitric oxide (NO) is synthesized by eNOS in the endothelial cells of the developing lung

and has been confirmed to play a role in angiogenesis (51). Many studies have confirmed that there is a great deal of cross talk occurring between the NO and the VEGF.
For instance, in vitro studies using human and bovine endothelial cells have found that
VEGF is able to increase eNOS mRNA and in turn increase the amount of NO being
produced (52,53). Additionally, NOS inhibition has been shown to block VEGF-
induced angiogenesis in vivo and in vitro (52–54). These studies demonstrate the
importance of cross talk between the epithelium and the endothelium for proper
development of the pulmonary vasculature. More recently, interactions between the
mesenchyme and the epithelium have also been shown to control growth of the capillary plexus through the regulation of VEGF-A. FGF-9 has been a candidate for a
regulatory molecule that leads to examine the potential affects of this growth factor on
formation of the capillary network. FGF-9$^{-/-}$ mice show a significant reduction in the
density of the distal capillary network, suggesting that it does play a role in the vascularization of the lung (16). To further validate this theory, the authors created an
inducible transgene system where FGF-9 could be induced at various developmental
windows. Using VEGF-A–LacZ lung, they found that FGF-9 expression caused an
increase in VEGF throughout the epithelium (16). SHH was shown to be at least one
downstream mediator of FGF-9 signaling that leads to the increase in VEGF, which in
turn leads to an increase in vascular growth (16). Finally, this effect was not found to be
mediated through the endothelial cells, supporting the role of mesenchymal-epithelial
interactions in vascular development.

VIII. Insulin-Like Growth Factors

The insulin-like growth factor (IGF) family is composed of two peptides, IGF-I and IGF-II,
which interact with two specific IGF receptors. The type 1 IGF receptor (IGFR-1) is
the primary receptor and transmits signals pertaining to differentiation and proliferation,
whereas the type 2 receptor has the more specialized function of internalizing and
transporting IGF-II to the lysozomes for degradation (55). IGF is synthesized by the
mesenchyme, especially the undifferentiated mesenchyme, and signals to the IGFR-1 in
the epithelium, where it plays a role in early branching morphogenesis (56,57). IGF-1
null mice show many developmental problems including growth retardation, delayed
brain development, and defects in muscle, bone, and lung, in addition to fertility issues,
demonstrating the importance of this growth factor for normal development (58). There
is evidence that IGF-binding proteins (IGFBPs) mediate the mitogenic effects of the
IGF, by enhancing or inhibiting their expression (55). The expression pattern of IGFBP
can determine which cell types can respond to paracrine/autocrine signaling of IGF. Six
IGFBPs have been characterized to date, and IGFBP-2 to -5 are expressed in the
developing lung. IGFBP-2 is preferentially expressed in the distal epithelium whereas
IGFBP-4 is confined to the mesenchyme throughout lung development. IGFBP-3 and -5
are expressed in a variety of cells with increasing levels as parturition approaches
(59,60). While the specific role of each IFGBP has yet to be elucidated, the general
expression patterns suggest that they control IGF signaling in a site-specific and time-
specific manner (Table 1).

Table 1 Expression Pattern of Growth Factors and Their Receptors in the Developing Mouse Lung

Growth factor	Expression pattern	Time of expression (mouse)	Receptor	Expression pattern of receptor
FGF-7	Mesenchyme	E11	FGFR-2-IIIb	Epithelial cells
FGF-9	Epithelium	E10.5	FGFR-2-b	Mesenchyme
FGF-10	Mesenchyme of distal buds	E9.5	FGFR-2-IIIb	Distal epithelial cells
BMP-4	Epithelium of distal buds	E11.5	BMPR	Distal mesenchyme
Spry2	Epithelium of growing bud tips	E10.5	FRS2 and Grb2 (MAP kinase/ ERK pathway)	N/A (MAP kinase pathway downstream of FGFR receptor)
SHH	Epithelium (highest at distal tips)	E9.5	Patched	Mesenchyme adjacent to SHH expression
RA	Fibroblasts in alveolar walls	E17	RAR-α	Epithelium
			RAR-β	Epithelium
			RAR-γ	Mesenchyme
VEGF	Epithelium of distal buds	E14.5	Flt (VEGFR-1)	Mesenchyme
			Flk (VEGFR-2)	Mesenchyme
IGF-I	Mesenchyme (undifferentiated)		IGFR-1	Epithelium
IGF-II		E12.5		
TGF-β1	Bronchiolar mesenchyme	E11	TGFBR-I	Epithelium lining bronchi
TGF-β2	Bronchiolar epithelium			
TGF-β3	Mesenchyme		TGFBR-II	Cuboidal epithelium
EGF	Mesenchyme	E11	EGFR	Epithelium
TGF-α	Mesenchyme	E11	EGFR	Epithelium
PDGF-α	Greater in epithelium	E12	PDGF-α	Mesenchyme
PDGF-β		E14	PDGF-β	Mesenchyme

IX. Transforming Growth Factor β

TGF-β is a part of the TGF-β superfamily, which also includes activins and BMPs. This family of cytokines is involved in regulating cell cycle progression, growth, differentiation, and extracellular matrix (ECM) deposition (61). The TGF-β peptide is composed of three subtypes, TGF-β1, -β2, and -β3, all of which have been found in the developing murine lung. Each of these isoforms is tightly regulated, and their expression is controlled spatially and temporally over the course of development (62). TGF-β1 is expressed primarily in the bronchiolar mesoderm. While its mRNA can be detected as early as E11, expression increases around E14 to E15 (63) and can be colocalized at this time with ECM proteins including type I and III collagen, glycosaminoglycans, and fibronectin (64). These colocalization sites coincide with the epithelial-mesenchymal interfaces of the clefts of the branching lung, and it has been postulated that TGF-β1 exerts its effect on branching morphogenesis by increasing cell-ECM interactions (64). TGF-β2 expression is localized to the bronchiolar epithelium and increases at later stages of development (63). TGF-β3 is found in the tracheal mesenchyme at earlier time points of development (E12.5), but around E14.5, the expression shifts to the epithelium of the bronchioles, and by E16.5, it is no longer detectable (63). Although all play roles in lung development, there is evidence that TGF-β2 has a critical role in branching. Rat lung explants treated with antisense oligonucleotides and neutralizing antibodies against TGF-β2 showed an inhibition of early lung branching. In addition, exogenously added TGF-β2 was able to rescue the effect. This effect was not seen with TGF-β1 and TGF-β3 (65). Overexpression of TGF-β1, by way of a chimeric SFPTC–TGF-β1 protein, results in arrested growth at the psuedoglandular phase of development (66). Lungs from these animals had fewer acinar buds, and also a reduction in epithelial cell differentiation, determined by a reduction in Clara cell secretory protein and SFPTC expression. Mice null for TGF-β2 are born cyanotic and die shortly after birth due to respiratory distress. Examination of the lungs of these pups revealed collapsed conducting airways (67). Mice null for TGF-β3 die within 20 hours of birth and become cyanotic and gasp for air prior to death (68). Lungs from these animals are hypoplastic and lack alveolar septation. In addition, there is mesenchymal thickening and hypercellularity, suggesting a role for TGF-β3 in regulating mesenchymal-epithelial interactions in the lung (68). TGF-β1 null mice are born with inflammatory disease accompanied by tissue necrosis, which leads to organ failure and death approximately 20 days after birth (69). The lack of overlapping phenotypes between these three knockout models suggests that each TGF-β isoform plays its own distinct role in lung-regulating development (67).

TGF-β signals through the TGF-β family of receptors (TBR), which consists of two subfamilies (I and II). TBRI and II form a heterodimeric complex that allow for the transduction of the TGF-β signal through the serine/threonine kinase activity of the receptors. The expression pattern of both receptors changes throughout development. TBRII can be detected in the cuboidal epithelium of the distal lung by E16, but is virtually undetectable in the proximal airway at this time. This has led to postulation that TBRII plays an important role in providing positional information to the cells it is expressed in (70). At E14, TBRI can be found in the epithelial lining of the bronchi and in the mesenchyme. By E16, a shift occurs and there is an upregulation of the receptor in the mesenchyme. In contrast to the TBRII, TBRI does not appear to have a proximal-distal gradient and may instead play a role in directing differentiation of target cells (62). Once the receptors are heterodimerized, the family of SMAD proteins transduce the TGF signal from the membrane-bound receptors to the nucleus. Smad2 and Smad3 bind to the TBR complex and are activated once phosphorylated by the activated TBRI. Once activated, Smad2 and Smad3 are able to bind Smad4, and this complex can now move into the nucleus where it can act as a transcription factor (71). Given the role of SMADs to transduce TGF-β signaling, it is no surprise that disruption of their normal signaling results in abnormal lung development. Inhibition of Smad2 and Smad3 with antisense oligonucleotides resulted in an increase in branching in lung explants (66,72). This was also seen when Smad4 alone was inhibited and could not be rescued by exogenous addition of TGF-β-1, confirming its downstream role in the signaling pathway (71).

X. Epidermal Growth Factor

Epidermal growth factor (EGF), TGF-α, and amphiregulin (AR) are all members of the EGF family that signals through the EGF receptor (EGFR). EGFR (also known as ErbB1) is a member of the ErbB family, a group of transmembrane tyrosine kinase receptors. These receptors are located in the basolateral side of the epithelium to allow for cross talk with the mesenchyme (73). Other members of this receptor family include ErbB2, ErbB3, and ErbB4. Both ErbB3 and ErbB4 are able to bind neuregulins, EGF-related proteins, and in addition, ErbB4 has been shown also to bind EGF. ErbB2 has no known high-affinity receptors, but is speculated to heterodimerize with the other ligand-bound ErbBs (74). EGF mRNA can be detected in the mouse lung between E11 and E17. EGF protein was found in the epithelium at these time points and found to colocalize with EGFR here (75). In both rats and human studies, EGF protein was expressed in the bronchial and bronchiolar epithelium and in the type II cells of the distal airway (76,77). TGF-α, AR, and EGF mRNA have been localized primarily to the mesenchymal cells (78), suggesting that these factors are acting in a paracrine fashion to signal to their receptors in the epithelial cells. EGFR has been localized to the epithelium in rat and mouse studies, but can also be detected in the surrounding mesenchyme (75,76). EGF, TGF-α, and AR have been shown to influence branching morphogenesis in the embryonic murine lung. Mesenchymal cells in the embryonic mouse lung have been shown to proliferate under the influence of exogenous AR, whereas antibodies against AR block the growth (79). This AR-mediated cell proliferation is thought to occur through heparin sulfate proteoglycan (HSPG), as antibodies against the AR-HSPG–binding site in lung explants inhibited branching morphogenesis (79). Addition of exogenous EGF and TGF-α to mouse lung explants stimulates proliferation of both the mesenchyme and the epithelium in addition to enhancing branching. TITF1 and SFPTC expression along with other markers of cellular differentiation were found to be stimulated (75). This effect was not seen in EGFR-deficient lung suggesting that the receptor plays a role in regulating expression of these genes in the lung (80). Blocking signaling through EGFR using inhibitors, EGFR null mice, an EGFR antisense gene knockdown, and EGF deficiency all resulted in deceased branching in concert with a downregulation of TITF1 and SFPTC (75,80–82). In the above-mentioned study, mice homozygous for EGFR null mutations died postnatally due to respiratory insufficiency (80). Of note, studies using mice of another genetic background did not display any lung abnormalities, implying that strain-specific modifiers of EGFR may be involved (83). ErbB2 and ErbB4 null mice die at E10.5 due to nervous system and cardiac malformations (84,85). ErbB4 downregulation using siRNA in E19 rat type II cells has been shown to impair surfactant synthesis (74).

XI. Platelet-Derived Growth Factor

Platelet-derived growth factor (PDGF) is a peptide containing two peptide chains, A and B, which can homodimerize into PDGF-AA and PDGF-BB, or it can heterodimerize to form a PDGF-AB subtype (86). Binding of these ligands to their cell surface receptors causes an intracellular signaling cascade that results in DNA synthesis and cell proliferation (87). PDGFs have been shown to bind to two receptors, PDGFR-α and PDGFR-β. PDGFR-α is able to bind all PDGF isoforms, whereas PDGFR-β can only bind PDGF-BB with high affinity (88). Each of the PDGF isoforms is differentially expressed in fetal lung epithelial and mesenchymal cells. Studies in rats have shown that expression of PDGF-AA and PDGF-BB is detectable in the airway epithelium as early as E12. While both isoforms are present in the mesenchyme, they are not detected until E14 (87). Protein concentrations of PDGF-AA and PDGF-BB are highest in the embryonic and pseudoglandular period and decrease as parturition approaches (87). Both receptors are found in greater concentrations in the mesenchyme, particularly at earlier gestational time points, making PDGF a candidate for mesenchymal-epithelial interactions involved in lung development. Studies have shown that using antisense oligonucleotides against PDGF-A in fetal rat lung explants produce a hypoplastic lung with decreased terminal buds. Addition of PDGF-AA, but not PDGF-BB, was able to moderate the effects (87). In contrast, antisense PDGF-B oligonucleotides inhibited DNA synthesis in the lung in a concentration-dependent manner, but had no significant effect on the number terminal lung buds (89). Overexpressing PDGF-B causes enlarged airspaces, inflammation, and thickened primary septa, a phenotype similar to that seen in emphysema and fibrotic lung disease (90). Null mutants for PDGF-B/PDGFR-β die perinatally from problems with angiogenic sprouting in many organs, including the kidney and lungs (91,92). This problem with angiogenesis could be caused by the lack of pericyte recruitment and proliferation, which is known to be affected by PDGF-B/PDGFR-β signaling (93). Mice null for PDGF-A lack alveolar smooth muscle cells, have a reduction in elastin fibers in the parenchyma, and do not undergo alveolarization (94). In these mice, there is also a failure of the PDGFR-α cells to proliferate and migrate from the distal epithelial tips to the terminal sac walls (95). Since these cells are progenitors for alveolar smooth muscle cells, this lack of recruitment caused by disruption of PDGF-A signaling could explain why alveolarization is absent in these animals (95).

XII. Conclusion

Proper development of the lung involves the temporal and spatial coordination of a number of transcription and growth factors. Cross talk between the tissue layers through soluble/diffusible factors allows the mesenchyme and epithelium to develop in concert and coordinate their actions to allow the mature lung to form correctly. The appositional placement of signaling molecules and receptors in the layers of lung tissue is vital for lung development to occur appropriately. While gain and loss of function and in vitro cell culture studies have provided great insight into the roles of various signaling molecules, the interplay between tissue layers and these molecules may be modulated in vivo in a distinct manner. Transgenic rodent models with the help of tissue-specific knockout studies have helped to supplement the in vitro data and provide novel insights into the interactions that are occurring during lung development. Further elucidation of the role of mesenchymal-epithelial interactions during fetal lung development can aid in better understanding human lung disease and malformation and can help in creating novel therapies for these problems.

References

1. Wessells NK. Mammalian lung development: interactions in formation and morphogenesis of tracheal buds. J Exp Zool 1970; 175(4):455–466.
2. Perl AK, Wert SE, Nagy A, et al. Early restriction of peripheral and proximal cell lineages during formation of the lung. Proc Natl Acad Sci U S A 2002; 99(16):10482–10487.
3. Igarashi M, Finch PW, Aaronson SA. Characterization of recombinant human fibroblast growth factor (FGF)-10 reveals functional similarities with keratinocyte growth factor (FGF-7). J Biol Chem 1998; 273(21):13230–13235.
4. Post M, Souza P, Liu J, et al. Keratinocyte growth factor and its receptor are involved in regulating early lung branching. Development 1996; 122(10):3107–3115.
5. Colvin JS, White AC, Pratt SJ, et al. Lung hypoplasia and neonatal death in Fgf9-null mice identify this gene as an essential regulator of lung mesenchyme. Development 2001; 128(11): 2095–2106.
6. Bellusci S, Grindley J, Emoto H, et al. Fibroblast growth factor 10 (FGF10) and branching morphogenesis in the embryonic mouse lung. Development 1997; 124(23):4867–4878.
7. Tichelaar JW, Lu W, Whitsett JA. Conditional expression of fibroblast growth factor-7 in the developing and mature lung. J Biol Chem 2000; 275(16):11858–11864.
8. Ware LB, Matthay MA. Keratinocyte and hepatocyte growth factors in the lung: roles in lung development, inflammation, and repair. Am J Physiol Lung Cell Mol Physiol 2002; 282(5): L924–L940.
9. Miki T, Bottaro DP, Fleming TP, et al. Determination of ligand-binding specificity by alternative splicing: two distinct growth factor receptors encoded by a single gene. Proc Natl Acad Sci U S A 1992; 89(1):246–250.
10. Guo L, Degenstein L, Fuchs E. Keratinocyte growth factor is required for hair development but not for wound healing. Genes Dev 1996; 10(2):165–175.
11. Panos RJ, Rubin JS, Csaky KG, et al. Keratinocyte growth factor and hepatocyte growth factor/scatter factor are heparin-binding growth factors for alveolar type II cells in fibroblast-conditioned medium. J Clin Invest 1993; 92(2):969–977.
12. Ulich TR, Yi ES, Longmuir K, et al. Keratinocyte growth factor is a growth factor for type II pneumocytes in vivo. J Clin Invest 1994; 93(3):1298–1306.
13. Chelly N, Henrion A, Pinteur C, et al. Role of keratinocyte growth factor in the control of surfactant synthesis by fetal lung mesenchyme. Endocrinology 2001; 142(5):1814–1819.
14. Colvin JS, Feldman B, Nadeau JH, et al. Genomic organization and embryonic expression of the mouse fibroblast growth factor 9 gene. Dev Dyn 1999; 216(1):72–88.
15. Del Moral PM, De Langhe SP, Sala FG, et al. Differential role of FGF9 on epithelium and mesenchyme in mouse embryonic lung. Dev Biol 2006; 293(1):77–89.
16. White AC, Lavine KJ, Ornitz DM. FGF9 and SHH regulate mesenchymal Vegfa expression and development of the pulmonary capillary network. Development 2007; 134(20):3743–3752.
17. Yamasaki M, Miyake A, Tagashira S, et al. Structure and expression of the rat mRNA encoding a novel member of the fibroblast growth factor family. J Biol Chem 1996; 271(27): 15918–15921.
18. Park WY, Miranda B, Lebeche D, et al. FGF-10 is a chemotactic factor for distal epithelial buds during lung development. Dev Biol 1998; 201(2):125–134.
19. Min H, Danilenko DM, Scully SA, et al. Fgf-10 is required for both limb and lung development and exhibits striking functional similarity to Drosophila branchless. Genes Dev 1998; 12(20):3156–3161.
20. Clark JC, Tichelaar JW, Wert SE, et al. FGF-10 disrupts lung morphogenesis and causes pulmonary adenomas in vivo. Am J Physiol Lung Cell Mol Physiol 2001; 280(4): L705–L715.

21. Hyatt BA, Shangguan X, Shannon JM. FGF-10 induces SP-C and Bmp4 and regulates proximal-distal patterning in embryonic tracheal epithelium. Am J Physiol Lung Cell Mol Physiol 2004; 287(6):L1116–L1126.

22. Nyeng P, Norgaard GA, Kobberup S, et al. FGF10 maintains distal lung bud epithelium and excessive signaling leads to progenitor state arrest, distalization, and goblet cell metaplasia. BMC Dev Biol 2008; 8:2.

23. Hacohen N, Kramer S, Sutherland D, et al. Sprouty encodes a novel antagonist of FGF signaling that patterns apical branching of the Drosophila airways. Cell 1998; 92(2):253–263.

24. Mailleux AA, Tefft D, Ndiaye D, et al. Evidence that SPROUTY2 functions as an inhibitor of mouse embryonic lung growth and morphogenesis. Mech Dev 2001; 102(1–2):81–94.

25. Weaver M, Yingling JM, Dunn NR, et al. Bmp signaling regulates proximal-distal differentiation of endoderm in mouse lung development. Development 1999; 126(18):4005–4015.

26. King JA, Marker PC, Seung KJ, et al. BMP5 and the molecular, skeletal, and soft-tissue alterations in short ear mice. Dev Biol 1994; 166(1):112–122.

27. Jena N, Martin-Seisdedos C, McCue P, et al. BMP7 null mutation in mice: developmental defects in skeleton, kidney, and eye. Exp Cell Res 1997; 230(1):28–37.

28. Winnier G, Blessing M, Labosky PA, et al. Bone morphogenetic protein-4 is required for mesoderm formation and patterning in the mouse. Genes Dev 1995; 9(17):2105–2116.

29. Bellusci S, Henderson R, Winnier G, et al. Evidence from normal expression and targeted misexpression that bone morphogenetic protein (Bmp-4) plays a role in mouse embryonic lung morphogenesis. Development 1996; 122(6):1693–1702.

30. Weaver M, Dunn NR, Hogan BL. Bmp4 and Fgf10 play opposing roles during lung bud morphogenesis. Development 2000; 127(12):2695–2704.

31. Litingtung Y, Lei L, Westphal H, et al. Sonic hedgehog is essential to foregut development. Nat Genet 1998; 20(1):58–61.

32. Bellusci S, Furuta Y, Rush MG, et al. Involvement of Sonic hedgehog (Shh) in mouse embryonic lung growth and morphogenesis. Development 1997; 124(1):53–63.

33. Miller LA, Wert SE, Whitsett JA. Immunolocalization of sonic hedgehog (Shh) in developing mouse lung. J Histochem Cytochem 2001; 49(12):1593–1604.

34. van TM. Lung Development: Vascular and Epithelial Branching Morphogenesis [PhD thesis]. University of Rotterdam, 2004.

35. Pepicelli CV, Lewis PM, McMahon AP. Sonic hedgehog regulates branching morphogenesis in the mammalian lung. Curr Biol 1998; 8(19):1083–1086.

36. van TM, Post M. From fruitflies to mammals: mechanisms of signalling via the Sonic hedgehog pathway in lung development. Respir Res 2000; 1(1):30–35.

37. Grindley JC, Bellusci S, Perkins D, et al. Evidence for the involvement of the Gli gene family in embryonic mouse lung development. Dev Biol 1997; 188(2):337–348.

38. McGowan SE, Harvey CS, Jackson SK. Retinoids, retinoic acid receptors, and cytoplasmic retinoid binding proteins in perinatal rat lung fibroblasts. Am J Physiol 1995; 269(4 pt 1): L463–L472.

39. Han GR, Dohi DF, Lee HY, et al. All-trans-retinoic acid increases transforming growth factor-beta2 and insulin-like growth factor binding protein-3 expression through a retinoic acid receptor-alpha-dependent signaling pathway. J Biol Chem 1997; 272(21):13711–13716.

40. Grummer MA, Thet LA, Zachman RD. Expression of retinoic acid receptor genes in fetal and newborn rat lung. Pediatr Pulmonol 1994; 17(4):234–238.

41. Mendelsohn C, Lohnes D, Decimo D, et al. Function of the retinoic acid receptors (RARs) during development (II). Multiple abnormalities at various stages of organogenesis in RAR double mutants. Development 1994; 120(10):2749–2771.

42. McGowan S, Jackson SK, Jenkins-Moore M, et al. Mice bearing deletions of retinoic acid receptors demonstrate reduced lung elastin and alveolar numbers. Am J Respir Cell Mol Biol 2000; 23(2):162–167.

43. Niederreither K, Subbarayan V, Dolle P, et al. Embryonic retinoic acid synthesis is essential for early mouse post-implantation development. Nat Genet 1999; 21(4):444–448.
44. Wang Z, Dolle P, Cardoso WV, et al. Retinoic acid regulates morphogenesis and patterning of posterior foregut derivatives. Dev Biol 2006; 297(2):433–445.
45. Neufeld G, Cohen T, Gengrinovitch S, et al. Vascular endothelial growth factor (VEGF) and its receptors. FASEB J 1999; 13(1):9–22.
46. Galambos C, deMello DE. Molecular mechanisms of pulmonary vascular development. Pediatr Dev Pathol 2007; 10(1):1–17.
47. Pauling MH, Vu TH. Mechanisms and regulation of lung vascular development. Curr Top Dev Biol 2004; 64:73–99.
48. Shalaby F, Ho J, Stanford WL, et al. A requirement for Flk1 in primitive and definitive hematopoiesis and vasculogenesis. Cell 1997; 89(6):981–990.
49. Fong GH, Rossant J, Gertsenstein M, et al. Role of the Flt-1 receptor tyrosine kinase in regulating the assembly of vascular endothelium. Nature 1995; 376(6535):66–70.
50. Acarregui MJ, Penisten ST, Goss KL, et al. Vascular endothelial growth factor gene expression in human fetal lung in vitro. Am J Respir Cell Mol Biol 1999; 20(1):14–23.
51. Zhang R, Wang L, Zhang L, et al. Nitric oxide enhances angiogenesis via the synthesis of vascular endothelial growth factor and cGMP after stroke in the rat. Circ Res 2003; 92(3): 308–313.
52. Hood JD, Meininger CJ, Ziche M, et al. VEGF upregulates ecNOS message, protein, and NO production in human endothelial cells. Am J Physiol 1998; 274(3 pt 2):H1054–H1058.
53. Papapetropoulos A, Garcia-Cardena G, Madri JA, et al. Nitric oxide production contributes to the angiogenic properties of vascular endothelial growth factor in human endothelial cells. J Clin Invest 1997; 100(12):3131–3139.
54. Babaei S, Stewart DJ. Overexpression of endothelial NO synthase induces angiogenesis in a co-culture model. Cardiovasc Res 2002; 55(1):190–200.
55. Jones JI, Clemmons DR. Insulin-like growth factors and their binding proteins: biological actions. Endocr Rev 1995; 16(1):3–34.
56. Moats-Staats BM, Retsch-Bogart GZ, Price WA, et al. Insulin-like growth factor-I (IGF-I) antisense oligodeoxynucleotide mediated inhibition of DNA synthesis by WI-38 cells: evidence for autocrine actions of IGF-I. Mol Endocrinol 1993; 7(2):171–180.
57. Stiles AD, Moats-Staats BM. Production and action of insulin-like growth factor I/somatomedin C in primary cultures of fetal lung fibroblasts. Am J Respir Cell Mol Biol 1989; 1(1):21–26.
58. Woods KA, Camacho-Hubner C, Savage MO, et al. Intrauterine growth retardation and postnatal growth failure associated with deletion of the insulin-like growth factor I gene. N Engl J Med 1996; 335(18):1363–1367.
59. Moats-Staats BM, Price WA, Xu L, et al. Regulation of the insulin-like growth factor system during normal rat lung development. Am J Respir Cell Mol Biol 1995; 12(1):56–64.
60. Retsch-Bogart GZ, Moats-Staats BM, Howard K, et al. Cellular localization of messenger RNAs for insulin-like growth factors (IGFs), their receptors and binding proteins during fetal rat lung development. Am J Respir Cell Mol Biol 1996; 14(1):61–69.
61. Kingsley DM. The TGF-beta superfamily: new members, new receptors, and new genetic tests of function in different organisms. Genes Dev 1994; 8(2):133–146.
62. Zhao Y, Young SL, McIntosh JC, et al. Ontogeny and localization of TGF-beta type I receptor expression during lung development. Am J Physiol Lung Cell Mol Physiol 2000; 278(6):L1231–L1239.
63. Schmid P, Cox D, Bilbe G, et al. Differential expression of TGF beta 1, beta 2 and beta 3 genes during mouse embryogenesis. Development 1991; 111(1):117–130.
64. Heine UI, Munoz EF, Flanders KC, et al. Colocalization of TGF-beta 1 and collagen I and III, fibronectin and glycosaminoglycans during lung branching morphogenesis. Development 1990; 109(1):29–36.

65. Liu J, Tseu I, Wang J, et al. Transforming growth factor beta2, but not beta1 and beta3, is critical for early rat lung branching. Dev Dyn 2000; 217(4):343–360.

66. Zhou L, Dey CR, Wert SE, et al. Arrested lung morphogenesis in transgenic mice bearing an SP-C-TGF-beta 1 chimeric gene. Dev Biol 1996; 175(2):227–238.

67. Sanford LP, Ormsby I, Gittenberger-de Groot AC, et al. TGFbeta2 knockout mice have multiple developmental defects that are non-overlapping with other TGFbeta knockout phenotypes. Development 1997; 124(13):2659–2670.

68. Kaartinen V, Voncken JW, Shuler C, et al. Abnormal lung development and cleft palate in mice lacking TGF-beta 3 indicates defects of epithelial-mesenchymal interaction. Nat Genet 1995; 11(4):415–421.

69. Shull MM, Ormsby I, Kier AB, et al. Targeted disruption of the mouse transforming growth factor-beta 1 gene results in multifocal inflammatory disease. Nature 1992; 359(6397): 693–699.

70. Zhao Y, Young SL. Expression of transforming growth factor-beta type II receptor in rat lung is regulated during development. Am J Physiol 1995; 269(3 pt 1):L419–L426.

71. Zhang Y, Feng X, We R, et al. Receptor-associated Mad homologues synergize as effectors of the TGF-beta response. Nature 1996; 383(6596):168–172.

72. Zhao J, Lee M, Smith S, et al. Abrogation of Smad3 and Smad2 or of Smad4 gene expression positively regulates murine embryonic lung branching morphogenesis in culture. Dev Biol 1998; 194(2):182–195.

73. Yarden Y, Sliwkowski MX. Untangling the ErbB signalling network. Nat Rev Mol Cell Biol 2001; 2(2):127–137.

74. Liu W, Zscheppang K, Murray S, et al. The ErbB4 receptor in fetal rat lung fibroblasts and epithelial type II cells. Biochim Biophys Acta 2007; 1772(7):737–747.

75. Warburton D, Seth R, Shum L, et al. Epigenetic role of epidermal growth factor expression and signalling in embryonic mouse lung morphogenesis. Dev Biol 1992; 149(1):123–133.

76. Strandjord TP, Clark JG, Madtes DK. Expression of TGF-alpha, EGF, and EGF receptor in fetal rat lung. Am J Physiol 1994; 267(4 pt 1):L384–L389.

77. Sannes PL, Burch KK, Khosla J. Immunohistochemical localization of epidermal growth factor and acidic and basic fibroblast growth factors in postnatal developing and adult rat lungs. Am J Respir Cell Mol Biol 1992; 7(2):230–237.

78. Ruocco S, Lallemand A, Tournier JM, et al. Expression and localization of epidermal growth factor, transforming growth factor-alpha, and localization of their common receptor in fetal human lung development. Pediatr Res 1996; 39(3):448–455.

79. Schuger L, Johnson GR, Gilbride K, et al. Amphiregulin in lung branching morphogenesis: interaction with heparan sulfate proteoglycan modulates cell proliferation. Development 1996; 122(6):1759–1767.

80. Miettinen PJ, Berger JE, Meneses J, et al. Epithelial immaturity and multiorgan failure in mice lacking epidermal growth factor receptor. Nature 1995; 376(6538):337–341.

81. Seth R, Shum L, Wu F, et al. Role of epidermal growth factor expression in early mouse embryo lung branching morphogenesis in culture: antisense oligodeoxynucleotide inhibitory strategy. Dev Biol 1993; 158(2):555–559.

82. Raaberg L, Nexo E, Jorgensen PE, et al. Fetal effects of epidermal growth factor deficiency induced in rats by autoantibodies against epidermal growth factor. Pediatr Res 1995; 37(2): 175–181.

83. Threadgill DW, Dlugosz AA, Hansen LA, et al. Targeted disruption of mouse EGF receptor: effect of genetic background on mutant phenotype. Science 1995; 269(5221):230–234.

84. Lee KF, Simon H, Chen H, et al. Requirement for neuregulin receptor erbB2 in neural and cardiac development. Nature 1995; 378(6555):394–398.

85. Gassmann M, Casagranda F, Orioli D, et al. Aberrant neural and cardiac development in mice lacking the ErbB4 neuregulin receptor. Nature 1995; 378(6555):390–394.

86. Ross R. Platelet-derived growth factor. Lancet 1989; 1(8648):1179–1182.
87. Han RN, Mawdsley C, Souza P, et al. Platelet-derived growth factors and growth-related genes in rat lung. III. Immunolocalization during fetal development. Pediatr Res 1992; 31(4 pt 1):323–329.
88. Souza P, Kuliszewski M, Wang J, et al. PDGF-AA and its receptor influence early lung branching via an epithelial-mesenchymal interaction. Development 1995; 121(8):2559–2567.
89. Souza P, Sedlackova L, Kuliszewski M, et al. Antisense oligodeoxynucleotides targeting PDGF-B mRNA inhibit cell proliferation during embryonic rat lung development. Development 1994; 120(8):2163–2173.
90. Hoyle GW, Li J, Finkelstein JB, et al. Emphysematous lesions, inflammation, and fibrosis in the lungs of transgenic mice overexpressing platelet-derived growth factor. Am J Pathol 1999; 154(6):1763–1775.
91. Lindahl P, Johansson BR, Leveen P, et al. Pericyte loss and microaneurysm formation in PDGF-B-deficient mice. Science 1997; 277(5323):242–245.
92. Soriano P. Abnormal kidney development and hematological disorders in PDGF beta-receptor mutant mice. Genes Dev 1994; 8(16):1888–1896.
93. Hellstrom M, Kalen M, Lindahl P, et al. Role of PDGF-B and PDGFR-beta in recruitment of vascular smooth muscle cells and pericytes during embryonic blood vessel formation in the mouse. Development 1999; 126(14):3047–3055.
94. Bostrom H, Willetts K, Pekny M, et al. PDGF-A signaling is a critical event in lung alveolar myofibroblast development and alveogenesis. Cell 1996; 85(6):863–873.
95. Lindahl P, Karlsson L, Hellstrom M, et al. Alveogenesis failure in PDGF-A-deficient mice is coupled to lack of distal spreading of alveolar smooth muscle cell progenitors during lung development. Development 1997; 124(20):3943–3953.

3

Basic Mechanisms of Alveolarization

JACQUES R. BOURBON and CHRISTOPHE DELACOURT
INSERM, Unité 955-Institut Mondor de Recherche Biomédicale, Faculté de Médecine, Université Paris 12, Créteil, France

OLIVIER BOUCHERAT
Centre de Recherche en Cancérologie de l'Université Laval, Centre Hospitalier Universitaire de Québec, L'Hôtel-Dieu de Québec, Québec, Canada

I. Introduction

The so-called "new" bronchopulmonary dysplasia (BPD) is characterized by a combination of alveolar simplification and decreased microvascular density (1,2). These reflect impairment of alveolar developmental mechanisms, a feature shared also by less frequent congenital lung development disorders. Better understanding of these mechanisms should help progressing in the treatment of these diseases.

The formation of alveoli, which constitute the mature gas-exchange units, initiates in utero around 35 weeks of pregnancy, but extends at least over the two first postnatal years (3,4). The major cause of BPD is preterm birth (1,5,6), and the latter seems to affect alveolarization even in the lungs of healthy infants who do not develop overt BPD features (7). Prematurely born infants have to face the challenge of breathing with lungs in the canalicular or early saccular stage of development (Fig. 1). Recent progress has allowed extremely low gestational age infants to survive, and despite the use of prenatal corticosteroids and exogenous surfactant, the incompletion of lung structures still necessitates to ventilate them mechanically with increased oxygen. Although less aggressive ventilation is presently used, these injurious treatments (5,6), along with infectious process (8), precipitate alveolar developmental arrest. Injuries are susceptible to interfere with developmental mechanisms at multiple levels. Alveolarization involves the regulated expression of a myriad of genes in various lung cell types that act cooperatively in an intricate and precisely timed cascade of events. A large number of investigations have tremendously increased knowledge about these mechanisms in the last decades, of which the present chapter tentatively presents an integrative view.

II. What Does "Alveolarization" Stand For?

A. Alveolarization Vs. Alveolar Septation

Alveolarization and synonymous terms alveolization and alveologenesis designate the process through which the developing lung acquires its fully mature structure. Alveoli are the hallmark of mammalian lungs. Their formation allows achievement of the

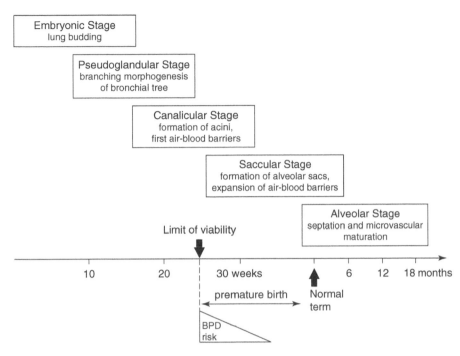

Figure 1 Stages of lung development and chronology in human species. The absolute limit of viability at about 24 weeks of amenorrhea corresponds to the appearance of first functional air-blood barriers. Alveolar development initiates in utero but extends at least until 18 months of postnatal life. The lung of prematurely delivered infants is in late canalicular or saccular stage. The risk of BPD decreases with gestational age.

extensive exchange area necessary to meet the respiratory needs of the organism. In man, postnatal alveolarization increases the number of alveoli in the lung from at most 50 millions at birth (3) to about 480 millions in the adult (9). Surface folding increases gas-exchange surface area 20-fold between birth and adulthood with much lower concomitant increase in chest size (10).

However, the presence of alveoli is not required at birth. In rodents, neonatal lungs only present undivided saccules (or alveolar sacs), and alveolarization is entirely postnatal (11–13). The limiting condition of respiratory gas-exchanges is the presence of air-blood barriers formed by tight apposition of type I alveolar epithelial cells (AECI) and capillary endothelial cells. These structures, about 0.2 μm thick, are ideally suited for gas diffusion (14). Their appearance in late canalicular stage in humans (3,15) marks the absolute limit of viability (Fig. 1). Their extension is pursued over the saccular and alveolar periods of development.

Through the saccular stage, lung morphogenesis proceeds by dichotomous branching of tubules (16,17). The extension of gas-exchange surface that characterizes alveolarization occurs through a different mechanism designated alveolar septation. Saccular walls (or primary septa) undergo subdivision by the protrusion of secondary

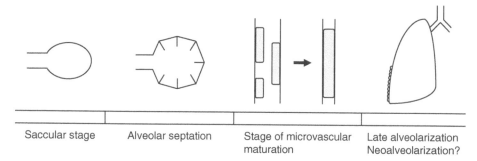

| Saccular stage | Alveolar septation | Stage of microvascular maturation | Late alveolarization Neoalveolarization? |

Figure 2 The successive steps of alveolarization. During alveolar septation, secondary septa subdivide alveolar sacs, and possibly new septa form from mature septa to create new alveoli. The stage of microvascular maturation that overlaps septation but extends beyond its termination is characterized by fusion of the double capillary layer (*gray tone*) of immature septa and thinning of septa. During late alveolarization and, possibly, already contemporaneous with secondary septation and in adult lung neoalveolarization, new alveoli would be added peripherally.

septa that grow perpendicularly (18) (Figs. 2 and 3). This distinctive mode of development designated secondary septation accounts for differences between control mechanisms of branching and alveolarization (19). However, septation of primary saccules may not be the unique mechanism of alveolar development. It has been proposed that alveoli would also be generated by newly formed septa at sites other than within preexisting saccules. More especially, in the rat, gas-exchange regions were shown to grow fastest in the subpleural areas that represent preferential sites for addition of new alveoli (20). It has been proposed that these are formed by subdivision of enlarging subpleural alveoli (20). In this species in which bulk alveolar formation takes place between 4 and 14 postnatal days (11), the major part of alveoli would not be formed by sudivision of primary saccules (21,22) but rather through this latter mechanism (20).

It should be emphasized that alveolarization largely encompasses the secondary septation process. The step of microvascular reshaping that follows septation is an integral part of alveolarization. Moreover, addition of alveoli appears to remain possible beyond postnatal septation. The terms alveolarization and septation must therefore be used distinctively.

B. Microvascular Growth and Remodeling

As the alveoli multiply, the capillary bed undergoes extensive expansion. This growth is intrinsic to alveolar development; preventing it leads to septation arrest (see sect. VI.A). In humans, capillary volume increases by over 35 times between birth and adulthood (4). In this period, angiogenesis appears to proceed principally by "intussusceptive microvascular growth," which designates subdivision of the capillary network by the interposition of newly formed intercapillary connective tissue pillars (23,24). In addition, the two capillary layers of the immature primary or secondary septa ensheathing a central interstitial tissue layer finally fuse into a single capillary layer that faces both lumens. This is designated microvascular maturation and confers to the alveolar wall its mature

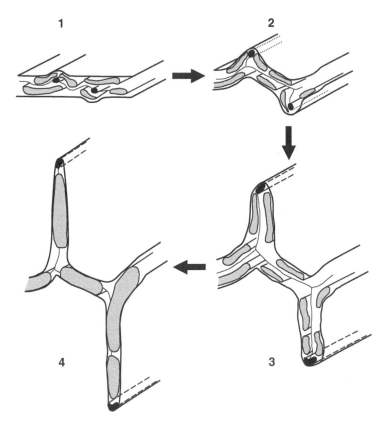

Figure 3 Three-dimensional scheme of formation of secondary septa. (1) Elastic fiber form deposits (*black*) in the thickness of primary septa between the two layers of capillary vessels (*gray tone*); crests appear at their level. (2) Crests elongate and lift capillary vessels. (3) Secondary septa have established but still display immature microvascular structure with bilayers of capillary vessels. Elastic fibers at the tip of septa form rings along their free edge and are interconnected together and with peripheral and axial elastic fiber systems. (4) Mature septa after capillary fusion into a single layer and thinning of alveolar walls.

adult morphology (25) (Fig. 2). It goes along with thinning of septa through reduction of interstitial tissue volume and fibroblast apoptosis (26,27), which represents the final step of alveolarization.

C. Late Alveolarization and Neoalveolarization

Determining when alveolarization is terminated is a difficult question. Whereas former studies fixed the end of alveolarization at 8 (28) or even 20 years (29), more recent studies indicated that bulk alveolarization in humans is more likely to be terminated by 18 to 24 months (3,4). However, it cannot be excluded that some alveolar formation is pursued during childhood and may even remain possible in the adult lung, which has been designated "late alveolarization" (10). This view is supported by observations in three different species. There is thus good evidence that alveoli in the rat are added beyond the early phase of bulk septation, when the lung parenchyma is already mature (20,21,30,31). This was also recently demonstrated in the mouse lung in which about 10% of the septa present in adulthood are formed prenatally, approximately 50% are generated postnatally before and approximately 40% after maturation of the alveolar microvasculature (32). The report that formation of alveoli continues until adulthood in a primate species, namely the rhesus monkey, although at a slower pace than during the first two years (33), suggests that late alveolarization is a general feature.

Formation of new septa involves deposition of elastic fibers in the wall thickness between the two capillary layers of immature septa and lifting of capillary vessels in the rising septa (see sect. "Elastic Fiber Formation Conditions Alveolar Septation"). It was therefore considered that once microvascular maturation was over, formation of new septa was no longer possible due to absence of the second capillary layer (12,34). How can this be reconciled with the observations of septa formation after microvascular maturation? First, in rat neonates treated with high doses of a glucocorticosteroid (GC), which induces precocious microvascular maturation and inhibits septation (see sect. IX.A), withdrawal of the drug was followed by a step-back in lung maturity with reappearance of double-layered septal capillaries and complete catch-up from the insult (35). This indicates that microvascular maturation is not irreversible. Moreover, recent stereological study of the alveolar capillary network using high-resolution synchrotron radiation X-ray tomographic microscopy revealed that new septa are formed at least until young adulthood in the rat and that about half of the new septa are lifted off from mature septa with single-layered capillary network (36). Remarkably, on the basis of newly forming septa, a local duplication of the capillary network was detected, allowing the new septa to be vascularized (36).

Contrary to previously prevailing opinion, the potential to form new alveoli may never be lost, even in adulthood. Loss of alveoli following food restriction has been observed in several rodent species (37–39) and in starved human beings (40,41). This loss is reversible since alveolar regeneration is observed following refeeding (39,42). Enhanced alveolar septal growth was similarly found in guinea pigs and dogs raised at high altitude to reduce oxygen availability (43,44). The alveolar surface area therefore adapts reversibly to the oxygen needs (45). Lastly, additional alveoli also appear to form during compensatory growth consecutive to lung resection. In adult mice, subpleural region of remaining lung showed higher proliferative activity like in development (46), and it was established that the number of alveoli was increased by about 50% 20 days after pneumonectomy (47). Compensatory growth therefore implies creating new alveoli, a process designated "neoalveolarization," and the adult lung is therefore able to recapitulate morphogenetic processes to face increased oxygen demand.

D. Relevance for BPD

As far as BPD of the premature newborn is concerned, it should be emphasized that developmental mechanisms that are impaired are those involved in early phases of alveolarization, including formation of saccules and secondary septation. In a therapeutic perspective, progress should be expected from better knowledge of these mechanisms and the search for methods to restore them. Nevertheless, the existence of late alveolarization and lung plasticity indicates that recovery may yet be expected to some extent beyond the period of bulk alveolarization.

III. Lung Interstitial Cells in Alveolarization

A. Fibroblast Proliferation

Lung interstitial cells play crucial roles in alveolarization. Peak alveolar formation is characterized by intense lung cell proliferation (48,49). Particularly, the number of fibroblasts is multiplied fourfold in rat lung, with 14% of proliferating cells during alveolarization versus less than 1% afterward (48). Moreover, apoptosis of lung cells that tremendously increases just after birth in the rat compared with fetal stages markedly declines next to fetal levels during alveolar septation (50).

B. Elastogenesis and Alveolar Septation

Elastic Fibers of Lung Parenchyma

The lung comprises three interconnected elastic fiber systems that form a "fibrous continuum" (51). Axial fibers originate from the bronchiolar wall and form an outline of alveolar ducts from which rings originate to enter the alveolar region. Peripheral fibers are connected to the pleura and form a felting beneath alveolar acini between which they penetrate. Delicate septal (or parenchymatous) fibers, which are anchored to both axial and peripheral fiber systems (52), form during late fetal and early postnatal development, contemporaneous with saccular and alveolar formation (12,53). Elastic fibers, which are associated with collagen fibers, are complex structures that contain amorphous insoluble elastin issued from cross-linkage of the soluble precursor tropoelastin by lysyl oxidase (LOX) and LOX-like (LOX-L) enzymes, and reticular microfibrils and associated glycoproteins including fibrillins, fibulins, and emilins. Tropoelastin monomers are assembled and cross-linked on preexisting microfibrillar scaffolds (54). Expression of these proteins must be coordinated, including LOX and LOX-L, so that the correct temporal sequence necessary to their assembly can be followed (55). Elastin is an exceedingly stable molecule; once the continuum of connective fibers is established, the components are meant to remain in that configuration (56).

Role of Fibroblasts in Septal Elastogenesis

The developing lung presents two subsets of interstitial cells designated myofibroblasts or nonlipid lung interstitial cells, and lipid interstitial cells or lipid-laden fibroblasts or lipofibroblasts (57–59). Although they are likely to derive from the same embryonic mesenchymal cells, they display different growth rates at any age and have been considered as separate populations (60,61). Lipofibroblasts, characterized by the presence of lipid droplets containing triglycerides, cholesterol esters, and retinyl esters (62–65), are present at the base of elongating septa (57). They may supply triglycerides for the synthesis of surfactant phospholipids (65) or to serve as antioxidants (66), and most importantly for alveolarization, they are the source of retinoic acid (RA) (see sect. VIII). Their existence in the human lung has recently been demonstrated (67). Myofibroblasts, which lack lipid droplets, express smooth muscle actin (αSMA), are contractile (59), and represent the source of septal elastin. When cultured on plastic in the presence of fetal bovine serum, isolated lung lipofibroblasts lose their lipid droplets and increase the production of elastin and αSMA (63,68), whereas reciprocally, factors that enhance lipid accumulation in vitro decrease tropoelastin and αSMA expression (68). Location of myofibroblasts in developing secondary crests and at septal tips (57,69–71) and dual immunostaining of the same cells for elastin and αSMA (72) also support their role in elastogenesis. Lastly, the areal density of αSMA almost doubles during alveolarization in the rat (71).

Elastic Fiber Formation Conditions Alveolar Septation

It is generally accepted, although not positively demonstrated, that the force necessary to raise alveolar crests is generated by septal elastic fibers. Elastic fiber deposits appear in the thickness of primary septa, and low ridges are formed next by lifting one of the capillary layers to grow upward into secondary septa (Fig. 3). Elastic fiber deposits present as a thickening of the elastic fiber network located at the tip of septa (Fig. 4) that forms a ring around the free edge of alveolar walls (Fig. 3). This represents a general feature in all examined species, including man (73). Mechanical stress applied to elastic fibers running along bends in alveolar walls may cause the fibers to pull away from walls, hence initiating the formation of a new septum (18,74). However, an alternative theoretical model has been proposed, which consists in the presence of a repulsive signal for epithelial cells in primary septum that could possibly push the secondary septum inward into the airspace, the capillaries and myofibroblasts following then (75). As a support for this theory, mice with targeted deletion of Roundabout (Robo), a receptor known to be involved in repellent signaling, have been reported to present impaired distal lung morphogenesis (76).

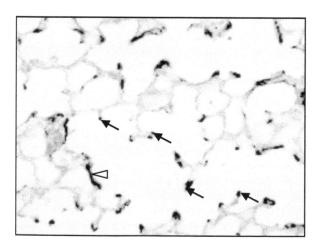

Figure 4 Aspect of elastic fibers in the developing lung parenchyma of 10-day-old rat (Weigert's coloration of elastin on a lung section). Elastin deposits are visible as black patches with typical location at the tip of growing secondary septa (*arrows*) and lining alveolar walls (*arrowhead*).

Developmental changes in tropoelastin expression correlate temporally with saccular and alveolar development (77–80). Consistently, cultured fibroblasts isolated from rat lung at various postnatal ages showed peak elastin expression coincidental with maxaimal septation (81). This increase was significantly reduced by exposure to hyperoxia (80), a classical model of arrested alveolarization (20,82). The pulmonary expression of fibrillins and fibulins is also upregulated during alveologenesis (83).

Results of various approaches support the essential role of elastic fibers in septation. Mice invalidated for the tropoelastin gene displayed dilated air saccules limited by attenuated walls at birth (84), which evidenced the importance of elastogenesis for saccular development already, but the animals died before the start of alveolar septation. Postnatal inhibition of LOX activity by β-amino propionitrile in the rat (85,86), which interferes with the synthesis of elastin and collagen, and the inactivation of LOX (87) or LOX L1 (88) genes in the mouse also led to airspace enlargement and reduced number of septa. Lastly, mice deficient in fibrillin 1, 4, or 5 have been reported to display defective elastic fiber assembly, impairment of alveolar septation, and later, emphysema-like phenotype (89–92). LOX-L1, which localizes specifically to sites of elastogenesis, has been shown to interact with fibulin 5 (88). Interestingly, elastogenesis was disrupted and elastic fibers displayed strikingly similar abnormal features in various pathological conditions with impaired alveolar development, including a premature lamb model of BPD (93,94), a transgenic model of arrested alveolar septation in mice (95), mechanically ventilated newborn mice (96), and congenital diaphragmatic hernia (CDH) (97,98). Thick and tortuous elastic fibers formed disorganized meshworks along walls instead of being located at septal tips. Moreover, mechanical ventilation of newborn mice uncoupled the expression of elastin, which was increased, and that of associated fibrils and LOX L1 that was unchanged (96). Altogether, these investigations demonstrate that elastic fiber formation is instrumental in alveolar septation and better support the "pull theory" of septa formation than the "repulsion theory."

Control of Myofibroblast Differentiation and Migration

Transforming growth factor β1 (TGF-β1) appears crucial for differentiation of lung myofibroblasts. TGF-β1 markedly stimulated the expression of αSMA in isolated lung fibroblasts (99), and both exogenous and endogenous TGF-β1 were shown to stimulate the expression of tropoelastin (100). Consistent with a physiological role in myofibroblast differentiation, active TGF-β1 (101) and TGF-β receptor (102) increase prior to septation in the rat, and most importantly, mice devoid of smad3, a major intracellular downstream signal transducer in the TGF-β1 pathway, present retarded alveolarization with decreased tropoelastin expression (103,104). Changes in expression and localization of the TGF-β family members, bone morphogenetic proteins (BMPs), contemporaneous with the onset of septation suggest that they are also involved (105). On the other hand, TGF-β is known to play a role in the development of lung fibrosis (106), and exposure to hyperoxia increases TGF-β expression (101,107) and induces excessive differentiation of myofibroblasts (108,109), but impairs BMP signaling (107). Excess of TGF-β is also involved in mediation of the inhibition of alveolar development in neonatal animals exposed to chronic hypoxia (110,111). A strict control of balance between TGF-β and BMP signalings appears therefore essential to septation. Because TGF-β is increased in BPD (112), it is likely to play a role in pathogenesis.

Most importantly, disruption of the platelet-derived growth factor A (PDGF-A) gene in surviving mice led to absence of elastic fiber deposition in saccular walls and to complete failure of secondary septation (113,114). Myofibroblasts, which express the PDGF-AA receptor PDGFRα, appeared to remain trapped around prospective bronchiolar walls, which was interpreted as a requirement for PDGF-AA produced by epithelial cells as a chemoattractant allowing myofibroblast precursors to migrate to the peripheral locations where septal elastic fibers are deposited (114). Discrete RDG-containing domains of fibrillins might mediate the PDGF-AA-induced migration of lung fibroblasts (115).

Another mediator released by epithelial cells, insulin-like growth factor I (IGF-I), is involved in myofibroblast proliferation, differentiation, and migration. Exogenous IGF-I enhanced migration and proliferation of fibroblasts in vitro (116), and the extent of alveolar development was shown to correlate with IGF-I level in models of stimulated or arrested septation (117). IGF-I enhanced α-SMA expression and collagen synthesis in developing lung fibroblasts by a mechanism mediated by PI3 kinase (118). Consistently, leprechaunism, a disease caused by genetic defect of the receptor IGF-1R, is associated with deficient alveolarization (119). Surprisingly, the expression of IGF-I, IGF-II, and IGF-1R is increased in experimentally impaired septation as well as in BPD (120–122), but this appears to be associated with epithelial repair process (123). Fibroblast growth factors (FGFs) are also involved in myofibroblasts differentiation and functions (see sect. "FGF Signaling Is Necessary in Alveolar Septation").

Impaired septation was also reported in mice mutated for the homeobox transcription factor, HOXA5, due to defective motility of alveolar myofibroblast progenitors associated with inappropriate localization of elastic fiber deposits (124). Together, these findings highlight the requirement of myofibroblast migration and positioning for alveolarization.

C. FGF Signaling in Alveolarization

FGF Signaling Is Necessary in Alveolar Septation

FGFs represent a wide family of heparin-binding growth factors (125) that play crucial roles in the various steps of lung development (126). Their effects are transduced by tyrosine kinase receptors (FGFRs) that are encoded by four genes designated *Fgfr 1* to *4* and present numerous isoforms generated by alternative splicing (125). Alveolarization coincides with increased FGFR3 and FGFR4 expression (127). This is clearly related to the control of septation, since the latter totally failed in the lungs of mice simultaneously devoid of both receptors (128). Nevertheless, myofibroblasts were present and elastogenesis occurred in this model, but elastin deposits never displayed the typical location at the tip of growing septa. Moreover, double-mutant lungs failed to downregulate elastin that continued to accumulate through adulthood (128). However, neither the synthesis of other elastic fiber components nor the ultrastructure of fibers have been studied in this model, and it cannot be ruled out that fibers with abnormal structure were produced that could not perform the function of rising septa.

FGFR2 is also involved. FGFR2IIIb and IIIc isoforms are expressed in lung epithelial and mesenchymal cells, respectively (129). FGFR2IIIb and FGF10 are required for early lung-branching morphogenesis (126) but do not appear to be involved in alveolar development since inhibition of FGFR2 activity in transgenic mice expressing an inducible soluble inactive receptor targeted on epithelial cells did not alter postnatal alveolarization (130). By contrast, alveolar septation was impaired in transgenic mice in which *Fgfr2IIIb* gene was expressed in mesenchymal tissue instead of *Fgfr2IIIc*, which was shown to result from prevented myofibroblast differentiation, due to establishment of an autocrine FGF10-FGFR2 signaling loop (131).

Involved FGFs

Because of its downregulating effects on elastin synthesis (132,133) and LOX activity (134), FGF2 is likely to be involved in the arrest of septal elastogenesis. The observations that EGF-like growth factor both downregulated elastin and increased FGF2 in cultured lung fibroblasts (135), and that FGF2 is an autocrine regulator of LOX expression in transformed fibroblasts (136) argue in favor of autocrine mechanism. However, epithelial cells also express FGF2 (137), and paracrine mechanism cannot be ruled out. FGF2 also appears to be involved in inducing rat lung cell apoptosis post-septation (138).

FGF18 might, by contrast, be involved in the induction of elastogenesis. In the rat lung, its transcript presents a twofold increase during prenatal saccular period and a sevenfold increase during postnatal alveolar septation (139). A rise coincident with the start of alveolar septation has also been reported in fetal human lung (98). Most importantly, FGF18 coordinately upregulated the expression of tropoelastin, LOX, and fibulins 1 and 5 in isolated rat lung fibroblasts (139). Consistently, fewer and larger air sacs were observed in *Fgf18*-deficient mouse fetuses (140), but lethality at birth prevented from studying consequences of secondary septation. Expressions of FGF18 and/ or FGFR3 and FGR4 were markedly diminished in septation arrest consecutive to neonatal exposure to hyperoxia (141–143). FGF18 expression was also reduced in the hypoplastic lung of human fetuses with CDH and in two experimental models of the disease (98). Two treatments that enhanced lung growth in CDH models simultaneously restored FGF18 expression, elastic fiber density and location, and alveolar septation (97,98). The presence of FGF18 transcripts (144) and of immunoreactive FGF18 (98) in interstitial cells of septa suggests possible autocrine mechanism, although endothelial cells also release FGF18 (145).

FGF7, otherwise known as keratinocyte growth factor, is expressed exclusively by interstitial cells (146), whereas its specific receptor FGFR2IIIb is found only in epithelial cells (129). FGF7 is accordingly involved in pulmonary mesenchymal-epithelial interactions (see sect. V.B), but was also reported recently to influence alveolar septation through enhanced growth of the vascular bed (147). Lastly, FGF9 controls mesenchymal cell proliferation, at least in the prenatal lung (148), and FGF9 signaling is necessary for distal lung capillary development, which appears to involve FGF9-regulated production of vascular endothelial growth factor (VEGF) by fibroblasts (149). The lung epithelium nevertheless appears to be the major source of VEGF (see sect. VI.A).

D. Identifying Alveolarization-Related Gene Expression in Fibroblasts

Recent investigations attempted identifying alveolarization-associated gene-expression changes in parenchymal wall fibroblasts through large-scale gene-profiling study.

Assuming that genes predominantly expressed in newly forming septa influence alveolarization, Foster et al. (150) isolated tips of growing mouse septa by laser capture microdissection and compared gene expression in tips to that in whole lung to characterize tip-specific expression. Among a variety of extracellular matrix (ECM) components or cell-matrix adhesion molecules of which tips were enriched, including tenascins (Tn) XB and C, developmentally regulated brain protein (drebrin), and laminin β2, they focused on galectin 1, a β-galactoside-binding protein involved in the regulation of cell proliferation, differentiation, and apoptosis. Galectin 1 indeed concentrated in myofibroblasts at the tips of septa with peak level at days 6 to 12 suggesting an important role in alveolarization. Because of known effects in transformation of dermal fibroblasts to myocytes (151), it might promote the differentiation of neonatal lung alveolar myofibroblasts but might also be involved in angiogenesis (152) or in apoptosis control (153).

Boucherat et al. (154), compared gene expression in fibroblasts isolated from developing rat lungs before alveolarization, within the peak of septation, and during the microvascular-maturation stage. Two groups of genes exhibited strikingly opposite expression profiles. First group gathered genes upregulated specifically during septation and downregulated afterward, including the transcription factors *Hoxa2, a4, a5*, and retinoid X receptor γ (*RXRγ*), and three genes involved in Wnt signaling, *Wnt5a*, Norriedisease protein (*Ndp*), and the receptor frizzled 1 (*Fzd1*). Their protein products were detected in the thickness and tip of growing septa. Interestingly, prenatal lung saccular development is delayed in *Wnt5a*$^{-/-}$ mice (155), and the involvement of WNT5a would therefore be pursued in alveolarization, possibly through proangiogenic effects (156). Data from previous investigations (157–159) suggest that *Fzd1* may be involved in myofibroblast proliferation and differentiation. The second group that gathered genes with lowered expression during septation and considerable upregulation thereafter included cartilage oligomeric protein, osteopontin, osteoactivin, *TnX*, and the negative proliferation regulator *schlafen 4*. Their expression profile suggests an involvement in the phase of alveolar wall thinning and microvascular maturation. Strikingly, the expression of genes up- and downregulated during septation was decreased or enhanced, respectively, in two models of arrested septation (154), suggesting that alveolar septation not only involves upregulation of specific genes but also necessitates downregulation of other sets of genes.

Another gene-profiling study identified genes downregulated by calorie restriction in adult mice and rapidly upregulated after refeeding (160). These include genes previously linked to septation, such as fibulins, RARγ, matrix metalloproteinases (MMPs), and galectin 1, or involved in angiogenesis during alveolarization such as VEGF and angiopoietin 2 (see sect. VI). This indicates that late alveolarization shares common molecular mechanisms with postnatal development.

IV. Extracellular Matrix Remodeling in Alveolarization

In addition to elastogenesis, alveolar septation involves the deposition of ECM components, including collagens, fibronectin, laminins, and proteoglycans. Corresponding genes are upregulated coincidentally with septation (79,83), and the relative fibronectin and collagen lung contents markedly increase during this stage (161,162). Laminin α5 is essential for normal alveolarization and epithelial cell differentiation and maturation

(163). Although the expression of these genes is almost ubiquitous, the contribution of myofibroblasts appears important (164).

In addition to deposition of ECM components, ECM remodeling appears to be crucial for alveolarization. Thus, up to 40% of newly formed collagen is rapidly degraded during septation period (165). Two MMPs appear particularly important. MMP2 (or gelatinase A) that presents maximal activity during the first 11 days of postnatal life in rats (165) showed impacted induction in septation arrest caused by hyperoxia (101). Moreover, *Mmp2*-null mice, in addition to defects in branching morphogenesis, exhibited abnormally large saccular spaces at birth (166). Similar although more pronounced features were found in mice devoid of the epidermal growth factor receptor (EGFR), which went along with lower proportion of active MMP2 (166). This was attributed to reduced expression of an activator enzyme of MMP2, membrane type 1 MMP (MT1-MMP) or MMP14, in $Egfr^{-/-}$ mice (166). Soon after, alveolarization was reported to be abolished in *Mmp14*-null mice (167–169), and contrary to $Mmp\text{-}2^{-/-}$ mice, there was no subsequent recovery, which suggests that MMP14 acts in alveolar septation via mechanisms largely independent of pro-MMP2 activation (167,168). The mechanism(s) of action of MMP14 is (are) not fully established, but endothelial cells from lungs of one-week-old $Mmp14^{-/-}$ mice displayed reduced in vitro migration and tube formation, suggesting defective angiogenesis (167). MMP14 expression increases fivefold in lung fibroblasts during septation (170), which indicates the probable role of fibroblasts also in alveolarization-related production of MMP14. Taking into account the variety of known functions and substrates of MMP14 in pericellular proteolysis (171), its involvement in fibroblast and endothelial cell migration through ECM is likely.

Late-gestation lung 1 (*Lgl1*), a developmentally regulated gene cloned as a glucocorticoid-inducible gene in rat lung fibroblasts, has been assumed to be involved in the regulation of ECM degradation (172). It seems to be involved in branching morphogenesis (173) and in mesenchymal-epithelial interactions (174), but maximal expression coincides with the onset of alveolar septation (175). LGL1 protein concentrates at the tips of budding secondary septa, and its expression is profoundly decreased by exposure to hyperoxia (175), which is suggestive of physiological involvement in septation although its mechanism of action remains to be defined.

V. Mesenchymal-Epithelial Cell Interrelationships in Alveolarization

A. Differentiated Alveolar Epithelial Cells Are Required for Alveolarization

Mesenchymal cells exert paracrine effects on the lung epithelium that are essential at all lung developmental steps, including for patterning of the organ and epithelial cell fate (126,176). Although maturation of type II alveolar epithelial cells (AECII), the source of pulmonary surfactant, occurs before birth and precedes alveolarization in all species, the integrity of involved control mechanisms seems necessary for alveolarization. Moreover, accurate course of a given developmental step is likely to be conditioned by that of the preceding one. Thus, when the gene of transcription factor Forkhead box (Fox) a2, which is required for AECII differentiation (177), is deleted in mice at the end of gestation, air-space enlargement and altered septation occur (178). Maintenance of elevated level of expression of the transcription factor GATA6, which is also required for differentiation of alveolar epithelial cells (179,180), similarly impaired alveolar septation (181). This may be related to disturbance in AECI differentiation because of sustained thyroid transcription factor-1 expression (181,182). Similarly, abrogation of TGF-β type 2 receptor in mouse lung epithelium resulted in retardation of postnatal lung alveolarization with markedly decreased AECI, while no abnormality in prenatal lung development was observed (183). Requirement of AECI differentiation for distal lung development and alveolar sac formation has indeed been demonstrated by inactivation of the gene of the type I cell marker T1α in mice (184). A strict control of differentiation of both alveolar cell types, which involves both up- and downregulation of implicated transcription factors, is therefore required for normal distal lung development.

B. Mesenchymal Mediators of Alveolar Epithelial Cell Differentiation and Maturation

One major mesenchymal mediator of AECII proliferation, differentiation, and maturation is FGF7 (185–190). Its effects are mediated by c-Jun N-terminal kinase (191). FGF7 mediates AECII-maturing effects of corticosteroids (192,193). FGF7 also protects the alveolar epithelium against injuries (reviewed in Ref. 194), which has considerable potential importance for the prevention of BPD. Consistent with animal investigations, low FGF7 level in tracheal aspirates from human neonates has been associated with increased risk of BPD (195). Leptin (196) and the EGFR ligand neuregulin 1β (197) are two other mesenchymal factors that relay glucocorticoid stimulation of AECII maturation. Lastly, hepatocyte growth factor (HGF), another heparin-binding growth factor produced by lung fibroblasts whereas its receptor is expressed in epithelial cells (198), is a growth factor for AECII (185,199) and seems necessary to compensatory lung growth (200) and alveolarization (201).

C. Mesenchymal-Epithelial Interactions Are Reciprocal

In addition to PDGF-AA and IGF-I involved in myofibroblasts differentiation and migration, AECII release factors that influence lipofibroblasts, namely prostaglandin E2 and parathyroid hormone-related protein (PTHrP). These have been shown in turn to stimulate surfactant synthesis through a positive regulation loop between AECII and lipofibroblasts, implying the secretion of leptin by the latter (196,202,203). The crucial importance of this mechanism is illustrated by impaired AECII differentiation in mice missing the PTHrP gene (204). Interestingly, PTHrP was lowered in tracheal aspirates of infants who developed BPD (205).

VI. Epithelial-Endothelial Interactions in Angiogenesis and Alveolarization

A. VEGF Signaling and Angiogenesis Are Required for Alveolar Septation

Impaired alveolar development in BPD is associated with arrested and dysmorphic vascular growth (206–208). This goes along with decreased levels of VEGF-A (thereafter designated simply VEGF) and its receptor Flt-1 (VEGFR1) (206). VEGF plays a key role for microvascular development of the lung (209). The requirement of VEGF signaling for normal alveolarization was demonstrated through blockade in the rat by use of VEGFR inhibitor (210,211) or neutralizing antibody (212), which markedly reduced septation and final alveolar number. Moreover, VEGF signaling was reduced by hyperoxic exposure (213,214), and enhancing angiogenesis by VEGF treatment promoted both vascular growth and alveolarization in this model (215–217).

The major source of VEGF for alveolarization appears to be AECII (218,219). VEGF exists as three isoforms designated VEGFs 120, 164, and 188 according to their molecular weight, which present different affinity for the various VEGF receptors. AECII produce high levels of VEGF188 (220). Total VEGF deletion induces precocious embryonic lethality (221), but targeted deletion of the VEGF gene that allowed only VEGF120 to be expressed supported development and survival of mice (220). These mice nevertheless displayed reduced pulmonary microvascular bed and fewer air-blood barriers, and had decreased airspace-parenchyma ratio (220,222). Furthermore, VEGF188 expression is developmentally regulated with strong increase shortly before birth when it becomes predominant (220,223,224). Lastly, selective inactivation of the VEGF-A gene in respiratory epithelium resulted in almost complete absence of pulmonary capillaries, demonstrating the dependence of their development on epithelium-derived VEGF (225). This was associated with a defect in primary septa formation and decreased HGF expression (225). Together, these data lead to ascribe to VEGF released by AECII, particularly the 188 isoform, a central role in the control of lung parenchymal angiogenesis, and hence of alveolarization. However, whereas being in close apposition to AECI, endothelial cells are relatively remote from type II cells. It was shown that fibroblasts establish contacts with epithelial and endothelial cells through interruptions in basement membrane, thus providing a bridge directly connecting AECII to endothelial cells, which is likely to facilitate molecular exchanges between the three cell types (226).

B. Other Pro- and Antiangiogenic Factors

Disordered expression of other angiogenesis-modulating factors including the angiopoietin 1 (Ang-1) receptor Tie2, Ang-2, and endostatin appear to be involved in the pathophysiology of BPD (206,227–229), which suggests their involvement in normal alveolar angiogenesis. Ang-1 plays a major role in maturation and maintenance of capillary vessels (230). By contrast, Ang2 and endostatin exert antiangiogenic signaling (231,232). Possible implication of Ang-2 in microvascular abnormalities of BPD is further supported by its role in acute injury and necrotic cell death in hyperoxia-exposed mouse lungs (233).

Another antiangiogenic factor, endothelial monocyte-activating polypeptide II (EMAP II), inhibited both developing-lung vascularization and AECII differentiation (234). A surge in expression that correlates with the stage of microvascular maturation when it was widely distributed in a perivascular fashion (235) suggests physiological role in downregulating microvascular growth when fusion of septal capillary occurs. EMAP II production appears to directly result from epithelial-mesenchymal cell interactions (236). Consistent with an involvement in precocious arrest of alveolarization in BPD, increased EMAP II was found in human BPD and in the premature baboon model

(237). All these findings suggest that imbalance between pro- and antiangiogenic factors accounts for disturbed angiogenesis in failing alveolar development in BPD.

VII. Role of Mechanical Factors in Alveolarization

A. Expansion-Induced Alveolar Development in The Sheep Fetus

Experiments in the sheep fetus demonstrated that lung growth, morphogenesis, and cell differentiation are critically dependent on the degree to which the lungs are expanded by fluid secreted by epithelial cells (238–240). Because alveolarization is a prenatal event in sheep (241), the models are suitable to evaluate consequences for this process. Clearly, lung distension consecutive to tracheal obstruction enhanced alveolar development (242), whereas sustained decrease in expansion consecutive to tracheal drainage reduced alveolar number and surface area (243). Consistently, tracheal obstruction elevated pulmonary elastin content, whereas it was strongly reduced by drainage (244,245). Moreover, secondary septation appeared to have failed and tissue location of elastin was altered in drained lung (244) with features reminiscent of the aspect displayed in models of BPD and diaphragmatic hernia (see sect. "Elastic Fiber Formation Conditions Alveolar Septation"). Tracheal obstruction partly restored lung structure and alveolar surface area in drained lung (243), and it reinitiated alveolar septation and restored elastin density and distribution in diaphragmatic hernia (98). Lastly, lung distension enhanced AECI differentiation (97,246).

Attempts have been made to identify molecular mechanisms underlying expansion-induced lung development. VEGF transcript was increased, whereas active TGF-β1 was decreased following tracheal obstruction, which, taking into account the central role of VEGF in alveolar angiogenesis and septation, points this factor as a likely candidate in enhanced alveolar development (247). Differential expression of various genes was determined between expanded and unexpanded lungs in a same sheep fetus through gene-profiling study (248). Further attention has been paid to vitamin D_3–upregulated protein 1 (VDUP1) that was reduced by lung expansion and increased by drainage. It was suggested that VDUP1 might be an important mediator of expansion-induced alveolar epithelial cell proliferation and differentiation (249). Thrombospondin-1 (TSP-1) was also enhanced by lung expansion and was speculated to play a significant role in regulating lung growth (250). AECI differentiation appears to involve control of entry of their AECII precursor in cell cycle through modulation by TGF-β (251).

B. Mechanical Forces and Alveolar Development in the Air-Breathing Lung

The forces applied to the air-filled lung are different and more complex, with constant changes in lung tension induced by the respiratory cycle. Little is known of how changing the mechanical environment of the lung influences its development after birth. This has however important implications for understanding the impact of mechanical ventilation on the developing lung, particularly in prematurely born infants. Although a positive internal distending pressure may support the mechanisms described above, it has been recognized for long that high positive airway pressure induced barotrauma that represented a major factor of injury.

Increased lung expansion by positive-end expiratory pressure in the mechanically ventilated neonatal lamb significantly increased the proportion of lung-proliferating cells consistently with prenatal findings, but did not affect AEC differentiation (252). Stretching the lung clearly influences behavior and fate of epithelial cells and fibroblasts. Continuous cycles of stretch-relaxation of mixed lung cells mimicking the respiratory cycle increased the expression of VEGF (253). Consistently, lung distension induced by tracheal occlusion in the rat fetus accelerated the maturational pattern of VEGF isoforms and increased lung VEGF contents (224). Mechanical strain also increased type I collagen expression in cultured pulmonary fibroblasts (254) and tropoelastin expression in cultures of mixed lung cells (255), which supports a putative role of respiratory cycle–induced cell distension in the regulation of expression of these proteins. Lastly, tonic distension of cultured AECII increased PTHrP production, while distension of cultured fibroblasts increased their PTHrP responsiveness, suggesting that stretching couples and coordinates the production and receptor-mediated action of PTHrP (256).

VIII. Retinoic Acid: A Major Player in Alveolarization Control

RA is derived from vitamin A (retinol) and binds to a group of heterodimerized transcription factors, the retinoic acid receptors (RARs) α, β, and γ and the retinoid X receptors (RXRs) α, β, and γ. Upon binding of all-*trans* RA (RARs) or 9-*cis* RA (RARs and RXRs), these receptors are activated and bind to their respective response elements (RAREs, RXREs) in the promoter region of their target genes (257). Through this mechanism, RA controls the transcription of a multitude of genes involved in development and homeostasis. The developing lung contains large supply of vitamin A stored in lipo-fibroblasts under the form of retinyl esters that are mobilized during the perinatal period and converted into RA (64,258,259). The enzymes of RA-synthesis pathway are upregulated during the period of alveolar septation (49). Both retinoid-binding proteins and RAR isoforms are temporally regulated, peaking from postnatal days 2 to 9 in the rat at the onset of septation, and were found within the septal regions during alveologenesis (64,260).

Numerous investigations have evidenced the crucial role of RA signaling in alveolarization. Mild vitamin A deficiency from fetal to neonatal life decreased the surface area of air spaces and accelerated vascular maturation in infant rats (261). Reciprocally, RA enhanced alveolar formation in postnatal rats (262) and rescued impaired alveolarization consecutive to dexamethasone treatment or hyperoxic exposure (262–264). Exogenous RA enhanced tropoelastin gene expression in cultured neonatal rat lung fibroblasts (265), and the role of endogenous retinoids in controlling tropoelastin expression has been demonstrated (266). RA also stimulated the expression of PDGF-A and PDGFRα in newborn rats in vivo (267) and in cultured lung fibroblasts (268), and the expression of Hoxa5 in fetal mouse lung fibroblasts (269). It is therefore likely to act upstream of myofibroblast proliferation, differentiation, and migration pathways mediated by PDGF-AA and the Hoxa5 transcription-control cascade. Furthermore, *RARγ* gene deletion in mice resulted in a decrease in the steady state level of tropoelastin transcript in lung fibroblasts, and a decrease in whole lung elastic tissue and alveolar number, which was further accentuated by the simultaneous deletion of *RXRα* (270). Expression of a dominant-negative *RARα* transgene reduced alveolar number and diminished alveolar surface area (271), but subsequent study in mice deleted for *RARα* gene suggested that

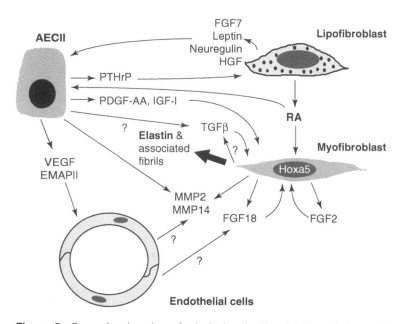

Figure 5 Comprehensive view of principal cell-cell and cell-matrix interactions and their diffusible mediators in the alveolarization process. *Abbreviations*: AECII, alveolar epithelial cell type II; RA, retinoic acid; FGF, fibroblast growth factor; TGF, transforming growth factor; VEGF, vascular endothelial growth factor; PDGF, platelet-derived growth factor; HGF, hepatocyte growth factor; EMAP, endothelial monocyte-activating polypetide; PTHrP, parathyroid hormone-related peptide; MMP, matrix metalloproteinase.

this receptor could be involved mostly in late alveolarization (272). The role of *RARβ* is less clear and debated. *RARβ* gene–deleted mice have been reported to present premature and accelerated septation, suggesting a role of this receptor as an inhibitor of septation (273). However, further investigation showed that *RARβ*-null mice had significant increase in the volume density of airspaces, reduced gas-exchange surface area, and impaired respiratory function in early adulthood starting from 28 days (274). Moreover, PDGF-A protein levels were significantly lowered in *RARβ*-null mice (274). *RARβ* may therefore have different functions during the period of bulk septation and in late alveolarization or alveolar maintenance. However, most of these data have been gained in rodents and may not necessarily be extendable to primates since retinoids failed to restore alveolar morphology and angiogenesis in premature ventilated baboons, despite enhanced elastin expression (275). Figure 5 integrates the various cell-cell interactions involved in alveolarization, including RA signaling.

IX. Hormonal Control of Alveolarization

A. Glucocorticosteroid Hormones

GCs have been repeatedly shown to inhibit outgrowth of new septa, to diminish fibroblast proliferation, to impair the transdifferentiation of alveolar type II into type I cells, and to accelerate alveolar wall thinning and capillary fusion, leading to early termination of alveolarization in rhesus monkeys (276), rats (277–280), or lambs (281,282). Their mechanism of action is very partially understood. Although they stimulate elastogenesis in the prenatal lung (283) and in cultured mixed lung cells (255), and LOX expression in cultured murine lungs (284), they prevent alveolar deposition of elastin (285). They also block microvascular growth due to downregulation of VEGFR2 (286). GCs are likely to be involved in negative regulation of cell proliferation since pulmonary expression of the negative regulator of the cell cycle p21 CIP1 was markedly reduced, whereas that of the lung growth factor midkine was strongly increased in mice with disruption of the gluco-corticoid receptor gene (287). Nevertheless, prenatal GC signaling appears necessary to structural saccular development and further alveolar development, as evidenced in this same mouse model that displayed increased thickness of lung interstitial tissue (288).

The serum concentration of active GC indeed displays a trough during lung septation, whether this takes place before (guinea pig) (289) or after (rat) (290) birth. It increases thereafter as septation ends and as thinning of alveolar walls occurs. The physiological role of GC therefore appears to be to control the final steps of alveola-rization, and their deleterious effects are likely to be the consequence of temporally inadapted play. When they occur in their normal temporal sequence of action, the roles of RA and GC should therefore be regarded as complementary rather than antagonist.

B. Other Hormones

The administration of thyroid hormone (thyroxine) or its active derivate triiodothyronine (T3) to newborn rats increased lung DNA synthesis, accelerated the pace of alveolar septation, and induced the formation of additional alveoli (291–293), whereas injection of propylthiouracil, a drug that blocks conversion of thyroxine to T3, impaired septation (293). In this species, serum thyroid hormone concentration (292) and thyroid hormone receptor density in the lung (294) start increasing just before the onset of septation. Thyroid hormones therefore appear as physiological stimuli of alveolar septation.

Early interest was spurred to the potential role of growth hormone (GH) in alveolar development because patients with acromegaly exhibited partially reversible increases in lung volume and distensibility (295–297). In the rat, however, exogenous GH given to young adult rats induced increases in lung volume and lung surface area proportional to the increase of body growth (298), suggesting primarily an effect on growth of the rib cage without specific enhancement of alveolar development. Reversibility in human lung changes nevertheless calls for further investigation to determine whether GH influences late alveolarization or neoalveolarization.

X. Conclusions

Although current findings render more and more complex the view of alveolarization mechanisms, considerable progress has undoubtedly been made in its understanding. Taking into account the large number of involved mediators and genes, it is clear that a strict control and integration of these mechanisms is required. Disorders that lead to impaired alveolarization in BPD are likely to result from ruptures in control pathways, leading to imbalanced interactions between cells and signal molecules. In addition to make the care of very low birth weight infants as little harmful as possible, it should become attainable soon to define specific therapeutic strategies to restore balanced mechanisms of alveolar development.

References

1. Husain AN, Siddiqui NH, Stocker JT. Pathology of arrested acinar development in post-surfactant bronchopulmonary dysplasia. Hum Pathol 1998; 29(7):710–717.
2. Jobe AJ. The new BPD: an arrest of lung development. Pediatr Res 1999; 46(6):641–643.
3. Langston C, Kida K, Reed M, et al. Human lung growth in late gestation and in the neonate. Am Rev Respir Dis 1984; 129(4):607–613.
4. Zeltner TB, Caduff JH, Gehr P, et al. The postnatal development and growth of the human lung. I. Morphometry. Respir Physiol 1987; 67(3):247–267.
5. Jobe AH, Bancalari E. Bronchopulmonary dysplasia. Am J Respir Crit Care Med 2001; 163(7):1723–1729.
6. Baraldi E, Filippone M. Chronic lung disease after premature birth. N Engl J Med 2007; 357(19):1946–1955.
7. Hjalmarson O, Sandberg K. Abnormal lung function in healthy preterm infants. Am J Respir Crit Care Med 2002; 165(1):83–87.
8. Watterberg KL, Demers LM, Scott SM, et al. Chorioamnionitis and early lung inflammation in infants in whom bronchopulmonary dysplasia develops. Pediatrics 1996; 97(2): 210–215.
9. Ochs M, Nyengaard JR, Jung A, et al. The number of alveoli in the human lung. Am J Respir Crit Care Med 2004; 169(1):120–124.
10. Burri PH. Structural aspects of postnatal lung development—alveolar formation and growth. Biol Neonate 2006; 89(4):313–322.
11. Burri PH, Dbaly J, Weibel ER. The postnatal growth of the rat lung. I. Morphometry. Anat Rec 1974; 178(4):711–730.
12. Burri PH. The postnatal growth of the rat lung. III. Morphology. Anat Rec 1974; 180(1):77–98.
13. Amy RW, Bowes D, Burri PH, et al. Postnatal growth of the mouse lung. J Anat 1977; 124(pt 1):131–151.
14. Weibel ER. Design and morphometry of the pulmonary gas exchanger. In: Crystal RG, West JB, eds. The Lung: Scientific Foundations. Vol 1. New York: Raven Press, 1991:795–805.
15. DiMaio M, Gil J, Ciurea D, et al. Structural maturation of the human fetal lung: a morphometric study of the development of air-blood barriers. Pediatr Res 1989; 26(2):88–93.
16. Hilfer SR. Morphogenesis of the lung: control of embryonic and fetal branching. Annu Rev Physiol 1996; 58:93–113.
17. Metzger RJ, Klein OD, Martin GR, et al. The branching programme of mouse lung development. Nature 2008; 453(7196):745–750.
18. Burri PH. Structural aspects of prenatal and postnatal development and growth of the lung. In: MacDonald JA, ed. Lung Growth and Development. New York: Marcel Dekker, 1997:1–35.
19. Roth-Kleiner M, Post M. Similarities and dissimilarities of branching and septation during lung development. Pediatr Pulmonol 2005; 40(2):113–134.
20. Massaro GD, Massaro D. Postnatal lung growth: evidence that the gas-exchange region grows fastest at the periphery. Am J Physiol Lung Cell Mol Physiol 1993; 265(4 pt 1): L319–L322.
21. Randell SH, Mercer RR, Young SL. Postnatal growth of pulmonary acini and alveoli in normal and oxygen-exposed rats studied by serial section reconstructions. Am J Anat 1989; 186(1):55–68.

22. Blanco LN, Massaro D, Massaro GD. Alveolar size, number, and surface area: developmentally dependent response to 13% O2. Am J Physiol 1991; 261(6):L370–L377.
23. Burri PH, Tarek MR. A novel mechanism of capillary growth in the rat pulmonary microcirculation. Anat Rec 1990; 228(1):35–45.
24. Burri PH, Djonov V. Intussusceptive angiogenesis—the alternative to capillary sprouting. Mol Aspects Med 2002; 23(suppl. 6):S1–S27.
25. Zeltner TB, Burri PH. The postnatal development and growth of the human lung. II. Morphology. Respir Physiol 1987; 67(3):269–282.
26. Schittny JC, Djonov V, Fine A, et al. Programmed cell death contributes to postnatal lung development. Am J Respir Cell Mol Biol 1998; 18(6):786–793.
27. Bruce MC, Honaker CE, Cross RJ. Lung fibroblasts undergo apoptosis following alveolarization. Am J Respir Cell Mol Biol 1999; 20(2):228–236.
28. Dunnill MS. Postnatal growth of the lung. Thorax 1962; 17:329–333.
29. Emery JL, Wilcock PF. The postnatal development of the lung. Acta Anat 1966; 65(1):10–29.
30. Massaro D, Teich N, Maxwell S, et al. Postnatal development of alveoli. Regulation and evidence for a critical period in rat. J Clin Invest 1985; 76(4):1297–1305.
31. Wood JP, Kolassa JE, McBride JT. Changes in alveolar septal border lengths with postnatal lung growth. Am J Physiol Lung Cell Mol Physiol 1998; 275(6 pt 1):L1157–L1163.
32. Mund SI, Stampanoni M, Schittny JC. Developmental alveolarization of the mouse lung. Dev Dyn 2008; 237(8):2108–2116.
33. Hyde DM, Blozis SA, Avdalovic MV, et al. Alveoli increase in number but not size from birth to adulthood in rhesus monkeys. Am J Physiol Lung Cell Mol Physiol 2007; 293(3): L570–L579.
34. Caduff JH, Fischer LC, Burri PH. Scanning electron microscopic study of the developing microvasculature in the postnatal rat lung. Anat Rec 1986; 216(2):154–164.
35. Tschanz SA, Makanya AN, Haenni B, et al. Effects of neonatal high-dose short-term glucocorticoid treatment on the lung: a morphometric study in the rat. Pediatr Res 2003; 53(1):72–80.
36. Schittny JC, Mund SI, Stampanoni M. Evidence and structural mechanism for late lung alveolarization. Am J Physiol Lung Cell Mol Physiol 2008; 294(2):L246–L254.
37. Sahebjami H, Wirman JA. Emphysema-like changes in the lungs of starved rats. Am Rev Respir Dis 1981; 124(5):619–624.
38. Karlinsky JB, Goldstein RH, Ojserkis B, et al. Lung mechanics and connective tissue levels in starvation-induced emphysema in hamsters. Am J Physiol 1986; 251(2 pt 2):R282–R288.
39. Massaro GD, Radaeva S, Clerch LB, et al. Lung alveoli: endogenous programmed destruction and regeneration. Am J Physiol Lung Cell Mol Physiol 2002; 283(2):L305–L309.
40. Fliderbaum J. Clinical aspects of hunger diseases in adults. In: Winick M, ed., Hunger Disease: Studies by the Jewish Physicians in the Warsaw Ghetto. New York: John Wiley and Sons, 1979:11–36.
41. Coxson HO, Chan IH, Mayo JR, et al. Early emphysema in patients with anorexia nervosa. Am J Respir Crit Care Med 2004; 170(7):748–752.
42. Massaro D, Massaro GD, Baras A, et al. Calorie-related rapid onset of alveolar loss, regeneration, and changes in mouse lung gene expression. Am J Physiol Lung Cell Mol Physiol 2004; 286(5):L896–L906.
43. Hsia CC, Carbayo JJ, Yan X, et al. Enhanced alveolar growth and remodelling in guinea pigs raised at high altitude. Respir Physiol Neurobiol 2005; 147(1):105–115.
44. Hsia CC, Johnson LR Jr., McDonough P, et al. Residence at 3,800-m altitude for 5 mo in growing dogs enhances lung diffusing capacity for oxygen that persists at least 2.5 years. J Appl Physiol 2007; 102(4):1448–1455.
45. Massaro D, Massaro GD. Pulmonary alveoli: formation, the "call for oxygen," and other regulators. Am J Physiol Lung Cell Mol Physiol 2002; 282(3):L345–L358.

46. Foster DJ, Yan X, Bellotto DJ, et al. Expression of epidermal growth factor and surfactant proteins during postnatal and compensatory lung growth. Am J Physiol Lung Cell Mol Physiol 2002; 283(5):L981–L990.

47. Fehrenbach H, Voswinckel R, Michl V, et al. Neoalveolarisation contributes to compensatory lung growth following pneumonectomy in mice. Eur Respir J 2008; 31(3):515–522.

48. Kauffman SL, Burri PH, Weibel ER. The postnatal growth of the rat lung. II. Autoradiography. Anat Rec 1974; 180(1):63–76.

49. Hind M, Corcoran J, Maden M. Alveolar proliferation, retinoid synthesizing enzymes, and endogenous retinoids in the postnatal mouse lung. Different roles for Aldh-1 and Raldh-2. Am J Respir Cell Mol Biol 2002; 26(1):67–73.

50. Kresch MJ, Christian C, Wu F, et al. Ontogeny of apoptosis during lung development. Pediatr Res 1998; 43(3):426–431.

51. Weibel ER. Functional morphology of lung parenchyma. In: Macklem PT, Mead J, eds. Handbook of Physiology. Section 3: The Respiratory System. Vol III. Part 1. Bethesda: American Physiological Society, 1986:89–111.

52. Weibel ER, Bachofen H. The fiber scaffold of lung parenchyma. In: Crystal RG, West JB, eds. The Lung: Scientific Foundations. Vol 1. New York: Raven Press, 1991:787–794.

53. Burri PH, Weibel, ER. Ultrastructure and morphometry of the developing lung. In: Hodson WA, ed. Lung biology in Health and Disease. Development of the Lung. Vol 6. New York: Marcel Dekker, 1977:215–268.

54. Wagenseil JE, Mecham RP. New insights into elastic fiber assembly. Birth Defects Res C Embryo Today 2007; 81(4):229–240.

55. Shifren A, Mecham RP. The stumbling block in lung repair of emphysema: elastic fiber assembly. Proc Am Thorac Soc 2006; 3(5):428–433.

56. Starcher BC. Elastin and the lung. Thorax 1986; 41(8):577–585.

57. Vaccaro C, Brody JS. Ultrastructure of developing alveoli. I. The role of the interstitial fibroblast. Anat Rec 1978; 192(4):467–479.

58. McGowan SE, Torday JS. The pulmonary lipofibroblast (lipid interstitial cell) and its contributions to alveolar development. Annu Rev Physiol 1997; 59:43–62.

59. Powell DW, Mifflin RC, Valentich JD, et al. Myofibroblasts. I. Paracrine cells important in health and disease. Am J Physiol Cell Physiol 1999; 277(1 pt 1):C1–C9.

60. Brody JS, Kaplan NB. Proliferation of alveolar interstitial cells during postnatal lung growth. Evidence for two distinct populations of pulmonary fibroblasts. Am Rev Respir Dis 1983; 127(6):763–770.

61. Awonusonu F, Srinivasan S, Strange J, et al. Developmental shift in the relative percentages of lung fibroblast subsets: role of apoptosis postseptation. Am J Physiol Lung Cell Mol Physiol 1999; 277(4 pt 1):L848–L859.

62. Maksvytis HJ, Vaccaro C, Brody JS. Isolation and characterization of the lipid-containing interstitial cell from the developing rat lung. Lab Invest 1981; 45(3):248–259.

63. Maksvytis HJ, Niles RM, Simanovsky L, et al. In vitro characteristics of the lipid-filled interstitial cell associated with postnatal lung growth: evidence for fibroblast heterogeneity. J Cell Physiol 1984; 118(2):113–123.

64. McGowan SE, Harvey CS, Jackson SK. Retinoids, retinoic acid receptors, and cytoplasmic retinoid binding proteins in perinatal rat lung fibroblasts. Am J Physiol Lung Cell Mol Physiol 1995; 269(4 pt 1):L463–L472.

65. Torday J, Hua J, Slavin R. Metabolism and fate of neutral lipids of fetal lung fibroblast origin. Biochim Biophys Acta 1995; 1254(2):198–206.

66. Torday JS, Torday DP, Gutnick J, et al. Biologic role of fetal lung fibroblast triglycerides as antioxidants. Pediatr Res 2001; 49(6):843–849.

67. Rehan VK, Sugano S, Wang Y, et al. Evidence for the presence of lipofibroblasts in human lung. Exp Lung Res 2006; 32(8):379–393.

68. McGowan SE, Jackson SK, Doro MM, et al. Peroxisome proliferators alter lipid acquisition and elastin gene expression in neonatal rat lung fibroblasts. Am J Physiol 1997; 273(6 pt 1): L1249–L1257.
69. Leslie KO, Mitchell JJ, Woodcock-Mitchell JL, et al. Alpha smooth muscle actin expression in developing and adult human lung. Differentiation 1990; 44(2):143–149.
70. Wright C, Strauss S, Toole K, et al. Composition of the pulmonary interstitium during normal development of the human fetus. Pediatr Dev Pathol 1999; 2(5):424–431.
71. Dickie R, Wang YT, Butler JP, et al. Distribution and quantity of contractile tissue in postnatal development of rat alveolar interstitium. Anat Rec (Hoboken) 2008; 291(1):83–93.
72. Noguchi A, Reddy R, Kursar JD, et al. Smooth muscle isoactin and elastin in fetal bovine lung. Exp Lung Res 1989; 15(4):537–552.
73. Nakamura Y, Fukuda S, Hashimoto T. Pulmonary elastic fibers in normal human development and in pathological conditions. Pediatr Pathol 1990; 10(5):689–706.
74. Ad hoc Statement Committee, American Thoracic Society. Mechanisms and limits of induced postnatal lung growth. Am J Respir Crit Care Med 2004; 170(3):319–343.
75. Prodhan P, Kinane TB. Developmental paradigms in terminal lung development. Bioessays 2002; 24(11):1052–1059.
76. Xian J, Clark KJ, Fordham R, et al. Inadequate lung development and bronchial hyperplasia in mice with a targeted deletion in the Dutt1/Robo1 gene. Proc Natl Acad Sci U S A 2001; 98(26):15062–15066.
77. Bruce MC. Developmental changes in tropoelastin levels in rat lung: evaluation by in situ hybridization. Am J Respir Cell Mol Biol 1991; 5(4):344–350.
78. Noguchi A, Samaha H. Developmental changes in tropoelastin gene expression in the rat lung studied by in situ hybridization. Am J Respir Cell Mol Biol 1991; 5(6):571–578.
79. Quaglino D, Fornieri C, Nanney LB, et al. Extracellular matrix modifications in rat tissues of different ages. Correlations between elastin and collagen type I mRNA expression and lysyl-oxidase activity. Matrix 1993; 13(6):481–490.
80. Bruce MC, Honaker CE. Transcriptional regulation of tropoelastin expression in rat lung fibroblasts: changes with age and hyperoxia. Am J Physiol 1998; 274(6 pt 1):L940–L950.
81. Noguchi A, Firsching K, Kursar JD, et al. Developmental changes of tropoelastin synthesis by rat pulmonary fibroblasts and effects of dexamethasone. Pediatr Res 1990; 28(4):379–382.
82. Bonikos DS, Bensch KG, Ludwin SK, et al. Oxygen toxicity in the newborn. The effect of prolonged 100 per cent O2 exposure on the lungs of newborn mice. Lab Invest 1975; 32(5): 619–635.
83. Mariani TJ, Reed JJ, Shapiro SD. Expression profiling of the developing mouse lung: insights into the establishment of the extracellular matrix. Am J Respir Cell Mol Biol 2002; 26(5):541–548.
84. Wendel DP, Taylor DG, Albertine KH, et al. Impaired distal airway development in mice lacking elastin. Am J Respir Cell Mol Biol 2000; 23(3):320–326.
85. Kida K, Thurlbeck WM. The effects of beta-aminopropionitrile on the growing rat lung. Am J Pathol 1980; 101(3):693–710.
86. Das RM. The effect of beta-aminopropionitrile on lung development in the rat. Am J Pathol 1980; 101(3):711–722.
87. Mäki JM, Sormunen R, Lippo S, et al. Lysyl oxidase is essential for normal development and function of the respiratory system and for the integrity of elastic and collagen fibers in various tissues. Am J Pathol 2005; 167(4):927–936.
88. Liu X, Zhao Y, Gao J, et al. Elastic fiber homeostasis requires lysyl oxidase-like 1 protein. Nat Genet 2004; 36(2):178–182.
89. Neptune ER, Frischmeyer PA, Arking DE, et al. Dysregulation of TGF-β activation contributes to pathogenesis in Marfan syndrome. Nat Genet 2003; 33(3):407–411.
90. Yanagisawa H, Davis EC, Starcher BC, et al. Fibulin-5 is an elastin-binding protein essential for elastic fibre development in vivo. Nature 2002; 415(6868):168–171.

91. Nakamura T, Lozano PR, Ikeda Y, et al. Fibulin-5/DANCE is essential for elastogenesis in vivo. Nature 2002; 415(6868):171–175.

92. McLaughlin PJ, Chen Q, Horiguchi M, et al. Targeted disruption of fibulin-4 abolishes elastogenesis and causes perinatal lethality in mice. Mol Cell Biol 2006; 26(5):1700–1709.

93. Albertine KH, Jones GP, Starcher BC, et al. Chronic lung injury in preterm lambs. Disordered respiratory tract development. Am J Respir Crit Care Med 1999; 159(3): 945–958.

94. Bland RD, Xu L, Ertsey R, et al. Dysregulation of pulmonary elastin synthesis and assembly in preterm lambs with chronic lung disease. Am J Physiol Lung Cell Mol Physiol 2007; 292(6):L1370–L1384.

95. Le Cras TD, Hardie WD, Deutsch GH, et al. Transient induction of TGF-alpha disrupts lung morphogenesis, causing pulmonary disease in adulthood. Am J Physiol Lung Cell Mol Physiol 2004; 287(4):L718–L729.

96. Bland RD, Ertsey R, Mokres LM, et al. Mechanical ventilation uncouples synthesis and assembly of elastin and increases apoptosis in lungs of newborn mice. Prelude to defective alveolar septation during lung development? Am J Physiol Lung Cell Mol Physiol 2008; 294(1):L3–L14.

97. Benachi A, Delezoide AL, Chailley-Heu B, et al. Ultrastructural evaluation of lung maturation in a sheep model of diaphragmatic hernia and tracheal occlusion. Am J Respir Cell Mol Biol 1999; 20(4):805–812.

98. Boucherat O, Benachi A, Barlier-Mur AM, et al. Decreased lung fibroblast growth factor 18 and elastin in human congenital diaphragmatic hernia and animal models. Am J Respir Crit Care Med 2007; 175(10):1066–1077.

99. Hashimoto S, Gon Y, Takeshita I, et al. Transforming growth Factor-beta1 induces phenotypic modulation of human lung fibroblasts to myofibroblast through a c-Jun-NH2-terminal kinase-dependent pathway. Am J Respir Crit Care Med 2001; 163(1):152–157.

100. McGowan SE, Jackson SK, Olson PJ, et al. Exogenous and endogenous transforming growth factors-beta influence elastin gene expression in cultured lung fibroblasts. Am J Respir Cell Mol Biol 1997; 17(1):25–35.

101. Buckley S, Warburton D. Dynamics of metalloproteinase-2 and -9, TGF-beta, and uPA activities during normoxic vs. hyperoxic alveolarization. Am J Physiol Lung Cell Mol Physiol 2002; 283(4):L747–L754.

102. Alejandre-Alcázar MA, Michiels-Corsten M, Vicencio AG, et al. TGF-beta signaling is dynamically regulated during the alveolarization of rodent and human lungs. Dev Dyn 2008; 237(1):259–269.

103. Bonniaud P, Kolb M, Galt T, et al. Smad3 null mice develop airspace enlargement and are resistant to TGF-beta-mediated pulmonary fibrosis. J Immunol 2004; 173(3):2099–2108.

104. Chen H, Sun J, Buckley S, et al. Abnormal mouse lung alveolarization caused by Smad3 deficiency is a developmental antecedent of centrilobular emphysema. Am J Physiol Lung Cell Mol Physiol 2005; 288(4):L683–L691.

105. Alejandre-Alcázar MA, Shalamanov PD, Amarie OV, et al. Temporal and spatial regulation of bone morphogenetic protein signaling in late lung development. Dev Dyn 2007; 236(10): 2825–2835.

106. Sime PJ, O'Reilly KM. Fibrosis of the lung and other tissues: new concepts in pathogenesis and treatment. Clin Immunol 2001; 99(3):308–319.

107. Alejandre-Alcázar MA, Kwapiszewska G, Reiss I, et al. Hyperoxia modulates TGF-beta/ BMP signaling in a mouse model of bronchopulmonary dysplasia. Am J Physiol Lung Cell Mol Physiol 2007; 292(2):L537–L549.

108. Boros LG, Torday JS, Paul Lee WN, et al. Oxygen-induced metabolic changes and transdifferentiation in immature fetal rat lung lipofibroblasts. Mol Genet Metab 2002; 77(3):230–236.

109. Rehan V, Torday J. Hyperoxia augments pulmonary lipofibroblast-to-myofibroblast transdifferentiation. Cell Biochem Biophy 2003; 38(3):239–250.

110. Vicencio AG, Eickelberg O, Stankewich MC, et al. Regulation of TGF-beta ligand and receptor expression in neonatal rat lungs exposed to chronic hypoxia. J Appl Physiol 2002; 93(3):1123–1130.

111. Ambalavanan N, Nicola T, Hagood J, et al. Transforming growth factor-beta signaling mediates hypoxia-induced pulmonary arterial remodeling and inhibition of alveolar development in newborn mouse lung. Am J Physiol Lung Cell Mol Physiol 2008; 295(1): L86–L95.

112. Bartram U, Speer CP. The role of transforming growth factor beta in lung development and disease. Chest 2004; 125(2):754–765.

113. Boström H, Willetts K, Pekny M, et al. PDGF-A signaling is a critical event in lung alveolar myofibroblast development and alveogenesis. Cell 1996; 85(6):863–873.

114. Lindahl P, Karlsson L, Hellström M, et al. Alveogenesis failure in PDGF-A-deficient mice is coupled to lack of distal spreading of alveolar smooth muscle cell progenitors during lung development. Development 1997; 124(20):3943–3953.

115. McGowan SE, Holmes AJ, Mecham RP, et al. Arg-Gly-Asp-containing domains of fibrillins-1 and -2 distinctly regulate lung fibroblast migration. Am J Respir Cell Mol Biol 2008; 38(4):435–445.

116. Chetty A, Faber S, Nielsen HC. Epithelial-mesenchymal interaction and insulin-like growth factors in hyperoxic lung injury. Exp Lung Res 1999; 25(8):701–718.

117. Liu H, Chang L, Rong Z, et al. Association of insulin-like growth factors with lung development in neonatal rats. J Huazhong Univ Sci Technolog Med Sci 2004; 24(2):162–165.

118. Chetty A, Cao GJ, Nielsen HC. Insulin-like Growth Factor-I signaling mechanisms, type I collagen and alpha smooth muscle actin in human fetal lung fibroblasts. Pediatr Res 2006; 60(4):389–394.

119. Thurlbeck WM, Cooney TP. Dysmorphic lungs in a case of leprechaunism: case report and review of literature. Pediatr Pulmonol 1988; 5(2):100–106.

120. Veness-Meehan KA, Moats-Staats BM, Price WA, et al. Re-emergence of a fetal pattern of insulin-like growth factor expression during hyperoxic rat lung injury. Am J Respir Cell Mol Biol 1997; 16(5):538–548.

121. Chetty A, Nielsen HC. Regulation of cell proliferation by insulin-like growth factor 1 in hyperoxia-exposed neonatal rat lung. Mol Genet Metab 2002; 75(3):265–275.

122. Chetty A, Andersson S, Lassus P, et al. Insulin-like growth factor-1 (IGF-1) and IGF-1 receptor (IGF-1R) expression in human lung in RDS and BPD. Pediatr Pulmonol 2004; 37(2):128–136.

123. Narasaraju TA, Chen H, Weng T, et al. Expression profile of IGF system during lung injury and recovery in rats exposed to hyperoxia: a possible role of IGF-1 in alveolar epithelial cell proliferation and differentiation. J Cell Biochem 2006; 97(5):984–998.

124. Mandeville I, Aubin J, LeBlanc M, et al. Impact of the loss of Hoxa5 function on lung alveogenesis. Am J Pathol 2006; 169(4):1312–1327.

125. Itoh N. The Fgf families in humans, mice, and zebrafish: their evolutional processes and roles in development, metabolism, and disease. Biol Pharm Bull 2007; 30(10):1819–1825.

126. Warburton D, Bellusci S. The molecular genetics of lung morphogenesis and injury repair. Paediatr Respir Rev 2004; 5(suppl A):S283–S287.

127. Powell PP, Wang CC, Horinouchi H, et al. Differential expression of fibroblast growth factor receptors 1 to 4 and ligand genes in late fetal and early postnatal rat lung. Am J Respir Cell Mol Biol 1998; 19(4):563–572.

128. Weinstein M, Xu X, Ohyama K, et al. FGFR-3 and FGFR-4 function cooperatively to direct alveogenesis in the murine lung. Development 1998; 125(18):3615–3623.

129. Orr-Urtreger A, Bedford MT, Burakova T, et al. Developmental localization of the splicing alternatives of fibroblast growth factor receptor-2 (FGFR2). Dev Biol 1993; 158(2):475–486.

130. Hokuto I, Perl AK, Whitsett JA. Prenatal, but not postnatal, inhibition of fibroblast growth factor receptor signaling causes emphysema. J Biol Chem 2003; 278(1):415–421.

131. De Langhe SP, Carraro G, Warburton D, et al. Levels of mesenchymal FGFR2 signaling modulate smooth muscle progenitor cell commitment in the lung. Dev Biol 2006; 299(1): 52–62.

132. Brettell LM, McGowan SE. Basic fibroblast growth factor decreases elastin production by neonatal rat lung fibroblasts. Am J Respir Cell Mol Biol 1994; 10(3):306–315.

133. Rich CB, Fontanilla MR, Nugent M, et al. Basic fibroblast growth factor decreases elastin gene transcription through an AP1/cAMP-response element hybrid site in the distal promoter. J Biol Chem 1999; 274(47):33433–33439.

134. Feres-Filho EJ, Menassa GB, Trackman PC. Regulation of lysyl oxidase by basic fibroblast growth factor in osteoblastic MC3T3-E1 cells. J Biol Chem 1996; 271(11):6411–6416.

135. Liu J, Rich CB, Buczek-Thomas JA, et al. Heparin-binding EGF-like growth factor regulates elastin and FGF-2 expression in pulmonary fibroblasts. Am J Physiol Lung Cell Mol Physiol 2003; 285(5):L1106–L1115.

136. Palamakumbura AH, Sommer P, Trackman PC. Autocrine growth factor regulation of lysyl oxidase expression in transformed fibroblasts. J Biol Chem 2003; 278(33):30781–30787.

137. Gonzalez AM, Hill DJ, Logan A, et al. Distribution of fibroblast growth factor (FGF)-2 and FGF receptor-1 messenger RNA expression and protein presence in the mid-trimester human fetus. Pediatr Res 1996; 39(3):375–385.

138. Yi M, Belcastro R, Shek S, et al. Fibroblast growth factor-2 and receptor-1alpha(IIIc) regulate postnatal rat lung cell apoptosis. Am J Respir Crit Care Med 2006; 174(5):581–589.

139. Chailley-Heu B, Boucherat O, Barlier-Mur AM, et al. FGF-18 is upregulated in the postnatal rat lung and enhances elastogenesis in myofibroblasts. Am J Physiol Lung Cell Mol Physiol 2005; 288(1):L43–L51.

140. Usui H, Shibayama M, Ohbayashi N, et al. Fgf18 is required for embryonic lung alveolar development. Biochem Biophys Res Commun 2004; 322(3):887–892.

141. Lopez E, Boucherat O, Franco-Montoya ML, et al. Nitric oxide donor restores lung growth factor and receptor expression in hyperoxia-exposed rat pups. Am J Respir Cell Mol Biol 2006; 34(6):738–745.

142. Wagenaar GT, ter Horst SA, van Gastelen MA, et al. Gene expression profile and histopathology of experimental bronchopulmonary dysplasia induced by prolonged oxidative stress. Free Radic Biol Med 2004; 36(6):782–801.

143. Park MS, Rieger-Fackeldey E, Schanbacher BL, et al. Altered expressions of fibroblast growth factor receptors and alveolarization in neonatal mice exposed to 85% oxygen. Pediatr Res 2007; 62(6):652–657.

144. Whitsett JA, Clark JC, Picard L, et al. Fibroblast growth factor 18 influences proximal programming during lung morphogenesis. J Biol Chem 2002; 277(25):22743–22749.

145. Antoine M, Wirz W, Tag CG, et al. Expression pattern of fibroblast growth factors (FGFs), their receptors and antagonists in primary endothelial cells and vascular smooth muscle cells. Growth Factors 2005; 23(2):87–95.

146. Aaronson SA, Bottaro DP, Miki T, et al. Keratinocyte growth factor. A fibroblast growth factor family member with unusual target cell specificity. Ann N Y Acad Sci 1991; 638:62–77.

147. Padela S, Yi M, Cabacungan J, et al. A critical role for fibroblast growth factor-7 during early alveolar formation in the neonatal rat. Pediatr Res 2008; 63(3):232–238.

148. Colvin JS, White AC, Pratt SJ, et al. Lung hypoplasia and neonatal death in Fgf9-null mice identify this gene as an essential regulator of lung mesenchyme. Development 2001; 128(11): 2095–2106.

149. White AC, Lavie KJ, Ornitz DM. FGF9 and SHH regulate mesenchymal VEGFA expression and development of the pulmonary capillary network. Development 2007; 134(20):3743–3752.

150. Foster JJ, Goss KL, George CL, et al. Galectin-1 in secondary alveolar septae of neonatal mouse lung. Am J Physiol Lung Cell Mol Physiol 2006; 291(6):L1142–L1149.
151. Goldring K, Jones GE, Thiagarajah R, et al. The effect of galectin-1 on the differentiation of fibroblasts and myoblasts in vitro. J Cell Sci 2002; 115(pt 2):355–366.
152. Sanford GL, Harris-Hooker S. Stimulation of vascular cell proliferation by beta-galactoside specific lectins. FASEB J 1990; 4(11):2912–2918.
153. Hsu DK, Liu FT. Regulation of cellular homeostasis by galectins. Glycoconj J 2004; 19(7-9): 507–515.
154. Boucherat O, Franco-Montoya ML, Thibault C, et al. Gene expression profiling in lung fibroblasts reveals new players in alveolarization. Physiol Genomics 2007; 32(1):128–141.
155. Li C, Xiao J, Hormi K, et al. Wnt5a participates in distal lung morphogenesis. Dev Biol 2002; 248(1):68–81.
156. Masckauchan TN, Agalliu D, Vorontchikhina M, et al. Wnt5a signaling induces proliferation and survival of endothelial cells in vitro and expression of MMP-1 and Tie-2. Mol Biol Cell 2006; 17(12):5163–5172.
157. Liu T, Dhanasekaran SM, Jin H, et al. FIZZ1 stimulation of myofibroblast differentiation. Am J Pathol 2004; 164(4):1315–1326.
158. Wang Z, Shu W, Lu MM, et al. Wnt7b activates canonical signaling in epithelial and vascular smooth muscle cells through interactions with Fzd1, Fzd10, and LRP5. Mol Cell Biol 2005; 25(12):5022–5030.
159. Shu W, Jiang YQ, Lu MM, et al. Wnt7b regulates mesenchymal proliferation and vascular development in the lung. Development 2002; 129(20):4831–4842.
160. Massaro D, Alexander E, Reiland K, et al. Rapid onset of gene expression in lung, supportive of formation of alveolar septa, induced by refeeding mice after calorie restriction. Am J Physiol Lung Cell Mol Physiol 2007; 292(5):L1313–L1326.
161. Plumb DJ, Dubaybo BA, Thet LA. Changes in lung tissue fibronectin content and synthesis during postnatal lung growth. Pediatr Pulmonol 1987; 3(6):413–419.
162. Thibeault DW, Mabry SM, Ekekezie II, et al. Collagen scaffolding during development and its deformation with chronic lung disease. Pediatrics 2003; 111(4 pt 1):766–776.
163. Nguyen NM, Kelley DG, Schlueter JA, et al Epithelial laminin alpha5 is necessary for distal epithelial cell maturation, VEGF production, and alveolization in the developing murine lung. Dev Biol 2005; 282(1):111–125.
164. Kaarteenaho-Wiik R, Pääkkö P, Herva R, et al. Type I and III collagen protein precursors and mRNA in the developing human lung. J Pathol 2004; 203(1):567–574.
165. Arden MG, Adamson IY. Collagen degradation during postnatal lung growth in rats. Pediatr Pulmonol 1992; 14(2):95–101.
166. Kheradmand F, Rishi K, Werb Z. Signaling through the EGF receptor controls lung morphogenesis in part by regulating MT1-MMP-mediated activation of gelatinase A/MMP2. J Cell Sci 2002; 115(pt 4):839–848.
167. Oblander SA, Zhou Z, Gálvez BG, et al. Distinctive functions of membrane type 1 matrix-metalloprotease (MT1-MMP or MMP-14) in lung and submandibular gland development are independent of its role in pro-MMP-2 activation. Dev Biol 2005; 277(1):255–256.
168. Atkinson JJ, Holmbeck K, Yamada S, et al. Membrane-type 1 matrix metalloproteinase is required for normal alveolar development. Dev Dyn 2005; 232(4):1079–1090.
169. Irie K, Komori K, Seiki M, et al. Impaired alveolization in mice deficient in membrane-type matrix metalloproteinase 1 (MT1-MMP). Med Mol Morphol 2005; 38(1):43–46.
170. Boucherat O, Bourbon JR, Barlier-Mur AM, et al. Differential expression of matrix metalloproteinases and inhibitors in developing rat lung mesenchymal and epithelial cells. Pediatr Res 2007; 62(1):20–25.
171. Barbolina MV, Stack MS. Membrane type 1-matrix metalloproteinase: substrate diversity in pericellular proteolysis. Semin Cell Dev Biol 2008; 19(1):24–33.

172. Kaplan F, Ledoux P, Kassamali FQ, et al. A novel developmentally regulated gene in lung mesenchyme: homology to a tumor-derived trypsin inhibitor. Am J Physiol Lung Cell Mol Physiol 1999; 276(6 pt 1):L1027–L1036.
173. Oyewumi L, Kaplan F, Gagnon S, et al. Antisense oligonucleotides decrease LGL1 mRNA and protein levels and inhibit branching morphogenesis in fetal rat lung. Am J Respir Cell Mol Biol 2003; 28(2):232–240.
174. Oyewumi L, Kaplan F, Sweezey NB. Lgl1, a mesenchymal regulator of early branching morphogenesis, is a secreted glycoprotein imported by late gestation lung epithelial cells. Biochem J 2003; 376(pt 1):61–69.
175. Nadeau K, Jankov RP, Tanswell AK, et al. Lgl1 is suppressed in oxygen toxicity animal models of bronchopulmonary dysplasia and normalizes during recovery in air. Pediatr Res 2006; 59(3):389–395.
176. Shannon JM, Hyatt BA. Epithelial-mesenchymal interactions in the developing lung. Annu Rev Physiol 2004; 66:625–645.
177. Wan H, Xu Y, Ikegami M, et al. Foxa2 is required for transition to air breathing at birth. Proc Natl Acad Sci U S A 2004; 101(40):14449–14454.
178. Wan H, Kaestner KH, Ang SL, et al. Foxa2 regulates alveolarization and goblet cell hyperplasia. Development 2004; 131(4):953–964.
179. Liu C, Morrisey EE, Whitsett JA. GATA-6 is required for maturation of the lung in late gestation. Am J Physiol Lung Cell Mol Physiol 2002; 283(2):L468–L475.
180. Yang H, Lu MM, Zhang L, et al. GATA6 regulates differentiation of distal lung epithelium. Development 2002; 129(9):2233–2246.
181. Liu C, Ikegami M, Stahlman MT, et al. Inhibition of alveolarization and altered pulmonary mechanics in mice expressing GATA-6. Am J Physiol Lung Cell Mol Physiol 2003; 285(6): L1246–L1254.
182. Wert SE, Dey CR, Blair PA, et al. Increased expression of thyroid transcription factor-1 (TTF-1) in respiratory epithelial cells inhibits alveolarization and causes pulmonary inflammation. Dev Biol 2002; 242(2):75–87.
183. Chen H, Zhuang F, Liu YH, et al. TGF-{beta} receptor II in epithelia versus mesenchyme plays distinct role in developing lung. Eur Respir J 2008 Mar 5 [Epub ahead of print].
184. Ramirez MI, Millien G, Hinds A, et al. T1alpha, a lung type I cell differentiation gene, is required for normal lung cell proliferation and alveolus formation at birth. Dev Biol 2003; 256(1):61–72.
185. Panos RJ, Rubin JS, Csaky KG, et al. Keratinocyte growth factor and hepatocyte growth factor/scatter factor are heparin-binding growth factors for alveolar type II cells in fibroblast-conditioned medium. J Clin Invest 1993; 92(2):969–977.
186. Ulich TR, Yi ES, Longmuir K, et al. Keratinocyte growth factor is a growth factor for type II pneumocytes in vivo. J Clin Invest 1994; 93(3):1298–1306.
187. Chelly N, Mouhieddine-Gueddiche OB, Barlier-Mur AM, et al. Keratinocyte growth factor enhances maturation of fetal rat lung type II cells. Am J Respir Cell Mol Biol 1999; 20(3): 423–432.
188. Shannon JM, Gebb SA, Nielsen LD. Induction of alveolar type II cell differentiation in embryonic tracheal epithelium in mesenchyme-free culture. Development 1999; 126(8): 1675–1688.
189. Isakson BE, Lubman RL, Seedorf GJ, et al. Modulation of pulmonary alveolar type II cell phenotype and communication by extracellular matrix and KGF. Am J Physiol Cell Physiol 2001; 281(4):C1291–C1299.
190. Mason RJ, Lewis MC, Edeen KE, et al. Maintenance of surfactant protein A and D secretion by rat alveolar type II cells in vitro. Am J Physiol Lung Cell Mol Physiol 2002; 282(2):L249–L258.

191. Qiao R, Yan W, Clavijo C, et al. Effects of KGF on alveolar epithelial cell transdifferentiation are mediated by JNK signaling. Am J Respir Cell Mol Biol 2008; 38(2):239–246.
192. Chelly N, Henrion A, Pinteur C, et al. Role of keratinocyte growth factor in the control of surfactant synthesis by fetal lung mesenchyme. Endocrinology 2001; 142(5):1814–1819.
193. Deimling J, Thompson K, Tseu I, et al. Mesenchymal maintenance of distal epithelial cell phenotype during late fetal lung development. Am J Physiol Lung Cell Mol Physiol 2007; 292(3):L725–L741.
194. Ray P. Protection of epithelial cells by keratinocyte growth factor signaling. Proc Am Thorac Soc 2005; 2(3):221–225.
195. Danan C, Franco ML, Jarreau PH, et al. High concentrations of keratinocyte growth factor in airways of premature infants predicted absence of bronchopulmonary dysplasia. Am J Respir Crit Care Med 2002; 165(10):1384–1387.
196. Torday JS, Sun H, Wang L, et al. Leptin mediates the parathyroid hormone-related protein paracrine stimulation of fetal lung maturation. Am J Physiol Lung Cell Mol Physiol 2002; 282(3):L405–L410.
197. Dammann CE, Nielsen HC, Carraway KL 3rd. Role of neuregulin-1 beta in the developing lung. Am J Respir Crit Care Med 2003; 167(12):1711–1716.
198. Sonnenberg E, Meyer D, Weidner KM, et al. Scatter factor/hepatocyte growth factor and its receptor, the c-met tyrosine kinase, can mediate a signal exchange between mesenchyme and epithelia during mouse development. J Cell Biol 1993; 123(1):223–235.
199. Mason RJ, Leslie CC, McCormick-Shannon K. Hepatocyte growth factor is a growth factor for rat alveolar type II cells. Am J Respir Cell Mol Biol 1994; 11(5):561–567.
200. Sakamaki Y, Matsumoto K, Mizuno S, et al. Hepatocyte growth factor stimulates proliferation of respiratory epithelial cells during postpneumonectomy compensatory lung growth in mice. Am J Respir Cell Mol Biol 2002; 26(5):525–533.
201. Padela S, Cabacungan J, Shek S, et al. Hepatocyte growth factor is required for alveologenesis in the neonatal rat. Am J Respir Crit Care Med 2005; 172(7):907–914.
202. Torday JS, Sun H, Qin J. Prostaglandin E2 integrates the effects of fluid distension and glucocorticoid on lung maturation. Am J Physiol 1998; 274(1 pt 1):L106–L111.
203. Torday JS, Torres E, Rehan VK. The role of fibroblast transdifferentiation in lung epithelial cell proliferation, differentiation, and repair in vitro. Pediatr Pathol Mol Med 2003; 22(3): 189–207.
204. Rubin LP, Kovacs CS, De Paepe ME, et al. Arrested pulmonary alveolar cytodifferentiation and defective surfactant synthesis in mice missing the gene for parathyroid hormone-related protein. Dev Dyn 2004; 230(2):278–289.
205. Rehan VK, Torday JS. Lower parathyroid hormone-related protein content of tracheal aspirates in very low birth weight infants who develop bronchopulmonary dysplasia. Pediatr Res 2006; 60(2):216–220.
206. Bhatt AJ, Pryhuber GS, Huyck H, et al. Disrupted pulmonary vasculature and decreased vascular endothelial growth factor, Flt-1, and TIE-2 in human infants dying with bronchopulmonary dysplasia. Am J Respir Crit Care Med 2001; 164(2):1971–1980.
207. Lassus P, Turanlahti M, Heikkilä P, et al. Pulmonary vascular endothelial growth factor and Flt-1 in fetuses, in acute and chronic lung disease, and in persistent pulmonary hypertension of the newborn. Am J Respir Crit Care Med 2001; 164(10 pt 1):1981–1987.
208. De Paepe ME, Mao Q, Powell J, et al. Growth of pulmonary microvasculature in ventilated preterm infants. Am J Respir Crit Care Med 2006; 173(10 pt 1):204–211.
209. Stenmark KR, Abman SH. Lung vascular development: implications for the pathogenesis of bronchopulmonary dysplasia. Annu Rev Physiol 2005; 67:623–661.
210. Jakkula M, Le Cras TD, Gebb S, et al. Inhibition of angiogenesis decreases alveolarization in the developing rat lung. Am J Physiol Lung Cell Mol Physiol 2000; 279(3):L600–L607.

211. Le Cras TD, Markham NE, Tuder RM, et al. Treatment of newborn rats with VEGF inhibitor causes pulmonary hypertension and abnormal lung structure. Am J Physiol Lung Cell Mol Physiol 2000; 283(3):L555–L562.

212. McGrath-Morrow SA, Cho C, Cho C, et al. Vascular endothelial growth factor receptor blockade disrupts postnatal lung development. Am J Respir Cell Mol Biol 2005; 32(5): 420–427.

213. Maniscalco WM, Watkins RH, D'Angio CT, et al. Hyperoxic injury decreases alveolar epithelial cell expression of vascular endothelial growth factor (VEGF) in neonatal rabbit lung. Am J Respir Cell Mol Biol 1997; 16(5):557–567.

214. Hosford GE, Olson DM. Effects of hyperoxia on VEGF, its receptors, and HIF-2alpha in the newborn rat lung. Am J Physiol Lung Cell Mol Physiol 2003; 285(1):L161–L168.

215. Thébaud B, Ladha F, Michelakis ED, et al. Vascular endothelial growth factor gene therapy increases survival, promotes lung angiogenesis and prevents alveolar damage in hyperoxia-induced lung injury: evidence that angiogenesis participates in alveolarization. Circulation 2005; 112(16):2477–2486.

216. Kunig AM, Balasubramaniam V, Markham NE, et al. Recombinant human VEGF treatment enhances alveolarization after hyperoxic lung injury in neonatal rats. Am J Physiol Lung Cell Mol Physiol 2005; 289(4):L529–L535.

217. Kunig AM, Balasubramaniam V, Markham NE, et al. Recombinant human VEGF treatment transiently increases lung edema but enhances lung structure after neonatal hyperoxia. Am J Physiol Lung Cell Mol Physiol 2006; 291(5):L1068–L1078.

218. Shifren JL, Doldi N, Ferrara N, et al. In the human fetus, vascular endothelial growth factor is expressed in epithelial cells and myocytes, but not vascular endothelium: implications for mode of action. J Clin Endocrinol Metab 1994; 79(1):316–322.

219. Acarregui MJ, Penisten ST, Goss KL, et al. Vascular endothelial growth factor gene expression in human fetal lung in vitro. Am J Respir Cell Mol Biol 1999; 20(1):14–23.

220. Ng YS, Rohan R, Sunday ME, et al. Differential expression of VEGF isoforms in mouse during development and in the adult. Dev Dyn 2001; 220(2):112–121.

221. Ferrara N, Carver-Moore K, Chen H, et al. Heterozygous embryonic lethality induced by targeted inactivation of the VEGF gene. Nature 1996; 380(6573):439–442.

222. Galambos C, Ng YS, Ali A, et al. Defective pulmonary development in the absence of heparin-binding vascular endothelial growth factor isoforms. Am J Respir Cell Mol Biol 2002; 27(2):194–203.

223. Watkins RH, D'Angio CT, Ryan RM, et al. Differential expression of VEGF mRNA splice variants in newborn and adult hyperoxic lung injury. Am J Physiol Lung Cell Mol Physiol 1999; 276(5 pt 1):L858–L867.

224. Hara A, Chapin CJ, Ertsey R, et al. Changes in fetal lung distension alter expression of vascular endothelial growth factor and its isoforms in developing rat lung. Pediatr Res 2005; 58(1):30–37.

225. Yamamoto H, Yun EJ, Gerber HP, et al. Epithelial-vascular cross talk mediated by VEGF-A and HGF signaling directs primary septae formation during distal lung morphogenesis. Dev Biol 2007; 308(1):44–53.

226. Sirianni FE, Chu FS, Walker DC. Human alveolar wall fibroblasts directly link epithelial type 2 cells to capillary endothelium. Am J Respir Crit Care Med 2003; 168(12):1532–1537.

227. Maniscalco WM, Watkins RH, Pryhuber GS, et al. Angiogenic factors and alveolar vasculature: development and alterations by injury in very premature baboons. Am J Physiol Lung Cell Mol Physiol 2002; 282(4):L811–L823.

228. Janér J, Andersson S, Haglund C, et al. Pulmonary endostatin perinatally and in lung injury of the newborn infant. Pediatrics 2007; 119(1):e241–e246.

229. Aghai ZH, Faqiri S, Saslow JG, et al. Angiopoietin 2 concentrations in infants developing bronchopulmonary dysplasia: attenuation by dexamethasone. J Perinatol 2008; 28(2): 149–155.
230. Makinde T, Agrawal DK. Intra and extra-vascular trans-membrane signaling of angiopoietin-1-Tie2 receptor in health and disease. J Cell Mol Med 2008; 12(3):810–828.
231. Maisonpierre PC, Suri C, Jones PF, et al. Angiopoietin-2, a natural antagonist for Tie2 that disrupts in vivo angiogenesis. Science 1997; 277(5322):55–60.
232. Abdollahi A, Hahnfeldt P, Maercker C, et al. Endostatin's antiangiogenic signaling network. Mol Cell 2004; 13(5):649–663.
233. Bhandari V, Choo-Wing R, Lee CG, et al. Hyperoxia causes angiopoietin 2-mediated acute lung injury and necrotic cell death. Nat Med 2006; 12(11):1286–1293.
234. Schwarz MA, Zhang F, Gebb S, et al. Endothelial monocyte activating polypeptide II inhibits lung neovascularization and airway epithelial morphogenesis. Mech Dev 2000; 95(1–2):123–132.
235. Schwarz M, Lee M, Zhang F, et al. EMAP II: a modulator of neovascularization in the developing lung. Am J Physiol 1999; 276(2 pt 1):L365–L375.
236. Schwarz MA, Wan Z, Liu J, et al. Epithelial-mesenchymal interactions are linked to neovascularization. Am J Respir Cell Mol Biol 2004; 30(6):784–792.
237. Quintos-Alagheband ML, White CW, Schwarz MA. Potential role for antiangiogenic proteins in the evolution of bronchopulmonary dysplasia. Antioxid Redox Signal 2004; 6(1):137–145.
238. Alcorn D, Adamson TM, Lambert TF, et al. Morphological effects of chronic ligation and drainage in the fetal lamb lung. J Anat 1977; 123(pt 3):649–660.
239. Adzick NS, Harrison MR, Glick PL, et al. Experimental pulmonary hypoplasia and oligohydramnios: relative contributions of lung fluid and fetal breathing movements. J Pediatr Surg 1984; 19(6):658–665.
240. Moessinger AC, Harding R, Adamson TM, et al. Role of lung fluid volume in growth and maturation of the fetal sheep lung. J Clin Invest 1990; 86(4):1270–1277.
241. Alcorn DG, Adamson TM, Maloney JE, et al. A morphologic and morphometric analysis of fetal lung development in the sheep. Anat Rec 1981; 201(4):655–667.
242. Hashim E, Laberge JM, Chen MF, et al. Reversible tracheal obstruction in the fetal sheep: effects on tracheal fluid pressure and lung growth. J Pediatr Surg 1995; 30(8): 1172–1177.
243. Davey MG, Hooper SB, Cock ML, et al. Stimulation of lung growth in fetuses with lung hypoplasia leads to altered postnatal lung structure in sheep. Pediatr Pulmonol 2001; 32(4): 267–276.
244. Joyce BJ, Wallace MJ, Pierce RA, et al. Sustained changes in lung expansion alter tropoelastin mRNA levels and elastin content in fetal sheep lungs. Am J Physiol Lung Cell Mol Physiol 2003; 284(4):L643–L649.
245. Boland R, Joyce BJ, Wallace MJ, et al. Cortisol enhances structural maturation of the hypoplastic fetal lung sheep. J Physiol 2004; 554(pt 2):505–517.
246. Flecknoe SJ, Wallace MJ, Harding R, et al. Determination of alveolar epithelial cell phenotypes in fetal sheep: evidence for the involvement of basal lung expansion. J Physiol 2002; 542(pt 1):245–253.
247. Wallace MJ, Thiel AM, Polglase GR, et al. Role of platelet-derived growth factor-B, vascular endothelial growth factor, insulin-like growth factor-II, mitogen-activated protein kinase and transforming growth factor-beta1 in expansion-induced lung growth in fetal sheep. Reprod Fertil Dev 2006; 18(6):655–665.
248. Sozo F, Wallace MJ, Zahra VA, et al. Gene expression profiling during increased fetal lung expansion identifies genes likely to regulate development of the distal airways. Physiol Genomics 2006; 24(2):105–113.

249. Filby CE, Hooper SB, Sozo F, et al. VDUP1: a potential mediator of expansion-induced lung growth and epithelial cell differentiation in the ovine fetus. Am J Physiol Lung Cell Mol Physiol 2006; 290(2):L250–L258.
250. Sozo F, Hooper SB, Wallace MJ. Thrombospondin-1 expression and localization in the developing ovine lung. J Physiol 2007; 584(pt 2):625–635.
251. Bhaskaran M, Kolliputi N, Wang Y, et al. Trans-differentiation of alveolar epithelial type II cells to type I cells involves autocrine signaling by transforming growth factor beta 1 through the Smad pathway. J Biol Chem 2007; 282(6):3968–3976.
252. Flecknoe SJ, Crossley KJ, Zuccal GM, et al. Increased lung expansion alters lung growth but not alveolar epithelial cell differentiation in newborn lambs. Am J Physiol Lung Cell Mol Physiol 2007; 292(2):L454–L461.
253. Muratore CS, Nguyen HT, Ziegler MM, et al. Stretch-induced upregulation of VEGF gene expression in murine pulmonary culture: a role for angiogenesis in lung development. J Pediatr Surg 2000; 35(6):906–912.
254. Breen EC. Mechanical strain increases type I collagen expression in pulmonary fibroblasts in vitro. J Appl Physiol 2000; 88(1):203–209.
255. Nakamura T, Liu M, Mourgeon E, et al. Mechanical strain and dexamethasone selectively increase surfactant protein C and tropoelastin gene expression. Am J Physiol Lung Cell Mol Physiol 2000; 278(5):L974–L980.
256. Torday JS, Sanchez-Esteban J, Rubin LP. Paracrine mediators of mechanotransduction in lung development. Am J Med Sci 1998; 316(3):205–208.
257. Bastien J, Rochette-Egly C. Nuclear retinoid receptors and the transcription of retinoid-target genes. Gene 2004; 1328:1–16.
258. Shenai JP, Chytil F. Vitamin A storage in lungs during perinatal development in the rat. Biol Neonate 1990; 57(2):126–132.
259. Dirami G, Massaro GD, Clerch LB, et al. Lung retinol storing cells synthesize and secrete retinoic acid, an inducer of alveolus formation. Am J Physiol Lung Cell Mol Physiol 2004; 286(2):L249–L256.
260. Hind M, Corcoran J, Maden M. Temporal/spatial expression of retinoid binding proteins and RAR isoforms in the postnatal lung. Am J Physiol Lung Cell Mol Physiol 2002; 282(3):L468–L476.
261. Frey G, Egli E, Chailley-Heu B, et al. Effects of mild vitamin a deficiency on lung maturation in newborn rats: a morphometric and morphologic study. Biol Neonate 2004; 86(4):259–268.
262. Massaro GD, Massaro D. Postnatal treatment with retinoic acid increases the number of pulmonary alveoli in rats. Am J Physiol 1996; 270(2 pt 1):L305–L310.
263. Massaro GD, Massaro D. Retinoic acid treatment partially rescues failed septation in rats and in mice. Am J Physiol Lung Cell Mol Physiol 2000; 278(5):L955–L960.
264. Veness-Meehan KA, Pierce RA, Moats-Staats BM, et al. Retinoic acid attenuates O2-induced inhibition of lung septation. Am J Physiol Lung Cell Mol Physiol 2002; 283(5):L971–L980.
265. Liu B, Harvey CS, McGowan SE. Retinoic acid increases elastin in neonatal rat lung fibroblast cultures. Am J Physiol 1993; 265(5 pt 1):L430–L437.
266. McGowan SE, Doro MM, Jackson SK. Endogenous retinoids increase perinatal elastin gene expression in rat lung fibroblasts and fetal explants. Am J Physiol Lung Cell Mol Physiol 1997; 273(2 pt 1):L410–L416.
267. Chen H, Chang L, Liu H, et al. Effect of retinoic acid on platelet-derived growth factor and lung development in newborn rats. J Huazhong Univ Sci Technolog Med Sci 2004; 24(3):226–228.
268. Liebeskind A, Srinivasan S, Kaetzel D, et al. Retinoic acid stimulates immature lung fibroblast growth via a PDGF-mediated autocrine mechanism. Am J Physiol Lung Cell Mol Physiol 2000; 279(1):L81–L90.

269. Kim C, Nielsen HC. Hoxa-5 in mouse developing lung: cell-specific expression and retinoic acid regulation. Am J Physiol Lung Cell Mol Physiol 2000; 279(5):L863–L871.
270. McGowan S, Jackson SK, Jenkins-Moore M, et al. Mice bearing deletions of retinoic acid receptors demonstrate reduced lung elastin and alveolar numbers. Am J Respir Cell Mol Biol 2000; 23(2):162–167.
271. Yang L, Naltner A, Yan C. Overexpression of dominant negative retinoic acid receptor alpha causes alveolar abnormality in transgenic neonatal lungs. Endocrinology 2003; 144(7):3004–3011.
272. Massaro GD, Massaro D, Chambon P. Retinoic acid receptor-alpha regulates pulmonary alveolus formation in mice after, but not during, perinatal period. Am J Physiol Lung Cell Mol Physiol 2003; 284(2):L431–L433.
273. Massaro GD, Massaro D, Chan WY, et al. Retinoic acid receptor-beta: an endogenous inhibitor of the perinatal formation of pulmonary alveoli. Physiol Genomics 2000; 4(1):51–57.
274. Snyder JM, Jenkins-Moore M, Jackson SK, et al. Alveolarization in retinoic acid receptor-beta-deficient mice. Pediatr Res 2005; 57(3):384–391.
275. Pierce RA, Joyce B, Officer S, et al. Retinoids increase lung elastin expression but fail to alter morphology or angiogenesis genes in premature ventilated baboons. Pediatr Res 2007; 61(6):703–709.
276. Bunton TE, Plopper CG. Triamcinolone-induced structural alterations in the development of the lung of the fetal rhesus macaque. Am J Obstet Gynecol 1984; 148(2):203–215.
277. Massaro D, Massaro GD. Dexamethasone accelerates postnatal alveolar wall thinning and alters wall composition. Am J Physiol Regul Integr Comp Physiol 1986; 251(2 pt 2):R218–R224.
278. Sahebjami H, Domino M. Effects of postnatal dexamethasone treatment on development of alveoli in adult rats. Exp Lung Res 1989; 15(6):961–973.
279. Tschanz S, Damke BM, Burri PH. Influence of postnatally administered glucocorticoids on rat lung growth. Biol Neonate 1995; 68(4):229–245.
280. Roth-Kleiner M, Berger TM, Tarek MR, et al. Neonatal dexamethasone induces premature microvascular maturation of the alveolar capillary network. Dev Dyn 2005; 233(4): 1261–1271.
281. Willet KE, McMenamin P, Pinkerton KE, et al. Lung morphometry and collagen and elastin content: changes during normal development and after prenatal hormone exposure in sheep. Pediatr Res 1999; 45(5 pt 1):615–625.
282. Willet KE, Jobe AH, Ikegami M, et al. Lung morphometry after repetitive antenatal glucocorticoid treatment in preterm sheep. Am J Respir Crit Care Med 2001; 163(6): 1437–1443.
283. Pierce RA, Mariencheck WI, Sandefur S, et al. Glucocorticoid upregulate tropoelastin gene expression during late stages of fetal lung development. Am J Physiol Lung Cell Mol Physiol 1995; 268(3 pt 1):L491–L500.
284. Chinoy MR, Zgleszewski SE, Cilley RE, et al. Dexamethasone enhances ras-recision gene expression in cultured murine fetal lungs: role in development. Am J Physiol Lung Cell Mol Physiol 2000; 279(2):L312–L318.
285. Blanco LN, Frank L. The formation of alveoli in rat lung during the third and fourth postnatal weeks: effect of hyperoxia, dexamethasone, and deferoxamine. Pediatr Res 1993; 34(3):334–340.
286. Clerch LB, Baras AS, Massaro GD, et al. DNA microarray analysis of neonatal mouse lung connects regulation of KDR with dexamethasone-induced inhibition of alveolar formation. Am J Physiol Lung Cell Mol Physiol 2004; 286(2):L411–L419.
287. Bird AD, Tan KH, Olsson PF, et al. Identification of glucocorticoid-regulated genes that control cell proliferation during murine respiratory development. J Physiol 2007; 585(pt 1): 187–201.

288. Nemati B, Atmodio W, Gagnon S, et al. Glucocorticoid receptor disruption delays structural maturation in the lungs of nemborn mice. Pediatr Pulmonol 2008; 43(2):125–133.
289. Jones CT. Corticosteroid concentrations in the plasma of fetal and maternal guinea pigs during gestation. Endocrinology 1974; 95(4):1129–1133.
290. Henning SJ. Plasma concentrations of total and free corticosterone during development in the rat. Am J Physiol 1978; 235(5):E451–E456.
291. Steele RE, Wekstein DR. Influence of thyroid hormone on homeothermic development of the rat. Am J Physiol 1972; 222(6):1528–1533.
292. Morishige WK, Joun NS, Guernsey DL. Thyroidal influence on postnatal lung development in the rat. Endocrinology 1982; 110(2):444–451.
293. Massaro D, Teich N, Massaro GD. Postnatal development of pulmonary alveoli: modulation in rats by thyroid hormones. Am J Physiol Regul Integr Comp Physiol 1986; 250(1 pt 2): R51–R55.
294. Ruel J, Coulombe P, Dussault JH. Characterization of nuclear 3,5,3'-triiodothyronine receptors in the developing rat lung: effects of hypo- and hyperthyroidism. Pediatr Res 1982; 16(3):238–242.
295. Brody JS, Fisher AB, Goemen A, et al. Acromegalic pneumonomegaly: lung growth in the adult. J Clin Invest 1970; 49:1051–1060.
296. Donnelly PM, Grunstein RR, Peat JK, et al. Large lungs and growth hormone: an increased alveolar number? Eur Respir J 1995; 8:939–947.
297. Garcia-Rio F, Pino JM, Diez JJ, et al. Reduction of lung distensibility in acromegaly after suppression of growth hormone hypersecretion. Am J Respir Crit Care Med 2001; 164: 852–857.
298. Bartlett D Jr. Postnatal growth of the mammalian lung: influence of excess growth hormone. Respir Physiol 1971; 12:297–304.

4

Lung Vascular Development

ALISON A. HISLOP
Institute of Child Health, University College London, London, U.K.

I. Introduction

Airway development and its control have been described in chapters 1 to 3. From the earliest stage of lung development, there is an accompanying pulmonary blood circulation. In the adult lung, the pulmonary arteries run alongside the branching airways distributing blood to the alveolar capillary bed. The pulmonary veins have a similar number of branches (tributaries) and return blood from the capillary bed to the heart. They are separated from the airways by alveolar parenchyma and connective tissue septa. The proximity and similarity of branching of the circulation to the airway system suggests that there is an interaction between them both during development and later. In this chapter, the development of the pulmonary circulation has been related to the traditional stages of human lung development since it is likely that there are changes in the mechanism of control as the lung changes its histological appearance and its function (Fig. 1). The stages are the following: (*i*) The *embryonic stage* (up to 7 weeks' gestation) when the lung primordium derives from the foregut and lobar airways lined with endoderm are established within the surrounding mesenchyme. (*ii*) The *pseudoglandular stage* (7–17 weeks' gestation) during which all preacinar airways are formed by progressive branching of epithelium-lined airways into the expanding mesenchyme. (*iii*) The *canalicular stage* (16–27 weeks' gestation) when intra-acinar airways branch and the peripheral airways enlarge and have a thinned epithelium that eventually forms type I and II pneumonocytes. (*iv*) The *saccular stage* (28–36 weeks' gestation) when the sac-shaped distal airways develop crests containing elastin and muscle, which cause shallow indentations in the walls. These crests extend to form cup-shaped alveoli. (*v*) The *alveolar stage* (36 weeks' gestation onward and into infancy and childhood) when alveoli multiply. They continue to increase in number during early childhood and increase in size until somatic growth is complete. The same stages of lung development are seen in other mammalian lungs but the timetable is different in them, and in most rodents the alveolar stage does not appear until after birth.

II. Origin of Pulmonary Vessels

Two opposing models of how blood vessels arise have been suggested; historically, the pulmonary arteries were thought to derive from the sixth branchial arches and to grow out alongside the branching airways into the surrounding mesenchyme. Serial reconstruction of injected arteries in human fetal lungs aged from 12 weeks of gestation showed that arteries

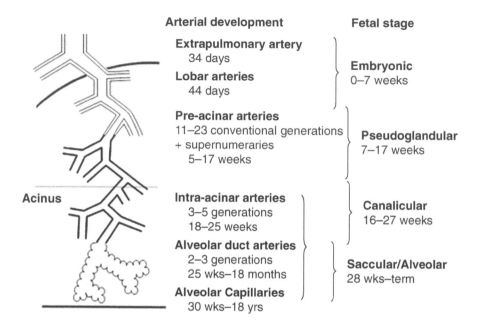

Figure 1   Diagram illustrating the stages of lung development with the development of arteries and airways. Preacinar arteries start as a capillary plexus around growing lung buds—vasculogenesis. Intra-acinar arteries grow by angiogenesis.

branched alongside airway branches, so-called conventional arteries (1). At the same time, additional small, patent supernumerary arteries branched from the main pathways; they would supply the alveolar region more directly when it formed later. This suggested genetic control of the branching pattern with angiogenic growth from hilum to periphery. Later using a casting technique in embryonic mouse lungs, deMello et al. (2) suggested that the proximal arteries did grow by angiogenesis, but that at the periphery of the lung, there was de novo formation of capillaries in the mesenchyme surrounding the lung buds. Eventually, these two types of vessel fused to form a completed circulation by E13 to E14. More recently, new immunostaining techniques have made it possible to trace more accurately the formation of the pulmonary circulation in man (3–5), mice (6,7), and chick (8). In all these studies, there was evidence of a patent circulation from the aorta via the lung mesenchyme to the sinus venosus of the heart by the time the first division of the lung bud had occurred.

Using serial reconstruction in a human embryo of 28 days of gestation, the single lung bud leading from the embryonic foregut was surrounded by mesenchyme that contained a number of cells staining positively for CD31, a marker for endothelial cells (3). By 34 days of gestation, a capillary network was seen around each prospective main bronchus. These connected with the aortic sac cranially by two pulmonary arteries lying on each side of the prospective trachea and to the left atrium caudally. Parera et al. (7) using serial reconstruction of mouse lungs showed that the pulmonary arteries were a coalescence of a vasculogenic plexus between E10.5 and E11.5 days and were connected to the dorsal aorta. A similar appearance of a completed circulation has been described in the mouse at E10.5 days using identification of endothelial cells by Flk-1, the specific receptor for vascular endothelial growth factor (VEGF) (6). In the human, there is evidence of circulating blood cells at this stage (4), and in the mouse, there was evidence that the erythrocytes came from the fetal liver showing the connection of the lung circulation to the rest of the body (7). Thus, it seems that the earliest pulmonary vessels have formed de novo in the mesenchyme by the process of *vasculogenesis*, that is, differentiation of cells to form single endothelial cells and then capillary tubes.

Study of older human fetuses showed that as each new airway buds into the mesenchyme a new plexus forms as a halo and adds to the peripheral circulation, extending the arteries and veins (Fig. 2). Thus, there is sustained addition of the newly formed tubules to the existing vessels, and the airways act as a template for the development of blood vessels (3). Formation of vessels by vasculogenesis occurs until about the 17th week of gestation in human (end of the pseudoglandular stage) when all preacinar airways and their accompanying arteries and veins have formed (1,9) and there is little undifferentiated mesenchyme left between the airway structures, and the capillaries are close to the epithelial cell basement membrane. The debate continues and Parera et al. (7) using the Tie-2 receptor and CD31 as markers for the endothelium in mice describe a similar development of the capillaries to Schachtner et al. (6). However, they have interpreted the appearance of the capillaries as a combination of vasculogenesis and angiogenesis since they have identified sprouting capillaries in whole mounts. It may be that the supernumerary arteries are formed in this way.

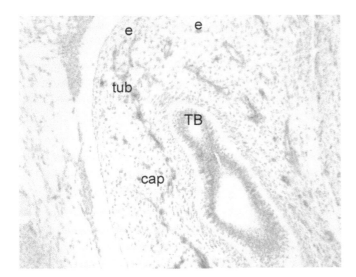

Figure 2 Photomicrograph of lung of an embryo at 44 days' gestation stained for CD31 demonstrating endothelial cells as darker gray. Endothelial cells (e) and capillary tubules (tub) are seen as a halo in the mesenchyme around the terminal bud (TB). These coalesce to form capillaries (cap).

III. Development of the Pulmonary Veins

Pulmonary veins also develop by vasculogenesis in the mesenchyme and from very early in development can be discriminated from the arteries. At 38 days of gestation, they were traced and found to be continuous with the arteries via the capillary bed (4). They are usually on the opposite side of the lung bud from the artery and soon become separated from the airway by a number of cell layers and are found running in an area of low cell density. A similar appearance has been described in the mouse by E13.5 when the veins have a wider lumen than the arteries (7), and in human lungs, they have less muscle and a wider lumen by eight weeks of gestation (4) It is likely that the lacunae and hematopoietic lakes as described by Schachtner et al. (6) and deMello et al. (2) are in fact veins. In mice, venous and arterial endothelial cells in the systemic bed are distinct with EphB4 expressed on venous endothelium and Ephrin B2 on the arteries (10). In the study by Hall et al. (4) on human lungs, these markers were not discriminatory in the systemic or pulmonary vessels. The complex regulation of angiogenesis by Eph and Ephrins has been reviewed recently by Kuijper et al. (11). After 12 weeks of gestation, large clear spaces lined by CD31 positive cells appeared adjacent to the veins two to three generations proximal to the capillary bed. These were lymphatic channels and there was a gradual appearance of connective tissue around them to form connective tissue septa. By term, lymphatic channels were found within the alveolar region (4).

IV. Control of Early Blood Vessel Development

Control of early airway development is by a panel of hox genes, transcription factors, and growth factors acting in an orchestrated manner (12–14). The control of the development of the pulmonary circulation has been less extensively studied, but it is apparent that there are interactions between the epithelium, the mesenchyme, and the blood vessels. The vascular tree is influenced at every branch by local factors; however, there is a similar branching pattern within each species suggesting genetic control. In a study on armadillos, a species in which littermates are genetically identical, Glenny et al. (15) showed a common control of the fractal geometry of the vascular tree and that blood flow was also strongly correlated between littermates. In a study on human lung arteriograms, a similarity between siblings of the hilar and segmental branching pattern was reported (16).

Endothelial precursor cells have been derived from the lung mesenchyme of fetal mice, and these form extensive capillary-like networks with a lumen when cultured (17). These cells expressed the RNA for the receptors for VEGF, the receptor tyrosine kinases Tie-1 and -2, and Angiopoietin 1 and 2 (Ang-1 and -2). The VEGF receptors Flt-1 and Flk-1 are expressed in the endothelium of capillaries in the mesenchyme from 38 days of gestation in human (3). Endothelial progenitor cells capable of de novo vasculogenesis have been isolated from the microvasculature of postnatal rat lungs (18).

The formation of new capillaries by vasculogenesis occurs at a similar distance from the epithelial buds at all ages. This suggests some control by the epithelial cells (Fig. 3). In a study of rat lung explants at fetal day 13, the presence of the epithelial cells was needed to maintain the presence of endothelial (Flk-1 positive) cells in the distal lung mesenchyme (19). VEGF is known to be involved in angiogenesis and

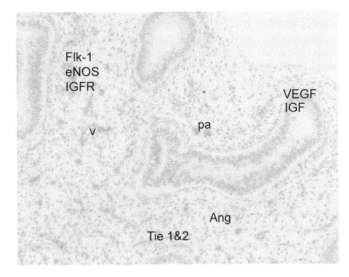

Figure 3 Photomicrograph of the periphery of an eight-week fetal lung immunostained with CD31 showing the location of factors involved in vasculogenesis. *Abbreviations*: VEGF, vascular endothelial growth factor; IGF, insulin-like growth factor; Flk-1, VEGF receptor; eNOS, endothelial nitric oxide synthase; IGFR, IGF receptor, Ang, Angiopoietin; Tie, receptor for Angiopoietin; v, vein between airways; pa, pulmonary artery alongside airway.

vasculogenesis and has been demonstrated in the epithelial cells of human fetuses both in the pseudoglandular phase and in the later phases (5,20,21). In cultured mouse lungs, most VEGF is found at the branching points of the peripheral airways (22), and grafting of VEGF-coated beads into cultured mouse lung leads to the production of an increased capillary bed. VEGF-deficient mice do not survive to term even in the presence of one allele and have defects in their vessel formation (23). Recent studies have shown that there is reciprocal control between blood vessels and airways in that overexpression of VEGF leads to disrupted vascular net assembly and arrested airway branching (24). Mice deficient in Flt-1 die between E8.5 and E9.5 due to a defect in angiogenesis (25), and mice deficient in Flk-1 have no blood vessel development (26). A comprehensive review on VEGF in the lung was published in 2006 (27).

In the relatively low-oxygen environment during fetal lung growth, the transcription factor hypoxia-inducible factor (HIF) for VEGF is upregulated. In the human lung at 8 to 14 weeks of gestation, HIF-1α colocalized with VEGF in the branching epithelial tubules and HIF-2α was found in both the epithelium and the vascular structures in the mesenchyme (28). Mouse lung buds reduce their branching rate in 20% oxygen and there is concomitant failure of blood vessel development. It is likely that the failure of airway growth is due to the lack of blood vessel development since VEGF is reduced in the relative hyperoxia (29).

Angiopoietin and the Tie receptors are also involved in vasculogenesis; Tie-2 is expressed on the endothelial cells in the mesenchyme. Null mice for Tie-2 and Ang-1 have abnormal vascular network formation (30), whereas those deficient in Tie-1 had a failure in the integrity of the endothelial layer resulting in edema (31). These factors are more involved in vessel assembly and stabilization of the network rather than its initial appearance and also in the formation of the vessel wall (see following text). In mice, Ang-2 is not required for embryonic blood vessel development but for later remodeling, and is also necessary for normal lymphatic development (32). More recently, it has been shown that Ang-1 actively promoted lymphatic enlargement in adult mouse tissues (33).

Another candidate for the activation of vascular cell differentiation is BMP-4, which acts as a stimulant for VEGF. High levels of BMP-4 are located at the tips of distal airways. Overexpression of the inhibitory vascular morphogen matrix GLA protein in mouse lungs disrupts BMP-4 and leads to failure of peripheral arterial branching (34).

A study on human lung tissue showed the presence of insulin-like growth factor (IGF) and its receptor from four weeks onward (35); both colocalized with endothelial markers during the embryonic and pseudoglandular stage. IGF receptors were also found on epithelial cells, and blockade of the receptor led to a reduction in production of endothelial tubules. Inactivation of the IGF receptor in the human lung explants led to loss of endothelial cells in existing capillaries by apoptosis, and this in turn led to an abnormal growth of the lung buds, suggesting that IGF receptors are involved in both airway and endothelium development (35). Rat pulmonary vascular endothelial cells respond to exogenous IGF-1 by a twofold increase in number (36). The endothelial cells produce substances that control tone and also cellular multiplication.

Endothelial nitric oxide synthase (eNOS) is expressed on the endothelium of arteries, capillaries, and veins throughout fetal life and was demonstrated in human lung by 38 days of gestation (3). Nitric oxide (NO) is known to stimulate endothelial proliferation, migration, and tube formation and inhibits apoptosis. It also controls airway branching in cultured rat lungs where there was an increase in airway branching within three days in the presence of an NO donor and decrease in presence of a NOS inhibitor (37). Cultured fetal ovine pulmonary artery endothelial cells have a twofold increase in tube formation in hypoxia rather than room air. This seems to depend on the presence of NO, and NO added to a room air will enhance angiogenesis and tube formation (38).

V. Canalicular Stage

The appearance of the lung changes in the canalicular stage (16–27 weeks' gestation in human) the respiratory airways form by branching, but the epithelium is now much thinner in the peripheral airways. Type I and type II pneumonocytes differentiate, and the airspaces enlarge. It is considered that at this stage there is a sudden expansion of the vascular bed. However, using a chemiluminescence technique to identify and quantify the relative amounts of endothelial cells to total protein in mouse lung, Schachtner et al. (6) found that there was a steady increase in the endothelium at the same rate as the total lung tissue from E13.5 day onward, that is, before the start of the canalicular phase. The increase in the capillary bed is likely now by sprouting angiogenesis, and cell division can be identified in the endothelial cells of the capillaries (4). The capillaries can now be identified close to the epithelium. We do not know what attracts the capillaries to underlie the epithelium, but once there they seem to be responsible for the thinning and stretching of the epithelium that in turn leads to the differentiation to type I and II pneumonocytes (39). In vitro studies have demonstrated that cell matrix produced by rat pulmonary vascular endothelial cells leads to differentiation of rat type II to type I cells (40). There is also increase in VEGF production that converts glycogen to surfactant in the type II cells (41). This would seem to be under the control of the transcription factor HIF-2α. HIF-2α knockout mice have a failure of maturation of surfactant (41), and HIF-1α knockout mice have a failure of angiogenesis via failure of VEGF.

There is a balance of factors both promoting and opposing angiogenesis in this phase of development. There is an increase in size of the peripheral airspaces, which maybe due to fluid production, stretching the epithelial cells. In human, there is also fetal breathing movement. In cultured bovine vascular smooth muscle cells, there is evidence that cyclic stretch upregulates myogenic differentiation and leads to an increase in VEGF mRNA, which in turn stimulates endothelial cell motility and an increase in capillary number via the Flk-1 receptor (42). Furthermore, stretch of smooth muscle cells from lambs increased first transforming growth factor (TGF)-β1 and then VEGF, TGF-β1 being required for the production of the VEGF (43). However, transgenic mice with an excess of TGF-β1 fail to differentiate peripheral epithelial cells to produce surfactant proteins in the canalicular phase, and in addition, the mRNAs for both VEGF and Flk-1 were decreased associated with a decrease in the number of alveolar capillaries (44). Further negative control is found by endothelial monocyte-activating polypeptide (EMAP) II, a potent tumor antiangiogenic factor (45), which if increased in mice reduced vessel density and alveolar type II cell formation and if blocked allowed an increase in vascularization together with increased expression of surfactant C in the distal epithelium (46).

VI. Saccular and Alveolar Stage

During the saccular stage, there is an increase in size of the peripheral airspaces and a decrease in the amount of mesenchyme between the airspaces, although there is still a capillary bed under each adjacent epithelial layer. The precursors of alveoli appear as low ridges or crests protruding from the saccular walls. Each has myofibroblasts and elastin within the tips of the crest. During the alveolar stage (from 36 weeks' gestation in human), the ridges elongate and extend into the airspaces with a capillary plexus lining on each side of the septum, forming a capillary loop. By this time, the alveoli appear cup shaped but have a relatively thick wall due to the double-capillary layer and the matrix between. In human, this appearance is present in the alveolar region until 18 months of age (47). The double-capillary layer coalesces to form a single-capillary sheet. The capillaries come into contact within the septa and the wall between them fuses and eventually breaks down (48). Burri and colleagues have shown that physically a double-capillary network is needed for the formation of alveolar septa (47). In rats, glucocorticoid treatment leads to premature fusion of the capillaries, which may explain the failure of alveolar development (48). There is downregulation of VEGF and Flk-1 in dexamethasone-treated mice (49). More recently, using high-resolution microscopy, Schittny et al. (50) have observed in rats that new septa can form due to uplifting from a mature single-layered alveolar wall that occurs via angiogenesis. This suggests that some regenerative alveolization can occur beyond the rapid early development. The capillary bed is also thought to increase by a process of intussusceptive microvascular growth. In this, there is repeated insertion of new transcapillary tissue pillars, which increase in size and allow an increase in capillary surface area (51).

By term, up to half the adult number of alveoli have formed in human (52), whereas mice and rats are born during the saccular phase and alveoli form entirely after birth (53). The interaction of the arteries with the airways continues into alveolar development. Experimental studies have shown in mice and rabbits that as alveoli form, type II pneumonocytes produce mRNA for VEGF (54,55). Both VEGF and its receptor Flk-1 have been shown to increase in perinatal mice during this period (56), and in a study on rat alveolar development, the inhibitor of Flk-1 (Su5416) reduced the number of arteries and alveoli as did antiangiogenic factors such as fumagillin and thalidomide (57). A similar study on mice showed that Flk-1 was essential for early alveolar and thus capillary development (58). Increasing VEGF leads to increase in capillaries and also alveoli in recovery of rat lungs after loss of both during hyperoxic exposure (59). There is continuing interaction of VEGF and NO and angiogenesis. Exposure of neonatal rats to hyperoxia reduces expression of VEGF, VEGF receptors, and eNOS while reducing alveolar multiplication. Inhaled NO enhanced recovery by increasing blood vessel development (60).

The transcription factors HIF-1α and -2α, which increase in hypoxic conditions, promote VEGF and angiogenesis. HIF-2α knockout mice have fewer blood vessels (41). In preterm baboons, an experimental increase in HIF-1α by reducing its breakdown by prolyl-hydroxylase domain (PHD)-containing protein leads to an increase in CD31, VEGF, and endothelial cells, and thus capillaries (61). Hypoxia also induces mitogenic factor coexpression with HIF-2α and has potent angiogenic properties (62). Hyperoxia conversely reduces vascular density and alveolar development with a reduction in VEGF (63). This study also showed the importance of endothelial progenitor cells. These cells are implicated in repair of vasculature; their role in vascular development is unknown. However, exposure of newborn mice (1-day-old) to hyperoxia reduced the number of circulating endothelial progenitor cells and their number in the bone marrow suggesting their importance (63).

VII. Development of the Vessel Wall

Once the newly formed vessels are present, they acquire a muscle wall. Muscle cells are not seen in mouse lung at E10.5 but are present in proximal structures including the pulmonary arteries by E11.5. Muscle is first seen in human fetal intrapulmonary arteries at 38 days. This is later than the first appearance in airway walls where mesenchymal cells expressing α–smooth muscle actins are seen in the walls of preterminal bud airways from 34 days' gestation. In human, from 6 to 14 weeks of gestation in the penultimate airway, there are four layers of muscle cells, the outer two layers being loosely packed. By 17 weeks of gestation, this thick layer is reduced to one layer. It seems that initially at the lung periphery, the pulmonary arterial muscle cells, which lie around the newly formed arteries, are derived from the bronchial smooth muscle of adjacent airways (3). Cytoplasmic processes from the outer layers of bronchial smooth muscle cells in the preterminal airway extend to the endothelial tubes and line up around the lumen (Fig. 4).

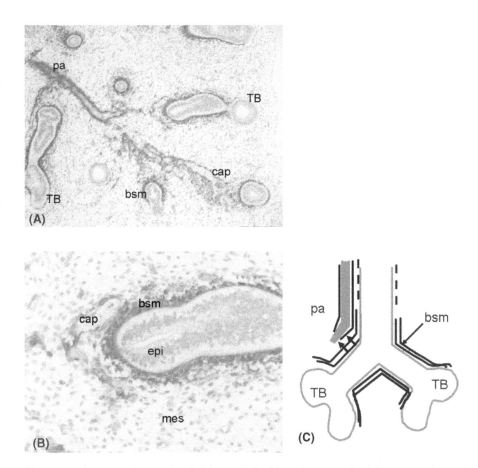

Figure 4 (**A**) Photomicrograph of eight-week fetal lung immunostained for α–smooth muscle actin. Smooth muscle cells (bsm) are seen around the penultimate airways and also around a coalescing capillary (cap). This is continuous with a single muscularized artery with a narrow lumen (pa). (**B**) High-power photomicrograph of an airway wall. Processes of smooth muscle cells can be seen between the airway smooth muscle (bsm) and the wall of a capillary (cap). (**C**) A diagram illustrating the derivation of the arterial smooth muscle cells from the bronchial smooth muscle. *Abbreviations:* TB, terminal bud; epi, epithelium; mes, mesenchyme.

Once the arteries have a layer of muscle cells, the endothelial cells protrude into the lumen suggesting some vasoconstriction. In more proximal vessels, the inner one to two layers of muscle cells are closely packed and brick shaped even in the newborn, and experimental studies in piglets suggest that even after birth their phenotype may be different (64). We do not know what stimulates the migration of smooth muscle cells from the bronchial smooth muscle; however, tenascin, versican, and fibronectin that are all involved in cell locomotion colocate only in this area (3). Later from eight weeks' gestation in the proximal arteries, the inner smooth muscle layers were surrounded by loosely packed layers of fusiform-shaped cells. The number of these layers increased with age and the size of the artery. Fibroblasts from the mesenchyme have lined up around the outer part of the arterial wall and then develop a smooth muscle cell phenotype expressing first α–smooth muscle actin and then gradual maturation of the cytoskeletal proteins SM-1, γ–smooth muscle actin, and caldesmon. Hypoxia induces differentiation of fibroblasts into myofibroblasts (65). Increased levels of hypoxia during fetal life as in sheep kept at high altitude leads to an increase in smooth muscle cell area in the peripheral pulmonary arteries (66), which is greater in male than in female animals.

The arterial smooth muscle is always more mature in the inner layers and less mature than adjacent bronchial smooth muscle. Elastic laminae form between the muscle layers to form the typical elastic arterial appearance. An elastic arterial wall is found to the same level in the arterial pathway as in the adult by 19 weeks of gestation though in much smaller arteries (1). A third source of arterial smooth muscle cells, the endothelial cell, is seen later in development for a short period. The capillary endothelial cells stain positively for α–smooth muscle actin and may give rise to smooth muscle cells by division (3).

In a study on human fetal lungs (4), venous smooth muscle appeared at eight weeks of gestation, later than arterial smooth muscle, and was of a layer of flattened cells closely adherent to the endothelial cells. Around these was a loose network of elongated mesenchymal cells, also α–smooth muscle actin positive. The veins did not derive any muscle cells from the bronchial smooth muscle but there was evidence that some muscle derived from the endothelial cells. Maturation of the smooth muscle cells followed a similar pattern to the arteries but without caldesmon being expressed. The veins did not constrict as the muscle surrounded them. Myocardial muscle-expressing desmin was present in the walls of the extrapulmonary veins from eight weeks' gestation (4). In human, it does not extend into the lung as it does in rats and mice.

The smooth muscle cells of the airways, arteries, and veins show progressive and gradual maturation of their cytoskeletal structure. Folkman and D'Amore (67) suggested that Angiopoietin produced by undifferentiated mesenchymal cells binds to and activates the Tie-2 receptor on the endothelial cells, resulting in a chemoattractant signal (platelet-derived growth factor or epidermal growth factor) for the fibroblasts. These are then attracted to the vessel wall and become committed to becoming smooth muscle cells as a result of further growth factors from the endothelial cells. Once the cells have been attracted they become differentiated. This may be controlled by TGF-β that inhibits endothelial and smooth muscle proliferation and migration and induces differentiation of mesenchymal cells into smooth muscle cells (68). Overexpression of angiopoietin in rats led to muscle hypertrophy and hyperplasia in pulmonary arteries (69). Angiopoietin knockout mice die in utero with no muscle cell encasement around their endothelial tubes (30).

VIII. Development of the Bronchial Circulation

In the human lung, the bronchial circulation carries systemic blood to the walls of the airways and the large pulmonary vessels. The bronchial arteries are found in adult airways as far to the periphery as the alveolar ducts. They form later than the pulmonary circulation and are first identified in the lungs around eight weeks of gestation (70). At this time, one or two small vessels extend from the dorsal aorta and enter the lung within the main bronchus alongside the cartilage plates. They extend to the periphery as the airways increase in size and the walls develop cartilage plates and submucosal glands. They eventually form a network throughout the airway wall both in the subepithelium and in the outer wall. In the adult, they extend as far as the respiratory bronchioli. They remain small relative to the adjacent pulmonary arteries and only increase in size in cases where there is a failure of development of the pulmonary circulation. Many of the small bronchial veins within the airway wall drain into the pulmonary veins. Bronchial veins are only seen close to the hilum and drain into the cardinal veins and the right atrium.

IX. Adaptation to Extrauterine Life

During fetal life, there is a high resistance in the pulmonary circulation diverting blood away from the lung. As the pulmonary arteries develop, they have a thick wall relative to the lumen that offers a high resistance to flow. At birth, the endothelial cells are squat with a narrow base on the basement membrane and low surface-to-volume ratio and the smooth muscle cells are brick shaped (71). Immediately after birth, the peripheral arteries thin rapidly and reach adult percentage wall thickness within three days (72). Using electron microscopy, it is apparent that there is not a loss of smooth muscle cells but a change in cell shape from brick shape to spindle shape and a spreading around the increasing lumen of both the smooth muscle cells and endothelial cells (71,73). This is facilitated in the smooth muscle cells by the rearrangement of the actin cytoskeleton allowed by an abrupt but transient decrease in total actin and an increase in the monomeric form of actin (74). There is also a paucity of fixed connective tissue in the arterial wall at this time. At birth, the actin filaments form a network and lack a specific orientation; by 14 days of age, the smooth muscle cells are spindle shaped and actin filaments form dense sheets along the longitudinal axis of the cell. At this time, there has been an increase in the relative amount of connective tissue between the muscle cells (75). During the transition period, the blood vessels are less responsive to contractile stimuli (76,77). Once the peripheral arteries have adapted, the more proximal arteries decrease their wall thickness by slower growth of the wall relative to the lumen and external diameter (72).

The mechanisms responsible for the postnatal fall in pulmonary vascular resistance (PVR) are still uncertain, but the initial rapid dilatation of the pulmonary vasculature is stimulated by ventilation, an increase in oxygen tension, and an increase in sheer stress. The sudden increase in flow and sheer stress leads to increased production of potent vasodilators such as NO and prostacyclin (PGI_2). NOS is present in utero and there is a surge in both protein and enzyme activity at birth (78,79). In vitro studies on isolated porcine and ovine pulmonary arteries have shown that endothelium-dependent and -independent relaxation in response to a variety of agonists is absent or poor immediately after birth (80), but increases rapidly in the first few days (81,82). By contrast, the pulmonary veins in piglets have a consistent amount of eNOS during fetal life and after birth and isolated veins relax well to acetylcholine, although the response does improve with age (83). The NO pathway is not the only one involved in adaptation since mice in which the eNOS gene has been knocked out still reduce their arterial wall thickness after birth (84). Of less importance is PGI_2 that is released by increased sheer stress and increased oxygen tension. Prostacyclin synthesis is higher in newborn than fetal ovine vessels (85) and PGI_2 synthase expression is low at birth and increases rapidly in the first week of life in piglets. Prostacyclin production in lambs decreases within hours after birth; however, hypoxia increases its production and gene expression (86).

The maintenance of the low-pressure system in the lung is a balance between the vasodilators and vasoconstrictors. Endothelin (ET-1) is a potent vasoconstrictor and growth factor produced by the endothelium. In experimental studies, ET-1 constricts fetal lamb arteries and veins and increases the pulmonary artery pressure in newborn lambs (86). It is probably an important player in maintaining the high PVR in fetal life since inhibition of the ET_A receptor leads to a decrease in basal PVR in sheep (87). Plasma ET is high in infants and in animal models at birth and in those with pulmonary hypertension (88). ET-1 is abundant in the pulmonary arteries of piglets at birth (89). Its expression decreases at 2 days of age and increases again by 10 days when it is less than in the fetus. ET-1 has two receptors: ET_A receptors are found on smooth muscle cells and their stimulation leads to vasoconstriction; ET_B receptors are found both on the smooth muscle cells, where their stimulation also leads to vasoconstriction, and on the endothelial cells, where they lead to release of NO or PGI_2 and thus vasodilatation. In a study on piglet lungs, ET_A and ET_B receptor-binding sites were densely distributed over smooth muscle cells of pulmonary arteries and veins at birth with an increase in the proportion of ET_B receptors with age. ET_B receptors transiently appeared on the pulmonary arterial endothelium one to three days after birth (90), and the vasodilator response to ET-1 increases in both pulmonary arteries and veins at this time (91).

X. Summary

In the adult lung, the arteries and veins have a similar branching pattern to the airways, and from the earliest stage of lung development, there is a circulation alongside the airways. During branching morphogenesis, the airways act as a template via a variety of growth factors for the vessels, which form by vasculogenesis. The interaction between airways and blood vessels continues throughout development. It is now apparent that airway development particularly of the alveoli is influenced by blood vessel growth. For the future, this interaction can be manipulated to aid recovery growth in the hypoplastic lungs of infants with bronchopulmonary dysplasia.

References

1. Hislop A, Reid L. Intrapulmonary arterial development during fetal life—branching pattern and structure. J Anat 1972; 113:35–48.
2. deMello D, Sawyer D, Galvin N, et al. Early fetal development of lung vasculature. Am J Resp Cell Mol Biol 1997; 16:568–581.
3. Hall SM, Hislop AA, Pierce CM, et al. Prenatal origins of human intrapulmonary arteries: formation and smooth muscle maturation. Am J Respir Cell Mol Biol 2000; 23(2):194–203.
4. Hall SM, Hislop AA, Haworth SG. Origin, differentiation, and maturation of human pulmonary veins. Am J Respir Cell Mol Biol 2002; 26(3):333–340.
5. Maeda S, Suzuki S, Suzuki T, et al. Analysis of intrapulmonary vessels and epithelial-endothelial interactions in the human developing lung. Lab Invest 2002; 82(3):293–301.
6. Schachtner SK, Wang Y, Scott BH. Qualitative and quantitative analysis of embryonic pulmonary vessel formation. Am J Respir Cell Mol Biol 2000; 22(2):157–165.

7. Parera MC, van DM, van KM, et al. Distal angiogenesis: a new concept for lung vascular morphogenesis. Am J Physiol Lung Cell Mol Physiol 2005; 288(1):L141–L149.
8. Anderson-Berry A, O'Brien EA, Bleyl SB, et al. Vasculogenesis drives pulmonary vascular growth in the developing chick embryo. Dev Dyn 2005; 233(1):145–153.
9. Hislop A, Reid L. Fetal and childhood development of the intrapulmonary veins in man—branching pattern and structure. Thorax 1973; 28:313–319.
10. Gale NW, Baluk P, Pan L, et al. Ephrin-B2 selectively marks arterial vessels and neovascularization sites in the adult, with expression in both endothelial and smooth-muscle cells. Dev Biol 2001; 230(2):151–160.
11. Kuijper S, Turner CJ, Adams RH. Regulation of angiogenesis by Eph-ephrin interactions. Trends Cardiovasc Med 2007; 17(5):145–151.
12. Warburton D, Schwarz M, Tefft D, et al. The molecular basis of lung morphogenesis. Mech Dev 2000; 92(1):55–81.
13. Minoo P. Transcriptional regulation of lung development: emergence of specificity (review). Respir Res 2000; 1:109–115.
14. Roth-Kleiner M, Post M. Genetic control of lung development. Biol Neonate 2003; 84(1):83–88.
15. Glenny R, Bernard S, Neradilek B, et al. Quantifying the genetic influence on mammalian vascular tree structure. Proc Natl Acad Sci U S A 2007; 104(16):6858–6863.
16. Hislop A, Reid L. The similarity of the pulmonary artery branching system in siblings. Forensic Sci 1973; 2:37–52.
17. Akeson AL, Wetzel B, Thompson FY, et al. Embryonic vasculogenesis by endothelial precursor cells derived from lung mesenchyme. Dev Dyn 2000; 217(1):11–23.
18. Alvarez DF, Huang L, King JA, et al. Lung microvascular endothelium is enriched with progenitor cells that exhibit vasculogenic capacity. Am J Physiol Lung Cell Mol Physiol 2008; 294(3):L419–L430.
19. Gebb SA, Shannon JM. Tissue interactions mediate early events in pulmonary vasculogenesis. Dev Dyn 2000; 217(2):159–169.
20. Acarregui MJ, Penisten ST, Goss KL, et al. Vascular endothelial growth factor gene expression in human fetal lung in vitro. Am J Respir Cell Mol Biol 1999; 20:14–23.
21. Shifren JL, Doldi N, Ferrara N, et al. In the human fetus, vascular endothelial growth factor is expressed in epithelial cells and myocytes, but not vascular endothelium: implications for mode of action. J Clin Endocrinol Metab 1994; 79(1):316–322.
22. Healy AM, Morgenthau L, Zhu X, et al. VEGF is deposited in the subepithelial matrix at the leading edge of branching airways and stimulates neovascularization in the murine embryonic lung. Dev Dyn 2000; 219(3):341–352.
23. Carmeliet P, Ferreira V, Breier G, et al. Abnormal blood vessel development and lethality in embryos lacking a single VEGF allele. Nature 1996; 380(6573):435–439.
24. Akeson AL, Greenberg JM, Cameron JE, et al. Temporal and spatial regulation of VEGF-A controls vascular patterning in the embryonic lung. Dev Biol 2003; 264(2):443–455.
25. Fong GH, Rossant J, Gertsenstein M, et al. Role of the Flt-1 receptor tyrosine kinase in regulating the assembly of vascular endothelium. Nature 1995; 376(6535):66–70.
26. Shalaby F, Rossant J, Yamaguchi TP, et al. Failure of blood-island formation and vasculogenesis in Flk-1-deficient mice. Nature 1995; 376(6535):62–66.
27. Voelkel NF, Vandivier RW, Tuder RM. Vascular endothelial growth factor in the lung. Am J Physiol Lung Cell Mol Physiol 2006; 290(2):L209–L221.
28. Groenman F, Rutter M, Caniggia I, et al. Hypoxia-inducible factors in the first trimester human lung. J Histochem Cytochem 2007; 55(4):355–363.
29. van Tuyl M, Liu J, Wang J, et al. Role of oxygen and vascular development in epithelial branching morphogenesis of the developing mouse lung. Am J Physiol Lung Cell Mol Physiol 2005; 288(1):L167–L178.

30. Suri C, Jones PF, Patan S, et al. Requisite role of angiopoietin-1, a ligand for the TIE2 receptor, during embryonic angiogenesis. Cell 1996; 87(7):1171–1180.

31. Sato TN, Tozawa Y, Deutsch U, et al. Disdinct roles of the receptor tyrosine kinases tie-1 and tie-2 in blood vessel formation. Nature 1995; 376:70–74.

32. Gale NW, Thurston G, Hackett SF, et al. Angiopoietin-2 is required for postnatal angiogenesis and lymphatic patterning, and only the latter role is rescued by Angiopoietin-1. Dev Cell 2002; 3(3):411–423.

33. Tammela T, Saaristo A, Lohela M, et al. Angiopoietin-1 promotes lymphatic sprouting and hyperplasia. Blood 2005; 105(12):4642–4648.

34. Yao Y, Nowak S, Yochelis A, et al. Matrix GLA protein, an inhibitory morphogen in pulmonary vascular development. J Biol Chem 2007; 282(41):30131–30142.

35. Han RN, Post M, Tanswell AK, et al. Insulin-like growth factor-I receptor-mediated vasculogenesis/angiogenesis in human lung development. Am J Respir Cell Mol Biol 2003; 28(2):159–169.

36. Tanswell AK, Han RN, Jassal D, et al. The response of small vessel endothelial cells from fetal rat lung to growth factors. J Dev Physiol 1991; 15(4):199–209.

37. Young SL, Evans K, Eu JP. Nitric oxide modulates branching morphogenesis in fetal rat lung explants. Am J Physiol Lung Cell Mol Physiol 2002; 282(3):L379–L385.

38. Balasubramaniam V, Maxey AM, Fouty BW, et al. Nitric oxide augments fetal pulmonary artery endothelial cell angiogenesis in vitro. Am J Physiol Lung Cell Mol Physiol 2006; 290 (6):L1111–L1116.

39. Gutierrez JA, Ertsey R, Scavo LM, et al. Mechanical distention modulates alveolar epithelial cell phenotypic expression by transcriptional regulation. Am J Respir Cell Mol Biol 1999; 21(2):223–229.

40. Adamson IY, Young L. Alveolar type II cell growth on a pulmonary endothelial extracellular matrix. Am J Physiol 1996; 270(6 pt 1):L1017–L1022.

41. Compernolle V, Brusselmans K, Acker T, et al. Loss of HIF-2alpha and inhibition of VEGF impair fetal lung maturation, whereas treatment with VEGF prevents fatal respiratory distress in premature mice. Nat Med 2002; 8(7):702–710.

42. Smith JD, Davies N, Willis AI, et al. Cyclic stretch induces the expression of vascular endothelial growth factor in vascular smooth muscle cells. Endothelium 2001; 8(1):41–48.

43. Mata-Greenwood E, Grobe A, Kumar S, et al. Cyclic stretch increases VEGF expression in pulmonary arterial smooth muscle cells via TGF-beta1 and reactive oxygen species: a requirement for NAD(P)H oxidase. Am J Physiol Lung Cell Mol Physiol 2005; 289(2): L288–L289.

44. Zeng X, Gray M, Stahlman MT, et al. TGF-beta1 perturbs vascular development and inhibits epithelial differentiation in fetal lung in vivo. Dev Dyn 2001; 221(3):289–301.

45. Schwarz MA, Zhang F, Gebb S, et al. Endothelial monocyte activating polypeptide II inhibits lung neovascularization and airway epithelial morphogenesis. Mech Dev 2000; 95(1–2): 123–132.

46. Schwarz MA, Zhang F, Lane JE, et al. Angiogenesis and morphogenesis of murine fetal distal lung in an allograft model. Am J Physiol Lung Cell Mol Physiol 2000; 278(5): L1000–L1007.

47. Zeltner TB, Burri PH. The postnatal development and growth of the human lung. II. Morphology. Respir Physiol 1987; 67(3):269–282.

48. Roth-Kleiner M, Berger TM, Tarek MR, et al. Neonatal dexamethasone induces premature microvascular maturation of the alveolar capillary network. Dev Dyn 2005; 233(4):1261–1271.

49. Clerch LB, Baras AS, Massaro GD, et al. DNA microarray analysis of neonatal mouse lung connects regulation of KDR with dexamethasone-induced inhibition of alveolar formation. Am J Physiol Lung Cell Mol Physiol 2004; 286(2):L411–L419.

50. Schittny JC, Mund SI, Stampanoni M. Evidence and structural mechanism for late lung alveolarization. Proc Am Thorac Soc 2008; 5(3):360.

51. Burri PH, Djonov V. Intussusceptive angiogenesis—the alternative to capillary sprouting. Mol Aspects Med 2002; 23(6S):S1–S27.

52. Hislop A, Wigglesworth JS, Desai R. Alveolar development in the human fetus and infant. Early Hum Dev 1986; 13(19):1–11.

53. Burri PH. Structural aspects of prenatal and postnatal development and growth of the lung. In: McDonald JA, ed. Lung Growth and Development. New York: Marcel Dekker, 1997:1–35.

54. Ng YS, Rohan R, Sunday ME, et al. Differential expression of VEGF isoforms in mouse during development and in the adult. Dev Dyn 2001; 220:112–121.

55. Maniscalco WM, Watkins RH, D'Angio CT, et al. Hyperoxic injury decreases alveolar epithelial cell expression of vascular endothelial growth factor (VEGF) in neonatal rabbit lung. Am J Respir Cell Mol Biol 1997; 16(5):557–567.

56. Bhatt AJ, Amin SB, Chess PR, et al. Expression of vascular endothelial growth factor and Flk-1 in developing and glucocorticoid-treated mouse lung. Pediatr Res 2000; 47(5):606–613.

57. Jakkula M, Le Cras TD, Gebb S, et al. Inhibition of angiogenesis decreases alveolarization in the developing rat lung. Am J Physiol Lung Cell Mol Physiol 2000; 279(3):L600–L607.

58. McGrath-Morrow SA, Cho C, Cho C, et al. Vascular endothelial growth factor receptor 2 blockade disrupts postnatal lung development. Am J Respir Cell Mol Biol 2005; 32(5):420–427.

59. Kunig AM, Balasubramaniam V, Markham NE, et al. Recombinant human VEGF treatment enhances alveolarization after hyperoxic lung injury in neonatal rats. Am J Physiol Lung Cell Mol Physiol 2005; 289(4):L529–L535.

60. Lin YJ, Markham NE, Balasubramaniam V, et al. Inhaled nitric oxide enhances distal lung growth after exposure to hyperoxia in neonatal rats. Pediatr Res 2005; 58(1):22–29.

61. Asikainen TM, Waleh NS, Schneider BK, et al. Enhancement of angiogenic effectors through hypoxia-inducible factor in preterm primate lung in vivo. Am J Physiol Lung Cell Mol Physiol 2006; 291(4):L588–L595.

62. Wagner KF, Hellberg AK, Balenger S, et al. Hypoxia-induced mitogenic factor has anti-apoptotic action and is upregulated in the developing lung: coexpression with hypoxia-inducible factor-2alpha. Am J Respir Cell Mol Biol 2004; 31(3):276–282.

63. Balasubramaniam V, Mervis CF, Maxey AM, et al. Hyperoxia reduces bone marrow, circulating, and lung endothelial progenitor cells in the developing lung: implications for the pathogenesis of bronchopulmonary dysplasia. Am J Physiol Lung Cell Mol Physiol 2007; 292(5):L1073–L1084.

64. Bailly K, Ridley AJ, Hall SM, et al. RhoA activation by hypoxia in pulmonary arterial smooth muscle cells is age and site specific. Circ Res 2004; 94(10):1383–1391.

65. Short M, Nemenoff RA, Zawada WM, et al. Hypoxia induces differentiation of pulmonary artery adventitial fibroblasts into myofibroblasts. Am J Physiol Cell Physiol 2004; 286(2): C416–C425.

66. Bixby CE, Ibe BO, Abdallah MF, et al. Role of platelet-activating factor in pulmonary vascular remodeling associated with chronic high altitude hypoxia in ovine fetal lambs. Am J Physiol Lung Cell Mol Physiol 2007; 293(6):L1475–L1482.

67. Folkman J, D'Amore PA. Blood vessel formation: what is its molecular basis? Cell 1996; 87 (7):1153–1155.

68. Frid MG, Kale VA, Stenmark KR. Mature vascular endothelium can give rise to smooth muscle cells via endothelial-mesenchymal transdifferentiation: in vitro analysis. Circ Res 2002; 90(11):1189–1196.

69. Chu D, Sullivan CC, Du L, et al. A new animal model for pulmonary hypertension based on the overexpression of a single gene, angiopoietin-1. Ann Thorac Surg 2004; 77(2):449–456.

70. Hislop AA. Airway and blood vessel interaction during lung development. J Anat 2002; 201 (4):325–334.

71. Haworth SG, Hall SM, Chew M, et al. Thinning of fetal pulmonary arterial wall and postnatal remodelling: ultrastructural studies on the respiratory unit arteries of the pig. Virchows Arch A Pathol Anat Histopathol 1987; 411(2):161–171.

72. Haworth SG, Hislop AA. Pulmonary vascular development: normal values of peripheral vascular structure. Am J Cardiol 1983; 52(5):578–583.

73. Hall SM, Haworth SG. Normal adaptation of pulmonary arterial intima to extrauterine life in the pig: ultrastructural studies. J Pathol 1986; 149(1):55–66.

74. Hall SM, Gorenflo M, Reader J, et al. Neonatal pulmonary hypertension prevents reorganisation of the pulmonary arterial smooth muscle cytoskeleton after birth. J Anat 2000; 196 (pt 3):391–403.

75. Kelly DA, Hislop AA, Hall SM, et al. Correlation of pulmonary arterial smooth muscle structure and reactivity during adaptation to extrauterine life. J Vasc Res 2002; 39(1):30–40.

76. Kelly DA, Hislop AA, Hall SM, et al. Relationship between structural remodeling and reactivity in pulmonary resistance arteries from hypertensive piglets. Pediatr Res 2005; 58(3): 525–530.

77. Schindler MB, Hislop AA, Haworth SG. Postnatal changes in response to norepinephrine in the normal and pulmonary hypertensive lung. Am J Respir Crit Care Med 2004; 170(6):641–646.

78. Hislop AA, Springall DR, Buttery LD, et al. Abundance of endothelial nitric oxide synthase in newborn intrapulmonary arteries. Arch Dis Child Fetal Neonatal Ed 1995; 73(1):F17–F21.

79. Arrigoni FI, Hislop AA, Pollock JS, et al. Birth upregulates nitric oxide synthase activity in the porcine lung. Life Sci 2002; 70(14):1609–1620.

80. Haworth SG. Pulmonary hypertension in the young. Heart 2002; 88(6):658–664.

81. Tulloh RM, Hislop AA, Boels PJ, et al. Chronic hypoxia inhibits postnatal maturation of porcine intrapulmonary artery relaxation. Am J Physiol 1997; 272(5 pt 2):H2436–H2445.

82. Abman SH, Chatfield BA, Rodman DM, et al. Maturational changes in endothelium-derived relaxing factor activity of ovine pulmonary arteries in vitro. Am J Physiol 1991; 260:L280–L285.

83. Arrigoni FI, Hislop AA, Haworth SG, et al. Newborn intrapulmonary veins are more reactive than intrapulmonary arteries in normal and hypertensive piglets. Am J Physiol 1999; 277(5): L887–L892.

84. Miller AA, Hislop AA, Vallance PJ, et al. Deletion of the eNOS gene has a greater impact on the pulmonary circulation of male than female mice. Am J Physiol Lung Cell Mol Physiol 2005; 289(2):L299–L306.

85. Shaul PW, Farrar MA, Magness RR. Pulmonary endothelial nitric oxide production is developmentally regulated in the fetus and newborn. Am J Physiol 1993; 265(4 pt 2):H1056–H1063.

86. Abman SH, Kinsella JP, Mercier J. Nitric oxide and endothelin in the developing pulmonary circulation: physiologic and clinical implications. In: Gaultier C, Bourbon JR, Post M, eds. Lung Development. New York: Oxford University Press, 1999:196–220.

87. Ivy DD, Parker TA, Ziegler JW, et al. Prolonged endothelin A receptor blockade attenuates chronic pulmonary hypertension in the ovine fetus. J Clin Invest 1997; 99(6):1179–1186.

88. Noguchi Y, Hislop AA, Haworth SG. Influence of hypoxia on endothelin-1 binding sites in neonatal porcine pulmonary vasculature. Am J Physiol 1997; 272(2 pt 2):H669–H678.

89. Levy M, Souil E, Sabry S, et al. Maturational changes of endothelial vasoactive factors and pulmonary vascular tone at birth. Eur Respir J 2000; 15(1):158–165.

90. Hislop AA, Zhao YD, Springall DR, et al. Postnatal changes in endothelin-1 binding in porcine pulmonary vessels and airways. Am J Respir Cell Mol Biol 1995; 12(5):557–566.

91. Schindler MB, Hislop AA, Haworth SG. Postnatal changes in pulmonary vein responses to endothelin-1 in the normal and chronically hypoxic lung. Am J Physiol Lung Cell Mol Physiol 2007; 292(5):L1273–L1279.

5

Oxidative and Nitrosative Stress and Bronchopulmonary Dysplasia

RICHARD L. AUTEN
Duke University Medical Center, Durham, North Carolina, U.S.A.

CARL WHITE
National Jewish Medical and Research Center, Denver, Colorado, U.S.A.

I. Introduction

Reactive oxygen species (ROS) and reactive nitrogen species (RNS) alter bio-molecular structure and function. Biochemical immaturity of the preterm newborn limits antioxidant defenses. ROS formation may be favored through sudden transition from the relatively hypoxic fetal environment to markedly increased oxygen. Resuscitation with 21% rather than 100% oxygen may minimize early oxidative stress (1). Intubation and mechanical ventilation are associated with inflammation and therefore additional oxidative (2) and nitrosative stress (3). Chorioamnionitis may contribute to early, even prenatal, oxidative stress in the preterm newborn (4). Likewise, the preterm newborn is predisposed to infection that can compound inflammation and oxidative stress.

To understand the mechanisms and design successful adaptive strategies aimed at preventing and treating bronchopulmonary dysplasia (BPD), it is necessary to understand how and where ROS and RNS are generated in newborns at risk to develop BPD, and to recognize that the timing and location of the generation of nitrogen oxides and ROS will have interdependent effects on their respective biological impacts (5). Superoxide and nitric oxide react at nearly diffusion limited rates to form peroxynitrite (6), so local generation of superoxide and nitric oxide in proximity will destroy NO biological activities that are mediated via effects on binding to the heme Fe(II) of guanylyl cyclase, or the formation of S-nitrosothiols, increasingly recognized to be critical to a number of pathways important to pulmonary homeostasis, like airway tone (7) and modulation of inflammation (8).

Likewise, hydrogen peroxide–dependent processes, which can depend on dismutation of superoxide, could also be affected. It is therefore critical to the understanding of the role of these reactive species that the location and the relative abundances of NO and superoxide accumulation are assessed, as depicted in Figure 1. These in turn will be influenced by the cellular, subcellular, and developmental stage–specific expression of NO synthases and antioxidant enzymes. This chapter will focus on the evidence supporting a role for these pathways in the pathogenesis of BPD.

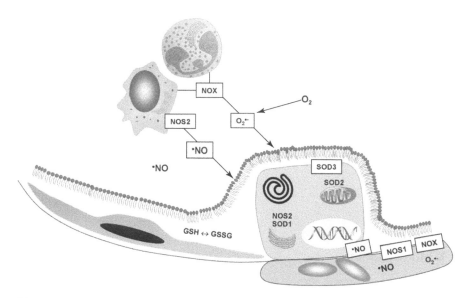

Figure 1 Reactive oxygen and nitrogen species sources and defenses in the alveolus. ROS/RNS can be generated by ambient gases in stochastic reactions and by NOX and NOS isoforms, among others. The generation of $^{\bullet}NO$ and $O_2^{\bullet-}$ occurs in proximity in many microenvironments within the alveolus.

II. Vulnerability to ROS/RNS and Bronchopulmonary Dysplasia

The lung is protected against these reactive species by a variety of enzymatic and nonenzymatic antioxidants. Many pulmonary antioxidant systems are developmentally regulated. As such, the preterm newborn has diminished lung activities or levels of a number of both types of these antioxidants (9–15). Further, the preterm newborn may also have a limited ability to elevate or induce the levels of these antioxidants in a timely fashion in response to the oxidative stress that is posed by preterm birth with respiratory distress (16).

A. Enzymatic Antioxidant Defenses and BPD

Superoxide and Superoxide Dismutases

Superoxide dismutases (SODs) "dismutate" (one oxidation and one reduction) two superoxides to dioxygen and hydrogen peroxide. SOD rate constants are almost diffusion limited. Copper-zinc SOD, also termed cytosolic SOD or SOD1, is present in the cytoplasm, nucleus, and mitochondrial intermembrane space. It constitutes about 85% to 90% of the intracellular SOD in lung. The manganese SOD, also known as mitochondrial SOD or SOD2, is present in the mitochondrial matrix. It has greater inducibility than SOD1: bacterial endotoxin, oxidative stresses, and inflammatory cytokines induce

SOD2 activity. In the baboon model of BPD induced by preterm delivery, mechanical ventilation and exposure to either "as needed" oxygen or 100% oxygen, the lung-specific activities of SOD1 and SOD2 do not increase, despite increased mRNA expression (17). Extracellular SOD (EC-SOD or SOD3) is present in the extracellular matrix in adults, especially in the vicinity of airways and blood vessels, and is present at high levels in macrophages. It is intracellular in alveolar epithelial and bronchiolar epithelial cells in newborns rabbits (18) and mice (19). SOD3 is equipped with a heparin-binding tail that tethers it to matrix and is required for normal protection. Lung-targeted transgenic overexpression of SOD3 protects newborn mice from hyperoxia effects on inflammation and alveolar development (20).

Hydrogen Peroxide, Peroxidases, and Catalase

There are multiple enzymatic defenses against hydrogen peroxide, a highly reactive and diffusible ROS. These include catalase, which is not dependent on other enzyme systems, but is highly compartmentalized. Catalase produces O_2 and water from hydrogen peroxide. Glutathione (GSH) peroxidases react with higher affinity for hydrogen peroxide and are dependent on the cofactor GSH, the most abundant intracellular antioxidant. GSH peroxidase is dependent on the enzyme GSH reductase and ultimately on its reduction by NAD(P)H, provided by the hexose monophosphate shunt. Most recently discovered are peroxiredoxins (21), making up $\sim 1\%$ of total cellular protein in some cell types. Peroxiredoxins are versatile, with various isoforms capable of detoxifying hydrogen peroxide, lipid hydroperoxides, and/or phospholipid hydroperoxides (21,22). In the baboon model of BPD, both peroxiredoxins and the related thioredoxin and thioredoxin reductase can be regulated by oxygen in a developmentally related manner (23,24). A shift of thioredoxin from reduced to oxidized during hyperoxia may indicate the inability of the system to maintain redox homeostasis under oxidative stress in the preterm newborn.

B. Nonenzymatic Antioxidant Defenses and BPD

A variety of nonenzymatic antioxidants are important, particularly in distal small airways in defense against both ROS and RNS. Among these are ascorbate, uric acid, GSH, and α-tocopherol. In addition to its antioxidant role (25), GSH is a principal storage pool for cysteine. Despite supplementation, preterm newborns are frequently hypocysteinemic relative to term newborns (26,27), potentially contributing to decreased ability to synthesize GSH, which can "detoxify" peroxynitrite and nitrogen dioxide. Treatment to replace or supplement relatively deficient α-tocopherol has not been shown to prevent BPD (28). Vitamin A (retinoic acid) is a low molecular weight antioxidant that is necessary for lung growth and integrity of respiratory epithelium (29), acting through the retinoic acid receptor. The best evidence suggests that vitamin A supplementation may have a role in BPD prevention (30), although the reported effects are relatively modest.

Other molecules that may have nonenzymatic antioxidant functions are found in distal airways. Thiols of albumin, mucins, and other proteins may react with ROS or RNS. In addition, proteins that transport and limit the reactivities of metals, such as ceruloplasmin, transferrin (31), ferritin, metallothioneins, and other chelators, may also be present, indirectly affecting ROS generation.

III. Sources of Oxidative Stress: Exogenous Oxygen → ROS

Increases in ROS production are oxygen concentration dependent over a wide range of oxygen tensions (0–100% oxygen). Mitochondria are a major source of ROS in hyperoxia, although other cell organelles and cytoplasmic enzyme systems also can contribute. ROS are normal by-products of cell metabolism, and uncoupling of electron transport enhances such production. Multiple enzyme systems such as those of the cytochrome P450 monooxygenase system, xanthine oxidoreductase, nitric oxide synthases, and several involved in arachidonic acid metabolism (cyclooxygenase, lipoxygenase) all can contribute to the burden of ROS, including cellular production of superoxide. Hydrogen peroxide can facilitate formation of the more toxic and reactive hydroxyl radical ($HO^{\bullet}$) in the presence of reduced transition metals. Importantly, superoxide reacts rapidly with nitric oxide to form peroxynitrite ($ONOO^{-}$), a strong nitrating and oxidizing compound (32). Formation of such highly reactive species as hydroxyl radical or peroxynitrite can react with membrane lipids to cause more complex radicals by initiating lipid peroxidation. The direct role of lipid peroxidation in BPD is unknown.

A. Oxygen Therapy and BPD

Oxidative stress is more easily prevented than treated. Premature babies at risk to develop BPD have demonstrated increased protein (33) and lipid oxidation products (34). Examinations of oxidant stress in accessible compartments (blood, tracheal aspirates/lung lavage, urine) in premature newborns at risk to develop BPD have yielded conflicting results (35). The local cellular and subcellular environments are dynamic, so choosing the right targets and achieving specific therapeutic goals with acceptable risks has been problematic. Clinical efforts aimed at addressing the reduction of oxidative stress have been focused on minimizing the use of supplemental inhaled oxygen and supplementation with antioxidants, considered in detail in other chapters of this book.

Choosing the "right" level for supplemental oxygen has been complicated by a lack of information on appropriate targets—S_pO_2, cytochrome *aa* 3—and monitoring of oxygen delivery, and by a shifting definition of BPD, originally defined by oxygen use rather than a specific clinical constellation. Recent efforts have been made to more narrowly define short- and long-term criteria defining BPD (36). Arbitrary limitation of supplemental oxygen >40 years ago, in an attempt to avoid retinopathy associated with unfettered oxygen use, unexpectedly increased mortality and neurocognitive impairment among sick newborns. Preclinical studies aimed at optimizing oxygen therapy to prevent BPD have been hampered by the complex problem of matching the oxidative stress with the species- and developmental stage–dependent antioxidant repertoire, as well as the species-specific aspects of developmental lung biology. Recent clinical trials aimed at optimizing oxygen therapy to avoid retinopathy of prematurity revealed significant effects of lowered supplemental oxygen exposure on the incidence of pulmonary complications of prematurity that included BPD (37).

Even relatively brief exposures to oxidative stress may have permanent effects on lung function. A series of cohort studies of children with relatively mild oxygen exposure, but who were born prematurely, had significant long-term decrements of airflow compared with non-oxygen-exposed cases at similar gestational ages (38). Whether these effects were mediated by impaired alveolar development is unknown.

IV. Oxidative Stress: Endogenous

Reducing exogenous ROS may be partly under the control of physicians trying to prevent BPD, but endogenously generated ROS are less prone to manipulation, and are used in a variety of biological functions. Low levels of superoxide are produced by NADPH oxidases (*NOX 1-3*) in nonphagocytic cells such as smooth muscle and vascular endothelium. Hydrogen peroxide is produced by SODs and by so-called dual oxidases (*DUOX 1, 2*) and *NOX 4* in epithelial cells (39). Reactive oxygen intermediates are used in signal transduction for the actions of growth factors, cytokines and calcium signaling, and in the regulation of nitric oxide bioavailability, among others (40).

Relatively high levels of superoxide are generated by NADPH oxidase in professional phagocytes, neutrophils and macrophages, at ~ 1000-fold higher levels in neutrophils than in nonphagocytes. Blocking neutrophil influx in hyperoxia-exposed newborn rats abrogates oxidative DNA damage (41), hydroxyl radical formation (42), superoxide accumulation (43), and protects alveolar development (43,44). In experimental lung injury models, genetic ablation of NADPH oxidase routinely reduces pulmonary ROS accumulation (45,46). Indirect evidence correlates high levels of neutrophils or neutrophil chemokine IL-8 in tracheal aspirates of babies with respiratory distress syndrome correlated with an increased risk to develop BPD (47).

Physiological generation of ROS or generation of ROS in association with inflammation can become pathological when increases occur in the presence of limited or impaired antioxidant defenses, generating oxidative stress. The burden of ROS can be further amplified by the presence of free metals like iron, copper, and manganese. Free iron has been documented in the circulating plasma of preterm newborns (15,48), but a role for free iron, or metals in general in BPD, if any, is yet to be firmly established. On the other hand, indirect evidence has linked the presence of free iron in association with increased protein carbonyls of patients treated with high supplemental oxygen. Failure to handle iron to maintain its sequestration/storage could be a developmental liability in premature babies with relative deficiencies in iron carriers like ceruloplasmin (49).

V. ROS and RNS: Interdependence

Nitric oxide (•NO)-mediated effects on BPD must be considered in the context of the local redox milieu, since NO and its higher order nitrogen oxides, as well as RNS, have been implicated in the pathogenesis of BPD: both alter biomolecular structure and function. The premature newborn at risk to develop BPD has demonstrated relative "deficiencies" in ROS detoxification and NO generation compared with term newborns or adults. To understand the mechanisms and design successful adaptive strategies aimed at preventing and treating BPD, it is necessary to understand how and where ROS and RNS are generated in newborns at risk to develop BPD, and to recognize that the timing and location of the generation of nitrogen oxides and ROS will have interdependent effects on their respective biological impacts (5). Superoxide and nitric oxide react at nearly diffusion limited rates to form peroxynitrite (6), so local generation of superoxide and nitric oxide in proximity will destroy NO biological activities that are mediated via effects on binding to the heme Fe(II) of guanylyl cyclase or the formation of *S*-nitrosothiols, increasingly recognized to be critical to a number of pathways important to pulmonary homeostasis, like airway tone (7) and modulation of inflammation (8).

Hydrogen peroxide–dependent processes, which can depend on dismutation of superoxide, could also be affected. It is therefore critical to the understanding of the role of these reactive species that the location and the relative abundances of NO and superoxide accumulation are assessed. These in turn will be influenced by the cellular, subcellular, and developmental stage–specific expression of NO synthases and antioxidant enzymes.

VI. Nitrosative Stress

A. Endogenous NO Formation

The potential for adverse RNS formation hinges on the developmental and disease-specific effects on endogenous NO production. NO is generated by several cell types using one or more of three isoforms of nitric oxide synthase: NOS1 (neuronal NOS), NOS2 (inducible NOS, iNOS), and NOS3 (endothelial NOS, eNOS). Human autopsy studies do not demonstrate gestational age-dependent effects on pulmonary NOS isoform abundance (50). Late gestation baboon lung contains all three NOS isoforms, with expression of each being greatest in the proximal airway epithelia (51). Increases in NOS2 activity (52) are shown during the development of BPD in baboons, and increased NOS2 expression has been shown in humans that developed BPD (50).

Endogenous production of NO may be limited by arginase that controls L-arginine, the indispensable substrate for NOSs. In vitro effects of NO inactivation of nuclear factor kappa B (NF-κB), which is critical to inflammation, are arginase dependent (53). Oxidative stress in immature newborn rats impairs airway smooth muscle relaxation in part through effects on the arginase-NOS-cGMP signaling pathway (54).

Inflammation is a key pathway implicated in the pathogenesis of BPD, and in other systems, also linked with increased generation of NO and RNS in part through increased NOS2 activity. This has been investigated in detail in allergic asthma, but evidence linking direct nitrogen-oxygen adducts with the development of BPD is very limited.

Nitrogen Oxide Reactions

Endogenously generated NO or its products may react with a variety of physiological or pathological targets. It is useful to keep in mind the definitions of some NO-related reactions. *Nitrosylation* is the addition of nitric oxide (•NO), *nitrosation* is the addition of the nitroso group (NO), and *nitration* is the addition of the nitro group (NO₂). Each of these categories of reactions has "preferred" targets. Heme proteins tend to undergo addition of nitric oxide (nitrosylation); thiols tend to add a nitroso (NO) group (nitrosation forming RSNOs), and protein tyrosine residues and DNA bases can undergo addition of a nitro group (NO_2), resulting in nitration. Nitrite can be converted into more toxic species like nitrogen dioxide in the presence of catalysts like myeloperoxidase, which may be present in an inflammatory milieu (55). Among all the free radical reactions undergone by nitric oxide and its products, including peroxynitrite and nitrogen dioxide, the most frequent (>90%) are oxidation reactions.

Protein Nitration Targets and BPD

Among the reaction products formed, 3-nitrotyrosine is the one that has been most studied. This product of protein tyrosine nitration provides a useful biological footprint of peroxynitrite. The nitration pathways seemingly involve all reactions by carbonate radicals and/or oxo-metal complexes causing oxidation of tyrosine to tyrosyl radical. This step is followed by a diffusion-limited reaction of nitrogen dioxide with the tyrosyl radical, resulting in nitrotyrosine formation. Nitrogen dioxide alone is inefficient in nitrotyrosine formation because it must first form tyrosyl radical from tyrosine, a slow process (56). Even in inflammation, nitrotyrosine is a rare event, affecting ~ 5 per 10,000 residues. Nevertheless, elevations of 3-nitrotyrosine in a number of compartments have been shown in clinical and pre-clinical studies of BPD (57–59).

The relevance of peroxynitrite formation to the evolution of CLD is difficult to disentangle. A few targets relevant to BPD that have shown nitration-dependent functional effects include SOD2 (60) and SOD3 (61). Others, such as nitration of surfactant protein A, while showing functional effects, are harder to link to the pathophysiology of BPD (62). Conditions that would disfavor nitration, such as treatment with exogenous NO or SOD, are likely to have effects through other pathways, such as the reduction of oxidative stress, or mitigation of inflammation.

Nitrite and nitrate anion effects on regulatory proteins have been proposed as yet another alternative pathway mediating NO-based pharmacological effects, since they can, under certain conditions, be "recycled" to form NO in vivo (63), particularly in hypoxic states. These pathways have been less extensively studied in models relevant to BPD. The relative contributions of the nitrogen-oxygen moieties have been difficult to disentangle because of the considerable challenges inherent in the analytical methods used to distinguish them.

Protein Nitrosation/Nitrosylation Targets and BPD

NO can react with the sulfur in cysteine residues positioned between acidic and basic amino acid residues to form S-nitrosothiol. This posttranslational protein modification has been linked to a number of processes relevant to lung biology (see Ref. 64 for review). One important S-nitrosothiol-dependent pathway of particular relevance to BPD is the activation of NF-κB. Inflammation is a central mechanism in the pathogenesis of BPD, and several pro-inflammatory cytokines and leukocyte chemokines are regulated through NF-κB-dependent pathways (65). Oxidative stress in hyperoxia-exposed newborn mice (66) and rats (67) increases NF-κB abundance. In vitro studies have shown that NO blocks NF-κB through S-nitrosothiol modifications of components required for activation of the NF-κB pathway (see Ref. 68 for review). It may be that oxidative stress inactivates endogenous NO via peroxynitrite formation and therefore allows NF-κB activation. Indirectly supplementing S-nitrosothiol formation through treatment with ethyl nitrite, which forms nitrosonium, $^+$NO $\longleftrightarrow$ HONO + H$^+$ (69), rather than $^•$NO, blocked NF-κB activation and prevented adverse hyperoxia effects in a newborn rat model of BPD (67).

Other systems that are relevant to BPD, in which S-nitrosation has been implicated include the antioxidant system (70) and apoptosis (71,72). Indeed, S-nitrosation and denitrosylation have been proposed as an analog to the more familiar phosphorylation-dephosphorylation scheme of enzyme activity regulation (73). How these reactions proceed in vivo and under which conditions remains to be established.

Lipid Nitration Products and BPD

Compared with protein modifications, lipid modifications by nitrogen oxides/nitrosative stress have been relatively less well understood. Unsaturated fatty acids undergo nitration via homolytic addition of NO$_2$ to the double bond, resulting in the formation of a variety of regio- and stereoisomers (74). Fatty acid nitroalkene derivatives reversibly form adducts with nucleophilic targets, such as protein cysteine and histidine residues, resulting in posttranslational modification of proteins. Oleic acid-NO$_2$ is a strong, dose-dependent activator for peroxisome proliferator–activated receptors (PPARs), most potently affecting PPAR-γ. Nitrolinoleic acid is present in blood of healthy individuals at about 500 nM and is a highly potent ligand for PPAR-γ, exceeding the potency of other endogenous PPAR agonists (75). Nitrolinoleic acid also activates the transcription factor, nuclear factor-erythroid 2-related factor (Nrf-2), and antioxidant-responsive element-driven gene activation by impairing Kelch-like ACH-associating protein 1 (Keap-1) (76). The Nrf-2 system is better known for its ability to upregulate expression of a variety of antioxidant enzymes and proteins. This relatively new family of nitric oxide lipid adducts is thus linked to a host of effects pertaining to cell differentiation, proliferation and signaling, anti-inflammation, and antioxidant defense. The potential actions of these compounds in BPD have not yet been reported.

B. Exogenous NO: Friend or Foe?

Inhaled NO gas is by far the best-studied exogenous source of nitrosative stress relevant to BPD (77). The rationale and evidence for and against its clinical use for the prevention of BPD is considered elsewhere in this book. Clinical studies have focused on minimizing the exposure to higher order nitrogen oxides, particularly NO$_2$, and delivery systems have been designed to monitor and minimize NO$_2$ exposure. As noted above, it is expected that the toxicities associated with exogenous NO gas treatment will depend on the local redox state, concentration of the nitrogen:oxygen moieties, and on the cumulative effects of NO exposure and the stability of its downstream reaction products.

Direct evidence of toxicity attributable to inhaled NO in the context of clinical BPD is scant. Methemoglobinemia (>4 g/dL), which results from NO-dependent oxidation of hemoglobin, was rarely reported in two large clinical trials (78,79). A few studies have identified the formation of 3-nitrotyrosine in patients at risk to develop BPD or with established BPD, as noted above, whether this signifies NO-driven toxicity is not clear (57). In contrast, treatment with inhaled nitric oxide does not increase 3-nitrotyrosine, whether in adult mice (80) or newborn rats (67) exposed to hyperoxia. The adverse effects, if any, of inhaled NO at currently used clinical doses are likely attributable to direct pharmacological effects rather than nitrosative stress/RNS per se.

Some of the "off target" effects of inhaled/exogenous NO or NO equivalents may depend on *S*-nitrosothiol uptake. The delivered "dose" of inhaled NO gas may also depend on other mechanisms besides diffusion. While NO gas has the theoretical capacity to diffuse easily across cell membranes, inhaled NO must first traverse the gauntlet of the air-liquid interface in the alveoli, including high levels of GSH with which it may react. The biological effects of NO may require breaching a second potential barrier, the amino acid transport system. Recent studies have described the dependence of exogenous NO signaling in some conditions on the transport of NO as an *S*-nitrosothiol through L-type amino acid transporters in vitro (81). Similar findings have been recently reported in rat alveolar epithelial cells (82), and a preliminary report showed parallel results in rat type I alveolar epithelium exposed to NO gas at air-liquid interface (83). It is not known whether the L-type amino acid transporters or other peptide transporters govern downstream biological effects attributed to NO signaling, but it is possible that *S*-nitrosothiol-dependent processes, including toxicities, could be dependent on the expression and function of these transport systems.

VII. Summary

Tightly controlled spatiotemporal regulation of endogenous ROS and RNS production in mammalian lung can be disrupted by premature birth, which overwhelms under-developed enzymatic and nonenzymatic antioxidants. Cellular injury that generates persistent maladaptive inflammation adds to the ROS/RNS burden, which can impair normal reciprocal signaling pathways among the cells in pulmonary alveoli. Clinical strategies that have aimed at reducing oxygen exposure or augmenting antioxidant capacity have had the best short-term success. Long-term, permanent effects on lung function among children exposed to relatively modest oxidative stress underscore the need to understand the challenges posed by ROS/RNS during vulnerable periods of lung development.

References

1. Solberg R, Andresen JH, Escrig R, et al. Resuscitation of hypoxic newborn piglets with oxygen induces a dose-dependent increase in markers of oxidation. Pediatr Res 2007; 62:559–563.
2. Syrkina O, Jafari B, Hales CA, et al. Oxidant stress mediates inflammation and apoptosis in ventilator-induced lung injury. Respirology 2008; 13:333–340.
3. Ridnour LA, Thomas DD, Mancardi D, et al. The chemistry of nitrosative stress induced by nitric oxide and reactive nitrogen oxide species. Putting perspective on stressful biological situations. Biol Chem 2004; 385:1–10.
4. Cheah FC, Jobe AH, Moss TJ, et al. Oxidative stress in fetal lambs exposed to intra-amniotic endotoxin in a chorioamnionitis model. Pediatr Res 2008; 63:274–279.
5. Lang JD, McArdle PJ, O'Reilly PJ, et al. Oxidant-antioxidant balance in acute lung injury. Chest 2002; 122:314S–320S.
6. Beckman JS, Koppenol WH. Nitric oxide, superoxide, and peroxynitrite: the good, the bad, and ugly. Am J Physiol 1996; 271:C1424–C1437.

7. Gaston B, Sears S, Woods J, et al. Bronchodilator S-nitrosothiol deficiency in asthmatic respiratory failure. Lancet 1998; 351:1317–1319.
8. Marshall HE, Stamler JS. Inhibition of NF-kappa B by S-nitrosylation. Biochemistry 2001; 40:1688–1693.
9. Frank L, Sosenko IR. Prenatal development of lung antioxidant enzymes in four species. J Pediatr 1987; 110:106–110.
10. Frank L, Groseclose EE. Preparation for birth into an O_2-rich environment: the antioxidant enzymes in the developing rabbit lung. Pediatr Res 1984; 18:240–244.
11. Tanswell AK, Freeman BA. Pulmonary antioxidant enzyme maturation in the fetal and neonatal rat. I. Developmental profiles. Pediatr Res 1984; 18:584–587.
12. Walther FJ, Wade AB, Warburton D, et al. Ontogeny of antioxidant enzymes in the fetal lamb lung. Exp Lung Res 1991; 17:39–45.
13. Asikainen TM, White CW. Pulmonary antioxidant defenses in the preterm newborn with respiratory distress and bronchopulmonary dysplasia in evolution: implications for antioxidant therapy. Antioxid Redox Signal 2004; 6:155–167.
14. Asikainen TM, White CW. Antioxidant defenses in the preterm lung: role for hypoxia-inducible factors in BPD? Toxicol Appl Pharmacol 2005; 203:177–188.
15. Saugstad OD. Bronchopulmonary dysplasia-oxidative stress and antioxidants. Semin Neonatol 2003; 8:39–49.
16. Frank L, Sosenko IR. Failure of premature rabbits to increase antioxidant enzymes during hyperoxic exposure: increased susceptibility to pulmonary oxygen toxicity compared with term rabbits. Pediatr Res 1991; 29:292–296.
17. Morton RL, Das KC, Guo XL, et al. Effect of oxygen on lung superoxide dismutase activities in premature baboons with bronchopulmonary dysplasia. Am J Physiol 1999; 276:L64–L74.
18. Nozik-Grayck E, Dieterle CS, Piantadosi CA, et al. Secretion of extracellular superoxide dismutase in neonatal lungs. Am J Physiol 2000; 279:L977–L984.
19. Auten RL, O'Reilly MA, Oury TD, et al. Transgenic extracellular superoxide dismutase protects postnatal alveolar epithelial proliferation and development during hyperoxia. Am J Physiol 2006; 290:L32–L40.
20. Ahmed MN, Suliman HB, Folz RJ, et al. Extracellular superoxide dismutase protects lung development in hyperoxia-exposed newborn mice. Am J Respir Crit Care Med 2003; 167:400–405.
21. Schremmer B, Manevich Y, Feinstein SI, et al. Peroxiredoxins in the lung with emphasis on peroxiredoxin VI. Subcell Biochem 2007; 44:317–344.
22. Rhee SG, Chae HZ, Kim K. Peroxiredoxins: a historical overview and speculative preview of novel mechanisms and emerging concepts in cell signaling. Free Radic Biol Med 2005; 38:1543–1552.
23. Das KC, Pahl PM, Guo XL, et al. Induction of peroxiredoxin gene expression by oxygen in lungs of newborn primates. Am J Respir cell Mol Biol 2001; 25:226–232.
24. Das KC, Guo XL, White CW. Induction of thioredoxin and thioredoxin reductase gene expression in lungs of newborn primates by oxygen. Am J Physiol 1999; 276:L530–L539.
25. Dickinson DA, Forman HJ. Cellular glutathione and thiols metabolism. Biochem Pharmacol 2002; 64:1019–1026.
26. White CW, Stabler SP, Allen RH, et al. Plasma cysteine concentrations in infants with respiratory distress. J Pediatr 1994; 125:769–777.
27. Stabler SP, Morton RL, Winski SL, et al. Effects of parenteral cysteine and glutathione feeding in a baboon model of severe prematurity. Am J Clin Nutr 2000; 72:1548–1557.
28. Phelps DL. The role of vitamin E therapy in high-risk neonates. Clin Perinatol 1988; 15:955–963.
29. Massaro GD, Massaro D, Chambon P. Retinoic acid receptor-alpha regulates pulmonary alveolus formation in mice after, but not during, perinatal period. Am J Physiol 2003; 284: L431–L433.

30. Darlow BA, Graham PJ. Vitamin A supplementation to prevent mortality and short and long-term morbidity in very low birthweight infants. Cochrane Database Syst Rev 2007: CD000501.
31. Yang F, Friedrichs WE, Coalson JJ. Regulation of transferrin gene expression during lung development and injury. Am J Physiol 1997; 273:L417–L426.
32. Beckman JS, Beckman TW, Chen J, et al. Apparent hydroxyl radical production by peroxynitrite: implications for endothelial injury from nitric oxide and superoxide. Proc Natl Acad Sci U S A 1990; 87:1620–1624.
33. Buss IH, Darlow BA, Winterbourn CC. Elevated protein carbonyls and lipid peroxidation products correlating with myeloperoxidase in tracheal aspirates from premature infants. Pediatr Res 2000; 47:640–645.
34. Pitkanen OM, Hallman M, Andersson SM. Correlation of free oxygen radical-induced lipid peroxidation with outcome in very low birth weight infants. J Pediatr 1990; 116:760–764.
35. Welty SE. Is oxidant stress in the causal pathway to bronchopulmonary dysplasia? Neo-Reviews 2000; 6:e1–e6.
36. Ehrenkranz RA, Walsh MC, Vohr BR, et al. Validation of the National Institutes of Health consensus definition of bronchopulmonary dysplasia. Pediatrics 2005; 116:1353–1360.
37. GROUP S-RS. Supplemental Therapeutic Oxygen for Prethreshold Retinopathy of Pre-maturity (STOP-ROP), a randomized, controlled trial. I: Primary outcomes. Pediatrics 2000; 105:295–310.
38. Halvorsen T, Skadberg BT, Eide GE, et al. Pulmonary outcome in adolescents of extreme preterm birth: a regional cohort study. Acta Paediatr 2004; 93:1294–1300.
39. van der Vliet A. NADPH oxidases in lung biology and pathology: host defense enzymes, and more. Free Rad Biol Med 2008; 44:938–955.
40. Lambeth JD. Nox enzymes, ROS, and chronic disease: an example of antagonistic pleiotropy. Free Rad Biol Med 2007; 43:332–347.
41. Auten RL, Whorton MH, Nicholas Mason S. Blocking neutrophil influx reduces DNA damage in hyperoxia-exposed newborn rat lung. Am J Respir Cell Mol Biol 2002; 26:391–397.
42. Liao L, Ning Q, Li Y, et al. CXCR2 blockade reduces radical formation in hyperoxia-exposed newborn rat lung. Pediatr Res 2006; 60:299–303.
43. Yi M, Jankov RP, Belcastro R, et al. Opposing effects of 60% oxygen and neutrophil influx on alveologenesis in the neonatal rat. Am J Respir Crit Care Med 2004; 170:1188–1196.
44. Auten RL Jr., Mason SN, Tanaka DT, et al. Anti-neutrophil chemokine preserves alveolar development in hyperoxia-exposed newborn rats. Am J Physiol 2001; 281:L336–L344.
45. Gao XP, Standiford TJ, Rahman A, et al. Role of NADPH oxidase in the mechanism of lung neutrophil sequestration and microvessel injury induced by gram-negative sepsis: studies in p47phox-/- and gp91phox-/- mice. J Immunol 2002; 168:3974–3982.
46. Yao H, Edirisinghe I, Yang SR, et al. Genetic ablation of NADPH oxidase enhances sus-ceptibility to cigarette smoke-induced lung inflammation and emphysema in mice. Am J Pathol 2008; 172:1222–1237.
47. Kotecha S, Chan B, Azam N, et al. Increase in interleukin-8 and soluble intercellular adhesion molecule-1 in bronchoalveolar lavage fluid from premature infants who develop chronic lung disease. Arch Dis Child 1995; 72:F90–F96.
48. Evans PJ, Evans R, Kovar IZ, et al. Bleomycin-detectable iron in the plasma of premature and full-term neonates. FEBS Lett 1992; 303:210–212.
49. Lindeman JH, Lentjes EG, van Zoeren-Grobben D, et al. Postnatal changes in plasma cer-uloplasmin and transferrin antioxidant activities in preterm babies. Biol Neonate 2000; 78:73–76.
50. Sheffield M, Mabry S, Thibeault DW, et al. Pulmonary nitric oxide synthases and nitro-tyrosine: findings during lung development and in chronic lung disease of prematurity. Pediatrics 2006; 118:1056–1064.

51. Shaul PW, Afshar S, Gibson LL, et al. Developmental changes in nitric oxide synthase isoform expression and nitric oxide production in fetal baboon lung. Am J Physiol 2002; 283: L1192–L1199.

52. Afshar S, Gibson LL, Yuhanna IS, et al. Pulmonary NO synthase expression is attenuated in a fetal baboon model of chronic lung disease. Am J Physiol 2003; 284:L749–L758.

53. Ckless K, van der Vliet A, Janssen-Heininger Y. Oxidative-nitrosative stress and post-translational protein modifications: implications to lung structure-function relations. Arginase modulates NF-kappaB activity via a nitric oxide-dependent mechanism. Am J Respir Cell Mol Biol 2007; 36:645–653.

54. Sopi RB, Haxhiu MA, Martin RJ, et al. Disruption of NO-cGMP signaling by neonatal hyperoxia impairs relaxation of lung parenchyma. Am J Physiol 2007; 293:L1029–L1036.

55. Eiserich JP, Hristova M, Cross CE, et al. Formation of nitric oxide-derived inflammatory oxidants by myeloperoxidase in neutrophils. Nature 1998; 391:393–397.

56. Radi R. Nitric oxide, oxidants, and protein tyrosine nitration. Proc Natl Acad Sci U S A 2004; 101:4003–4008.

57. Lorch SA, Banks BA, Christie J, et al. Plasma 3-nitrotyrosine and outcome in neonates with severe bronchopulmonary dysplasia after inhaled nitric oxide. Free Radic Biol Med 2003; 34:1146–1152.

58. Banks BA, Seri I, Ischiropoulos H, et al. Changes in oxygenation with inhaled nitric oxide in severe bronchopulmonary dysplasia. Pediatrics 1999; 103:610–618.

59. Banks BA, Ischiropoulos H, McClelland M, et al. Plasma 3-nitrotyrosine is elevated in premature infants who develop bronchopulmonary dysplasia. Pediatrics 1998; 101:870–874.

60. Demicheli V, Quijano C, Alvarez B, et al. Inactivation and nitration of human superoxide dismutase (SOD) by fluxes of nitric oxide and superoxide. Free Radic Biol Med 2007; 42:1359–1368.

61. Mamo LB, Suliman HB, Giles BL, et al. Discordant extracellular superoxide dismutase expression and activity in neonatal hyperoxic lung. Am J Respir Crit Care Med 2004; 170: 313–318.

62. Zhu S, Haddad IY, Matalon S. Nitration of surfactant protein A (SP-A) tyrosine residues results in decreased mannose binding ability. Arch Biochem Biophys 1996; 333:282–290.

63. Lundberg JO, Weitzberg E, Gladwin MT. The nitrate-nitrite-nitric oxide pathway in physiology and therapeutics. Nat Rev 2008; 7:156–167.

64. Gaston B, Singel D, Doctor A, et al. S-nitrosothiol signaling in respiratory biology. Am J Respir Crit Care Med 2006; 173:1186–1193.

65. Park GY, Christman JW. Nuclear factor kappa B is a promising therapeutic target in inflammatory lung disease. Curr Drug Targets 2006; 7:661–668.

66. Yang G, Abate A, George AG, et al. Maturational differences in lung NF-kappaB activation and their role in tolerance to hyperoxia. J Clin Invest 2004; 114:669–678.

67. Auten RL, Mason SN, Whorton MH, et al. Inhaled ethyl nitrite prevents hyperoxia-impaired postnatal alveolar development in newborn rats. Am J Respir Crit Care Med 2007; 176: 291–299.

68. Marshall HE, Hess DT, Stamler JS. S-nitrosylation: physiological regulation of NF-kappaB. Proc Natl Acad Sci U S A 2004; 101:8841–8842.

69. Moya MP, Gow AJ, McMahon TJ, et al. S-nitrosothiol repletion by an inhaled gas regulates pulmonary function. Proc Natl Acad Sci U S A 2001; 98:5792–5797.

70. Foster MW, Stamler JS. New insights into protein S-nitrosylation. Mitochondria as a model system. J Biol Chem 2004; 279:25891–25897.

71. Benhar M, Forrester MT, Hess DT, et al. Regulated protein denitrosylation by cytosolic and mitochondrial thioredoxins. Science 2008; 320:1050–1054.

72. Benhar M, Stamler JS. A central role for S-nitrosylation in apoptosis. Nat Cell Biol 2005; 7:645–646.

73. Hess DT, Matsumoto A, Kim SO, et al. Protein S-nitrosylation: purview and parameters. Nat Rev Mol Cell Biol 2005; 6:150–166.
74. Freeman BA, Baker PR, Schopfer FJ, et al. Nitro-fatty acid formation and signaling. J Biol Chem 2008; 283:15515–15519.
75. Schopfer FJ, Lin Y, Baker PR, et al. Nitrolinoleic acid: an endogenous peroxisome proliferator-activated receptor gamma ligand. Proc Natl Acad Sci U S A 2005; 102:2340–2345.
76. Villacorta L, Zhang J, Garcia-Barrio MT, et al. Nitro-linoleic acid inhibits vascular smooth muscle cell proliferation via the Keap1/Nrf2 signaling pathway. Am J Physiol Heart Circ Physiol 2007; 293:H770—H776.
77. Barrington KJ, Finer NN. Inhaled nitric oxide for preterm infants: a systematic review. Pediatrics 2007; 120:1088–1099.
78. Ballard RA, Truog WE, Cnaan A, et al. Inhaled nitric oxide in preterm infants undergoing mechanical ventilation. N Engl J Med 2006; 355:343–353.
79. Kinsella JP, Cutter GR, Walsh WF, et al. Early inhaled nitric oxide therapy in premature newborns with respiratory failure. N Engl J Med 2006; 355:354–364.
80. Lorch SA, Foust R III, Gow A, et al. Immunohistochemical localization of protein 3-nitrotyrosine and S-nitrosocysteine in a murine model of inhaled nitric oxide therapy. Pediatr Res 2000; 47:798–805.
81. Li S, Whorton AR. Functional characterization of two S-nitroso-L-cysteine transporters, which mediate movement of NO equivalents into vascular cells. Am J Physiol Cell Physiol 2007; 292:C1263–C1271.
82. Granillo OM, Brahmajothi MV, Li S, et al. Pulmonary alveolar epithelial uptake of S-nitrosothiols is regulated by L-type amino acid transporter. Am J Physiol 2008; 295: L38–L43.
83. Auten RL, Brahmajothi MV, Mason SN. L-type amino acid transporter regulates nitric oxide gas uptake by type 1 & 2 rat alveolar epithelium and alveolar macrophages. E-PAS 2008; 43304.

6

Prenatal Inflammation and Immune Responses of the Preterm Lung

SUHAS KALLAPUR and ALAN H. JOBE
University of Cincinnati, Cincinnati, Ohio, U.S.A.

BORIS W. KRAMER
Academisch Ziekenhuis Maastricht, Maastricht, The Netherlands

I. Bronchopulmonary Dysplasia and the Fetal Lung: An Overview

Bronchopulmonary dysplasia (BPD) results from acute and chronic interactions between lung developmental, injury, and repair pathways that interfere with airspace septation and microvascular development. The major postnatal associations with BPD in very low birth weight infants are supplemental oxygen, mechanical ventilation, sepsis, and patent ductus arteriosis (1). Other variables that are less defined clinically, but that cause BPD-type changes in animal models, are corticosteroids and nutritional deficiency (2,3). Our thesis is that prenatal exposures can inform us about postnatal associations with BPD. Postnatal associations such as oxygen and mechanical ventilation are complex and interdependent, and similarities with and differences from prenatal exposures can provide some insights into the pathophysiology of BPD. Preterm infants are not born with BPD, but clinical information supports prenatal events as promoting progression to BPD after very preterm birth, suggesting a sequential hit pathophysiology. Studies of prenatal exposures in animal models that may promote BPD are in their infancy compared with postnatal lung injury studies of the pathogenesis of BPD. Our goal is to link prenatal exposures with airway septation abnormalities and abnormal microvascular development.

II. Clinical Associations with BPD

A. Chorioamnionitis: The Syndromes

Fetal exposures to infectious agents are relatively common and are associated with specific syndromes (e.g., congenital cytomegalovirus or toxoplasmosis) that do not result in BPD. The acute chorioamnionitis frequently encountered in late preterm or term deliveries may be caused by highly pathogenic organisms and is associated with sepsis and pneumonia syndromes, but not BPD. When organisms such as *Escherichia coli* or group B streptococcus do infect the preterm fetus, stillbirth or severe sepsis/pneumonia is the likely outcome (4). We will focus on the more frequent occurrence of the chorioamnionitis that is highly associated with very preterm labor, rupture of membranes, and preterm delivery (5). Clinical chorioamnionitis is diagnosed by maternal findings such as fever, elevated white blood count, and uterine tenderness associated with preterm labor. These clinical findings occur in perhaps 10% to 20% of deliveries prior to 32 weeks' gestation and are quite nonspecific. However, 50% or more of infants delivered prior to 32-week gestational age have been exposed to a chronic and asymptomatic inflammation, and the frequency of exposure increases as gestational age decreases (6). This asymptomatic inflammation can be detected by increased white blood cells or cytokines such as interleukin-6 (IL-6) in amniotic fluid, by positive bacterial culture or polymerase chain reaction (PCR) for organisms in amniotic fluid, by white cells in the chorioamnion after delivery (histologic chorioamnionitis), by white blood cell infiltration of the fetal cord (funisitis), or by elevations of cytokines such as IL-6 in the cord blood (7). Funisitis and elevated IL-6 in cord blood are thought to reflect direct fetal involvement with inflammation, termed the fetal inflammatory response syndrome (8). There is no uniform or satisfactory diagnostic approach to this indolent chorioamnionitis associated with prematurity because each evaluation will identify overlapping, but distinct, patient populations. Amniotic fluids are most often positive for *Ureaplasma* or *Mycoplasma*, but amniotic fluid may be culture positive for multiple other low pathogenic organisms or there may be more than one organism identified (9,10). The fetal inflammatory response syndrome indicates fetal inflammation, and although this diagnosis can be made retrospectively by pathology of the cord or cord plasma IL-6 measurements, it is seldom made in clinical practice. A higher grade of histologic chorioamnionitis implies increased severity of inflammation. However, there is no good quantification of severity, location, or duration of fetal exposures. In clinical practice, specific organisms are not normally identified, nor is fetal exposure to inflammation assessed soon after birth.

The duration of fetal exposure is unknown in virtually all early gestation deliveries associated with inflammation. Endometrial cultures were positive for about 80% of nonpregnant women, and the percent positive was not different for women who had delivered very preterm or term infants in a prior pregnancy (11). These results suggest that the uterine cavity was not sterile at conception and during early embryonic development. In PCR studies with amniotic fluid from normal pregnancies sampled for genetic analysis at 15- to 19-week gestation, about 12% were positive for *Ureaplasma* and 6% for *Mycoplasma* (12–14). The majority of women with PCR-positive amniotic fluid did *not* deliver preterm. These results suggest that some pregnancies can carry organisms chronically without any apparent adverse effects. However, the association of very preterm delivery with organisms/infection is compelling (5). Diagnostic problems are the duration and range of fetal effects of these exposures. As many as 50% of very preterm deliveries are associated with *Ureaplasma* and *Mycoplasma*, and *Ureaplasma*-positive amniotic fluid had high IL-6 and white cell counts indicating robust inflammatory responses in the fetuses (15,16). Perhaps *Ureaplasma*, *Mycoplasma*, and other organisms are tolerated by some pregnancies whereas others have inflammatory responses. The diagnosis of the chorioamnionitis associated with preterm birth is imprecise in the extreme and generally does not contribute to clinical management because the diagnosis is either seldom made or made retrospectively.

B. Associations of Chorioamnionitis with the Preterm Lung

Given the limitations of the diagnosis of chorioamnionitis, the associations of cho-rioamnionitis with lung outcomes of preterm infants are problematic. There are multiple reports that preterm rupture of membranes is associated with less respiratory distress syndrome (RDS), and membrane rupture in preterms is a surrogate for chorioamnionitis (17). Watterberg et al. (18) reported in 1996 the counterintuitive observation that the *histologic* chorioamnionitis and increased proinflammatory mediators in tracheal aspi-rates soon after birth were associated with less RDS, but more BPD in *ventilated* preterm infants. However, others reported increased RDS following *clinical* chorioamnionitis (19), increased RDS with elevated levels of tumor necrosis factor α (TNF-α) in amniotic fluid (20), or increased IL-6 levels in cord blood (8). Two recent reports from the Alabama Preterm Birth Study illustrate the problem of definition of the populations at risk for the outcome RDS. RDS was decreased significantly in 446 consecutive deliv-eries at <32 weeks' gestation if there was histologic chorioamnionitis with neutrophils in the membranes, fetal plate, or cord (*p* values < 0.01) (21). However, for the 23% of the infants from the same population with cord blood cultures positive for *Ureaplasma*, RDS was not decreased (22). The clinical information is inconsistent about the asso-ciation of chorioamnionitis with decreased RDS, however diagnosed. RDS is also an imprecise diagnosis that can be altered by early postnatal management such as con-tinuous positive airway pressure or superimposed inflammation (23). An explanation for the inconsistency may be that severe inflammation can cause an Acute Respiratory Distress Syndrome that may be indistinguishable clinically from RDS, whereas less inflammation for the right interval may induce lung maturation and decrease RDS. The vagaries of the diagnosis of chorioamnionitis and RDS and variable clinical manage-ment of differing populations of infants confound the clinical correlations.

The diagnosis BPD has also been evaluated relative to chorioamnionitis in many studies, again with inconsistent outcomes. As noted earlier, Watterberg et al. (18) reported that histologic chorioamnionitis was associated with an increase in BPD. Yoon and colleagues found that BPD was increased for infants with amniotic fluid that con-tained increased TNF-α, IL-1β, and IL-8 (24). Fetal inflammatory response syndrome diagnosed by either funisitis or elevated cord blood levels of IL-6 also predicted more BPD in comparison to infants without signs of systemic inflammation (25–27). How-ever, BPD was not increased for infants exposed to histologic chorioamnionitis for the 446 consecutive preterm deliveries in the Alabama Preterm Delivery Study (21). Using the same delivery cohort, BPD was increased for infants with cord blood cultures positive for *Ureaplasma* (22). These variable associations likely are explained, in part, by postnatal interventions. Van Marter et al. (28) reported that histologic cho-rioamnionitis decreased the risk of BPD unless the infants were ventilated for more than seven days or had postnatal sepsis, which together with histologic chorioamnionitis increased the risk of BPD. Perhaps a more consistent observation is that the severity of the chorioamnionitis as graded histologically predicts the occurrence/severity of BPD (29). The difficulty remains the quantification of the severity and duration of cho-rioamnionitis, and the identification of the organisms associated with the prenatal inflammation. The lack of consistent associations of BPD with chorioamnionitis prob-ably just reflects the multifactorial etiology of BPD and the poorly refined diagnoses of chorioamnionitis and BPD.

C. Chorioamnionitis and Lung Inflammation in the Newborn

However diagnosed, chorioamnionitis has been associated with multiple indicators of inflammation in tracheal aspirates of preterm infants. Proinflammatory mediators in tracheal aspirates are increased on day 1 of life, following histologic chorioamnionitis (18). The converse is also true. Tracheal aspirate IL-8 levels on day 1 of life predicted histologic chorioamnionitis (30), and microbial colonization of tracheal aspirates were associated with increased proinflammatory mediators, neutrophils, and chemotactic activity (31). Inflammation in the lungs soon after birth indicates fetal exposure to inflammation, although this information is not routinely available clinically. The characteristics and extent of the inflammation have not been well quantified.

D. The Special Case of *Ureaplasma*

Ureaplasma serovars are the most frequent class of organisms associated with chorioamnionitis. The clinical reports linking *Ureaplasma* with BPD are not consistent, despite culture positivity representing a refining of the diagnosis of chorioamnionitis (22). A number of reports indicate no compelling association between *Ureaplasma* and BPD (32,33). In contrast, Colaizy et al. (34) detected *Ureaplasma* by PCR and, after controlling for confounding factors, reported an odds ratio of 4.2 for BPD and death in association with *Ureaplasma*. A recent meta-analysis of 23 studies found that *Ureaplasma* increased the risk for BPD defined as oxygen need at 28 days, and 8 studies showed a similar association for BPD defined as oxygen need at 36 weeks (35). A cautionary note was that the smaller studies showed larger effects than the larger studies. To further refine the analysis, Castro-Alcaraz et al. (36) carefully documented the patterns of colonization of preterm infants with *Ureaplasma* and found that culture positivity only after birth was not associated with BPD. In contrast, persistently positive *Ureaplasma* cultures were associated with BPD with an odds ratio of 34 by multivariant analysis. Prenatal treatments with antibiotics that should eradicate *Ureaplasma* or postnatal antibiotic treatments of infants with *Ureaplasma* have not been successful. The weight of evidence is that *Ureaplasma* colonization/infection of the fetal lung can increase the risk of BPD. We suspect that the variable outcomes reported clinically result from different serovars of the organism with different pathogenicities, an unknown and variable duration of fetal exposure prior to delivery, and postnatal exposures (oxygen, sepsis, and mechanical ventilation).

III. Proof of Principal: Animal Models

A. Lung Maturation

Animal models of fetal inflammation permit experimental control of the inflammatory mediator and the duration of exposure, and provide access to multiple tissues to explore what can occur after fetal exposures. These models imprecisely mimic chorioamnionitis in the human because the early phases of the development of the chronic asymptomatic chorioamnionitis that is associated with early preterm labor are just not understood. Although the effects of experimental inflammation on the fetus are striking, their implications for diseases of the preterm and long-term outcomes remain poorly defined (37). In studies of preterm labor, Bry et al. (38) noted that intra-amniotic injections of

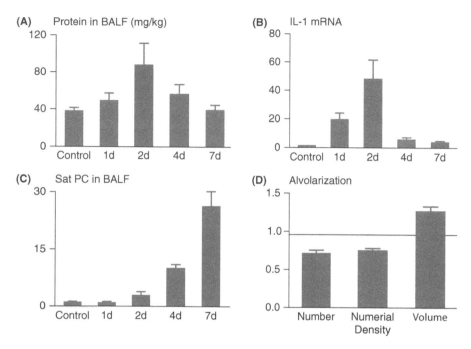

Figure 1 Inflammation, maturation, and alveolarization effects of intra-amniotic endotoxin on the fetal lung. Fetal sheep were exposed to intra-amniotic endotoxin for the intervals indicated on the horizontal axis prior to preterm delivery at 124 days' gestation. (**A**) Protein increases in BALF indicating injury at two days when (**B**) IL-1β mRNA is maximally expressed in the fetal lung. IL-1β mRNA values are expressed relative to a normalized control value of 1. (**C**) The amount of saturated phosphatidylcholine (Sat PC) increases in BALF indicating increased surfactant. Values are normalized to a control value of 1. (**D**) Morphometric measurements demonstrate decreased alveolarization as estimated by alveolar number, numerical density, and volume of the alveoli seven days after the intra-amniotic endotoxin. Values are expressed relative to the normalized controls of 1. *Abbreviation*: BALF, bronchoalveolar lavage fluid. *Source*: Data redrawn from Refs. 41, 60, and 66.

IL-1α into the amniotic fluid of rabbit fetuses caused lung maturation. Subsequently, the complex effects of inflammation on the fetal lungs have become apparent. Much of the focus of the research has been on the lung maturational effects of fetal exposure to inflammation. Intra-amniotic endotoxin, IL-1, or live *Ureaplasma* induced the surfactant protein mRNAs, and surfactant proteins increased in the fetal lung in parallel with increases in surfactant lipids (39–41) (Fig. 1). Fetal lung maturation occurred without increases in fetal plasma cortisol (40), but did not occur if the monocyte and neutrophil components of the inflammatory response to intra-amniotic endotoxin were blocked with an anti-CD-18 antibody (42). Maternal corticosteroid treatments augmented the functional lung maturation induced by intra-amniotic endotoxin (43). The lung maturation was induced when the inflammatory mediators were given by intra-amniotic injection or by fetal tracheal infusion five to seven days before the assessments (44,45).

The fetus responded to inflammation/chorioamnionitis at a very early gestational age. Intra-amniotic injections of endotoxin or live *Ureaplasma* at about 60-day gestational age resulted in increased surfactant at preterm delivery at 125 days' gestation (term is 150 days) (46,47). Endotoxin given between the uterine wall and the chorion did not induce chorioamnionitis or lung maturation (48). These results demonstrate that experimental intra-amniotic inflammation can cause fetal lung inflammation and induced lung maturation, which clinically should decrease the incidence and severity of RDS with preterm birth.

B. Septation Abnormalities

This inflammation-induced lung maturation at early gestational ages is not normal lung maturation. The lung inflammation is characterized by an increased expression of heat-shock protein 70 in the airways within hours, large increases in lung tissue expressions of IL-1β, IL-8, IP-10, and monocyte chemoattractant protein that peak at one to two days in association with increased protein in fetal lung fluid (fetal pulmonary edema/permeability abnormality) (49–51) (Fig. 1). Within seven days of the intra-amniotic endotoxin, the mesenchyme in the fetal lung decreases and the amount of potential airspace increases, but there are fewer and larger distal airspaces (alveoli and saccules), indicative of an arrest in septation (52). These changes also occur after a 28-day continuous infusion of endotoxin prior to preterm delivery (47). The effects of endotoxin exposure on elastin have not been assessed. The anatomic changes of inflammation-induced lung maturation in the fetus resemble a mild form of BPD. Antenatal corticosteroids cause a similar decreased septation in the fetal sheep (52).

The effects of proinflammatory mediators on the fetal lung seem to depend on developmental stage. In lung explants from preterm rabbits, IL-1 upregulated the expression of SP-A and SP-B, but IL-1, endotoxin, and TNF-α suppressed the surfactant proteins at term (53). Intra-amniotic endotoxin also increased the numbers of type II cells in fetal mouse lungs and their explants by a nuclear factor-kappa B (NF-κB)-dependent mechanism (54). As with the sheep, these maturational signals were accompanied by indicators of disrupted development. In mice, intra-amniotic endotoxin increased airspace luminal volume density, an effect that was also observed with explants in vitro as decreased distal airway branching (55). Inhibition of fibroblast growth factor-10 in mouse lung explants by the Toll-like receptor (TLR)-4 agonist endotoxin or a TLR2 agonist caused abnormal saccular airway morphogenesis and disrupted myofibroblast positioning (56). Epithelial overexpression of IL-1β in the fetal mouse lung disrupted alveolar septation and caused abnormal elastin deposition (57). The epithelial expression of proinflammatory mediators such as IL-6, TNF-α, and IL-13 during fetal development also caused inhibition of saccular septation and an emphysematous lung phenotype in transgenic mice (58). The observations are not uniformly congruent. For example, endotoxin disrupted septation in mouse lung explants (55), whereas it did not in sheep in vivo if inflammatory cell recruitment to the lungs was inhibited (42). Also, IL-1 caused septation abnormalities in mice that were not apparent with the intratracheal infusion of IL-1 in sheep (45). These differences may result from differences in dose, duration of exposure, or growth rates of the fetal lungs between species. However, the general conclusion is that the fetal lung inflammation from any source is associated with abnormal septation, the principal anatomic finding in the new BPD.

C.   Vascular Injury

Preterm infants with BPD have the arrest in airspace septation as well as decreased microvascular development that seems to track in parallel with the septation abnormalities (59). Vascularization abnormalities have not been evaluated as extensively as the septation abnormalities in animal models of fetal lung inflammation. However, chorioamnionitis does acutely interfere with lung microvascular development (Fig. 2). The lung inflammation caused by intra-amniotic endotoxin was associated with decreased eNOS protein expression in the pulmonary endothelium (60). Concurrently,

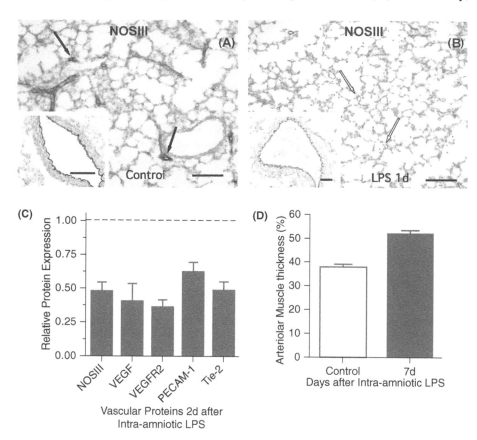

Figure 2   Intra-amniotic endotoxin-induced chorioamnionitis causes vascular injury in fetal lung. Preterm fetal sheep were given intra-amniotic endotoxin (LPS) and delivered one to seven days after exposures. NOSIII (eNOS) expression by immunohistology in (**A**) control and (**B**) one day after LPS. NOSIII expression decreased more in the distal vascular endothelium compared with pulmonary artery (compare panels A and B, inset shows pulmonary artery, *arrows* point to NOSIII in vascular endothelium). (**C**) Expression of vascular proteins by Western blot decreased two days after intra-amniotic LPS relative to control (*dashed line*). (**D**) Distal arteriolar smooth muscle thickness increased seven days after intra-amniotic LPS compared with controls. *Abbreviation*: LPS, lipopolysaccharide. *Source*: Data redrawn from Ref. 60.

vascular endothelial growth factor (VEGF) isoforms 165 and 188 decreased, as did platelet endothelial cell adhesion molecule-1, Tie-2, and VEGF-receptor 2. An increase in arteriolar thickness with increased adventitial fibrosis then became apparent. The potent cytokine inhibitor of vascular development IP-10 was expressed intensely in the bronchioles and vasculature (50). Another inhibitor of vascular development, monokine induced by interferon-γ (MIG), was highly expressed by the inflammatory cells that had been recruited to the fetal lungs. Connective tissue growth factor (CTGF) also is involved in angiogenesis and lung development. CTGF was markedly reduced in the lungs of chorioamnionitis-exposed animals, suggesting both alveolar and vascular injury, which may contribute to the anatomic changes of BPD (61). The endotoxin response by the fetal lung does not generate indicators of an oxidant injury until days after the initial inflammatory response (62). Inflammation of the fetal lungs results in an acute lung injury that includes vascular injury.

D. Fetal Models of *Ureaplasma*

The *Ureaplasma* associated with preterm labor and delivery may have been in the fetal compartment for months (5,12). Although infants exposed to *Ureaplasma* are not easily identified at birth, they do have an increased risk of BPD if colonization persists (34–36). Fetal baboons have been exposed to intra-amniotic injections of live *Ureaplasma* several days prior to preterm delivery (63). Animals that have persistent colonization with mechanical ventilation have more lung disease and inflammation at autopsy. The persistently colonized baboon lungs had more fibroses and profibrotic responses with elevated TGF-β (64). In more chronic models, fetal sheep exposed to live *Ureaplasma* at 80 days' gestation remain colonized at term (150 days) (39). Following intra-amniotic injections of live *Ureaplasma* at intervals from 3 to 10 weeks prior to preterm delivery, the lamb lung contains increased numbers of inflammatory cells, increased protein in the alveolar lavages, increased IL-8, and increased surfactant. Although the *Ureaplasma* is present in the lungs, they are minimally inflamed and their structures appear normal (46). Chronic colonization of the fetal sheep lung with *Ureaplasma* does not cause the lung structural changes of BPD. However, we anticipate that the fetal exposure may modulate postnatal lung responses to oxygen and mechanical ventilation.

E. Repeated Endotoxin Exposures

Clinical chorioamnionitis may be present for weeks or months prior to preterm delivery. While acute inflammatory exposures cause a mild BPD phenotype of decreased septation and vascular injury in the fetal sheep lung, chronic or repetitive exposures do not cause the progressive anatomic changes of BPD in fetal sheep models of chorioamnionitis. Fetal exposures to four weekly intra-amniotic doses of endotoxin or to a 28 days endotoxin infusion in the amniotic fluid at early gestation resulted in a low-grade persistent inflammation in the fetal lung and increased surfactant pools near term (65). However, no septation abnormalities or alterations of markers of vascular development persisted. The fetal lung can be injured and recovered with normal development despite persistent inflammation. Fetuses exposed to intra-amniotic endotoxin had normal lung function and anatomy at two months of age (66). Therefore, the fetal lung has a remarkable ability to adapt to chronic chorioamnionitis/inflammation without progressive injury. In contrast, overexpression of proinflammatory cytokines in fetal mouse lungs does disrupt saccular septation, which persists after birth (57,58). However, this focal epithelial overexpression does not reflect the clinical syndrome of chronic, indolent chorioamnionitis.

IV. Immune Modulation in the Fetus

The ability of the fetal lung to suppress progressive inflammation despite persistent (and presumably increasing) inflammatory mediators in amniotic fluid in clinical cho-rioamnionitis provokes a number of questions about fetal inflammatory responses. The fetal lung has a brisk inflammatory cytokine response to intra-amniotic endotoxin that disappears by about four days (67). Monocytes and neutrophils are recruited to the fetal lung tissue and airspaces, but not in the large numbers characteristic of a pneumonic response. This initial inflammatory response must differ from what occurs in the mature postnatal lung because the sentinel inflammatory cell, the alveolar macrophage, is not in the fetal lung and the monocytes that are present are immature and respond poorly to challenge with TLR agonists, IL-1, or TNF-α (68,69). Also, the fetal lung lacks or has very low amounts of modulators of inflammatory responses such as lysosome, SP-A, SP-D, and lipopolysaccharide (LPS)-binding protein.

We think that proinflammatory mediators such as endotoxin or IL-1 in amniotic fluid initiate lung inflammation via signaling by the epithelium of the airspace. The innate immune responses to that initial inflammatory response are profound. Following intra-amniotic endotoxin or IL-1, the fetal airspaces that were essentially free of inflammatory cells now contain large numbers of neutrophils and increasing numbers of immature monocytes (51). The fetal lung monocytes that were unresponsive prior to proin-flammatory exposure become as responsive by seven days to endotoxin challenge in vitro as alveolar macrophages from adult sheep (70). The fetal lung expresses granulocyte macrophage colony-stimulating factor (GM-CSF), and fetal neutrophils and monocytes express PU.1 indicating maturation (69) (Fig. 3). The alveolar monocytes have trans-formed their appearance to alveolar macrophages in seven days. The same functional maturation occurs for blood monocytes. Therefore, fetal exposure to endotoxin induces maturation of immature monocytes to become responsive alveolar macrophages. There are simultaneous increases in modulator proteins such as endotoxin-binding protein, SP-A, and SP-D.

This maturation of immature monocytes to functional monocytes/alveolar mac-rophages could prime the lung for progressive inflammation. However, a second dose of intra-amniotic endotoxin given five days after the first dose with assessment two days later causes no increase in proinflammatory cytokines and no increase in recruitment of inflammatory cells in the fetal lungs (37). When challenged with endotoxin in vitro, both blood monocytes and lung monocytes/macrophages are again unresponsive with low secretion of IL-6 and TNF-α (Fig. 4). These cells are now in a state of endotoxin tolerance, although the initial endotoxin dose had matured their ability to respond. This remarkable result also occurs if the second in vivo endotoxin dose was given seven days after the initial dose and the assessment was done seven days later (70). These endotoxin tolerance responses seem to be mediated by downregulation of IRAK-4 and upregulation of IRAK-M to modulate NF-κB signaling (37).

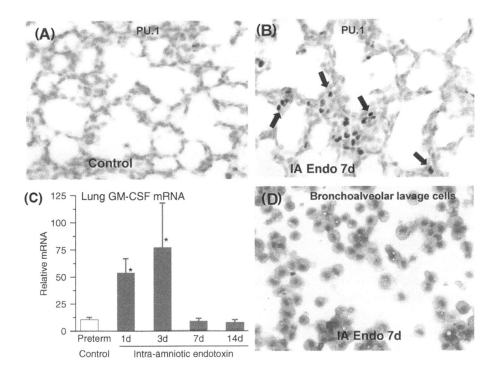

Figure 3 Response of fetal lung monocytes to intra-amniotic endotoxin. (**A**) Control lung with no cells staining for the transcription factor PU.1. (**B**) The monocytes/macrophage stain intensely for PU.1 seven days after the intra-amniotic endotoxin (*arrows*). (**C**) GM-CSF mRNA is expressed in response to intra-amniotic endotoxin. (**D**) A cytospin of a bronchoalveolar lavage done seven days after intra-amniotic endotoxin shows mature appearing alveolar macrophages. *Abbreviation*: GM-CSF, granulocyte macrophage colony-stimulating factor. *Abbreviation*: GM-CSF, granulocyte macrophage colony-stimulating factor. *Source*: Data from animals reported in Ref. 68.

In the clinical scenario, fetuses with preterm labor and exposed to chorioamnionitis are also exposed to maternal corticosteroids. Maternal corticosteroids also "mature" the function of blood monocytes in fetal sheep, although effects on lung monocytes have not been evaluated (71). In the endotoxin-induced chorioamnionitis model in fetal sheep, simultaneous exposure of the fetus to intra-amniotic endotoxin and maternal betamethasone resulted in an initial suppression of lung inflammation, but increased inflammation 5 or 15 days later (72). Therefore, the interactive effects of maternal corticosteroids and chorioamnionitis may be important clinically.

V. Fetal Lung Inflammation and BPD

The relationships between fetal inflammation from chorioamnionitis and an outcome such as BPD are complex. Fetal lung inflammation can induce a mild BPD-like phenotype with vascular injury and decreased septation. Perhaps more importantly, the

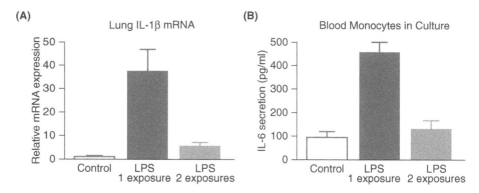

Figure 4 Repeated exposures to intra-amniotic endotoxin (LPS) decrease inflammatory responses: Preterm fetal sheep were exposed to either one or two injections of intra-amniotic LPS. (A) Lung IL-1β mRNA was induced after one exposure but not after the two exposures to LPS. (B) Blood monocytes were isolated after one or two exposures to intra-amniotic LPS and challenged with LPS in vitro. Monocytes from the single LPS group but not the LPS-2 exposure group responded to in vitro LPS challenge. *Abbreviation*: LPS, lipopolysaccharide. *Source*: Data redrawn from Ref. 37.

associated immune modulation can mature inflammatory responses such that the pre-term newborn lung could respond to oxygen or mechanical ventilation with an amplified inflammatory response. However, endotoxin tolerance could initially delay and change lung responses to oxygen or ventilation, in ways that can only be speculation at this point. This fetal tolerance response may contribute to other adverse events such as nosocomial sepsis that contribute to BPD. Antenatal corticosteroid effects on innate immune responses further cloud our understanding of the relationship of fetal exposures to BPD. Thus, there may be multiple pathways from fetal lung inflammation to BPD—some protective such as less RDS and some that prime or promote the postnatal insults that result in BPD. The fetal lung may receive "hits" that may ultimately progress to BPD. The primary injury may be less important than altered inflammatory responses to postnatal interventions (oxygen, ventilation) or occurrences (PDA, sepsis) that correlate with the development of BPD.

Acknowledgments

This work was supported in part by the National Institutes of Health, HL-65397 to A.H.J. and K08 HL70711 to S.G.K.

References

1. Bancalari E, Claure N, Sosenko IR. Bronchopulmonary dysplasia: changes in pathogenesis, epidemiology and definition. Semin Neonatol 2003; 8:63–71.
2. Massaro D, Massaro GD. Dexamethasone accelerates postnatal alveolar wall thinning and alters wall composition. Am J Physiol 1986; 251:R218–R224.

3. Massaro D, Massaro GD, Baras A, et al. Calorie-related rapid onset of alveolar loss, regeneration, and changes in mouse lung gene expression. Am J Physiol Lung Cell Mol Physiol 2004; 286:L896–L906.
4. Barton L, Hodgman JE, Pavlova Z. Causes of death in the extremely low birth weight infant. Pediatrics 1999; 103:446–451.
5. Goldenberg RL, Hauth JC, Andrews WW. Intrauterine infection and preterm delivery. N Engl J Med 2000; 342:1500–1507.
6. Lahra MM, Jeffery HE. A fetal response to chorioamnionitis is associated with early survival after preterm birth. Am J Obstet Gynecol 2004; 190:147–151.
7. Romero R, Espinoza J, Chaiworapongsa T, et al. Infection and prematurity and the role of preventive strategies. Semin Neonatol 2002; 7:259–274.
8. Gomez R, Romero R, Ghezzi F, et al. The fetal inflammatory response syndrome. Am J Obstet Gynecol 1998; 179:194–202.
9. Goldenberg RL, Andrews WW, Faye-Petersen OM, et al. The Alabama Preterm Birth Study: intrauterine infection and placental histologic findings in preterm births of males and females less than 32 weeks. Am J Obstet Gynecol 2006; 195:1533–1537.
10. Onderdonk AB, Delaney ML, DuBois AM, et al. Detection of bacteria in placental tissues obtained from extremely low gestational age neonates. Am J Obstet Gynecol 2008; 198:110. e1–110.e7.
11. Andrews WW, Goldenberg RL, Hauth JC, et al. Endometrial microbial colonization and plasma cell endometritis after spontaneous or indicated preterm versus term delivery. Am J Obstet Gynecol 2005; 193:739–745.
12. Gerber S, Vial Y, Hohlfeld P, et al. Detection of Ureaplasma urealyticum in second-trimester amniotic fluid by polymerase chain reaction correlates with subsequent preterm labor and delivery. J Infect Dis 2003; 187:518–521.
13. Perni SC, Vardhana S, Korneeva I, et al. Mycoplasma hominis and Ureaplasma urealyticum in midtrimester amniotic fluid: association with amniotic fluid cytokine levels and pregnancy outcome. Am J Obstet Gynecol 2004; 191:1382–1386.
14. Nguyen DP, Gerber S, Hohlfeld P, et al. Mycoplasma hominis in mid-trimester amniotic fluid: relation to pregnancy outcome. J Perinat Med 2004; 32:323–326.
15. Yoon BH, Romero R, Park JS, et al. Microbial invasion of the amniotic cavity with Ureaplasma urealyticum is associated with a robust host in fetal, amniotic, and maternal compartments. Am J Obstet Gynecol 1998; 179:1254–1260.
16. Yoon BH, Romero R, Lim JH, et al. The clinical significance of detecting Ureaplasma urealyticum by the polymerase chain reaction in the amniotic fluid of patients with preterm labor. Am J Obstet Gynecol 2003; 189:919–924.
17. Elimian A, Verma U, Beneck D, et al. Histologic chorioamnionitis, antenatal steroids, and perinatal outcomes. Obstet Gynecol 2000; 96:333–336.
18. Watterberg KL, Demers LM, Scott SM, et al. Chorioamnionitis and early lung inflammation in infants in whom bronchopulmonary dysplasia develops. Pediatrics 1996; 97:210–215.
19. Alexander JM, Gilstrap LC, Cox SM, et al. Clinical chorioamnionitis and the prognosis for very low birth weight infants. Obstet Gynecol 1998; 91:725–729.
20. Hitti J, Krohn MA, Patton DL, et al. Amniotic fluid tumor necrosis factor-alpha and the risk of respiratory distress syndrome among preterm infants. Am J Obstet Gynecol 1997; 177:50–56.
21. Andrews WW, Goldenberg RL, Faye-Petersen O, et al. The Alabama Preterm Birth Study: polymorphonuclear and mononuclear cell placental infiltrations, other markers of inflammation, and outcomes in 23- to 32-week preterm newborn infants. Am J Obstet Gynecol 2006; 195:803–808.
22. Goldenberg RL, Andrews WW, Goepfert AR, et al. The Alabama Preterm Birth Study: umbilical cord blood Ureaplasma urealyticum and Mycoplasma hominis cultures in very preterm newborn infants. Am J Obstet Gynecol 2008; 198:43.e1–43.e5.

23. Ammari A, Suri MS, Milisavljevic V, et al. Variables associated with the early failure of nasal CPAP in very low birth weight infants. J Pediatr 2005; 147:341–347.

24. Yoon BH, Romero R, Jun JK, et al. Amniotic fluid cytokines (interleukin-6, tumor necrosis factor-alpha, interleukin-1 beta, and interleukin-8) and the risk for the development of bronchopulmonary dysplasia. Am J Obstet Gynecol 1997; 177:825–830.

25. Matsuda T, Nakajima T, Hattori S, et al. Necrotizing funisitis: clinical significance and association with chronic lung disease in premature infants. Am J Obstet Gynecol 1997; 177:1402–1407.

26. Yoon BH, Romero R, Kim KS, et al. A systemic fetal inflammatory response and the development of bronchopulmonary dysplasia. Am J Obstet Gynecol 1999; 181:773–779.

27. Goepfert AR, Andrews WW, Carlo W, et al. Umbilical cord plasma interleukin-6 concentrations in preterm infants and risk of neonatal morbidity. Am J Obstet Gynecol 2004; 191:1375–1381.

28. Van Marter LJ, Dammann O, Allred EN, et al. Chorioamnionitis, mechanical ventilation, and postnatal sepsis as modulators of chronic lung disease in preterm infants. J Pediatr 2002; 140:171–176.

29. Viscardi RM, Muhumuza CK, Rodriguez A, et al. Inflammatory markers in intrauterine and fetal blood and cerebrospinal fluid compartments are associated with adverse pulmonary and neurologic outcomes in preterm infants. Pediatr Res 2004; 55:1009–1017.

30. De Dooy J, Colpaert C, Schuerwegh A, et al. Relationship between histologic chorioamnionitis and early inflammatory variables in blood, tracheal aspirates, and endotracheal colonization in preterm infants. Pediatr Res 2003; 54:113–119.

31. Groneck P, Goetze-Speer B, Speer CP. Inflammatory bronchopulmonary response of preterm infants with microbial colonization of the airways at birth. Arch Dis Child 1996; 74: F51–F55.

32. van Waarde WM, Brus F, Okken A, et al. Ureaplasma urealyticum colonization, prematurity and bronchopulmonary dysplasia. Eur Respir J 1997; 10:886–890.

33. Jonsson B, Karell AC, Ringertz S, et al. Neonatal Ureaplasma urealyticum colonization and chronic lung disease. Acta Paediatr 1994; 83:927–930.

34. Colaizy TT, Morris CD, Lapidus J, et al. Detection of ureaplasma DNA in endotracheal samples is associated with bronchopulmonary dysplasia after adjustment for multiple risk factors. Pediatr Res 2007; 61:578–583.

35. Schelonka RL, Katz B, Waites KB, et al. Critical appraisal of the role of Ureaplasma in the development of bronchopulmonary dysplasia with meta-analytic techniques. Pediatr Infect Dis J 2005; 24:1033–1039.

36. Castro-Alcaraz S, Greenberg EM, Bateman DA, et al. Patterns of colonization with Ureaplasma urealyticum during neonatal intensive care unit hospitalizations of very low birth weight infants and the development of chronic lung disease. Pediatrics 2002; 110:e45.

37. Kallapur SG, Jobe AH, Ball MK, et al. Pulmonary and systemic endotoxin tolerance in preterm fetal sheep exposed to chorioamnionitis. J Immunol 2007; 179:8491–8499.

38. Bry K, Lappalainen U, Hallman M. Intra-amniotic interleukin-1 accelerates surfactant protein synthesis in fetal rabbits and improves lung stability after premature birth. J Clin Invest 1997; 99:2992–2999.

39. Moss TJM, Knox CL, Kallapur SG, et al. Experimental amniotic fluid infection in sheep: effects of Ureaplasma parvum serovars 3 and 6 on preterm or term fetal sheep. Am J Obstet Gynecol 2008; 198:e1–e8.

40. Jobe AH, Newnham JP, Willet KE, et al. Endotoxin induced lung maturation in preterm lambs is not mediated by cortisol. Am J Respir Crit Care Med 2000; 162:1656–1661.

41. Willet K, Kramer BW, Kallapur SG, et al. Intra-amniotic injection of IL-1 induces inflammation and maturation in fetal sheep lung. Am J Physiol 2002; 282:L411–L420.

42. Kallapur SG, Moss JTM, Newnham JP, et al. Recruited inflammatory cells mediate endotoxin-induced lung maturation in preterm fetal lambs. Am J Respir Crit Care Med 2005; 172:1315–1321.
43. Newnham JP, Moss TJ, Padbury JF, et al. The interactive effects of endotoxin with prenatal glucocorticoids on short-term lung function in sheep. Am J Obstet Gynecol 2001; 185: 190–197.
44. Moss TJ, Nitsos I, Kramer BW, et al. Intra-amniotic endotoxin induces lung maturation by direct effects on the developing respiratory tract in preterm sheep. Am J Obstet Gynecol 2002; 187:1059–1065.
45. Sosenko IR, Kallapur SG, Nitsos I, et al. IL-1a causes lung inflammation and maturation by direct effects on preterm fetal lamb lungs. Pediatr Res 2006; 60:294–298.
46. Moss TJM, Nitsos I, Ikegami M, et al. Experimental intra-uterine Ureaplasma infection in sheep. Am J Obstet Gynecol 2005; 192:1179–1186.
47. Moss TM, Newnham J, Willet K, et al. Early gestational intra-amniotic endotoxin: lung function, surfactant and morphometry. Am J Respir Crit Care Med 2002; 165:805–811.
48. Newnham J, Moss TJ, Kramer BW, et al. The fetal maturational and inflammatory responses to different routes of endotoxin infusion in sheep. Am J Obstet Gynecol 2001; 186:1062–1068.
49. Kramer BW, Kramer S, Ikegami M, et al. Injury, inflammation and remodeling in fetal sheep lung after intra-amniotic endotoxin. Am J Physiol Lung Cell Mol Physiol 2002; 283: L452–L459.
50. Kallapur SG, Jobe AH, Ikegami M, et al. Increased IP-10 and MIG expression after intra-amniotic endotoxin in preterm lamb lung. Am J Respir Crit Care Med 2003; 167:779–786.
51. Kramer BW, Moss TJ, Willet K, et al. Dose and time response after intra-amniotic endotoxin in preterm lambs. Am J Respir Crit Care Med 2001; 164:982–988.
52. Willet KE, Jobe AH, Ikegami M, et al. Antenatal endotoxin and glucocorticoid effects on lung morphometry in preterm lambs. Pediatr Res 2000; 48:782–788.
53. Vayrynen O, Glumoff V, Hallman M. Regulation of surfactant proteins by LPS and proinflammatory cytokines in fetal and newborn lung. Am J Physiol Lung Cell Mol Physiol 2002; 282:L803–L810.
54. Prince LS, Okoh VO, Moninger TO, et al. Lipopolysaccharide increases alveolar type II cell number in fetal mouse lungs through Toll-like receptor 4 and NF-kappaB. Am J Physiol Lung Cell Mol Physiol 2004; 287:L999–L1006.
55. Prince LS, Dieperink HI, Okoh VO, et al. Toll-like receptor signaling inhibits structural development of the distal fetal mouse lung. Dev Dyn 2005; 233:553–561.
56. Benjamin JT, Smith RJ, Halloran BA, et al. FGF-10 is decreased in bronchopulmonary dysplasia and suppressed by Toll-like receptor activation. Am J Physiol Lung Cell Mol Physiol 2007; 292:L550–L558.
57. Bry K, Whitsett JA, Lappalainen U. IL-1beta disrupts postnatal lung morphogenesis in the mouse. Am J Respir Cell Mol Biol 2007; 36:32–42.
58. Jobe AH. The New BPD: an arrest of lung development. Pediatr Res 1999; 46:641–643.
59. Thebaud B, Abman SH. Bronchopulmonary dysplasia: where have all the vessels gone? Roles of angiogenic growth factors in chronic lung disease. Am J Respir Crit Care Med 2007; 175:978–985.
60. Kallapur SG, Bachurski C, Le Cras TD, et al. Vascular injury and remodeling following intra-amniotic endotoxin in the preterm lamb lung. Am J Physiol Lung Cell Mol Physiol 2004; 287:L1178–L1185.
61. Kunzmann S, Speer CP, Jobe AH, et al. Antenatal inflammation induced TGF-beta1 but suppressed CTGF in preterm lungs. Am J Physiol Lung Cell Mol Physiol 2007; 292:L223–L231.
62. Cheah FC, Jobe AH, Moss TJ, et al. Oxidative stress in fetal lambs exposed to intra-amniotic endotoxin in a chorioamnionitis model. Pediatr Res 2008; 63:1–5.

63. Yoder BA, Coalson JJ, Winter VT, et al. Effects of antenatal colonization with ureaplasma urealyticum on pulmonary disease in the immature baboon. Pediatr Res 2003; 54:797–807.
64. Viscardi RM, Atamas SP, Luzina IG, et al. Antenatal Ureaplasma urealyticum respiratory tract infection stimulates proinflammatory, profibrotic responses in the preterm baboon lung. Pediatr Res 2006; 60:141–146.
65. Kallapur SG, Nitsos I, Moss TJM, et al. Chronic endotoxin exposure does not cause sustained structural abnormalities in the fetal sheep lungs. Am J Physiol Lung Cell Mol Physiol 2005; 288:L966–L974.
66. Moss TJ, Davey MG, Harding R, et al. Effects of intra-amniotic endotoxin on lung structure and function two months after term birth in sheep. J Soc Gynecol Investig 2002; 9:220–225.
67. Kallapur SG, Willet KE, Jobe AH, et al. Intra-amniotic endotoxin: chorioamnionitis precedes lung maturation in preterm lambs. Am J Physiol 2001; 280:L527–L536.
68. Kramer BW, Jobe AH, Ikegami M. Monocyte function in preterm, term, and adult sheep. Pediatr Res 2003; 54:52–57.
69. Kramer BW, Joshi SN, Moss TJ, et al. Endotoxin-induced maturation of monocytes in preterm fetal sheep lung. Am J Physiol Lung Cell Mol Physiol 2007; 293:L345–L353.
70. Kramer BW, Ikegami M, Moss TJ, et al. Endotoxin-induced chorioamnionitis modulates innate immunity of monocytes in preterm sheep. Am J Respir Crit Care Med 2005; 171: 73–77.
71. Kramer BW, Ikegami M, Moss TJ, et al. Antenatal betamethasone changes cord blood monocyte responses to endotoxin in preterm lambs. Pediatr Res 2004; 55:764–768.
72. Kallapur SG, Kramer BW, Moss TJ, et al. Maternal glucocorticoids increase endotoxin-induced lung inflammation in preterm lambs. Am J Physiol Lung Cell Mol Physiol 2003; 284:L633–L642.

7
Inflammatory Mechanisms in Bronchopulmonary Dysplasia

CHRISTIAN P. SPEER
University Children's Hospital, Würzburg, Germany

I. Introduction

Bronchopulmonary dysplasia (BPD) is an evolving process of lung injury that can result in chronic impairment of lung function and may have lifelong consequences for the infant. Pre- and postnatal factors have been shown to induce an injurious inflammatory response in the immature airways and the pulmonary interstitium of preterm infants, which may subsequently affect normal alveolarization and pulmonary vascular development. More than half of very immature infants may have been exposed to chorioamnionitis, and a considerable number of them are born with inflamed lungs and signs of fetal inflammatory response. In addition, various postnatal factors such as resuscitation, high airway concentrations of inspired oxygen, mechanical ventilation, and pulmonary as well as systemic infections may perpetuate or even amplify an injurious inflammatory response in the airways and interstitium. The etiology of BPD is definitely multifactoral, and the multiple-hit theory offers a plausible concept that can help to explain the complex pathogenetic mechanisms involved in this chronic lung disease of very immature preterm infants (1,2). This actualized chapter summarizes, in a condensed form, the current pathogenetic concepts on the possible role of inflammation in the evolution of BPD and expands on previously published review articles (3–6).

II. Inflammatory Cells

There is general agreement that neutrophils and macrophages have a pivotal and crucial role in acute and chronic stages of pulmonary inflammation. During the evolution of inflammation, much higher and persisting numbers of inflammatory cells were detected in bronchoalveolar lavage fluid of preterm infants with BPD when compared with infants who recovered from respiratory distress syndrome (RDS) (7–9). The predominant cell identified in the early phase of inflammation was the neutrophil (7–11). Immediately after initiation of mechanical ventilation, a neutrophil influx into the airways was observed in animals as well as in preterm infants, and this inflammatory reaction was associated with a decrease in the number of circulating neutrophils (12,13). This phenomenon was shown to correlate with the extent of pulmonary edema formation and an increased risk of developing BPD (2,14,15). Moreover, circulating neutrophils and monocytes—as reflected by CD11b expression—became activated within one to three hours after initiation of mechanical ventilation (16). Most recently, a prolonged survival of neonatal neutrophils due to an inappropriate suppression of neutrophil apoptosis has been reported (17). Since apoptosis of inflammatory neutrophils and their timely removal by resident macrophages are critical to the resolution of inflammation, neonatal neutrophils with prolonged survival may have the functional capacity to perpetuate inflammation. Apoptotic cells per se were shown to induce inflammatory and fibrotic pulmonary responses (18). Alveolar and pulmonary tissue macrophages play a central role in the inflammatory event. Following their activation, macrophages secrete numerous cytokines and proinflammatory mediators that orchestrate the inflammatory response, particularly neutrophil recruitment. In lung tissues of preterm infants who had died during the early stages of RDS, the interstitial density of CD68-positive macrophages and neutrophils was at least 10- to 15-fold higher than in stillborn infants of equivalent age (19).

A. Cellular and Endothelial Interaction

Before inflammatory cells leave the circulation via a one-way exit into the extravascular space, cellular attachment to endothelial cells is mediated through a complex interaction with adhesion molecules. Increased concentrations of various soluble adhesion molecules on neutrophils and endothelium such as selectins and intercellular adhesion molecules (ICAM-1) have been detected in airway secretions and the circulation of infants with BPD, reflecting greater shedding of these molecules in response to inflammation (20). These data provide indirect evidence for an effective recruitment of circulating neutrophils and monocytes into the airways and the pulmonary tissue. In addition, a strong upregulation of ICAM-1 on endothelial cord cells and increased serum levels of soluble ICAM-1 in preterm infants exposed to chorioamnionitis have been described (20).

B. Chemotactic and Chemokinetic Factors

Airway secretions of infants with BPD have been shown to contain high concentrations of well-defined chemotactic factors that are responsible for the recruitment of inflammatory cells: C5a, tumor-necrosis factor α (TNF-α), interleukin (IL)-1, IL-8, IL-16, lipoxygenase products, leukotriene B$_4$, elastin fragments, metalloproteases fibronectin, and others (3,4,6,7). IL-8 is involved in the initiation of cellular endothelial interactions and is probably the most important chemotactic factor in the lung. In addition, potent β-chemokines that induce chemotaxis of monocytes and macrophages have been detected in the airway secretion of infants with RDS and BPD, such as monocyte chemotactic protein, macrophage inflammatory protein, and growth-related protein (3,4,6). The chemotactic activity and the concentrations of numerous chemotactic and chemokinetic factors were considerably higher in infants with BPD when compared with babies who recovered from RDS, and preceded the marked neutrophil influx in infants with BPD (7). Application of a selective chemokine receptor antagonist was recently shown to inhibit neutrophil influx into the rat lung, suppress pulmonary inflammation, and enhance lung growth (21). Most recently, inhibition of phosphodiesterase-4 similarly decreased influx of monocytes and macrophages in the airways of preterm infants and positively affected the extent of lung injury (22,23).

C. Pro- and Anti-Inflammatory Cytokines

TNF-α, IL-1, IL-6, and IL-8 play a crucial role in the early inflammatory response and the evolution of the injurious events. These proinflammatory cytokines are synthesized by various inflammatory and pulmonary cells on stimulation by hyperoxia, microorganisms, endotoxin [lipopolysaccharide (LPS)], other bacterial cell wall constituents, and biophysical factors such as volutrauma and barotrauma (4) (Fig. 1). Cytokines bind to specific cell surface receptors and act as mediators in an immune response via intracellular signaling, which includes the upregulation and/or downregulation of genes and their transcription factor (24). Recent findings suggest that IL-1 present in the airway secretions of ventilated preterm infants is inducing IL-8 expression of epithelial cells by way of a nuclear transcription factor (NF-κB)-dependent pathway, which is thought to be essential in the regulation of the cellular inflammatory reaction following activation by LPS. NF-κB activation has been reported in airway neutrophils and macrophages as well as in tracheobronchial secretions from infants with RDS (25,26). It has clearly been shown that proinflammatory cytokines do not cross the placenta (27). Increased protein levels and high mRNA expression of these proinflammatory cytokines

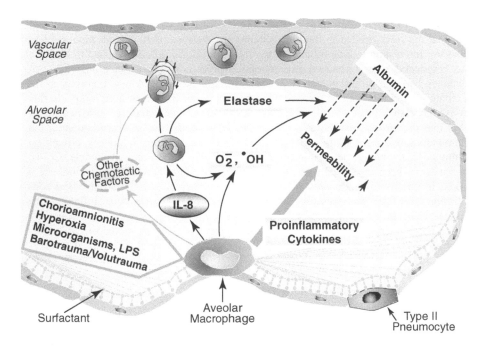

Figure 1 Postnatal risk factors such as chorioamnionitis, hyperoxia, microorganisms, LPS, and volutrauma induce the generation and secretion of proinflammatory cytokines by pulmonary or inflammatory cells that are responsible, in part, for the upregulation of endothelial and cellular adhesion molecules and for the recruitment and influx of neutrophils into the airways. Various inflammatory mediators induce an increased alveolar-capillary permeability. As a consequence, plasma proteins entering the airways contribute to the inactivation of the surfactant system.

have been detected in airway secretions, bronchoalveolar and pulmonary cells, and, moreover, in the systemic circulation of infants with evolving BPD (3,4,28).

The influx of TNF-α-positive macrophages in pulmonary tissue of preterm infants who had died of severe RDS was found to be associated with a loss of endothelial basement membrane and a destruction of interstitial glycosaminoglycanes (29). Furthermore, a transient overexpression of IL-1 in rat lungs by adenoviral gene transfer has recently been found to be accompanied by a local increase in TNF-α and IL-6 expression and a vigorous acute inflammatory reaction with evidence of profound tissue injury and fibrotic changes (30). Most recently, perinatal expression of IL-1-β in pulmonary epithelial cells of a bitransgenic mouse model was shown to induce a lung disease that was clinically and histologically similar to BPD (31). In contrast, treatment of surfactant-depleted rabbits with aerosolized IL-1 receptor antagonist before the induction of experimental lung injury clearly decreased inflammation and lung damage (32).

There is convincing experimental and clinical data that indicate that the profound proinflammatory cytokines response present in the airways and pulmonary tissue of preterm infants may reflect an inability to regulate inflammation through an adequate expression of the anti-inflammatory cytokines IL-4, IL-10, IL-11, IL-12, IL-13, IL-18, or IL-1 receptor antagonist (3,4,33–35). Cellular IL-10 mRNA was undetectable in most airway samples of preterm infants with BPD, but it was expressed in all term infants with respiratory failure (33). In general, monocytes of newborns seem to produce IL-10 far below the level needed to inhibit a submaximal release of IL-8 from mononuclear cells (36). Interestingly, lung inflammatory cells of preterm infants exposed to IL-10 in vitro responded with a reduced expression of proinflammatory cytokines (37). An imbalance between proinflammatory and anti-inflammatory cytokines, favoring proinflammatory cytokines, can be considered as an important feature of lung injury. In this context, substances that exert anti-inflammatory effects or interfere with neutrophil influx into the airways and lung tissue may be of potential use in downregulating the inflammatory response. Clara cell protein (CC-10) has various inhibitory effects on inflammation including the inhibition of phospholipase A_2. In animal models, CC-10 deficiency has been associated with high expression of proinflammatory cytokines and a marked infiltration of pulmonary tissue by inflammatory cells (38); a decreased concentration of CC10 was identified in premature infants with a fetal inflammatory response (39). In addition, bombesin-like peptide, a strong promoter of fetal lung development, has been shown to mediate lung injury in a baboon model of BPD; anti-bombesin antibodies, however, effectively reduced lung injury and promoted alveolarization (40).

D. Oxidative and Proteolytic Damage

Exposure to high inspiratory oxygen concentrations causes direct oxidative cell damage through increased production of reactive oxygen species (ROS). ROS are not only released by neutrophils and macrophages at sites of inflammation but also generated under hyperoxic conditions and reoxygenation injury by the cell-bound xanthine-oxidase system and free iron. Free iron was detected in the vast majority of ventilated preterm infants with RDS (41). Oxygen radicals have clearly been shown to exert direct toxic effects on bronchoalveolar structures by induction of inflammation, by lipid peroxidation, by oxidative inactivation of protective antiproteases, and by upregulation of metalloproteinases (41,42). Animal experiments indicate that oxidative stress as reflected by generation of toxic oxygen radicals is a very early and crucial event in the initiation of pulmonary inflammation (43). In mature infants, antioxidant enzymes such as superoxide dismutase, catalase, and glutathion peroxidase have protective activities against oxygen radicals. Very immature preterm infants, however, are particularly susceptible to hyperoxia and damage caused by ROS since the antioxidant system has yet to mature. As a consequence, preterm infants will be deficient in antioxidant enzyme activity at the time when they are receiving high inspiratory oxygen and are most likely exposed to hyperoxemia (42).

At sites of tissue injury, neutrophils and macrophages release various potent proteases that are thought to play an essential role in the destruction of the alveolar-capillary unit and the extracellular matrix, among them are elastase, β-glucoronidase, myeloperoxidase, cathepsin, metalloproteinase, and others. An imbalance between elastase—a powerful neutral protease—and α_1-proteinase inhibitor (α_1-PI) within the airway of preterm infants with RDS and BPD has clearly been demonstrated (7,44). α_1-PI is presumably functionally inactivated by oxygen intermediates. Various markers of destruction of elastase have been identified in airway secretions and urine of infants with free elastase activity, and moreover, alveolar septation has been shown to be markedly reduced in lungs of infants with BPD (2). In addition, elastase and other neutral proteases were shown to prime macrophages for an increased release of toxic oxygen metabolites (45). Furthermore, an imbalance between cysteine proteases and their inhibitors has recently been described (46). Similarly, high concentrations of different matrix metalloproteinases that are involved in remodeling throughout all stages of lung development have been identified in airway secretions of infants with BPD, and when overexpressed might cause disruption of the extracellular matrix. Protective levels of tissue inhibitors of metalloproteinases were rather low in these infants, also suggesting an imbalance within the metalloproteinase system (47,48). Blocking matrix metalloprotease-9 activity has recently been shown to reduce oxidative injury–mediated lung damage in mice (49).

E. Increased Alveolar-Capillary Permeability

The increased alveolar-capillary permeability is pathognomonic for the early stages of inflammation, and it is clearly associated with a deterioration of lung function (3,4). Various inflammatory mediators and cells, which have been addressed, have detrimental effects on the microvascular integrity. In addition, a variety of lipid mediators, present in airways of infants with BPD, have direct effects on the alveolar-capillary unit including leukotrienes, prostacyclin, platelet-derived factor, and endothelin-1. Protein leakage into the alveoli and airways of preterm infants was shown to take place within one hour after initiation of mechanical ventilation (14). At a postnatal age of 10 to 14 days, preterm infants who later developed BPD had a drastic increase of albumin concentrations in their airway secretions; albumin and other serum proteins profoundly contribute to alveolar edema, to the inactivation of the surfactant system and a deterioration of lung function (7). Using magnetic resonance imaging, infants with BPD showed an increased lung water content and were susceptible to gravity-induced collapse of the lung (50). In mechanically ventilated infants with RDS, a simultaneous activation of clotting, fibrinolysis, kinin-kallikrein and the complement system has been observed (4). These findings indicate that injury to the pulmonary vascular endothelium may subsequently promote neutrophil and platelet activation, and may induce pulmonary as well as systemic inflammation and activation of the clotting system (51,52).

F. Repair Mechanisms and Growth Factors

Inflammation-induced tissue injury is normally followed by a phase of repair, which has only partially been studied in BPD. Lung injury and the associated inflammatory process leads to an induction of transforming growth factor β (TGF-β) that limits some of the inflammatory reactions and plays a key role in mediating tissue remodeling and repair (51). However, if reparative processes are exaggerated, as indicated by increased expression of TGF-β in lungs of preterm animals, normal lung development may be inhibited, and fibrosis may ensue (4). One might speculate that overexpression of TGF-β as observed in preterm infants with BPD (53–55) together with low or suboptimal levels of various pulmonary and vascular growth factors could add to the pathogenesis of BPD. Recently, a reduced expression of connective tissue growth factor, which is responsible for various downstream actions of TGF-β and which is a second important key mediator in the induction of pulmonary fibrosis, has been found in a sheep model (56). Overexpression of TGF-β and subsequent downregulation of connective tissue growth factor together with suboptimal levels of various growth factors may partially explain the pathogenesis of the "new BPD," which is characterized by growth arrest of lung tissue and pulmonary vessels rather than by fibrosis. Low concentrations of hypoxic-inducible factor and keratinocyte and hepatocyte growth factors that are thought to participate in normal lung development and tissue regeneration after lung injury have been detected in infants with BPD (57–59). Similarly, impaired expression of vascular endothelial growth factor, its angiogenic receptors, and angiopoetin (60) in lungs from extremely preterm animals developing BPD were shown to contribute to dysmorphic microvasculature and disrupted alveolarization (61). Postnatal administration of intratracheally adenovirus-mediated vascular endothelial growth factor gene therapy improved survival and promoted lung capillary formation; the alveolar development was preserved in the rat model of irreversible lung injury (61).

III. Factors Inducing Pulmonary Inflammation

A. Chorioamnionitis

Epidemiological data suggest a strong association between chorioamnionitis, funisitis, and the development of BPD, and increased concentrations of proinflammatory cytokines in human amniotic fluid and fetal cord blood, indicating a systemic inflammatory response during chorioamnionitis, were shown to be independent risk factors of BPD (3,4,6). A pronounced infiltration of inflammatory cells, an increased expression of cytokines and markers of endothelial activation, as well as a large number of apoptotic airway cells has been observed in lung tissues of human fetuses with funisitis that have been exposed to chorioamnionitis (28,62,63). In addition, the presence of proteomic biomarkers characteristic of inflammation in the amniotic fluid was associated with an increased fetal inflammatory response at birth (64).

Very recently, in 23% of very immature preterm infants enrolled in the Alabama Preterm Birth Study, *Ureaplasma urealyticum* (Uu) and *Mycoplasma hominis* were detected in cord blood cultures: These infants were more likely to have neonatal systemic inflammatory response syndrome and probably BPD (65). The authors of an editorial note found compelling evidence that congenital fetal infection is more frequent than was previously realized: "Whatever the explanation is how such microorganisms gain access to the amniotic cavity, it is now clear that these microorganisms can induce cavity, fetus and mother" (66). The role of genetic predisposition is currently under investigation and has not provided conclusive data by now (24,67,68).

B. Infection

Early onset sepsis and systemic nosocomial infections have clearly been identified as individual risk factors of BPD (3,4,6,69–72). Besides direct effects of microorganisms, inflammatory cells, and mediators on endothelial and bronchoalveolar cells, hemodynamic changes in the vascular bed associated with persistent ductus arteriosus seem to play an essential role in the development of BPD (73). Most likely, vasoactive prostaglandin mediators released during septicemia prevent ductal closure or induce reopening of the duct (74). However, the potential role of Uu in the evolution of BPD is controversial. Uu is the microorganism most frequently isolated from the amniotic fluid in preterm births and a predominant pathogen detected in airway secretions immediately after birth (70,75). Animal experiments strongly indicate that a prolonged proinflammatory response initiated by antenatal Uu infection contributes to early fibrosis and altered developmental signaling in the immature lung (76). Moreover, the presence of Uu in the respiratory tract of preterm infants—even without clinical or laboratory signs of infection—has been correlated with elevated cellular and molecular markers of inflammation and associated with an increased risk of BPD (77–79). In baboons, antenatally and intra-amniotically colonized with Uu, two different patterns of disease were observed: One group with persistently Uu-positive tracheal cultures manifested continuously elevated proinflammatory cytokine levels and significantly worse lung function and pulmonary morphology than control animals. The other group that cleared Uu from the trachea by 72 hour of postnatal age showed a reduction in airway cytokine levels and white blood cell numbers, and this was associated with significantly improved lung function and morphology (75). Inherent responses of the maternal-fetal immune system to antenatal Uu, which have not been understood yet, most likely determine the pulmonary outcome of Uu colonization (75).

C. Mechanical Ventilation

A considerable number of animal experiments have clearly shown that any ventilatory trauma of the immature lung may be injurious to airways and lung tissue. An excessive tidal volume (volutrauma), rather than high inspiratory pressure (barotraumas), is the primary determinant of lung injury. Overdistension of the lungs or cyclic opening and closing of lung units causes disruption of structural elements and a release of proinflammatory mediators with subsequent leukocyte influx (3,4,6,80–86). The strongest inflammatory reaction was observed in those ventilatory strategies with high peak pressure and no positive end-expiratory pressure. If animals were pretreated with LPS, bronchoalveolar lavage fluid levels of proinflammatory cytokines were impressively increased even with a "less injurious" ventilation strategy (87). "Priming" of the fetal lung by LPS is a considerable pathogenetic factor in the initiation of the inflammatory reaction, and basically every form of mechanical ventilation may act as a "second strike" that can amplify or aggravate the inflammatory response (84).

D. Hyperoxia and Hypoxia

Very immature preterm infants with their reduced antioxidant defense system are at high risk of suffering from potential detrimental effects of hyperoxia and hyperoxemia (42,88). In preterm and full-term animals, hyperoxia has clearly been shown to be a strong and independent inductor of various mediators involved in pulmonary inflammation (89,90). Recently, differential gene expression with DNA microarray analysis in premature rat lungs exposed to prolonged hyperoxia during the saccular stage has been studied; this developmental stage closely resembles the pulmonary development of preterm infants receiving intensive care treatment. Oxidative stress affected a complex orchestra of genes involved in inflammation, extracellular matrix turnover, coagulation, and other events (91). The majority of proinflammatory genes was considerably upregulated. These findings were associated with an increased influx of inflammatory cells especially macrophages in pulmonary tissue. Moreover, hyperoxia resulted in progressive lung disease, which strongly reminded of BPD. Current knowledge about the role of hypoxia in pulmonary inflammation is limited. A recent animal study demonstrated that hypoxia had a substantial effect on LPS-induced pulmonary inflammation by increasing the magnitude of lung injury reflected by increased expression of inflammatory mediators, excessive neutrophil accumulation, and increased vascular permeability (92).

IV. Conclusion

There is growing evidence that BPD results, at least in part, from an imbalance between proinflammatory and anti-inflammatory mechanisms, with a persistent imbalance that favors proinflammatory mechanisms. The inflammatory response is characterized by a rapid accumulation of neutrophils and macrophages in the airways and pulmonary tissue of mechanically ventilated preterm infants and, moreover, by an arsenal of inflammatory mediators that might directly affect the alveolar-capillary unit and tissue integrity. During the last decade, it has become evident that there are multiple pre- and postnatal events that contribute in sense of multiple-hit scenario to the development of BPD in preterm infants. Chorioamnionitis and cytokine exposure in utero plus sequential lung injury caused by individual risk factors such as oxygen toxicity, resuscitation, volutrauma, barotrauma, and infection, all lead to a pulmonary inflammatory response that is most likely associated with aberrant wound healing. As a devastating consequence, normal alveolarization as well as vascular development can be compromised with life-long consequences for the infant. However, we have to realize that the exact pathogenetic sequence of acute and chronic inflammation is mainly hypothetical and speculative since the possible interaction between inflammatory cells and humoral mediators as well as regulatory aspects of inflammation in tissue injury and repair are largely descriptive, and the molecular basis of these events have only been partially defined yet. Moreover, most of the reported findings reflect associations of in vitro experiments, animal studies, and clinical observations in preterm infants with RDS and BPD rather than causal relationships. Especially in preterm babies with the burden of numerous pre- and post-natal risk factors and a considerable heterogeneity in disease severity as well as the limitations in study design, it seems impossible to define the significance of an individual risk factor in the pathogenesis of pulmonary inflammation. Many studies have examined mediators at single or very few time points and may have missed the phasic nature of the inflammatory process; others may have investigated an insufficient number of mediators to draw reasonable conclusions about the interaction between pro- and anti-inflammatory mechanisms (24). Nevertheless, our current understanding of the inflammatory mechanisms has opened up avenues that will allow to get a deeper insight into the pathogenesis of inflammatory events, and thus, allow strategies that will help to prevent or ameliorate BPD in high-risk infants to be defined (93).

References

1. Walsh MC, Szefler S, Davis J, et al. Summary proceedings from the bronchopulmonary dysplasia group. Pediatrics 2006; 117:52–56.
2. Bland RD. Neonatal chronic lung disease in the post-surfactant era. Biol Neonate 2005; 88(3):181–191.
3. Speer CP. Role of inflammation in the evolution of bronchopulmonary dysplasia. Drug Discov Today Dis Mech 2006; 3:409–414.
4. Speer CP. Inflammation and bronchopulmonary dysplasia: a continuing story. Semin Fetal Neonatal Med 2006; 11:354–362.
5. Speer CP. Pulmonary inflammation and bronchopulmonary dysplasia. J Perinatol 2006; 26: S57–S62.
6. Speer CP. Role of inflammation in the evolution of bronchopulmonary dysplasia. Drug Discovery Today: Disease Mechanisms 2006; 3(4):409–414.
7. Groneck P, Goetze-Speer B, Oppermann M, et al. Association of pulmonary inflammation and increased microvascular permeability during the development of bronchopulmonary dysplasia: a sequential analysis of inflammatory mediators in respiratory fluids of high risk preterm infants. Pediatrics 1994; 93:712–718.
8. Merritt TA, Cochrane CG, Holcomb K, et al. Elastase and α_1-proteinase inhibitor activity in tracheal aspirates during respiratory distress syndrome. J Clin Invest 1983; 72:656–666.
9. Ogden BE, Murphy SA, Saunders GC, et al. Neonatal lung neutrophils and elastase/proteinase inhibitor imbalance. Am Rev Respir Dis 1984; 130:817–821.
10. Arnon S, Grigg J, Silverman M. Pulmonary inflammatory cells in ventilated preterm infants: effect of surfactant treatment. Arch Dis Child 1993; 69:44–48.
11. Kotecha S, Chan B, Azam N, et al. Increase in interleukin-8 and soluble intercellular adhesion molecule-1 in bronchoalveolar lavage of premature infants with chronic lung disease. Arch Dis Child 1995; 72:F90–F96.
12. Ferreira PJ, Bunch TJ, Albertine KH, et al. Circulating neutrophil concentration and respiratory distress in premature infants. J Pediatr 2000; 136:466–472.
13. Carlton DP, Albertine KH, Cho SC, et al. Role of neutrophils in lung vascular injury and edema after premature birth in lambs. J Appl Physiol 1997; 83:1307–1317.
14. Jaarsma A, Braaksma MA, Geven WB, et al. Activation of the inflammatory reaction within minutes after birth in ventilated preterm lambs with neonatal respiratory distress syndrome. Biol Neonate 2004; 86:1–5.

15. Palta M, Sadek-Badawi M, Carlton DP. Association of BPD and IVH with early neutrophil and white counts in VLBW neonates with gestational age <32 weeks. J Perinatol 2008; 28:604–610.

16. Turunen R, Nupponen I, Siitonen S, et al. Onset of mechanical ventilation is associated with rapid activation of circulating phagocytes in preterm infants. Pediatrics 2006; 117:448–454.

17. Hanna N, Vasquez P, Pham P, et al. Mechanisms underlying reduced apoptosis in neonatal neutrophils. Pediatr Res 2005; 57:56–62.

18. Wang L, Scabilloni JF, Antonini JM, et al. Induction of secondary apoptosis, inflammation, and lung fibrosis after intratracheal instillation of apoptotic cells in rats. Am J Physiol Lung Cell Mol Physiol 2006; 290:L695–L702.

19. Murch SH, Costeloe K, Klein NJ, et al. Early production of macrophage inflammatory protein-1α occurs in respiratory distress syndrome and is associated with poor outcome. Pediatr Res 1996; 40:490–497.

20. d'Alquen D, Kramer BW, Seidenspinner S, et al. Activation of umbilical cord endothelial cells and fetal inflammatory response in preterm infants with chorioamnionitis and funisitis. Pediatr Res 2005; 57:263–269.

21. Yi M, Jankov RP, Belcastro R, et al. Opposing effect of 60% oxygen and neutrophil influx on alveologenesis in the neonatal rat. Am J Respir Crit Care Med 2004; 170:1188–1196.

22. de Visser YP, Walther FJ, Laghmani EH, et al. Phosphodiesterase 4 inhibition attenuates pulmonary inflammation in neonatal lung injury. Eur Respir J 2008; 31:633–644.

23. Woyda K, Koebrich S, Reiss I, et al. Inhibition of PDE4 enhances lung alveolarisation in neonatal mice exposed to hyperoxia. Eur Respir J 2009; 33:861–870.

24. Bose CL, Dammann CEL, Laughon MM. Bronchopulmonary dysplasia and inflammatory biomarkers in the premature neonate. Arch Dis Child Fetal Neonatal Ed 2008; 93:F455–F461.

25. Cao L, Liu C, Cai B, et al. Nuclear factor-kappa B expression in alveolar macrophages of mechanically ventilated neonates with respiratory distress syndrome. Biol Neonate 2004; 86:116–123.

26. Cheah FC, Winterbourn CC, Darlow BA, et al. Nuclear factor κB activation in pulmonary leukocytes from infants with hyaline membrane disease: associations with chorioamnionitis and Ureaplasma urealyticum colonization. Pediatr Res 2005; 57:616–623.

27. Aaltonen R, Heikkinen T, Hakala K, et al. Transfer of proinflammatory cytokines across term placenta. Obstet Gynecol 2005; 106:802–807.

28. Schmidt B, Cao L, Mackensen-Haen S, et al. Chorioamnionitis and inflammation of the fetal lung. Am J Obstet Gynecol 2001; 185:173–177.

29. Murch SH, Costeloe K, Klein NJ, et al. Mucosal tumor necrosis factor-α production and extensive disruption of sulfated glycosaminglycans begin within hours of birth in neonatal respiratory distress syndrome. Pediatr Res 1996; 40:484–489.

30. Kolb M, Margetts PJ, Anthony DC, et al. Transient expression of IL-1β induces acute lung injury and chronic repair leading to pulmonary fibrosis. J Clin Invest 2001; 107:1529–1536.

31. Bry K, Whitsett JA, Lappalainen U. IL-1 {beta} disrupts postnatal lung morphogenesis in the mouse. Am J Respir Cell Mol Biol 2007; 36:32–42.

32. Narimanbekov IO, Rozyiki HL. Effect of IL-1 blockade on inflammatory manifestations of acute ventilator-induced lung injury in a rabbit model. Exp Lung Res 1995; 21:239–254.

33. Jones CA, Cayabyab RG, Kwong KY, et al. Undetectable interleukin (IL)-10 and persistent IL-8 expression early in hyaline membrane disease: a possible developmental basis for the predisposition to chronic lung inflammation in preterm newborns. Pediatr Res 1996; 39:966–975.

34. Kakkera DK, Siddiq MM, Parton LA, et al. Interleukin-1 balance in the lungs of preterm infants who develop bronchopulmonary dysplasia. Biol Neonate 2004; 87:82–90.

35. Chetty A, Cao G-J, Manzo N, et al. The role of IL-6 and IL-11 in hyperoxic injury in developing lung. Pediatr Pulmonol 2008; 43:297–304.

36. Davidson D, Miskolci V, Clark DC, et al. Interleukin-10 production after pro-inflammatory stimulation of neutrophils and monocytic cells of the newborn. Comparison to exogenous interleukin-10 and dexamethasone levels needed to inhibit chemokine release. Neonatology 2007; 92:127–133.
37. Kwong KYC, Jones CA, Cayabyab R, et al. The effects of IL-10 on proinflammatory cytokine expression (IL-1β and IL-8) in hyaline membrane disease (HMD). Clin Immunol Immunopathol 1998; 88:105–113.
38. Miller TL, Shashikant BN, Pilan AL, et al. Effects of an intratracheally delivered anti-inflammatory protein (rhCC10) on physiological and lung structural indices in a juvenile model of acute lung injury. Biol Neonate 2005; 89:159–170.
39. Thomas W, Seidenspinner S, Kawczynska-Leda N, et al. CC10 in airways and umbilical cord serum of premature infants with systemic inflammation. Neonatology 2009 (in press).
40. Sunday ME, Yoder BA, Cuttitta F, et al. Bombesin-like peptide mediates lung injury in a baboon model of bronchopulmonary dysplasia. J Clin Invest 1998; 102:584–594.
41. Gerber CE, Bruchelt G, Stegmann H, et al. Presence of bleomycin-detectable free iron in the alveolar system of preterm infants. Biochem Biophys Res Commun 1999; 257:218–222.
42. Saugstad OD. Oxidative stress in the newborn—a 30 years perspective. Biol Neonate 2005; 88:228–236.
43. Kramer BW, Kramer S, Ikegami M, et al. Injury inflammation and remodelling in fetal sheep lung after intraamniotic endotoxin. Am J Physiol Lung Cell Mol Physiol 2002; 283: L452–L459.
44. Speer CP, Ruess D, Harms K, et al. Neutrophil elastase and acute pulmonary damage in neonates with severe respiratory distress syndrome. Pediatrics 1993; 91:794–799.
45. Speer CP, Pabst M, Hedegaard HB, et al. Enhanced release of oxygen metabolites by monocyte-derived macrophages exposed to proteolytic enzymes: activity of neutrophil elastase and cathepsin G. J Immunol 1994; 133:2151–2156.
46. Altiok O, Ysumatsu R, Bingol-Karakoc G. Imbalance between cysteine proteases and inhibitors in a baboon model of bronchopulmonary dysplasia. Am J Respir Crit Care Med 2006; 173:318–326.
47. Schock BC, Sweet DG, Ennis M, et al. Oxidative stress and increased type-IV collagenase levels in bronchoalveolar lavage fluid from newborn babies. Pediatr Res 2001; 50:29–33.
48. Cederquist K, Sorsa T, Tervahartiala T, et al. Matrix metalloproteinases-2, -8, and -9 and TIMP-2 in tracheal aspirates from preterm infants with respiratory distress. Pediatrics 2001; 108:686–692.
49. Chetty A, Cao GJ, Severgnini M, et al. Role of matrix metalloprotease-9 (MMP-9) in hyperoxic injury in developing lung. Am J Physiol Lung Cell Mol Physiol 2008; 29:L584–L592.
50. Adams EW, Harrison MC, Counsell SJ, et al. Increased lung water and tissue damage in bronchopulmonary dysplasia. J Pediatr 2004; 145:503–507.
51. Bartram U, Speer CP. The role of transforming growth factor β in lung development and disease. Chest 2004; 125:754–765.
52. Sitaru AG, Holzhauer S, Speer CP, et al. Neonatal platelets from cord blood and peripheral blood. Platelets 2005; 16:203–210.
53. Kotecha S, Wangoo A, Silverman M, et al. Increase in the concentration of transforming growth factor-β1 in bronchoalveolar lavage fluid before the development of chronic lung disease of prematurity. J Pediatr 1996; 128:464–469.
54. Lecart C, Cayabyab R, Bockley S, et al. Bioactive transforming growth factor-β in the lungs of extremely low birthweight neonates predicts the need for home oxygen supplementation. Biol Neonate 2000; 77:217–223.
55. Jónsson B, Li Y-H, Noack G, et al. Downregulatory cytokines in tracheobronchial aspirate fluid from infants with chronic lung disease of prematurity. Acta Paediatr 2000; 89:1375–1380.

56. Kunzmann S, Seher A, Kramer BW, et al. Connective tissue growth factor does not affect transforming growth factor beta 1-induced smad3 phosphorylation and T-lymphocyte proliferation. Int Arch Allergy Immunol 2008; 147:152–160.

57. Danan C, Franco ML, Jarreau PH, et al. High concentrations of keratinocyte growth factor in airways of premature infants predicted absence of bronchopulmonary dysplasia. Am J Respir Crit Care Med 2002; 165:1384–1387.

58. Lassus P, Heikkila P, Andersson LC, et al. Lower concentration of pulmonary hepatocyte growth factor is associated with more severe lung disease in preterm infants. J Pediatr 2003; 143:199–202.

59. Asikainen TM, Ahmad A, Schneider BK, et al. Effect of preterm birth on hypoxia-inducible factors and vascular endothelial growth factor in primate lungs. Pediatr Pulmonol 2005; 40:538–546.

60. Thomas W, Seidenspinner S, Kawczynska-Leda N, et al. Systemic fetal inflammation and reduced concentrations of macrophage migration inhibitory factor (MIF) in airways of extremely premature infants. Am J Obstet Gynecol 2008; 64:e1–e4.

61. Thébaud B, Ladha F, Michelakis ED, et al. Vascular endothelial growth factor gene therapy increases survival, promotes lung angiogenesis, and prevents alveolar damage in hyperoxia-induced lung injury: Evidence that angiogenesis participates in alveolarization. Circulation 2005; 112:2477–2486.

62. May M, Marx A, Seidenspinner S, et al. Apoptosis and proliferation in lungs of human fetuses exposed to chorioamnionitis. Histopathology 2004; 45:283–290.

63. Wirbelauer J, Schmidt B, Klingel K, et al. Serum and glucocorticoid inducible kinase in pulmonary tissue of preterm fetuses exposed to chorioamnionitis. Neonatology 2007; 93:257–262.

64. Buhimschi CS, Dulay AT, Abdel-Razeq S, et al. Fetal inflammatory response in women with proteomic biomarkers characteristic of intra-amniotic inflammation and preterm birth. BJOG 2009; 116:257–267.

65. Goldenberg RL, Andrews WW, Goepfert AR, et al. The Alabama Preterm Birth Study: umbilical cord blood Ureaplasma urealyticum and Mycoplasma hominis cultures in very preterm newborn infants. Am J Obstet Gynecol 2008; 198:43.e1–43.e5.

66. Romero R, Garite TJ. Twenty percent of very preterm neonates (23–32 weeks of gestation) are born with bacteremia caused by genital mycoplasmas. Am J Obstet Gynecol 2008; 198:1–3.

67. Lin HC, Su BH, Chang JS, et al. Nonassociation of interleukin 4 intron 3 and 590 promoter polymorphisms with bronchopulmonary dysplasia for ventilated preterm infants. Biol Neonate 2005; 87:181–186.

68. Kwinta P, Bik-Multanowski M, Mitkowska Z, et al. Genetic risk factors of bronchopulmonary dysplasia. Pediatr Res 2008; 64:682–688.

69. Van Marter LJ, Dammann O, Allred EN, et al. Chorioamnionitis, mechanical ventilation, and postnatal sepsis as modulators of chronic lung disease in preterm infants. J Pediatr 2002; 140:171–176.

70. Groneck P, Götze-Speer B, Speer CP. Inflammatory bronchopulmonary response of preterm infants with microbial colonisation of the airways at birth. Arch Dis Child Fetal Neonatal Ed 1996; 74:F51–F55.

71. Cordero L, Ayers LW, Davis K. Neonatal airway colonization with Gram-negative bacilli: association with severity of bronchopulmonary dysplasia. Pediatr Infect Dis J 1997; 16:18–23.

72. Rojas MA, Gonzalez A, Bancalari E, et al. Changing trends in the epidemiology and pathogenesis of neonatal chronic lung disease. J Pediatr 1995; 126:605–610.

73. Bancalari E, Claure N, Gonzalez A. Patent ductus arteriosus and respiratory outcome in premature infants. Biol Neonate 2005; 88:192–201.

74. Gonzales A, Sosenko IRS, Chandar J, et al. Influence of infection on patent ductus arteriosus and chronic lung disease in premature infants weighing 1000 grams or less. J Pediatr 1996; 128:470–478.
75. Yoder BA, Coalson JJ, Winter VT, et al. Effects of antenatal colonization with Ureaplasma urealyticum on pulmonary disease in the immature baboon. Pediatr Res 2003; 54:797–807.
76. Viscardi RM, Atamas SP, Luzina IG, et al. Antenatal Ureaplasma urealyticum respiratory tract infection stimulates proinflammatory, profibrotic responses in the preterm baboon lung. Pediatr Res 2006; 60:141–146.
77. Groneck P, Schmale J, Soditt V, et al. Bronchoalveolar inflammation following airway infection in preterm infants with chronic lung disease. Pediatr Pulmonol 2001; 31:331–338.
78. Kotecha S, Hodge R, Schaber JA, et al. Pulmonary Ureaplasma urealyticum is associated with the development of acute lung inflammation and chronic lung disease in preterm infants. Pediatr Res 2004; 55:61–68.
79. Schelonka RL, Katz B, Waites KB, et al. Critical appraisal of the role of Ureaplasma in the development of bronchopulmonary dysplasia with meta-analytic techniques. Pediatr Infect Dis J 2005; 12:1033–1039.
80. Muscedere JG, Mullen JBM, Gan K, et al. Tidal ventilation at low airway pressures can augment lung injury. Am J Respir Crit Care Med 1994; 149:1327–1334.
81. Dreyfuss D, Saumon G. Ventilator-induced lung injury: lessons from experimental studies. Am J Respir Crit Care Med 1998; 157:294–323.
82. Albertine KH, Jones GP, Starcher BC, et al. Chronic lung injury in preterm lambs. Disordered respiratory tract development. Am J Respir Crit Care Med 1999; 159:945–958.
83. Tremblay L, Valenza F, Ribeiro SP, et al. Injurious ventilatory strategies increase cytokines and c-fos m-RNA expression in an isolated rat lung model. J Clin Invest 1997; 99:944–952.
84. Thome U, Goetze-Speer B, Speer CP, et al. Comparison of pulmonary inflammatory mediators in preterm infants treated with intermittent positive pressure ventilation or high frequency oscillatory ventilation. Pediatr Res 1998; 44:330–337.
85. May M, Ströbel P, Seidenspinner S, et al. Apoptosis and proliferation in lungs of stillborn fetuses and ventilated preterm infants with respiratory distress syndrome. Eur Respir J 2004; 23:113–121.
86. Copland IB, Martinez F, Kavanagh BP, et al. High tidal volume ventilation causes different inflammatory responses in newborn versus adult lung. Am J Respir Crit Care Med 2004; 169:739–748.
87. Ricard JD, Dreyfuss D, Saumon G. Production of inflammatory cytokines in ventilator-induced lung injury: a reappraisal. Am J Respir Crit Care Med 2001; 163:1176–1180.
88. Saugstad OD. Bronchopulmonary dysplasia and oxidative stress: are we closer to an understanding of the pathogenesis of BPD? Acta Paediatr 1997; 86:1277–1282.
89. Coalson JJ. Experimental models of bronchopulmonary dysplasia. Biol Neonate 1997; 71:35–38.
90. Bonikos DS, Bensch KG, Ludwin SK, et al. Oxygen toxicity in the new born: the effect of prolonged 100% O_2 exposure on the lungs of new born mice. Lab Invest 1975; 32:619–635.
91. Wagenaar GT, ter Horst SA, van Gastelen MA, et al. Gene expression profile and histopathology of experimental bronchopulmonary dysplasia induced by prolonged oxidative stress. Free Radic Biol Med 2004; 36:782–801.
92. Vuichard D, Ganter MT, Schimmer RC, et al. Hypoxia aggravates lipopolysaccharide-induced lung injury. Clin Exp Immunol 2005; 141:248–260.
93. Thomas W, Speer CP. Nonventilatory strategies for prevention and treatment of bronchopulmonary dysplasia—what is the evidence? Neonatology 2008; 94:150–159.

8

Disruption of Lung Vascular Development

WILLIAM M. MANISCALCO
University of Rochester School of Medicine, Rochester, New York, U.S.A.

VINEET BHANDARI
Yale University School of Medicine, New Haven, Connecticut, U.S.A.

I. Introduction

Coordinated development of the alveolar microvasculature and alveolar airspaces is critical for normal gas exchange at birth. Both processes are complex, interactive, and disrupted in bronchopulmonary dysplasia (BPD). Much is known about distal lung epithelial development; however, the development of the microvasculature and alterations resulting from BPD are poorly understood. The potential for innovative therapeutic approaches to BPD may result from investigating mechanisms of lung microvascular development and its interaction with the distal epithelium. The following sections will briefly review normal lung vascular development and its regulation, critically evaluate evidence for interdependence of distal microvascular and epithelial development, describe changes that occur in BPD, and introduce potential therapies for BPD.

II. Lung Vascular Development

Vascular development requires the coordination of several processes, including differentiation of endothelial cell (EC) precursors, EC proliferation and migration, tube formation and branching, EC sprouting from existing vessels, attraction of perivascular supporting cells, and maturation of the endothelial lining. Two general mechanisms of primitive vessel formation contribute to lung vascular development: vasculogenesis and angiogenesis. Vasculogenesis is the in situ formation of primitive vessels by differentiation of angioblasts, the mesenchymal precursors of EC. Angiogenesis is the sprouting of new vessels from preexisting vessels. Conflicting data suggest that the embryonic lung vasculature arises by vasculogenesis (1,2), angiogenesis (3), or differing contributions of both processes to the proximal and distal vasculature (4–6).

A. Mechanisms of Lung Vascular Development

Vasculogenesis as the primary initial process of lung vascular formation requires coalescence of mesenchymal EC precursors into primitive vessels (2,7). As new peripheral lung buds form, a primitive capillary bed coalesces around the developing

Table 1 Stages of Lung Development

Stage	Mouse (days)	Rat (days)	Human (wk)
Embryonic	E8–E9	E10–E13	3–6
Pseudoglandular	E9–E16	E13.5–E18	6–16
Canalicular	E16–E18	E18–E20	16–26
Saccular	E18/birth	E21/birth	26–36
Alveolar	Postnatal	Postnatal	36+

tubule. In embryonic lung, EC progenitor cells are in close apposition to the developing epithelium where they form both proximal and distal capillaries (1,8). EC progenitor cells that form the proximal and distal vasculature may arise from distinct populations of stem cells (9). Through the pseudoglandular stage (Table 1), the vascular tree forms by fusion of the primitive capillaries. During the canalicular and saccular stages, sprouting and proliferation of the existing capillaries result in vascular expansion (2).

An alternative hypothesis of lung vascular development is that the proximal vessels develop by angiogenesis and the distal capillaries develop by vasculogenesis. Sprouting hilar vessels can be identified in the early pseudoglandular stage (4). By this time, the distal mesenchyme has vascular lakes lined with ECs that arise from hemangioblasts, precursors to both ECs and hematopoietic cells (9). In human fetal lung, channels between the nascent pulmonary artery and the peripheral vascular lakes are evident by 16 weeks' gestation (5). Identification of distal EC progenitors supports concurrent proximal angiogenesis and distal vasculogenesis in fetal lung (10). In the canalicular phase, the mesenchyme thins and the distal vascular lakes remodel into a capillary bed. Expansion of the distal microvasculature during the saccular stage is probably by angiogenesis (2,4).

In either model, distal vasculogenesis implies differentiation of EC progenitors in the distal mesenchyme. Mesenchymal cells in mid-pseudoglandular human lung express CD34, an early EC marker, and form tubelike structures around budding branches of airways (6). Putative EC precursors isolated from developing lung can form branching tubular networks, suggesting vasculogenic potential of the mesenchyme (11). The epithelium is necessary for survival and patterning of the primitive distal vasculature in vitro (8). EC progenitors can be identified in all phases of lung development, including the alveolar stage (12–14), suggesting they contribute to both fetal and postnatal development. Distinct populations of EC precursors may give rise to endothelial heterogeneity of the capillary bed (9,11).

Angiogenesis as the sole mechanism of lung vascular development is supported by analysis of murine lung in which the distal primitive vessels contain hematopoietic cells produced only in the yolk sac (3). These findings imply early continuity of the proximal and distal vessels. Because EC progenitor cells were not identified in the mesenchyme, "distal angiogenesis" may be the mechanism of capillary formation.

In later stages of lung development, when extrauterine survival is possible, the distal capillary bed undergoes substantial expansion and remodeling so that capillaries are in close apposition to the thinning epithelium (15,16). In the saccular stage, 90% of lung ECs are associated with terminal saccules (6). By the late canalicular–early saccular stage, the capillary-epithelial barrier thins to nearly adult values (17). As secondary septa form, expansion of the microvasculature appears coordinated with secondary septation (18). Secondary septation may require "folding up" of capillaries into double lumen septal vessels. As secondary septa thin, the dual capillaries fuse, split, and grow by differential expansion, a process termed intussusceptive angiogenesis, resulting in a single septal capillary (19,20). Therefore, secondary septation may be mechanistically dependent on vascular expansion and remodeling (15).

B. Regulation of Lung Vascular Development

Many growth factors, morphogens, and transcription factors regulate angiogenesis and vasculogenesis. In the developing lung, the vascular endothelial growth factor (VEGF) family is the most widely studied. The VEGF family currently has seven members (VEGF-A to VEGF-F, and placental growth factor or PlGF). VEGF-A is the best studied and is commonly known as VEGF. VEGF is critical for several steps in vessel formation, including differentiation of angioblasts, EC migration, tube formation, and capillary basement membrane remodeling (21). Embryos lacking a single *VEGF* allele die with defective vessel formation (22). VEGF is also essential for EC pattern formation (23). Conditional deletion of *VEGF* results in EC apoptosis (24,25). EC survival is enhanced by VEGF through induction of antiapoptotic factors (26). Nitric oxide (NO) is a downstream mediator of several VEGF actions, including EC survival and pulmonary vasodilation (27). The primary VEGF transcript is alternatively spliced to produce at least three protein isoforms, named for the number of amino acids (VEGF$_{121}$, VEGF$_{165}$, and VEGF$_{189}$). An important difference among the isoforms is their affinity for heparin and the extracellular matrix (ECM). VEGF$_{121}$ lacks a heparin-binding domain and is freely diffusible, whereas VEGF$_{165}$ is partially heparin-bound and VEGF$_{189}$ is highly bound to the ECM. The most commonly expressed isoforms are VEGF$_{120}$ and VEGF$_{164}$, but the lung has increased VEGF$_{189}$ compared with other organs (28). Both ECM-bound and diffusible VEGF may be necessary for vascular patterning (29).

In embryonic lung, VEGF is located in the primitive airway epithelium and the surrounding mesenchyme (6,8,30). By the pseudoglandular stage, VEGF is expressed mainly by epithelial cells of branching airways, and its expression increases in parallel with its receptors as development advances (8,30,31). In more mature lung, type II epithelial cells express VEGF (32–34). VEGF regulates vascularization in lung development, as shown by increased vessel density in embryonic lung explants exposed to VEGF$_{164}$ (30). Protein isoforms of VEGF are developmentally regulated in lung and may have specific developmental roles. VEGF$_{189}$ increases during development and is expressed primarily by type II cells (28,35).

VEGF actions are mediated by two high-affinity tyrosine kinase receptors, VEGFR1 (Flt-1) and VEGFR2 (Flk-1). VEGF binds to other receptors, but their roles in signaling are not clear (36). VEGFR2 is primarily on EC and mediates the major VEGF actions including differentiation, proliferation, migration and survival of EC, and vasodilation. Null mutants of VEGFR2 are embryo-lethal and fail to generate EC (37). VEGFR2 expression on EC progenitor cells is essential for primitive vessels organization (23,38). Embryonic lung epithelium is required for the differentiation of VEGFR2-expressing cells in the primitive mesenchyme, underscoring the importance of tissue interactions for pulmonary vascular development (8). Inhibition of VEGFR2 in embryonic lung results in decreased EC proliferation and decreased capillary branching (39).

Signaling through VEGFR2 induces NO production, which is essential for VEGF angiogenic and EC survival actions (40–42). Distal lung epithelial cells may also express VEGFR2 (43).

The role of VEGFR1 in vascular development is less clear. Null mutants of VEGFR1 are embryo-lethal, but increased ECs are present and the vasculature is poorly formed (44). However, VEGF ligation to VEGFR1 does not result in signal transduction or induce mitogenesis (45). In developing vessels, VEGFR1 may negatively modulate VEGF action by competing with VEGFR2 for ligand (46,47). VEGFR1 is expressed in lung later than VEGFR2 and may regulate vessel sprouting (48). In canalicular lung, enhancing VEGFR1 reduces EC proliferation but increases capillary network formation (39). A soluble form of VEGFR1 (termed sFlt-1) may be a dominant negative receptor and modulate embryonic vessel formation (48). It is highly expressed in late canalicular and saccular lung and may promote capillary network maturation (39). These data indicate that tight control of VEGF signaling by complex interactions with cell-bound and soluble receptors is essential for normal vascular morphogenesis.

Regulation of VEGF

Regulation of VEGF is complex and governed by hypoxia, growth factors, and morphogens (Table 2). VEGF gene transcription is strongly upregulated by hypoxia (49–51). The VEGF promoter binds hypoxia-inducible factor 1 (HIF-1), a transcription factor that is stabilized by hypoxia (52). HIF-1 is found in human fetal lung, and fetal lung explants cultured in 3% O_2 have increased VEGF and vascular development (34,53,54). Animals lacking HIF-2, a member of the HIF family, die shortly after birth and have decreased VEGF (43). Hyperoxia for several days decreases VEGF in lung and retina, but the molecular mechanism is not known (55–57). VEGF is also regulated by several growth factors and chemokines that are important for lung development (Table 2) (51,58–60). Lung VEGF expression is increased in fetal rats with high lung distension in the final two days of gestation (61). These animals also had a more mature

Table 2 Regulators of VEGF Expression

Growth factors	Cytokines
• PDGF	• TNF-α
• TGF-α, TGF-β	• COX-2/prostaglandins
• IGF	• IL-1β
• HGF	• IL-6
• EGF	Transcription factors
• FGF2	• HIF-1, HIF-2
• KGF	• NF-κB
Tumor suppressor genes	• AP-1
• P53, P73	Miscellaneous
• VHL	• Estrogen
	• Endotoxin

Source: Adapted from Ref. 60.

distribution of VEGF splice variants and advanced lung morphology. The cell-specific regulators of lung epithelial VEGF expression in development or injury are not known.

The Angiopoietin Family

The human angiopoietin (Ang) family consists of the ligands Ang1, Ang2, and Ang4 (62). Their receptor, Tie2, is mainly expressed by EC but has been identified on smooth muscle cells, fibroblasts, and lung epithelial cells (62–64). Ang1 binding to Tie2 transduces a signal, while Ang2 ligation does not, thereby acting as an antagonist of Ang1 (65). Ang1 is not mitogenic but mediates vascular remodeling, interactions of vessels with supporting cells, and vessel sprouting (65). In quiescent vessels, Ang1 stabilizes vessels, whereas Ang2 is induced during angiogenesis to loosen EC association with the ECM, thereby promoting VEGF-induced angiogenesis (66). Ang2 is expressed at sites of vascular remodeling where it may block the constitutive stabilizing action of Ang1. In some contexts, however, Ang2 may activate Tie2 while Ang1 isoforms inactivate the receptor (63,67–69). Embryos lacking Ang1 or Tie2 die with extensive vascular disorganization (65,70). Ang2 may also have Tie2-independent actions, including MMP2 expression and activation of the mitogen-activated protein kinase (MAPK) pathway (63,71,72). Ang1 and Ang2 are expressed in lung from the embryonic stage until term (73).

Interactions Between Angiopoietins and VEGF

Ang1, Ang2, and VEGF have complementary and coordinated roles in vascular development (74,75). Whereas VEGF induces primitive vessel formation, Ang1 promotes remodeling and stabilization of primitive vessels through interactions between EC and support cells (76). VEGF and Ang1 induce migration and sprouting; however, a combination of the two is more potent than either alone (77). Ang1 can counter the permeability effects of VEGF (78,79) and is anti-inflammatory when colocalized with VEGF (63). Interactions between VEGF and Ang family members may be necessary for normal pulmonary vascular development (76,80).

The Epithelium Is Critical for Distal Lung Vascular Development

Correlations between distal epithelial development and microvascular development implicate critical epithelial-mesenchymal interactions for normal lung morphogenesis, particularly distal epithelial VEGF expression. For example, fetal lung mesenchyme cultured without the epithelium develops few ECs (8). When cultured with the epithelium, the mesenchymal distribution of EC mimics lung in vivo. FGF9 and sonic hedgehog (SHH), which are required for normal lung branching morphogenesis, contribute to normal capillary plexus patterning by induction of spatially specific VEGF expression (81). Animals that are hypomorphic for FGF10 or that lack TTF-1 (NKX2.1) die shortly after birth with hypoplastic lungs, defective formation of distal lung vessels, and abnormal VEGF expression (82,83). Poor capillary and distal epithelial developments are found in both null mutants of IGF-I and animals with impaired IGF-IR signaling (10,84). Conditional ablation of epithelial laminin-α5 causes a reduction in type II cells, dilated distal airspaces, decreased capillary density, and decreased VEGF expression (85). Overexpression of matrix GLA protein (MGP), which antagonizes BMP-2, results in poor lung epithelial development, decreased epithelial VEGF, and abnormal vascular branching (86). Macrophage migration inhibitory factor (MIF), which induces VEGF, is expressed by the bronchial epithelium and vascular smooth muscle cells in the saccular stage. Animals lacking MIF have impaired lung maturation, including vascular development and septal thinning, associated with decreased VEGF (87). These data show a critical role for the distal epithelium in microvascular development.

III. Vascular Development Is Critical for Lung Epithelial Development

Normal vascular development may provide developmental signals for lung organogenesis, as has been documented for the liver and pancreas (88,89). Precise timing and location of VEGF expression may have a pivotal role in both early and later lung development, as suggested by studies that alter or block VEGF signaling. For example, overexpression or ectopic expression of VEGF results in both disrupted airspace and vascular development, implying precise temporal and spatial expression of VEGF are necessary for normal branching morphogenesis and vascular development (90–92). When lung allographs are treated with a decoy VEGF receptor, both capillary and epithelial morphogenesis are disrupted, even though the epithelium lacked VEGF receptors (93). Branching morphogenesis is impaired in lung explants treated with antisense oligonucleotides for VEGF or HIF-1 (54). However, inhibition of VEGFR2 signaling in embryonic lung explants maintained in hypoxic conditions abolished vascular development but only retarded branching morphogenesis, questioning a tight link between vascular and epithelial development at this stage (94).

VEGF$_{164}$ and VEGF$_{189}$ may be critical for development of both the distal vasculature and airspaces. Animals that express only VEGF$_{120}$ die shortly after birth with severe lung vascular defects and delayed airspace maturation (35,95). VEGF$_{164}$ increased epithelial branching, but this effect required mesenchyme (96), suggesting that VEGF does not directly affect lung epithelial cells. Conditional ablation of VEGF in lung results in death shortly after birth, poor primary septation, and deficient distal capillary formation (97). In these animals, epithelial proliferation is reduced, probably a result of decreased EC expression of hepatocyte growth factor (HGF), a lung epithelial morphogen that is implicated in the pathogenesis of BPD (98,99). Rather than a direct effect of VEGF on the epithelium, EC may be a source of a critical epithelial growth factor. Although VEGF increases epithelial proliferation in lung explants (100), the effect is likely indirect (101). Epithelial development is affected by inhibiting vascular development using methods that do not directly manipulate VEGF signaling. For example, endothelial monocyte activating polypeptide II (EMAP II) inhibits both vascularization and epithelial morphogenesis in fetal lung allographs (102). Ang1 and FGF2 can restore vascular and epithelial development in SHH-deficient lung explants (103). These data suggest that blocking vascular development, with or without affecting VEGF, may have major effects on epithelial development.

In murine species, secondary septation occurs mainly in the postnatal period and is disrupted by blocking VEGF signaling. In neonatal rats, blockade of angiogenesis or

VEGFR1/2 signaling with SU5416 results in poor secondary septation and vessel density, effects that persist into adulthood (104,105). Similarly, inhibition of VEGF signaling by soluble VEGF receptors impairs both alveolization and capillary density in postnatal rats (106). Antibody blockade of VEGFR2, but not VEGFR1, results in increased mortality and transient disruption of postnatal alveolization (107). As noted previously, NO is a downstream mediator of VEGF actions on angiogenesis and EC survival. VEGF receptor blockade decreases eNOS expression and results in EC apoptosis that precedes alveolar and vascular dysmorphogenesis (108,109). These effects are ameliorated by inhaled NO administered after receptor blockade (109). Impaired VEGF signaling is implicated in glucocorticoid inhibition of postnatal alveolization (110).

IV. Lung Microvascular Development in BPD

An important component of BPD is arrest of lung development, particularly diminished alveologenesis (111,112). Animal models of BPD suggest that impaired distal microvascular development is intimately linked to poor alveolar development. Studies of human autopsy specimens from premature infants dying with BPD suggest abnormal microvascular development of variable severity and timing (113–116).

A. Animal Models of BPD

Murine models of BPD have important limitations including lack of premature birth and reliance on interventions applied mainly in the alveolar stage of lung development. Alveolization is largely postnatal in these species, so postnatal hyperoxia can mimic some aspects of BPD, particularly impaired secondary septation (117). These models also suggest that postnatal hyperoxia results in impaired microvascular development. For example, hyperoxia in newborn rats and mice results in decreased capillary density and impaired alveologenesis (13,106,118–120). Most of these studies used at least 70% oxygen for exposures of 6 to 14 days. Other BPD models, such as premature lambs and baboons that are delivered at earlier stages of development, also show disrupted microvascular and alveolar development, as detailed below (121–126).

Because VEGF has a central role in lung microvascular development, it has been examined in various models of BPD. In models that employ postnatal hyperoxia, disrupted microvascular and alveolar development may be due to decreased lung VEGF or VEGF receptors. Evidence supporting this hypothesis comes from studies documenting decreased VEGF in hyperoxia and amelioration of the hyperoxic injury with VEGF treatment. These data are particularly interesting given the potential therapeutic roles of VEGF in BPD (127). In neonatal rabbits, decreased alveolar epithelial VEGF expression and a relative decrease in $VEGF_{189}$ are found at nine days of hyperoxia (28,55). Neonatal rats and piglets exposed to hyperoxia have decreased VEGF mRNA by 5 to14 days (106,128–130), but a transient increase in VEGF protein at earlier periods of hyperoxia (28,129). VEGFR1/2 and HIF-2 messages are also decreased by 9 to 12 days of hyperoxia. In adult animals, 1 to 3 days of hyperoxia results in decreased lung VEGF and VEGFR1/2 (55,131). Decreased VEGF and VEGFR2 messages are found in neonatal mice subjected to mechanical ventilation and 40% oxygen for 8 hours, while

24 hours treatment decreases the corresponding proteins (132). Gene expression profiling of neonatal rats exposed to 100% oxygen for 10 days shows downregulation of VEGFR2, PECAM-1 (an EC marker), and TIE-1 (an orphan EC receptor important in vascular development), coincident with impaired alveologenesis (133). Recovery from hyperoxia is associated with increased distal epithelial VEGF in neonates and adults. (32).

Premature baboons and lambs delivered during the late canalicular–early saccular stages and supported with variable oxygen and ventilation also have poor secondary septation (134,135). In the premature baboon model, animals are delivered at 125 days gestation (~25 weeks in the human) and supported with oxygen and ventilation to maintain normal blood gases for 14 days. Compared with gestational controls, they have dysmorphic capillaries, decreased PECAM-1 abundance, decreased type II cell VEGF, and decreased VEGFR1 (Fig. 1) (125). Consistent with arrested development, VEGF message did not increase above 125-day gestation levels. Blunted capillary growth into secondary septae is also characteristic of this model (136). The mechanism of decreased VEGF in these animals may be decreased HIF-1, which is coincident with decreased VEGF mRNA (137). HIF-2 is not changed. One study found increased VEGF protein by ELISA in whole lung homogenate at 14 days in this model (138), but VEGF ELISA may be falsely elevated in homogenates with small amounts of blood (139). Lambs delivered at 115 days gestation (term = 145 days) and treated with mechanical ventilation and

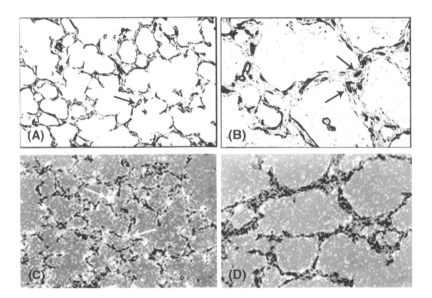

Figure 1 PECAM-1 immunostaining and VEGF in situ hybridization in baboons born at 125 days' gestation and treated with oxygen and ventilation for 14 days. (**A**) Black immunostaining (*black, arrow*) in 140-day gestational controls shows an extensive network of capillaries in close apposition to the epithelium. (**B**) In BPD animals, PECAM-1 immunostaining (*arrows*) shows dysmorphic capillaries that are imbedded in a thickened interstitium. (**C**) VEGF mRNA (*white grains, arrows*) is located in alveolar epithelial cells in gestational controls. (**D**) In BPD animals, there is a paucity of VEGF mRNA. 40× magnification. *Source*: Adapted from Ref. 125.

oxygen for 4 hours have decreased VEGF and HIF-1 (140). Ventilation and oxygen treatment of preterm (125 days) and term lambs for three weeks result in decreased VEGF message and protein compared with gestational controls (141). An additional premature lamb BPD model uses intra-amniotic endotoxin at 119 days gestation, which results in decreased alveolar number at 125 days without prolonged ex-utero exposure to oxygen or ventilation (142). These animals have decreased lung PECAM-1 protein and messages for $VEGF_{165}$, VEGFR2, eNOS, and TIE-2 (143). The effects are transient, but lung tissue VEGF protein remains depressed at seven days after endotoxin treatment. Fetal lung explants also have decreased VEGF when exposed to hyperoxic conditions. Pseudoglandular human lung cultured in 95% oxygen for 24 hours has decreased VEGF mRNA (56). Compared with embryonic mouse lung explants cultured in 3% oxygen, explants cultured for two days in relative hyperoxia (20% oxygen) have decreased VEGF and VEGFR2 (54). Although exceptions exist, the majority of studies on fetal lung models of BPD show impaired microvascular development and decreased VEGF signaling.

Some studies report an initial increase in VEGF protein in lung tissue or lavage during the early phases of hyperoxia (129,130,144). These data correspond to an increased VEGF secretion by A549 epithelial cells at 48 hours of hyperoxia (145). The mechanism was attributed to a posttranslational process. The early spike in VEGF expression may contribute to pulmonary edema resulting from hyperoxia (146). Recovery from several days of hyperoxia is associated with increased VEGF (32).

B. Human BPD

Studies of microvascular development in human BPD rely mainly on autopsy specimens or analysis of angiogenic factors in tracheal aspirates. Interpretation of autopsy material is hindered by many factors including small numbers, lack of appropriate controls, tissue sampling biases, disease heterogeneity, and use of archival autopsy tissues with variable tissue preservation. Despite these difficulties, most studies have shown disrupted microvascular development in BPD, although timing and severity are variable. In one study, lungs from premature infants with BPD were compared with controls who died from nonrespiratory causes at the same postconceptional age (114). The lungs were inflation fixed and processed by a single investigator in an average of six hours after death to preserve protein and mRNA. The BPD lungs had dysmorphic alveolar capillaries, decreased PECAM-1, and diminished VEGF and VEGFR1 mRNAs (Fig. 2). Archived autopsy samples from premature infants who died from BPD had VEGF immunostaining in type II cells, suggesting concurrent alveolar capillary repair (147). Immunostaining for endostatin, an antiangiogenic factor that inhibits VEGF signaling, is increased in archived lungs of premature infants who die with BPD (148), underscoring the importance of a balance between angiogenic and antiangiogenic factors.

Quantitative morphometrics of archived BPD and control lungs collected over 11 years showed a wide variation in capillary morphology in the patients with BPD (115). When compared with control lungs of various gestational ages, the BPD lungs of patients dying before 34 weeks' postmenstrual age had fewer air-blood barriers, less capillary load, and stunted secondary septation. The BPD patients who died after 34 weeks had evidence of adaptation involving vascularization of the primary septa. Contrary data were obtained from quantitative sterology of PECAM-1 staining and

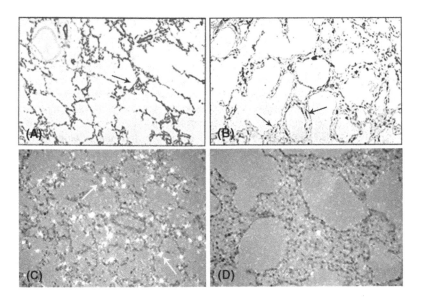

Figure 2 PECAM-1 immunostaining and VEGF in situ hybridization from infants of similar postmenstrual ages who died without lung disease or with BPD. (**A**) Extensive PECAM-1 immunostaining (*black, arrow*) in the control infants. (**B**) The BPD infants had disrupted capillary network formation with some capillaries imbedded in the thickened interstitium. (**C**): VEGF mRNA (*white grains, arrows*) is located in individual epithelial cells in patients without lung disease. (**D**) Decreased VEGF mRNA in the BPD patients. 20× magnification. *Source*: Adapted from Ref. 114.

PECAM-1 Western blotting in archived samples from ventilated premature infants obtained at an average of 15 to 18 hours postmortem (116). Long-term ventilated infants had expansion of the microvasculature compared with nonventilated controls. Growth in the capillary network may have been from increased EC proliferation. Although expanded, the pattern of capillary branching was immature in the BPD patients, as indicated by retention of a dual capillary pattern and poor network formation. Taken together, studies of human BPD using diverse methodologies display spectrum results ranging from decreased to increased microvasculature. Conflicting findings may be due to prolonged time from death to tissue processing, tissue degradation, inconsistencies in preservation of archived samples, and heterogeneity of human BPD. These issues notwithstanding, abnormalities in septal microvascular development and patterning are associated with BPD.

Interpretation of tracheal aspirates is complicated by several factors including VEGF expression by pulmonary macrophages and sampling distant from alveolar sources of VEGF (149). Tracheal aspirates from premature infants who developed BPD had lower VEGF levels during the first four to seven days than infants who did not develop BPD (150). Similarly, premature infants with severe RDS had lower tracheal aspirate VEGF levels than premature infants without severe RDS, suggesting that early lung injury impairs VEGF expression and is linked to development of BPD (147).

Decreased alveolar-lining fluid VEGF is also found in adults with ARDS (149). Soluble VEGFR1 (sFlt-1) is increased in ARDS, which results in lower bioactive VEGF (151). A phasic pattern of tracheal aspirate VEGF concentration was found in premature infants who developed BPD or died (144). In these patients, VEGF spiked at 12 hours, declined at 3 to 5 days, and increased at 28 days, compared with patients without BPD. In a trial of early glucocorticoids to ameliorate BPD, patients who received dexamethasone had increased deep lung lavage VEGF at seven days compared with controls (152). However, too few patients remained intubated at later times for meaningful comparisons of patients with and without BPD. Although differences in timing and methodology may account for variable tracheal aspirate VEGF concentrations, heterogeneity of BPD, including a complex pattern of injury and repair, probably contributes to the variable findings.

V. Potential BPD Therapies That Target Vascular Development

The concept that dysregulated vascular development and decreased VEGF contribute to poor alveolization in BPD (127) has sparked interest in manipulating VEGF, its upstream regulators, or its downstream mediators as potential BPD therapies. After 14 days of 75% oxygen, exogenous rhVEGF was given to neonatal rats for seven days of room air recovery (120). The VEGF-treated animals had improved lung structure and alveolization, comparable with nonhyperoxic animals, and increased vessel density. When used during a 14-day hyperoxic exposure, VEGF improved alveolization and eNOS expression, but also increased lung capillary permeability and lung edema (153,154). These concerns led to the treatment of hyperoxic newborn rats with adenovirus-mediated VEGF combined with Ang1 to counter the permeability effects of VEGF (106). This combination, delivered during hyperoxic exposure, resulted in preservation of alveolar development, matured new vasculature, and reduced vascular leakage seen in VEGF-only treatment (Fig. 3). Premature mice treated immediately after birth with VEGF had improved survival and lung maturation (43). VEGF induces NO production, which is a downstream mediator of important VEGF actions (108,155,156). Neonatal animals subjected to VEGFR2 blockade and treated with inhaled NO have improved alveolization, possibly secondary to reduced EC apoptosis (108,109). NO treatment of premature human neonates to ameliorate BPD remains controversial (157).

HIFs are important upstream transcriptional regulators of VEGF. HIF-1α is downregulated in experimental RDS and in the baboon model of BPD (137,140,158). HIFs can be stabilized by inhibiting prolyl hydroxylase domain–containing proteins (PHDs), which degrade HIFs. Pharmacologic stabilization of HIFs in the baboon model of BPD increases VEGF, VEGFR1, and PECAM-1 expression (137). This treatment also increases alveolar surface area and improves oxygenation compared with control animals (158).

In the human neonate, increased concentrations of Ang2 have been noted in the tracheal aspirates of infants who developed BPD or died (64,159). While the first study noted increased tracheal aspirate Ang2 concentrations in the first 24 hours (64), the latter noted the same over the first week of life, over multiple time points (159). Ang2 concentrations and birth weight were independent predictors of adverse outcome (BPD

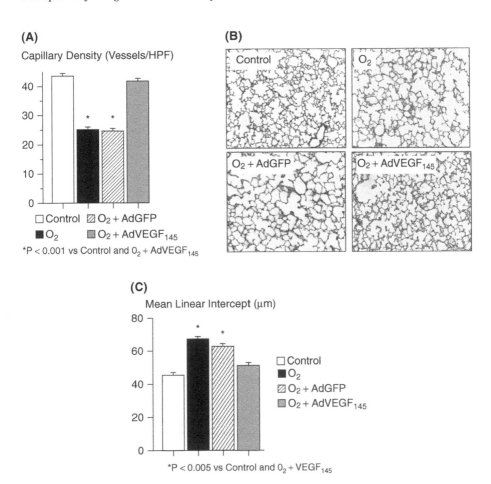

Figure 3 Adenovirus-mediated VEGF therapy in neonatal rats during hyperoxia. (**A**) AdVEGF improved capillary density compared with untreated oxygen-exposed animals or adenovirus controls (AdGFP). (**B**) Decreased alveolization in the oxygen-exposed animals is improved with AdVEGF. (**C**) Quantification of mean linear intercept confirms that AdVEGF improved alveolization in hyperoxic animals. *Source*: Adapted from Ref. 106.

and/or death), suggesting that inhibition of Ang2 may be a novel approach to ameliorate BPD.

VI. Conclusions

The interactions between alveolar epithelial and microvascular development are likely extensive and complex. The distal epithelium is a major source of VEGF, and distal ECs may express epithelial morphogens. Human BPD is associated with an abnormal alveolar microvasculature, but the timing, extent, and capacity for ongoing repair are not known. Novel therapeutic interventions that augment microvascular development in BPD hold promise to restore alveolar growth, morphology, and function.

References

1. Anderson-Berry A, O'Brien EA, Bleyl SB, et al. Vasculogenesis drives pulmonary vascular growth in the developing chick embryo. Dev Dynamics 2005; 233(1):145–153.
2. Hall SM, Hislop AA, Haworth SG. Origin, differentiation, and maturation of human pulmonary veins. Am J Respir Cell Mol Biol 2002; 26(3):333–340.
3. Parera MC, van Dooren M, van Kempen M, et al. Distal angiogenesis: a new concept for lung vascular morphogenesis. Am J Physiol: Lung Cell Mol Physiol 2005; 288(1):L141–L149.
4. deMello DE, Sawyer D, Galvin N, et al. Early fetal development of lung vasculature. Am J Respir Cell Mol Biol 1997; 16(5):568–581.
5. deMello DE, Reid LM. Embryonic and early fetal development of human lung vasculature and its functional implications. Pediatr Dev Pathol 2000; 3(5):439–449.
6. Maeda S, Suzuki S, Suzuki T, et al. Analysis of intrapulmonary vessels and epithelial-endothelial interactions in the human developing lung. Lab Invest 2002; 82(3):293–301.
7. Hall SM, Hislop AA, Pierce CM, et al. Prenatal origins of human intrapulmonary arteries: formation and smooth muscle maturation. Am J Respir Cell Mol Biol 2000; 23(2):194–203.
8. Gebb SA, Shannon JM. Tissue interactions mediate early events in pulmonary vasculogenesis. Dev Dynamics 2000; 217(2):159–169.
9. Fisher KA, Summer RS. Stem and progenitor cells in the formation of the pulmonary vasculature. Curr Topics Dev Biol 2006; 74:117–131.
10. Han RNN, Post M, Tanswell AK, et al. Insulin-like growth factor-I receptor-mediated vasculogenesis/angiogenesis in human lung development [see comment]. Am J Respir Cell Mol Biol 2003; 28(2): 159–169.
11. Akeson AL, Wetzel B, Thompson FY, et al. Embryonic vasculogenesis by endothelial precursor cells derived from lung mesenchyme. Dev Dyn 2000; 217(1):11–23.
12. Schachtner SK, Wang Y, Scott Baldwin H. Qualitative and quantitative analysis of embryonic pulmonary vessel formation. Am J Respir Cell Mol Biol 2000; 22(2):157–165.
13. Irwin D, Helm K, Campbell N, et al. Neonatal lung side population cells demonstrate endothelial potential and are altered in response to hyperoxia-induced lung simplification. Am J Physiol: Lung Cell Mol Physiol 2007; 293(4):L941–L951
14. Balasubramaniam V, Mervis CF, Maxey AM, et al. Hyperoxia reduces bone marrow, circulating, and lung endothelial progenitor cells in the developing lung: implications for the pathogenesis of bronchopulmonary dysplasia. Am J Physiol: Lung Cell Mol Physiol 2007; 292(5): L1073–L1084.
15. Burri PH. Fetal and postnatal development of the lung. Annu Rev Physiol 1984; 46:617–628.
16. Hislop AA. Airway and blood vessel interaction during lung development. J Anat 2002; 201(4): 325–334.
17. Burri PH, Dbaly J, Weibel ER. The postnatal growth of the rat lung. I. Morphometry. Anat Rec 1974; 178(4):711–730.
18. Moschopulos M, Burri PH. Morphometric analysis of fetal rat lung development. Anat Rec 1993; 237(1): 38–48.
19. Burri PH, Tarek MR. A novel mechanism of capillary growth in the rat pulmonary microcirculation. Anat Record 1990; 228(1): 35–45.
20. Roth-Kleiner M, Berger TM, Tarek MR, et al. Neonatal dexamethasone induces premature microvascular maturation of the alveolar capillary network. Dev Dyn 2005; 233(4): 1261–1271.

21. Ferrara N, Gerber HP, LeCouter J. The biology of VEGF and its receptors. Nat Med 2003; 9(6):669–676.
22. Ferrara N, Carver-Moore K, Chen H, et al. Heterozygous embryonic lethality induced by targeted inactivation of the VEGF gene. Nature 1996; 380(6573):439–442.
23. Ambler CA, Schmunk GM, Bautch VL. Stem cell-derived endothelial cells/progenitors migrate and pattern in the embryo using the VEGF signaling pathway. Dev Biol 2003; 257(1):205–219.
24. Tang K, Breen EC, Gerber HP, et al. Capillary regression in vascular endothelial growth factor-deficient skeletal muscle. Physiol Genomics 2004; 18(1):63–69.
25. Gerber HP, McMurtrey A, Kowalski J, et al. Vascular endothelial growth factor regulates endothelial cell survival through the phosphatidylinositol 3'-kinase/Akt signal transduction pathway. Requirement for Flk-1/KDR activation. J Biol Chem 1998; 273(46):30336–30343.
26. Nor JE, Christensen J, Mooney DJ, et al. Vascular endothelial growth factor (VEGF)-mediated angiogenesis is associated with enhanced endothelial cell survival and induction of Bcl-2 expression. Am J Pathol 1999; 154(2):375–384.
27. Grover TR, Zenge JP, Parker TA, et al. Vascular endothelial growth factor causes pulmonary vasodilation through activation of the phosphatidylinositol-3-kinase-nitric oxide pathway in the late-gestation ovine fetus. Pediatr Res 2002; 52(6):907–912.
28. Watkins RH, D'Angio CT, Ryan RM, et al. Differential expression of VEGF mRNA splice variants in newborn and adult hyperoxic lung injury. Am J Physiol: Lung Cell Mol Physiol 1999; 276(5 pt 1):L858–L867.
29. Bautch VL, Ambler CA. Assembly and patterning of vertebrate blood vessels. Trends Cardiovasc Med 2004; 14(4):138–143.
30. Healy AM, Morgenthau L, Zhu X, et al. VEGF is deposited in the subepithelial matrix at the leading edge of branching airways and stimulates neovascularization in the murine embryonic lung. Dev Dyn 2000; 219(3):341–352.
31. Bhatt AJ, Amin SB, Chess PR, et al. Expression of vascular endothelial growth factor and Flk-1 in developing and glucocorticoid-treated mouse lung. Pediatr Res 2000; 47(5):606–613.
32. Maniscalco WM, Watkins RH, Finkelstein JN, et al. Vascular endothelial growth factor mRNA increases in alveolar epithelial cells during recovery from oxygen injury. Am J Respir Cell Mol Biol 1995; 13(4):377–386.
33. Monacci WT, Merrill MJ, Oldfield EH. Expression of vascular permeability factor/vascular endothelial growth factor in normal rat tissues. Am J Physiol 1993; 264(4,pt 1):C995–C1002.
34. Acarregui MJ, Penisten ST, Goss KL., et al. Vascular endothelial growth factor gene expression in human fetal lung in vitro. Am J Respir Cell Mol Biol 1999; 20:14–23.
35. Ng YS, Rohan R, Sunday ME, et al. Differential expression of VEGF isoforms in mouse during development and in the adult. Dev Dyn 2001; 220:112–121.
36. Rossant J, Howard L. Signaling pathways in vascular development. Annu Rev Cell Dev Biol 2002; 18:541–573.
37. Shalaby F, Rossant J, Yamaguchi TP, et al. Failure of blood-island formation and vasculogenesis in Flk-1-deficient mice. Nature 1995; 376(6535):62–66.
38. Yamashita J, Itoh H, Hirashima M, et al. Flk1-positive cells derived from embryonic stem cells serve as vascular progenitors. Nature 2000; 408(6808):92–96.
39. Yamamoto Y, Shiraishi I, Dai P, et al. Regulation of embryonic lung vascular development by vascular endothelial growth factor receptors, Flk-1 and Flt-1. Anat Rec 2007; 290(8): 958–973.
40. Ziche M, Morbidelli L, Masini E, et al. Nitric oxide mediates angiogenesis in vivo and endothelial cell growth and migration in vitro promoted by substance P. J Clin Invest 1994; 94(5):2036–2044.

41. Shen BQ, Lee DY, Zioncheck TF. Vascular endothelial growth factor governs endothelial nitric-oxide synthase expression via a KDR/Flk-1 receptor and a protein kinase C signaling pathway. J Biol Chem 1999; 274(46):33057–33063.
42. Feng Y, Venema VJ, Venema RC, et al. VEGF induces nuclear translocation of Flk-1/KDR, endothelial nitric oxide synthase, and caveolin-1 in vascular endothelial cells. Biochem Biophys Res Commun 1999; 256(1):192–197.
43. Compernolle V, Brusselmans K, Acker T, et al. Loss of HIF-2alpha and inhibition of VEGF impair fetal lung maturation, whereas treatment with VEGF prevents fatal respiratory distress in premature mice [comment]. Nat Med 2002; 8(7):702–710.
44. Fong GH, Rossant J, Gertsenstein M, et al. Role of the flt-1 receptor tyrosine kinase in regulating the assembly of vascular endothelium. Nature 1995; 376(6535):66–70.
45. Seetharam L, Gotoh N, Maru Y, et al. A unique signal transduction from flt tyrosine kinase, a receptor for vascular endothelial growth factor VEGF. Oncogene 1995; 10(1):135–147.
46. Roberts DM, Kearney JB, Johnson JH, et al. The vascular endothelial growth factor (VEGF) receptor Flt-1 (VEGFR-1) modulates Flk-1 (VEGFR-2) signaling during blood vessel formation. Am J Pathol 2004; 164(5):1531–1535.
47. Rahimi N, Dayanir V, Lashkari K. Receptor chimeras indicate that the vascular endothelial growth factor receptor-1 (VEGFR-1) modulates mitogenic activity of VEGFR-2 in endothelial cells. J Biol Chem 2000; 275(22):16986–16992.
48. Kearney JB, Kappas NC, Ellerstrom C, et al. The VEGF receptor flt-1 (VEGFR-1) is a positive modulator of vascular sprout formation and branching morphogenesis. Blood 2004; 103(12):4527–4535.
49. Ikeda E, Achen MG, Brier G, et al. Hypoxia-induced transcriptional activation and increased mRNA stability of vascular endothelial growth factor in C6 glioma cells. J Biol Chem 1995; 270(34):19761–19766.
50. Tuder RM, Flook BE, Voelkel NF. Increased gene expression for VEGF and the VEGF receptors KDR/Flk and Flt in lungs exposed to acute or to chronic hypoxia. Modulation of gene expression by nitric oxide. J Clin Invest 1995; 95(4):1798–1807.
51. Boussat S, Eddahibi S, Coste A, et al. Expression and regulation of vascular endothelial growth factor in human pulmonary epithelial cells. Am J Physiol Lung Cell Mol Physiol 2000; 279(2):L371–L378.
52. Forsythe JA, Jiang BH, Iyer NV, et al. Activation of vascular endothelial growth factor gene transcription by hypoxia-inducible factor 1. Mol Cell Biol 1996; 16(9):4604–4613.
53. Groenman F, Rutter M, Caniggia I, et al. Hypoxia-inducible factors in the first trimester human lung. J Histochem Cytochem 2007; 55(4):355–363.
54. van Tuyl M, Liu J, Wang J, et al. Role of oxygen and vascular development in epithelial branching morphogenesis of the developing mouse lung. Am J Physiol: Lung Cell Mol Physiol 2005; 288(1):L167–L178.
55. Maniscalco WM, Watkins RH, Dangio CT, et al. Hyperoxic injury decreases alveolar epithelial cell expression of vascular endothelial growth factor (VEGF) in neonatal rabbit lung. Am J Respir Cell Mol Biol 1997; 16(5):557–567.
56. Bustani P, Hodge R, Tellabati A, et al. Differential response of the epithelium and interstitium in developing human fetal lung explants to hyperoxia. Pediatr Res 2006; 59(3):383–388.
57. Yamada H, Yamada E, Hackett SF, et al. Hyperoxia causes decreased expression of vascular endothelial growth factor and endothelial cell apoptosis in adult retina. J Cell Physiol 1999; 179(2):149–156.
58. Gille J, Swerlick RA, Caughman SW. Transforming growth factor-alpha-induced transcriptional activation of the vascular permeability factor (VPF/VEGF) gene requires AP-2-dependent DNA binding and transactivation. EMBO J 1997; 16(4):750–759.

59. Frank S, Hubner G, Breier G, et al. Regulation of vascular endothelial growth factor expression in cultured keratinocytes. Implications for normal and impaired wound healing. J Biol Chem 1995; 270(21):12607–12613.

60. Lahm T, Crisostomo PR, Markel TA, et al. The critical role of vascular endothelial growth factor in pulmonary vascular remodeling after lung injury. Shock 2007; 28(1):4–14.

61. Hara A, Chapin CJ, Ertsey R, et al. Changes in fetal lung distension alter expression of vascular endothelial growth factor and its isoforms in developing rat lung. Pediatr Res 2005; 58(1):30–37.

62. Shim WS, Ho IA, Wong PE. Angiopoietin: a TIE(d) balance in tumor angiogenesis. Mol Cancer Res 2007; 5(7):655–665.

63. Makinde T, Agrawal DK. Intra and extra-vascular trans-membrane signaling of Angiopoietin-1-Tie2 receptor in health and disease. J Cell Mol Med 2008; 12(3):810–828.

64. Bhandari V, Choo-Wing R, Lee CG, et al. Hyperoxia causes angiopoietin 2-mediated acute lung injury and necrotic cell death. Nat Med 2006; 12(11):1286–1293.

65. Suri C, Jones PF, Patan S, et al. Requisite role of angiopoietin-1, a ligand for the TIE2 receptor, during embryonic angiogenesis. Cell 1996; 87(7):1171–1180.

66. Oh H, Takagi H, Suzuma K, et al. Hypoxia and vascular endothelial growth factor selectively up-regulate angiopoietin-2 in bovine microvascular endothelial cells. J Biol Chem 1999; 274(22):15732–15739.

67. Davis S, Papadopoulos N, Aldrich TH, et al. Angiopoietins have distinct modular domains essential for receptor binding, dimerization and superclustering. Nat Struct Biol 2003; 10(1):38–44.

68. Huang YQ, Li JJ, Karpatkin S. Identification of a family of alternatively spliced mRNA species of angiopoietin-1. Blood 2000; 95(6):1993–1999.

69. Daly C, Pasnikowski E, Burova E, et al. Angiopoietin-2 functions as an autocrine protective factor in stressed endothelial cells. Proc Nat Acad Sci U S A 2006; 103(42):15491–15496.

70. Sato TN, Tozawa Y, Deutsch U, et al. Distinct roles of the receptor tyrosine kinases Tie-1 and Tie-2 in blood vessel formation. Nature 1995; 376(6535):70–74.

71. Hu B, Jarzynka MJ, Guo P, et al. Angiopoietin 2 induces glioma cell invasion by stimulating matrix metalloprotease 2 expression through the alphavbeta1 integrin and focal adhesion kinase signaling pathway. Cancer Res 2006; 66(2):775–783.

72. Carlson TR, Feng Y, Maisonpierre PC, et al. Direct cell adhesion to the angiopoietins mediated by integrins. J Biol Chem 2001; 276(28):26516–26525.

73. Colen KL, Crisera CA, Rose MI, et al. Vascular development in the mouse embryonic pancreas and lung. J Pediatr Surg 1999; 34(5):781–785.

74. Maisonpierre PC, Suri C, Jones PF, et al. Angiopoietin-2, a natural antagonist for Tie2 that disrupts in vivo angiogenesis. Science 1997; 277(5322):55–60.

75. Holash J, Maisonpierre PC, Compton D, et al. Vessel cooption, regression, and growth in tumors mediated by angiopoietins and VEGF. Science 1999; 284(5422):1994–1998.

76. Papapetropoulos A, Garcia-Cardena G, Dengler TJ, et al. Direct actions of angiopoietin-1 on human endothelium: evidence for network stabilization, cell survival, and interaction with other angiogenic growth factors. Lab Invest 1999; 79(2):213–223.

77. Chae JK, Kim I, Lim ST, et al. Coadministration of angiopoietin-1 and vascular endothelial growth factor enhances collateral vascularization. Arterioscler Thromb Vasc Biol 2000; 20(12):2573–2578.

78. Larcher F, Murillas R, Bolontrade M, et al. VEGF/VPF overexpression in skin of transgenic mice induces angiogenesis, vascular hyperpermeability and accelerated tumor development. Oncogene 1998; 17(3):303–311.

79. Thurston G, Rudge JS, Ioffe E, et al. Angiopoietin-1 protects the adult vasculature against plasma leakage. Nat Med 2000; 6(4):460–463.

80. Gale NW, Yancopoulos GD. Growth factors acting via endothelial cell-specific receptor tyrosine kinases: VEGFs, angiopoietins, and ephrins in vascular development. Genes Dev 1999; 13(9):1055–1066.

81. White AC, Lavine KJ, Ornitz DM. FGF9 and SHH regulate mesenchymal VEGFA expression and development of the pulmonary capillary network. Development 2007; 134(20): 3743–3752.

82. Yuan B, Li C, Kimura S, et al. Inhibition of distal lung morphogenesis in Nkx2.1(-/-) embryos. Dev Dyn 2000; 217(2):180–190.

83. Ramasamy SK, Mailleux AA, Gupte VV, et al. Fgf10 dosage is critical for the amplification of epithelial cell progenitors and for the formation of multiple mesenchymal lineages during lung development. Dev Biol 2007; 307(2):237–247.

84. Moreno-Barriuso N, Lopez-Malpartida AV, de Pablo F, et al. Alterations in alveolar epithelium differentiation and vasculogenesis in lungs of LIF/IGF-I double deficient embryos. Dev Dyn 2006; 235(8):2040–2050.

85. Nguyen NM, Kelley DG, Schlueter JA, et al. Epithelial laminin alpha5 is necessary for distal epithelial cell maturation, VEGF production, and alveolization in the developing murine lung. Dev Biol 2005; 282(1):111–125.

86. Yao Y, Nowak S, Yochelis A, et al. Matrix GLA protein, an inhibitory morphogen in pulmonary vascular development. J Biol Chem 2007; 282(41):30131–30142.

87. Kevill KA, Bhandari V, Kettunen M, et al. A role for macrophage migration inhibitory factor in the neonatal respiratory distress syndrome. J Immunol 2008; 180(1):601–608.

88. Matsumoto K, Yoshitomi H, Rossant J, et al. Liver organogenesis promoted by endothelial cells prior to vascular function. Science 2001; 294(5542):559–563.

89. Lammert E, Cleaver O, Melton D, et al. Induction of pancreatic differentiation by signals from blood vessels. Science 2001; 294(5542):564–567.

90. Zeng X, Wert SE, Federici R, et al. VEGF enhances pulmonary vasculogenesis and disrupts lung morphogenesis in vivo. Dev Dyn 1998; 211:215–227.

91. Akeson AL, Greenberg JM, Cameron JE, et al. Temporal and spatial regulation of VEGF-A controls vascular patterning in the embryonic lung. Dev Biol 2003; 264(2):443–455.

92. Akeson AL, Cameron JE, Le Cras TD, et al. Vascular endothelial growth factor-A induces prenatal neovascularization and alters bronchial development in mice. Pediatr Res 2005; 57(1): 82–88.

93. Zhao L, Wang K, Ferrara N, et al. Vascular endothelial growth factor co-ordinates proper development of lung epithelium and vasculature. Mech Dev 2005; 122(7–8):877–886.

94. Groenman FA, Rutter M, Wang J, et al. Effect of chemical stabilizers of hypoxia-inducible factors on early lung development. Am J Physiol Lung Cell Mol Physiol 2007; 293(3): L557–L567.

95. Galambos C, Ng YS, Ali A, et al. Defective pulmonary development in the absence of heparin-binding vascular endothelial growth factor isoforms. Am J Respir Cell Mol Biol 2002; 27(2):194–203.

96. Del Moral PM, Sala FG, Tefft D, et al. VEGF-A signaling through Flk-1 is a critical facilitator of early embryonic lung epithelial to endothelial crosstalk and branching morphogenesis. Dev Biol 2006; 290(1):177–188.

97. Yamamoto H, Yun EJ, Gerber H-P, et al. Epithelial-vascular cross talk mediated by VEGF-A and HGF signaling directs primary septae formation during distal lung morphogenesis. Dev Biol 2007; 308(1):44–53.

98. Ohmichi H, Koshimizu U, Matsumoto K, et al. Hepatocyte growth factor (HGF) acts as a mesenchyme-derived morphogenic factor during fetal lung development. Development 1998; 125(7):1315–1324.

99. Lassus P, Heikkila P, Andersson LC, et al. Lower concentration of pulmonary hepatocyte growth factor is associated with more severe lung disease in preterm infants. J Pediatr 2003; 143(2):199–202.

100. Brown KR, England KM, Goss KL, et al. VEGF induces airway epithelial cell proliferation in human fetal lung in vitro. Am J Physiol Lung Cell Mol Physiol 2001; 281(4): L1001–L1010.

101. Raoul W, Chailley-Heu B, Barlier-Mur AM, et al. Effects of vascular endothelial growth factor on isolated fetal alveolar type II cells. Am J Physiol Lung Cell Mol Physiol 2004; 286(6): L1293–L1301.

102. Schwarz MA, Zhang F, Gebb S, et al. Endothelial monocyte activating polypeptide II inhibits lung neovascularization and airway epithelial morphogenesis. Mech Dev 2000; 95(1–2):123–132.

103. van Tuyl M, Groenman F, Wang J, et al. Angiogenic factors stimulate tubular branching morphogenesis of sonic hedgehog-deficient lungs. Dev Biol 2007; 303(2):514–526.

104. Jakkula M, Le Cras TD, Gebb S, et al. Inhibition of angiogenesis decreases alveolarization in the developing rat lung. Am J Physiol Lung Cell Mol Physiol 2000; 279(3):L600–L607.

105. Le Cras TD, Markham NE, Tuder RM, et al. Treatment of newborn rats with a VEGF receptor inhibitor causes pulmonary hypertension and abnormal lung structure. Am J Physiol Lung Cell Mol Physiol 2002; 283(3):L555–L562.

106. Thebaud B, Ladha F, Michelakis ED, et al. Vascular endothelial growth factor gene therapy increases survival, promotes lung angiogenesis, and prevents alveolar damage in hyperoxia-induced lung injury: evidence that angiogenesis participates in alveolarization. Circulation 2005; 112(16):2477–2486.

107. McGrath-Morrow SA, Cho C, Cho C, et al. Vascular endothelial growth factor receptor 2 blockade disrupts postnatal lung development. Am J Respir Cell Mol Biol 2005; 32(5): 420–427.

108. Tang JR, Markham NE, Lin YJ, et al. Inhaled nitric oxide attenuates pulmonary hypertension and improves lung growth in infant rats after neonatal treatment with a VEGF receptor inhibitor. Am J Physiol Lung Cell Mol Physiol 2004; 287(2):L344–L351.

109. Tang J-R, Seedorf G, Balasubramaniam V, et al. Early inhaled nitric oxide treatment decreases apoptosis of endothelial cells in neonatal rat lungs after vascular endothelial growth factor inhibition. Am J Physiol Lung Cell Mol Physiol 2007; 293(5):L1271–L1280.

110. Clerch LB, Baras AS, Massaro GD, et al. DNA microarray analysis of neonatal mouse lung connects regulation of KDR with dexamethasone-induced inhibition of alveolar formation. Am J Physiol Lung Cell Mol Physiol 2004; 286(2):L411–L419.

111. Husain AN, Siddiqui NH, Stocker JT. Pathology of arrested acinar development in post-surfactant bronchopulmonary dysplasia. Hum Pathol 1998; 29(7):710–717.

112. Coalson J. Pathology of new bronchopulmonary dysplasia. Semin Neonatol 2003; 8(1): 73–81.

113. Coalson J. Pathology of chronic lung disease in early infancy. In: Bland RD, Coalson JJ, eds. Chronic Lung Disease in Early Infancy. New York: Marcel Dekker, 2000:85–124.

114. Bhatt AJ, Pryhuber GS, Huyck H, et al. Disrupted pulmonary vasculature and decreased vascular endothelial growth factor, Flt-1, and TIE-2 in human infants dying with bronchopulmonary dysplasia. Am J Respir Crit Care Med 2001; 164(10):1971–1980.

115. Thibeault DW, Mabry SM, Norberg M, et al. Lung microvascular adaptation in infants with chronic lung disease. Biol Neonate 2004; 85(4):273–282.

116. De Paepe ME, Mao Q, Powell J, et al. Growth of pulmonary microvasculature in ventilated preterm infants. Am J Respir Crit Care Med 2006; 173(2):204–211.

117. Warner BB, Stuart LA, Papes RA, et al. Functional and pathological effects of prolonged hyperoxia in neonatal mice. Am J Physiol Lung Cell Mol Physiol 1998; 275(1 pt 1): L110–L117.

118. Roberts RJ, Weesner KM, Bucher JR. Oxygen-induced alterations in lung vascular development in the newborn rat. Pediatr Res 1983; 17(5):368–375.

119. Boros V, Burghardt JS, Morgan CJ, et al. Leukotrienes are indicated as mediators of hyperoxia-inhibited alveolarization in newborn rats. Am J Physiol Lung Cell Mol Physiol 1997; 272(3 pt 1):L433–L441.

120. Kunig AM, Balasubramaniam V, Markham NE, et al. Recombinant human VEGF treatment enhances alveolarization after hyperoxic lung injury in neonatal rats. Am J Physiol Lung Cell Mol Physiol 2005; 289(4):L529–L535.

121. Bland RD, Albertine KH, Carlton DP, et al. Chronic lung injury in preterm lambs: abnormalities of the pulmonary circulation and lung fluid balance. Pediatr Res 2000; 48(1): 64–74.

122. Bland RD, Albertine KH, Carlton DP, et al. Inhaled nitric oxide effects on lung structure and function in chronically ventilated preterm lambs. Am J Respir Crit Care Med 2005; 172(7): 899–906.

123. Coalson JJ, Winter VT, Gerstmann DR, et al. Pathophysiologic, morphometric, and biochemical studies of the premature baboon with bronchopulmonary dysplasia. Am Rev Respir Dis 1992; 145(4 pt 1):872–881.

124. Coalson JJ, Winter VT, Siler-Khodr T, et al. Neonatal chronic lung disease in extremely immature baboons. Am J Respir Crit Care Med 1999; 160(4):1333–1346.

125. Maniscalco WM, Watkins RH, Pryhuber GS, et al. Angiogenic factors and alveolar vasculature: development and alterations by injury in very premature baboons. Am J Physiol Lung Cell Mol Physiol 2002; 282(4):L811–L823.

126. Maniscalco WM, Watkins RH, Roper JM, et al. Hyperoxic ventilated premature baboons have increased p53, oxidant DNA damage and decreased VEGF expression. Pediatr Res 2005; 58(3):549–556.

127. Thebaud B, Abman SH. Bronchopulmonary dysplasia: where have all the vessels gone? Roles of angiogenic growth factors in chronic lung disease. Am J Respir Crit Care Med 2007; 175(10):978–985.

128. Lin YJ, Markham NE, Balasubramaniam V, et al. Inhaled nitric oxide enhances distal lung growth after exposure to hyperoxia in neonatal rats. Pediatr Res 2005; 58(1):22–29.

129. Hosford GE, Olson DM. Effects of hyperoxia on VEGF, its receptors, and HIF-2alpha in the newborn rat lung. Am J Physiol Lung Cell Mol Physiol 2003; 285(1):L161–L168.

130. Ekekezie II, Thibeault DW, Rezaiekhaligh MH, et al. Endostatin and vascular endothelial cell growth factor (VEGF) in piglet lungs: effect of inhaled nitric oxide and hyperoxia. Pediatr Res 2003; 53(3):440–446.

131. Klekamp JG, Jarzecka K, Perkett EA. Exposure to hyperoxia decreases the expression of vascular endothelial growth factor and its receptors in adult rat lungs. Am J Pathol 1999; 154(3):823–831.

132. Bland RD, Mokres LM, Ertsey R, et al. Mechanical ventilation with 40% oxygen reduces pulmonary expression of genes that regulate lung development and impairs alveolar septation in newborn mice. Am J Physiol Lung Cell Mol Physiol 2007; 293(5):L1099–L1110.

133. Wagenaar GT, ter Horst SA, van Gastelen MA, et al. Gene expression profile and histopathology of experimental bronchopulmonary dysplasia induced by prolonged oxidative stress. Free Radic Biol Med 2004; 36(6):782–801.

134. Coalson JJ, Winter V, deLemos RA. Decreased alveolarization in baboon survivors with bronchopulmonary dysplasia. Am J Respir Crit Care Med 1995; 152(2):640–646.

135. Albertine KH, Jones GP, Starcher BC, et al. Chronic lung injury in preterm lambs. Disordered respiratory tract development. Am J Respir Crit Care Med 1999; 159(3):945–958.

136. Subramaniam M, Bausch C, Twomey A, et al. Bombesin-like peptides modulate alveolarization and angiogenesis in bronchopulmonary dysplasia. Am J Respir Crit Care Med 2007; 176(9):902–912.

137. Asikainen TM, Waleh NS, Schneider BK, et al. Enhancement of angiogenic effectors through hypoxia-inducible factor in preterm primate lung in vivo. Am J Physiol Lung Cell Mol Physiol 2006; 291(4):L588–L595.
138. Asikainen TM, Ahmad A, Schneider BK, et al. Effect of preterm birth on hypoxia-inducible factors and vascular endothelial growth factor in primate lungs. Pediatr Pulmonol 2005; 40(6):538–546.
139. Tambunting F, Beharry K, Waltzman J, et al. Impaired lung vascular endothelial growth factor in extremely premature baboons developing bronchopulmonary dysplasia/chronic lung disease. J Invest Med 2005; 53(5):253–262.
140. Grover TR, Asikainen TM, Kinsella JP, et al. Hypoxia-inducible factors HIF-1alpha and HIF-2alpha are decreased in an experimental model of severe respiratory distress syndrome in preterm lambs. Am J Physiol Lung Cell Mol Physiol 2007; 292(6):L1345–L1351.
141. Bland RD, Xu L, Ertsey R, et al. Dysregulation of pulmonary elastin synthesis and assembly in preterm lambs with chronic lung disease. Am J Physiol Lung Cell Mol Physiol 2007; 292(6):L1370–L1384.
142. Willet KE, Jobe AH, Ikegami M, et al. Antenatal endotoxin and glucocorticoid effects on lung morphometry in preterm lambs. Pediatr Res 2000; 48(6):782–788.
143. Kallapur SG, Bachurski CJ, Le Cras TD, et al. Vascular changes after intra-amniotic endotoxin in preterm lamb lungs. Am J Physiol Lung Cell Mol Physiol 2004; 287(6): L1178–L1185.
144. Bhandari V, Choo-Wing R, Lee CG, et al. Developmental regulation of NO-mediated VEGF-induced effects in the lung. Am J Respir Cell Mol Biol 2008; 39(4):420–430.
145. Shenberger JS, Zhang L, Powell RJ, et al. Hyperoxia enhances VEGF release from A549 cells via post-transcriptional processes. Free Radic Biol Med 2007; 43(5):844–852.
146. Kaner RJ, Ladetto JV, Singh R, et al. Lung overexpression of the vascular endothelial growth factor gene induces pulmonary edema. Am J Respir Cell Mol Biol 2000; 22(6):657–664.
147. Lassus P, Turanlahti M, Heikkila P, et al. Pulmonary vascular endothelial growth factor and Flt-1 in fetuses, in acute and chronic lung disease, and in persistent pulmonary hypertension of the newborn. Am J Respir Crit Care Med 2001; 164(10 pt 1):1981–1987.
148. Janer J, Andersson S, Haglund C, et al. Pulmonary endostatin perinatally and in lung injury of the newborn infant. Pediatrics 2007; 119(1):e241–e246.
149. Thickett DR, Armstrong L, Millar AB. A role for vascular endothelial growth factor in acute and resolving lung injury. Am J Respir Crit Care Med 2002; 166(10):1332–1337.
150. Lassus P, Ristimaki A, Ylikorkala O, et al. Vascular endothelial growth factor in human preterm lung. Am J Respir Crit Care Med 1999; 159(5 Pt 1):1429–1433.
151. Perkins GD, Roberts J, McAuley DF, et al. Regulation of vascular endothelial growth factor bioactivity in patients with acute lung injury. Thorax 2005; 60(2):153–158.
152. Dangio CT, Maniscalco WM, Ryan RM, et al. Vascular endothelial growth factor in pulmonary lavage fluid from premature infants: effects of age and postnatal dexamethasone. Biol Neonate 1999; 76(5):266–273.
153. Kunig AM, Balasubramaniam V, Markham NE, et al. Recombinant human VEGF treatment transiently increases lung edema but enhances lung structure after neonatal hyperoxia. Am J Physiol Lung Cell Mol Physiol 2006; 291(5):L1068–L1078.
154. Thickett DR, Armstrong L, Christie SJ, et al. Vascular endothelial growth factor may contribute to increased vascular permeability in acute respiratory distress syndrome. Am J Respir Crit Care Med 2001; 164(9):1601–1605.
155. Papapetropoulos A, Garcia-Cardena G, Madri JA, et al. Nitric oxide production contributes to the angiogenic properties of vascular endothelial growth factor in human endothelial cells. J Clin Invest 1997, 100(12):3131–3139.

156. Bhandari V, Choo-Wing R, Chapoval SP, et al. Essential role of nitric oxide in VEGF-induced, asthma-like angiogenic, inflammatory, mucus, and physiologic responses in the lung. Proc Nat Acad Sci U S A 2006; 103(29):11021–11026.
157. Barrington KJ, Finer NN. Inhaled nitric oxide for preterm infants: a systematic review. Pediatrics 2007; 120(5):1088–1099.
158. Asikainen TM, Chang LY, Coalson JJ, et al. Improved lung growth and function through hypoxia-inducible factor in primate chronic lung disease of prematurity. FASEB J 2006; 20(10): 1698–1700.
159. Aghai ZH, Faqiri S, Saslow JG, et al. Angiopoietin 2 concentrations in infants developing bronchopulmonary dysplasia: attenuation by dexamethasone. J Perinatol 2008; 28(2): 149–155.

9

Pulmonary Endothelial Progenitor Cells and Bronchopulmonary Dysplasia

REBECCA S. ROSE
Indiana University, Indianapolis, Indiana, U.S.A.

DAVID A. INGRAM and MERVIN C. YODER
Herman B Wells Center for Pediatric Research, Indianapolis, Indiana, U.S.A.

I. Introduction

The new bronchopulmonary dysplasia (BPD) is a disorder characterized by a failure of alveolarization. Alveolarization and angiogenesis are closely linked. If we can determine how to improve angiogenesis in the setting of prematurity and hyperoxia-induced lung disease, we may be able to prevent the development of or modulate the severity of BPD. Recently, it has become clear that postnatal vasculogenesis can occur via circulating endothelial precursor cells (EPCs). A better understanding of the origin and regulation of EPCs may lead to new therapies for prevention and treatment of BPD.

II. Characteristics of Endothelium

Endothelial cells form an important barrier lining for all blood vessels. This monolayer is responsible for maintaining a highly selective interface between the circulating blood and perfused tissues. The endothelial intima participates in controlling vasomotor tone, regulating immune responses, and initiating repair after injury (1). Endothelial cells are metabolically active and must respond to changing environmental signals in developmentally regulated and tissue-specific fashions. In fact, loss of the ability of the endothelium to respond to changes in the environment is frequently associated with disease development (2).

Endothelium arises from mesodermal precursors that emigrate from the primitive streak. The angioblasts emerging from the mesoderm migrate into regions where hypoxia and local growth factor gradients promote the formation of a primitive capillary plexus in a process referred to as vasculogenesis. Earlier, it was thought that vasculogenesis occurred only in the embryo. The description of "putative progenitor endothelial cells" isolated from adult peripheral blood and the report that these cells participate in neoangiogenesis in nude mice (3) have suggested a new paradigm for vascular regeneration. Thousands of papers have been published to describe the role of circulating EPCs in normal growth and development, disease development, and attempts to prevent vascular damage or regenerate vessels through EPC administration (4,5). More recently,

EPCs have been isolated directly from the endothelium removed from blood vessels (6). These resident endothelial cells with proliferative potential likely play a significant role in vascular maintenance and repair.

Repair and maintenance of vascular integrity is critical in the lung where a breakdown in endothelial repair may cause lethal hypoxia. Understanding circulating and resident EPCs and how they maintain and contribute to vascular function may help us to understand many disease processes of the lung. This chapter attempts to discuss the controversy in EPC definition and the role of vascular wall resident EPCs in lung vascular heterogeneity. This could have major implications for improving angiogenesis and alveolarization in the setting of prematurity and for preventing BPD.

III. Lung Vascular Development

Lung vascular development is complex. There is controversy about the mechanism of distal lung vascular development. Since this topic was discussed in detail in chapter 4, only a few key points relevant to the topic of this chapter are highlighted here. There are three paradigms for blood vessel formation: vasculogenesis, angiogenesis, and arteriogenesis. Vasculogenesis, as mentioned earlier, is the de novo formation of capillary tubules from EPCs, called angioblasts. Vasculogenesis is prominent during early embryonic development and is the mechanism for the formation of the heart and aorta (7). Vascular endothelial growth factor (VEGF) is a potent endothelial mitogen (8) and is important for vasculogenesis (9,10). Angiogenesis is the remodeling of existing capillaries into more organized, larger vessels. This occurs by sprouting of endothelial cells from existing capillaries, or by intussusception (11). Angiogenesis creates a more mature vascular network and appears to be dependent on *Notch-Jagged* signaling (12,13). Arteriogenesis is the formation of collateral vessels from an artery, usually in an attempt to provide alternative conduit flow for an area of obstruction in the parent vessel. For more detail on these processes, there are several recent reviews (14–17).

In lung development, it is likely that both vasculogenesis and angiogenesis participate in pulmonary vascular establishment. deMello and Reid (18) used the tools of electron microscopy and vascular casting to examine samples of human fetal lung at various embryonic stages from the Carnegie collection. They identified vascular lakes in the lung bud mesenchyme with aggregates of red blood cells surrounded by endothelium, suggesting that the distal airways are formed by vasculogenesis in a process reminiscent of blood island formation in the extraembryonic yolk sac. At the same Carnegie stage of development, there were solid cords of cells without lumens that were continuous with the extrapulmonary artery. These cords developed a lumen later in development, and later still, fusion of the vessels from the pulmonary artery occurred with the capillaries formed from the blood lakes. These observations suggested that the more proximal vasculature was formed by angiogenesis. Some investigators have recently suggested that the distal airway vascular supply may arise via angiogenesis rather than vasculogenesis (19). Other investigators have used molecular approaches to support a site-specific difference in the mechanisms of vascular development of the lung (20). For more detail on the controversies surrounding lung vascular development, please see chapter 4.

Given that the distal airway capillaries are likely formed by vasculogenesis and the proximal airways are formed by angiogenesis, it makes sense that the angioblasts that form these vessels may also be different. The differences in these precursors may account for the documented differences between the pulmonary macrovasculature and the pulmonary microvasculature (21) and may serve to explain the recent reported differences in the proliferative potential of the EPCs resident in the microvasculature compared with the macrovasculature of the lung (22,23).

IV. Endothelial Progenitor Cells Defined

In 1997, Asahara reported the isolation of putative progenitor endothelial cells (3) from human peripheral blood mononuclear cells (MNCs). Since that landmark paper, research on EPCs has flourished. A search for "endothelial progenitor cells" in PubMed yields over 7400 matches. Unfortunately, the literature surrounding EPCs suggests contradictory and confusing physiological roles for EPCs largely because of the multiple methods used to identify these cells. EPCs are very rare in adult peripheral blood making them difficult to isolate (24). Furthermore, there are no specific markers that define an EPC. Endothelial-specific markers, such as E-selectin and vascular endothelial-cadherin, are thought to be present only on differentiated mature endothelial cells (4). Many of the markers expressed by less mature endothelial cells, such as Flk-1/KDR (VEGF receptor-2) and von Willebrand factor, are also seen on immature cells of the hematopoietic lineage (25,26). Thus, authors have used various methods both to isolate and to define EPCs.

In the original paper, Asahara isolated cells that expressed cell surface CD34, a marker that is detected on both immature endothelial cells and immature hematopoietic cells (3). The CD34+ cells were also selected for Flk-1/KDR (VEGF receptor-2) expression. The double positive cells were then cultured on fibronectin, yielding a central core of round cells with spindle-shaped cells in the periphery. The spindle-shaped cells took up acetylated low-density lipoprotein (Ac-LDL), a characteristic of endothelial cells (27). When the spindle-shaped cells were injected into nude mice after hind limb ischemia, several of these cells were observed to engraft in newly formed vessels. Thus, Asahara et al. suggested that the circulating cells must be progenitors for the endothelial lineage and that these cells participate in neoangiogenesis (3). While these data generated significant interest in the field, a closer examination of the paper suggests some unanswered questions.

In the original paper (3), only 15% of the cells were positive for CD34 expression. Thus, 85% of the cells were undefined. To eliminate the mature endothelial cells that may have been present in the population of circulating CD34-expressing cells, Peichev et al. (28) suggested fractionating cells for CD133 and/or KDR expression in addition to CD34. Cells isolated by this method were cultured and were morphologically similar to the cells described by Asahara et al. (3), and they migrated toward stromal-derived factor-1, a characteristic displayed by endothelial cells. Following this report (28), CD34+CD133+KDR+ cells became accepted as a population of cells displaying features of EPCs. Subsequently, this phenotypic profile has been used for many studies examining the role of circulating cells in neovascularization and in studies using EPC enumeration as a biomarker for a cardiovascular or metabolic disease (29–51).

Further functional analysis of EPCs has shown that using surface antigen expression alone is not a reliable method to confirm that cells are specified to the endothelial lineage (25). Many of the "endothelial-specific proteins" such as CD31, KDR, and von Willebrand factor are also expressed on monocyte/macrophage cells (4,5,25,52–56). Although cells that are CD34+, CD133+, and/or KDR+ were thought to be endothelial in origin, several recent reports have questioned whether this method selects cells that truly are EPCs. Timmermans et al. (57) showed that with the use of very precise FACS (fluorescence activated cell sorting) analysis, all of the cells that were CD34+CD133+ were also positive for CD45, a pan leukocyte marker exclusively expressed on cells of the hematopoietic lineage. Culture of the CD34+CD133+CD45+ cells in vitro revealed adherent cells displaying features similar to those reported by Asahara et al. (3), suggesting that the cells defined by Asahara may have been derived from the hematopoietic system. Timmerman et al. also found that none of the cells that were CD34+CD45− (that gave rise to highly proliferative endothelial colony-forming cells) expressed CD133 (formerly thought to be a marker for EPCs).

Case et al. also noted that CD34+CD133+ cells express CD45 (58). They also performed multiple functional studies to determine whether these cells displayed properties of EPCs. When freshly isolated CD34+CD133+ cells were plated on the extracellular matrix material called Matrigel, Case et al. (58) failed to observe any tube-like structures formed in vitro. In contrast, the same population of double positive cells readily formed hematopoietic colony-forming cells in vitro (56). Thus, the vast majority of CD34+CD133+ cells are hematopoietic progenitor cells. Case et al. (58) further demonstrated that cells expressing CD34 but not CD45 were enriched for endothelial colony-forming cells with in vivo vessel-forming potential.

CD34+CD133+ cells circulate in the blood in much higher concentration than CD34+CD45− cells (24). Not surprisingly then, CD34+CD133+ can be more accurately and reproducibly quantified from a fresh blood sample than CD34+CD45− cells (52), and quantification of these cells does correlate with severity of a number of cardiovascular disease states. Thus, the field is left with a difficult paradox, where a circulating cell population identified by CD34 and CD133 expression is a robust measure as a biomarker for cardiovascular disease, but this population is largely functionally composed of hematopoietic progenitor cells and not endothelial colony-forming cells with in vivo vascular potential (58).

V. Culture of EPCs

EPC identification may also be performed by in vitro culture of peripheral blood or umbilical cord blood MNCs. Ito et al. (42) modified the original EPC isolation method of Asahara et al. (3) to plate low-density MNCs, obtained from centrifugation of the blood cells through Ficoll separation medium, on fibronectin-coated dishes. After 24 hours of in vitro culture, nonadherent cells were removed and replated on fibronectin-coated dishes. The adherent cells that emerged displayed KDR, Tie-2 (the receptor for angiopoeitin-1), and CD31 (platelet endothelial cell adhesion molecule-1), and these data were used to validate that the adherent cells isolated by this method differentiated into endothelial cells. This method was then modified by Hill (40), who used a 48-hour preplating step and then recovered the nonadherent cells. The replated nonadherent population subsequently gave rise to a colony within four to nine days in which the center of the colony is composed of a cluster of round cells, and adherent spindle-shaped cells emerge from the edges of this cluster. Hill et al. (40) reported that the circulating concentration of the cells giving rise to the colonies correlates very well with the Framingham risk score in predicting the severity of cardiovascular disease. This assay has become commercially available and the colonies enumerated are referred to as CFU-Hill. More recent analyses of the cellular composition and function of the cells comprising the CFU-Hill have questioned whether these cells represent EPCs.

Hur et al. (59) cultured MNCs on gelatin-coated plates and noted the early formation of colonies that were morphologically similar to CFU-Hill colonies. These cells were initially CD45+, but with time, in vitro, the level of CD45 and CD31 expression waned, while the adherent cells gained low-level expression of KDR and vascular endothelial-cadherin. With prolonged culture of the peripheral blood MNCs on the gelatin-coated dishes, Hur et al. (59) noted the appearance of another type of colony of cells. Functional testing of these late outgrowth colony-forming cells revealed a cell surface antigen profile similar to human umbilical vein endothelial cells (HUVECs) (59). These late outgrowth EPCs displayed a higher level of expression of vascular endothelial-cadherin than the earlier formed colonies. They suggested that both types of colony-forming cells might be important for neoangiogenesis (59). Hur et al. hypothesized that the early outgrowth colonies of cells may secrete the necessary growth factors that support the emergence and/or expansion of the later outgrowth colony-forming cells that may represent the actual cells necessary for incorporation into new vessels. Further work by the same group indicates that the central round cells from the CFU-Hill assay are CD3+CD31+CXCR4+ T cells (60). These cells secrete growth factors that improve angiogenesis and are necessary for the growth of the adherent spindle cells in the CFU-Hill assay.

Others have also questioned the type of cells obtained by the culture of MNCs on fibronectin-coated dishes (54,55,61). The adherent cells obtained by this method reportedly ingest Ac-LDL and are *Ulex europeus* lectin positive, characteristics previously thought to define a cell as belonging to the endothelial lineage (27,62). However, these adherent cells ingest India ink (a feature of phagocytic macrophages), do not proliferate significantly or grow to confluence, and express CD14, a well-recognized monocyte marker (61). Others have demonstrated that these cells are CD45+ and secrete multiple angiogenic growth factors (53). Therefore, Rehman has suggested that the adherent cells emerging from peripheral blood MNCs plated on fibronectin should be called circulating angiogenic cells (53). This term recognizes the fact that they do play a role in angiogenesis, but does not give them the designation of endothelial cell lineage.

Another method for culturing EPCs involves plating MNCs on type 1 collagen-coated dishes and discarding the nonadherent cells. Using this method, Ingram et al. (63) developed a clonogenic assay to define EPCs. They plated umbilical cord or adult peripheral blood MNCs and when adherent endothelial colony-forming cells emerged, the colonies were plucked and single cells replated and quantified for evidence of clonal colony-forming ability. A complete hierarchy of endothelial cells with varying levels of proliferative potential, similar to the hierarchy described for hematopoietic cells, was determined. Ingram et al. isolated single cells from the umbilical cord blood colonies, which formed colonies containing greater than 10,000 progeny within 14 days of culture in vitro and formed secondary colonies upon replating. Given that the frequency of the highly proliferative colony-forming cells was enriched compared to adult peripheral blood, umbilical cord blood may be a rich resource for further research.

VI. Source of EPCs

Recently, Ingram et al. cultured human aortic endothelial cells (6) and using their previously developed clonogenic assay reported that single endothelial cells gave rise to the complete hierarchy of endothelial colony-forming cells. While the turnover of endothelial cells within vessels is generally thought to be minimal, numerous papers have demonstrated that endothelial cells divide at varying rates depending on the vessel examined and the species (64–73). Schwartz and Benditt (74) demonstrated that endothelial cells incorporate radioactive thymidine and utilized this technique to determine whether endothelial turnover was a property of all endothelium or was restricted to a subpopulation. They reported endothelial replication occurred in clusters within the aorta and was highest in areas known to be at risk for injury (74). It is likely that these areas of replicating cells are the areas containing high-proliferative potential EPCs (HPP-EPCs); however, proof will require identification of a specific marker for human EPCs.

VII. Heterogeneity of Lung Endothelium

As mentioned earlier in the chapter, the more proximal lung vessels are thought to emerge via angiogenesis, whereas the distal microvascular vessels are thought to emerge via vasculogenesis (18). It is quite possible that these differences in mechanism of origin might reflect different precursor populations and may account for the known heterogeneity in structure, function, and gene expression of the endothelial cells isolated from these vascular beds. King et al. studied pulmonary artery endothelial cells (PAECs) and compared them with pulmonary microvascular endothelial cells (PMVECs) (75). They reported that PMVECs bound different lectins than PAECs, suggesting different sugars forming the glycocalyx on the endothelial cell surface. Interestingly, this characteristic persisted even after culturing the cells in similar culture mediums in vitro, suggesting a persistent epigenetic difference in the two types of cells. They also described morphological differences in the distance between the plasmalemma and the rough endoplasmic reticulum between PMVECs and PAECs. This difference likely contributes to the enhanced barrier function known to be displayed by PMVECs. In addition, PMVECs grew at a faster rate than PAECs, although the mechanism for this difference in proliferation was not determined.

Recently, Alvarez et al. (22) postulated that the more rapid growth of PMVECs was due to a higher percentage of resident EPCs among PMVECs compared with the percentage of resident EPCs among PAECs. They used a single-cell clonogenic assay and reported that 50% of the cells in the PMVEC population displayed characteristics of HPP-EPCs. They labeled an enriched population of these cells, resident microvascular endothelial progenitor cells (RMEPCs). These HPP-EPCs were able to form vessels both in vitro and in vivo but maintained their different lectin binding and barrier properties compared with the PAEC cells. The authors concluded that the higher percentage of RMEPCs among PMVECs may be an important characteristic of these vessels that allows rapid repair of the endothelial barrier in the setting of pulmonary microvascular injury (22).

The ability to rapidly repair this barrier function in the pulmonary microvascular system requires rapid proliferation in hypoxic conditions. PMVECs have increased cyclin D1 levels when compared with PAECs (76). This may account for the finding that PMVECs proliferate to a state of confluence even in the absence of serum containing growth factors in vitro. However, once confluence is reached, the cells have an increase in p27Kip expression and appropriately enter G0G1 arrest. Thus, PMVECs have a novel mechanism to maintain readiness for rapid proliferation in case of injury.

Clark et al. (23) showed that both PMVECs and RMEPCs expressed higher concentrations of nucleosome-associated protein-1 (NAP1) when compared with PAECs. Overexpression of NAP1 in PAECs in vitro was associated with an increase in PAEC proliferation to levels similar to PMVECs. They further showed that inhibition of NAP1 expression (using small hairpin RNA) in PMVECs slowed their in vitro growth to levels similar to PAECs. Thus, NAP1 may be an important regulator of growth in the resident EPCs within the pulmonary microvasculature. Novel methods of influencing the level of NAP1 in vivo may be a mechanism for increasing endothelial proliferation and improving endothelial repair.

VIII. EPCs and BPD

Decreased endothelial repair of injured peripheral pulmonary vasculature may be a mechanism for the development of BPD. Several authors have reported decreased vascular development in neonatal rodents that were exposed to hyperoxia (77–80). Increased numbers of colonies of CFU-Hill cells correlate with survival in human adults after acute lung injury (31). Patients with newly diagnosed pneumonia have increased numbers of CFU-Hill colonies compared with that after eight weeks of therapy (81). In the same study, patients who had lower CFU levels at the beginning of the study were more likely to have fibrotic changes on high-resolution CT scans eight weeks after therapy. This suggests that these cells may be important for recovery from disease states.

Infants born prematurely are often exposed to both hyperoxia and ventilator trauma. Extrapolating from the previous studies, high levels of circulating angiogenic cells and EPCs should help with repair after lung injury in these patients. Unfortunately, a recent study showed that neonatal mice exposed to hyperoxia had decreased levels of circulating EPCs (82). These mice developed a decreased pulmonary vascular density and simplified lung architecture, similar to descriptions of human BPD (83–85). This suggests that decreased levels of EPCs in premature infants may lead to the impaired angiogenesis seen in BPD. Therefore, a better understanding of EPCs and their role in angiogenesis in the setting of prematurity and hyperoxia may lead to novel therapies for prevention and treatment of BPD.

References

1. Aird WC. Phenotypic heterogeneity of the endothelium: I. Structure, function, and mechanisms. Circ Res 2007; 100(2):158–173.
2. Aird WC. Spatial and temporal dynamics of the endothelium. J Thromb Haemost 2005; 3(7):1392–1406.
3. Asahara T, Murohara T, Sullivan A, et al. Isolation of putative progenitor endothelial cells for angiogenesis. Science 1997; 275(5302):964–967.
4. Khakoo AY, Finkel T. Endothelial progenitor cells. Annu Rev Med 2005; 56:79–101.
5. Rafii S, Lyden D. Therapeutic stem and progenitor cell transplantation for organ vascularization and regeneration. Nat Med 2003; 9(6):702–712.
6. Ingram DA, Mead LE, Moore DB, et al. Vessel wall-derived endothelial cells rapidly proliferate because they contain a complete hierarchy of endothelial progenitor cells. Blood 2005; 105(7):2783–2786.
7. Laudy JA, Wladimiroff JW. The fetal lung. 1: Developmental aspects. Ultrasound Obstet Gynecol 2000; 16(3):284–290.
8. Ferrara N. Molecular and biological properties of vascular endothelial growth factor. J Mol Med 1999; 77(7):527–543.
9. Shalaby F, Rossant J, Yamaguchi TP, et al. Failure of blood-island formation and vasculogenesis in Flk-1-deficient mice. Nature 1995; 376(6535):62–66.
10. Carmeliet P, Ferreira V, Breier G, et al. Abnormal blood vessel development and lethality in embryos lacking a single VEGF allele. Nature 1996; 380(6573):435–439.
11. Risau W. Mechanisms of angiogenesis. Nature 1997; 386(6626):671–674.
12. Xue Y, Gao X, Lindsell CE, et al. Embryonic lethality and vascular defects in mice lacking the Notch ligand Jagged1. Hum Mol Genet 1999; 8(5):723–730.
13. Taichman DB, Loomes KM, Schachtner SK, et al. Notch1 and Jagged1 expression by the developing pulmonary vasculature. Dev Dyn 2002; 225(2):166–175.
14. Carmeliet P. Angiogenesis in health and disease. Nat Med 2003; 9(6):653–660.
15. Semenza GL. Vasculogenesis, angiogenesis, and arteriogenesis: mechanisms of blood vessel formation and remodeling. J Cell Biochem 2007; 102(4):840–847.
16. Simons M. Angiogenesis: where do we stand now? Circulation 2005; 111(12):1556–1566.
17. Skalak TC. Angiogenesis and microvascular remodeling: a brief history and future roadmap. Microcirculation 2005; 12(1):47–58.
18. deMello DE, Reid LM. Embryonic and early fetal development of human lung vasculature and its functional implications. Pediatr Dev Pathol 2000; 3(5):439–449.
19. Parera MC, van Dooren M, van Kempen M, et al. Distal angiogenesis: a new concept for lung vascular morphogenesis. Am J Physiol Lung Cell Mol Physiol 2005; 288(1):L141–149.
20. Han RN, Post M, Tanswell AK, et al. Insulin-like growth factor-I receptor-mediated vasculogenesis/angiogenesis in human lung development. Am J Respir Cell Mol Biol 2003; 28(2):159–169.
21. Gebb S, Stevens T. On lung endothelial cell heterogeneity. Microvasc Res 2004; 68(1):1–12.
22. Alvarez DF, Huang L, King JA, et al. Lung microvascular endothelium is enriched with progenitor cells that exhibit vasculogenic capacity. Am J Physiol Lung Cell Mol Physiol 2008; 294(3):L419–L430.
23. Clark J, Alvarez DF, Alexeyev M, et al. Regulatory role for nucleosome assembly protein-1 in the proliferative and vasculogenic phenotype of pulmonary endothelium. Am J Physiol Lung Cell Mol Physiol 2008; 294(3):L431–L439.
24. Prater DN, Case J, Ingram DA, et al. Working hypothesis to redefine endothelial progenitor cells. Leukemia 2007; 21(6):1141–1149.

25. Schmeisser A, Garlichs CD, Zhang H, et al. Monocytes coexpress endothelial and macro-phagocytic lineage markers and form cord-like structures in Matrigel under angiogenic conditions. Cardiovasc Res 2001; 49(3):671–680.
26. Shizuru JA, Negrin RS, Weissman IL. Hematopoietic stem and progenitor cells: clinical and preclinical regeneration of the hematolymphoid system. Annu Rev Med 2005; 56:509–538.
27. Voyta JC, Via DP, Butterfield CE, et al. Identification and isolation of endothelial cells based on their increased uptake of acetylated-low density lipoprotein. J Cell Biol 1984; 99(6):2034–2040.
28. Peichev M, Naiyer AJ, Pereira D, et al. Expression of VEGFR-2 and AC133 by circulating human CD34(+) cells identifies a population of functional endothelial precursors. Blood 2000; 95(3):952–958.
29. Influence of pravastatin and plasma lipids on clinical events in the West of Scotland Coronary Prevention Study (WOSCOPS). Circulation 1998; 97(15):1440–1445.
30. Bertolini F, Mancuso P, Shaked Y, et al. Molecular and cellular biomarkers for angiogenesis in clinical oncology. Drug Discov Today 2007; 12:806–812.
31. Burnham EL, Taylor WR, Quyyumi AA, et al. Increased circulating endothelial progenitor cells are associated with survival in acute lung injury. Am J Respir Crit Care Med 2005; 172(7):854–860.
32. Capillo M, Mancuso P, Gobbi A, et al. Continuous infusion of endostatin inhibits differen-tiation, mobilization, and clonogenic potential of endothelial cell progenitors. Clin Cancer Res 2003; 9(1):377–382.
33. Eizawa T, Murakami Y, Matsui K, et al. Circulating endothelial progenitor cells are reduced in hemodialysis patients. Curr Med Res Opin 2003; 19(7):627–633.
34. Fadini GP, Miorin M, Facco M, et al. Circulating endothelial progenitor cells are reduced in peripheral vascular complications of type 2 diabetes mellitus. J Am Coll Cardiol 2005; 45(9):1449–1457.
35. Fadini GP, Schiavon M, Cantini M, et al. Circulating progenitor cells are reduced in patients with severe lung disease. Stem Cells 2006; 24(7):1806–1813.
36. George J, Herz I, Goldstein E, et al. Number and adhesive properties of circulating endo-thelial progenitor cells in patients with in-stent restenosis. Arterioscler Thromb Vasc Biol 2003; 23(12):e57–e60.
37. Gill M, Dias S, Hattori K, et al. Vascular trauma induces rapid but transient mobilization of VEGFR2(+)AC133(+) endothelial precursor cells. Circ Res 2001; 88(2):167–174.
38. Grisar J, Aletaha D, Steiner CW, et al. Endothelial progenitor cells in active rheumatoid arthritis: effects of tumour necrosis factor and glucocorticoid therapy. Ann Rheum Dis 2007; 66(10):1284–1288.
39. Guven H, Shepherd RM, Bach RG, et al. The number of endothelial progenitor cell colonies in the blood is increased in patients with angiographically significant coronary artery disease. J Am Coll Cardiol 2006; 48(8):1579–1587.
40. Hill JM, Zalos G, Halcox JP, et al. Circulating endothelial progenitor cells, vascular function, and cardiovascular risk. N Engl J Med 2003; 348(7):593–600.
41. Hristov M, Fach C, Becker C, et al. Reduced numbers of circulating endothelial progenitor cells in patients with coronary artery disease associated with long-term statin treatment. Atherosclerosis 2007; 192(2):413–420.
42. Ito H, Rovira, II, Bloom ML, et al. Endothelial progenitor cells as putative targets for angiostatin. Cancer Res 1999; 59(23):5875–5877.
43. Kim HK, Song KS, Kim HO, et al. Circulating numbers of endothelial progenitor cells in patients with gastric and breast cancer. Cancer Lett 2003; 198(1):83–88.
44. Rauscher FM, Goldschmidt-Clermont PJ, Davis BH, et al. Aging, progenitor cell exhaustion, and atherosclerosis. Circulation 2003; 108(4):457–463.

45. Shintani S, Murohara T, Ikeda H, et al. Mobilization of endothelial progenitor cells in patients with acute myocardial infarction. Circulation 2001; 103(23):2776–2779.
46. Simper D, Wang S, Deb A, et al. Endothelial progenitor cells are decreased in blood of cardiac allograft patients with vasculopathy and endothelial cells of noncardiac origin are enriched in transplant atherosclerosis. Circulation 2003; 108(2):143–149.
47. Tepper OM, Galiano RD, Capla JM, et al. Human endothelial progenitor cells from type II diabetics exhibit impaired proliferation, adhesion, and incorporation into vascular structures. Circulation 2002; 106(22):2781–2786.
48. Vasa M, Fichtlscherer S, Adler K, et al. Increase in circulating endothelial progenitor cells by statin therapy in patients with stable coronary artery disease. Circulation 2001; 103(24):2885–2890.
49. Vasa M, Fichtlscherer S, Aicher A, et al. Number and migratory activity of circulating endothelial progenitor cells inversely correlate with risk factors for coronary artery disease. Circ Res 2001; 89(1):E1–E7.
50. Werner N, Kosiol S, Schiegl T, et al. Circulating endothelial progenitor cells and cardio-vascular outcomes. N Engl J Med 2005; 353(10):999–1007.
51. Yip HK, Chang LT, Chang WN, et al. Level and value of circulating endothelial progenitor cells in patients after acute ischemic stroke. Stroke 2008; 39(1):69–74.
52. Fadini GP, Baesso I, Albiero M, et al. Technical notes on endothelial progenitor cells: Ways to escape from the knowledge plateau. Atherosclerosis 2008; 197(2):496–503.
53. Rehman J, Li J, Orschell CM, et al. Peripheral blood "endothelial progenitor cells" are derived from monocyte/macrophages and secrete angiogenic growth factors. Circulation 2003; 107(8):1164–1169.
54. Rohde E, Malischnik C, Thaler D, et al. Blood monocytes mimic endothelial progenitor cells. Stem Cells 2006; 24(2):357–367.
55. Rohde E, Bartmann C, Schallmoser K, et al. Immune cells mimic the morphology of endothelial progenitor colonies in vitro. Stem Cells 2007; 25(7):1746–1752.
56. Yoder MC, Mead LE, Prater D, et al. Redefining endothelial progenitor cells via clonal analysis and hematopoietic stem/progenitor cell principals. Blood 2007; 109(5):1801–1809.
57. Timmermans F, Van Hauwermeiren F, De Smedt M, et al. Endothelial outgrowth cells are not derived from CD133+ cells or CD45+ hematopoietic precursors. Arterioscler Thromb Vasc Biol 2007; 27(7):1572–1579.
58. Case J, Mead LE, Bessler WK, et al. Human CD34+AC133+VEGFR-2+ cells are not endothelial progenitor cells but distinct, primitive hematopoietic progenitors. Exp Hematol 2007; 35(7):1109–1118.
59. Hur J, Yoon CH, Kim HS, et al. Characterization of two types of endothelial progenitor cells and their different contributions to neovasculogenesis. Arterioscler Thromb Vasc Biol 2004; 24(2):288–293.
60. Hur J, Yang HM, Yoon CH, et al. Identification of a novel role of T cells in postnatal vasculogenesis: characterization of endothelial progenitor cell colonies. Circulation 2007; 116(15):1671–1682.
61. Zhang SJ, Zhang H, Wei YJ, et al. Adult endothelial progenitor cells from human peripheral blood maintain monocyte/macrophage function throughout in vitro culture. Cell Res 2006; 16(6):577–584.
62. Holthofer H, Virtanen I, Kariniemi AL, et al. Ulex europaeus I lectin as a marker for vascular endothelium in human tissues. Lab Invest 1982; 47(1):60–66.
63. Ingram DA, Mead LE, Tanaka H, et al. Identification of a novel hierarchy of endothelial progenitor cells using human peripheral and umbilical cord blood. Blood 2004; 104(9):2752–2760.
64. Craig LE, Spelman JP, Strandberg JD, et al. Endothelial cells from diverse tissues exhibit differences in growth and morphology. Microvasc Res 1998; 55(1):65–76.

65. Grafe M, Graf K, Auch-Schwelk W, et al. Cultivation and characterization of micro- and macrovascular endothelial cells from the human heart. Eur Heart J 1993; 14(suppl 1):74–81.
66. Jaffe EA, Nachman RL, Becker CG, et al. Culture of human endothelial cells derived from umbilical veins. Identification by morphologic and immunologic criteria. J Clin Invest 1973; 52(11):2745–2756.
67. Kuzu I, Bicknell R, Harris AL, et al. Heterogeneity of vascular endothelial cells with relevance to diagnosis of vascular tumours. J Clin Pathol 1992; 45(2):143–148.
68. McCarthy SA, Kuzu I, Gatter KC, et al. Heterogeneity of the endothelial cell and its role in organ preference of tumour metastasis. Trends Pharmacol Sci 1991; 12(12):462–467.
69. Lang I, Pabst MA, Hiden U, et al. Heterogeneity of microvascular endothelial cells isolated from human term placenta and macrovascular umbilical vein endothelial cells. Eur J Cell Biol 2003; 82(4):163–173.
70. Nishida M, Carley WW, Gerritsen ME, et al. Isolation and characterization of human and rat cardiac microvascular endothelial cells. Am J Physiol 1993; 264(2 pt 2):H639–H652.
71. Plendl J, Neumuller C, Vollmar A, et al. Isolation and characterization of endothelial cells from different organs of fetal pigs. Anat Embryol (Berl) 1996; 194(5):445–456.
72. Thorin E, Shreeve SM. Heterogeneity of vascular endothelial cells in normal and disease states. Pharmacol Ther 1998; 78(3):155–166.
73. Thorin E, Shatos MA, Shreeve SM, et al. Human vascular endothelium heterogeneity. A comparative study of cerebral and peripheral cultured vascular endothelial cells. Stroke 1997; 28(2):375–381.
74. Schwartz SM, Benditt EP. Clustering of replicating cells in aortic endothelium. Proc Natl Acad Sci U S A 1976; 73(2):651–653.
75. King J, Hamil T, Creighton J, et al. Structural and functional characteristics of lung macro- and microvascular endothelial cell phenotypes. Microvasc Res 2004; 67(2):139–151.
76. Solodushko V, Fouty B. Proproliferative phenotype of pulmonary microvascular endothelial cells. Am J Physiol Lung Cell Mol Physiol 2007; 292(3):L671–L677.
77. Massaro GD, Olivier J, Massaro D. Short-term perinatal 10% O_2 alters postnatal development of lung alveoli. Am J Physiol 1989; 257(4 pt 1):L221–L225.
78. Roberts RJ, Weesner KM, Bucher JR. Oxygen-induced alterations in lung vascular development in the newborn rat. Pediatr Res 1983; 17(5):368–375.
79. Shaffer SG, O'Neill D, Bradt SK, et al. Chronic vascular pulmonary dysplasia associated with neonatal hyperoxia exposure in the rat. Pediatr Res 1987; 21(1):14–20.
80. Wilson WL, Mullen M, Olley PM, et al. Hyperoxia-induced pulmonary vascular and lung abnormalities in young rats and potential for recovery. Pediatr Res 1985; 19(10):1059–1067.
81. Yamada M, Kubo H, Ishizawa K, et al. Increased circulating endothelial progenitor cells in patients with bacterial pneumonia: evidence that bone marrow derived cells contribute to lung repair. Thorax 2005; 60(5):410–413.
82. Balasubramaniam V, Mervis CF, Maxey AM, et al. Hyperoxia reduces bone marrow, circulating, and lung endothelial progenitor cells in the developing lung: implications for the pathogenesis of bronchopulmonary dysplasia. Am J Physiol Lung Cell Mol Physiol 2007; 292(5):L1073–L1084.
83. Abman SH. Bronchopulmonary dysplasia: "a vascular hypothesis". Am J Respir Crit Care Med 2001; 164(10 pt 1):1755–1756.
84. Bhatt AJ, Pryhuber GS, Huyck H, et al. Disrupted pulmonary vasculature and decreased vascular endothelial growth factor, Flt-1, and TIE-2 in human infants dying with bronchopulmonary dysplasia. Am J Respir Crit Care Med 2001; 164(10 pt 1):1971–1980.
85. Jobe AH, Bancalari E. Bronchopulmonary dysplasia. Am J Respir Crit Care Med 2001; 163(7): 1723–1729.

10
Effects of Mesenchymal Stem Cell Therapy in BPD

BERNARD THÉBAUD
University of Alberta, Edmonton, Alberta, Canada

STELLA KOUREMBANAS
Harvard Medical School, Boston, Massachusetts, U.S.A.

I. Introduction

Continuous improvements in perinatal care have shifted the limits of viability every five years or so toward lower gestational ages and have made the task of protecting the more premature lung from injury increasingly challenging. Premature infants at risk of developing chronic lung disease of prematurity or bronchopulmonary dysplasia (BPD) are now born between 23 to 28 weeks' gestation (or 500–1000 g birth weight) (1,2), that is, at the late canalicular stage of lung development, just when the airways become juxtaposed to the lung vasculature and when gas exchange becomes possible. This suggests that the limit of viability has now been reached with today's resuscitation technology (ventilation and oxygenation) and that some progress in improving survival free of morbidity can be expected even with readily available strategies: improved antenatal management (education, regionalization, steroids, and antibiotics) together with prophylactic surfactant and early noninvasive ventilatory support targeting lower oxygen saturations will likely decrease the incidence/severity of BPD over the next few years.

Nonetheless, the long-term consequences of early interference with lung development still remain unknown. Alarming reports of irreversible arrested alveolar development at adult age in former premature infants with BPD are surfacing (3,4) and mirror results from experimental models of BPD (5). Consequently, much more needs to be learned about the mechanisms of lung development, injury, and repair to prevent lung injury and/or promote lung development/regeneration. Exciting discoveries in stem cell biology over recent years may offer new insight into the pathogenesis of BPD and open new therapeutic avenues. This chapter summarizes our current knowledge on the therapeutic potential of mesenchymal stem cells (MSCs) in lung injury.

II. Definition of Stem Cells

A. Definition

Stem cells are undifferentiated cells that retain the ability to divide throughout life and give rise to differentiated cells to replace cells that die or are lost to maintain organ integrity (6,7). Thus, stem cells contribute to the body's ability to renew and repair its tissues. Unlike mature cells, which are permanently committed to their fate, stem cells can both renew themselves and create new cells of whatever tissue they belong to.

B. Embryonic Vs. Adult Stem Cells

Stem cells are classically divided into two categories: embryonic stem cells and adult (postnatal) stem cells. Embryonic stem cells are pluripotent cells derived from the inner cell mass of blastocyst-stage embryos (8). They are able to form tissues within each of the germ layers (the endoderm, the mesoderm, and the ectoderm) and thus have enormous therapeutic potential to regenerate any damaged tissue, but embryonic stem cells are also mired in great controversy because of the present need of destroying an embryo to harvest these pluripotent cells (9). Adult stem cells are undifferentiated cells found in a differentiated tissue that can renew itself and differentiate (with certain limitations) to give rise to all the specialized cell types of the tissue from which it originated. Hematopoietic, endothelial, and MSCs are multipotent bone marrow (BM)-derived cells that can be mobilized to distal sites of injury and participate in remodeling and repair. Hematopoietic stem cells (HSCs) that give rise to blood cells and move between the BM and peripheral blood are the best-characterized adult stem cells in humans. HSC transplantation is performed since the late 1950s to treat various blood cell disorders. In the last decade, transplantation of endothelial progenitor and MSCs is being tested with promising therapeutic effects in animal models of cardiovascular and pulmonary diseases and in human trials after myocardial infarction (10,11).

C. Stem Cell Potency

Some stem cells are more *pluri*potent than others; for example, a fertilized egg is *toti*potent (i.e., can give rise to any cell type, including all cells of the embryo, and extraembryonic tissues including the placenta). Adult stem cells, although *pluri*potent, have been thought to have more limited differentiation ability and to be organ specific. For example, gastrointestinal crypt cells or oval cells of the liver contribute to local tissue regeneration. Thus, within their own specific tissue, these cells are capable of maintaining, generating, and replacing terminally differentiated cells as a consequence of physiological turnover or tissue injury (12). In the lung, tracheal epithelial basal cells are putative progenitor cells in the upper airways (13), whereas a subset of type II alveolar epithelial cells (AECs) (14) or recently described bronchioalveolar stem cells (15) are putative distal damage-resistant progenitor cells responsible for the repair of the alveolar interface after injury (16,17). While further characterization of resident lung stem cells (14,18) hold promise for novel therapeutic approaches for lung diseases, this chapter addresses the therapeutic potential of exogenous administration of BM-derived stem cells, focusing primarily on MSCs.

III. Mesenchymal Stem Cells

Traditionally, stem cells were believed to be lineage restricted and organ specific. However, recent data have challenged the hematopoietic specificity of BM-derived stem cells. Animal and human studies suggest that adult stem cells can generate differentiated tissue beyond their own tissue boundaries to form functional components of other tissues, expressing tissue-specific proteins in organs such as heart, liver, brain, skeletal muscle, and vascular endothelium (7). This developmental plasticity of stem cells bears an enormous therapeutic potential to repair irreversibly damaged tissue and seems to lie within the so-called stromal or MSC.

The existence of stromal cells in the BM with osteogenic potential was first suggested in the 19th century: transplantation of BM to heterotopic anatomical sites resulted in de novo generation of ectopic bone and marrow. In the 1970s, Friedenstein et al. characterized plastic adherent cells that were distinguishable from the majority of hematopoietic cells by their fibroblast-like appearance and had the ability to form cells within the osteogenic, chondrogenic, and adipogenic lineages (19). On the basis of multilineage differentiation capacity, Caplan introduced the term MSCs. It was not until over 20 years after Friedenstein's report that the multilineage potential of adult human MSCs was made apparent to investigators outside the hematopoietic field (20). In 2001, Krause et al. reported that a single BM-derived stem cell had the ability to engraft into numerous organs as well as having a "tremendous differentiative capacity" by adopting the phenotype of epithelial cells within the liver, lung, GI tract, and skin (21). To date, systemically injected BM-derived stem cells of mouse have been demonstrated to differentiate into parenchymal cells of various nonhematopoietic tissues including muscle, cartilage, bone, liver, heart, brain, intestine, and lung (21–24). The engrafted marrow cells are able to adopt the morphological and molecular phenotype of their new resident organ. But because investigators used different methods of isolation and expansion, and different approaches to characterizing these cells, the Mesenchymal and Tissue Stem Cell Committee of the International Society for Cellular Therapy proposed minimal criteria to define human MSCs (25). These included (*i*) plastic adherence, (*ii*) cell surface marker expression of CD105, CD73, and CD90, and lack of expression of CD45, CD34, CD14 or CD11b, CD79α or CD19, and HLA-DR surface molecules, and (*iii*) differentiation into osteoblasts, adipocytes, and chondroblasts in vitro. While these criteria will evolve as new knowledge unfolds, this minimal set of standard criteria will foster a more uniform characterization of MSCs and facilitate the exchange of data among investigators.

Despite the controversy around the true characteristics of MSCs, their therapeutic potential has been harnessed to treat a wide variety of diseases in the laboratory and is now being investigated in patients (26). In comparison, relatively little information is available on the therapeutic potential of MSCs in lung diseases (reviewed in Refs. 27–29) and whether MSCs can reside in the lung and participate in processes of cell renewal and repair. A recent report by Hennrick et al. identified resident MSCs in tracheal aspirates from ventilated human preterm infants that expressed MSC markers, but were negative for hematopoietic or endothelial cell markers and correlated with prolonged ventilator dependence and oxygen requirement (30). Lama et al. reported successful isolation of MSCs from the bronchoalveolar lavage of adult lung of transplant patients (31), and showed that in seven sex-mismatched transplant recipients, the MSCs were donor-derived up to 11 years post-transplantation, suggesting that the connective tissue cell progenitors reside in the lung.

IV. Therapeutic Potential of BM-Derived Stem Cells to Prevent/Regenerate the Damaged Lung

In the adult lung, most studies have focused on proof of principle that BM stem cells can home to the lung and adopt various lung cell phenotypes in various injury models, although these data are sometimes conflicting. Conversely, in all of these models, exogenous administration of MSCs showed therapeutic benefit in preventing lung injury (reviewed in Refs. 27–29). Relatively little information about the therapeutic potential of MSCs exist in the developing lung.

A. Engraftment of Stem Cells in the Lung

The 2001 report by Krause et al. opened the door to the potential that there may be an ethically appealing option in using nonembryonic stem cells for tissue replacement. On the basis of their previous work showing the potential of $CD34^+$ lin^- for hepatocyte regeneration (32), Krause et al. extended their observation to the lung. $CD34^+$ lin^- cells from male donor mice were administered intravenously (IV) to irradiated female recipients, and fluorescent in situ hybridization (FISH) to track the Y chromosome showed 20% of AEC being derived from a donor animal persisting up to 11 months posttransplant (21). Consistent with this first observation, other investigators reported that various preparations of BM-derived cells were able to engraft and adopt the phenotype of distal lung cells including type I (33) and type II AECs (34) as well as lung fibroblasts (35) in a variety of experimental models. These studies demonstrate the potential of BM-derived cells to home to the injured lung, engraft, and adopt the phenotype of one or many of the lung cells. Also, prior injury amplifies stem cell engraftment, as observed in other tissues (36).

Conversely, more recent studies do not support adult stem cell plasticity in the lung. Engraftment was assessed in chimeric animals (BM ablation and reconstituted with GFP HSCs) and in parabiotic animals (created by joining the circulation of a transgenic GFP mouse with the circulation of a wild-type mouse) (37). While the BM-ablated group showed robust reconstitution of circulating HSCs, and the parabiotic animals had robust hematopoietic chimerism, there was little evidence for stem cell engraftment and transdifferentiation in the brain and the liver and none in the lung (37). Two other studies investigated lungs of recipient mice transplanted with BM from transgenic mice that ubiquitously express eGFP or LacZ: engrafted cells displayed type II AEC characteristics (38). Deconvolution microscopy however—generating a three-dimensional image of the lung—determined that the coexpression of surfactant protein-C (SP-C) and eGFP was a false positive: the SP-C signal resided just outside the eGFP+ cells (38). This highlights the need for precise tools to assess stem cell engraftment including confocal microscopy (39). BM-reconstituted mice with BM-derived cells from SP-C-eGFP donor mice showed no evidence of donor cells becoming type II AECs using three antibody-independent assays, fluorescent-activated cell sorting (FACS), fluorescent microscopy, and real-time polymerase chain reaction (40). In humans, BM-MSC repopulation also seems to contribute minimally to the type II AECs after cross-gender lung transplantation (41).

Despite the controversy about stem cell engraftment, evidence suggests that BM-derived cells contribute to lung repair.

B. BM Stem Cell Therapy in Experimental Adult Lung Injury Models

In mouse models of acute lipopolysaccharide (LPS, a component of gram-negative bacterial cell walls)-induced lung inflammation, fibrosis, and emphysema, MSCs appear to abrogate lung injury.

LPS-Induced Lung Injury

Intratracheal LPS injection causes a rapid mobilization of BM cells into the circulation (42). BM cells accumulate within the inflammatory site and differentiate to become endothelial and epithelial cells. The suppression of BM cells by sublethal irradiation before intrapulmonary LPS leads to emphysema-like changes; reconstitution of the BM prevents these changes (42). Likewise, exogenous intratracheal administration of MSCs improves survival and attenuates lung inflammation and permeability (43). MSCs transfected with the vasculoprotective gene angiopoietin 1 and injected IV seem to provide additional protection against inflammation and lung permeability (44).

Bleomycin-Induced Lung Fibrosis

IV-injected BM-MSCs engraft to areas of fibrosis and exhibit an epithelium-like morphology (45). Immediate MSC administration, but not one week following bleomycin, attenuates lung inflammation and fibrosis (45). In the same model, myelosuppression increases the susceptibility to injury, and IV MSC administration improves survival and attenuates fibrosis (46).

Elastase- and Smoke-Induced Emphysema

Adipose tissue-derived stromal cells induce alveolar regeneration and improve lung function in elastase-induced emphysema in rats (47). Likewise, sex-mismatched BM-MSC transplantation in irradiated female rats improved lung architecture, and FISH for Y chromosome and immunohistochemical staining for SP-C confirmed that MSCs engrafted in recipient lungs and differentiated into type II alveolar epithelial cells (48).

All together, these observations suggest that an intact BM serves to limit the extent of lung injury, that exogenous administered MSCs home preferentially to sites of injury, can adopt distal lung cell phenotypes, and can prevent lung injury. In all these studies, however, the low numbers of engrafted stem cells seems insufficient to account for the therapeutic response.

Paracrine Effect of MSCs

Increasing evidence suggest that soluble factors secreted by the MSCs account for some of the beneficial effects. In vitro, cells from bleomycin-injured mouse, but not from normal mouse lung, produce soluble factors that cause BM-MSC proliferation and migration toward the injured lung (46). Furthermore, conditioned media obtained from MSCs blocks the proliferation of an interleukin-1α-dependent T-cell line and inhibits production of tumor necrosis factor α by activated macrophages in vitro (49). In endotoxin-induced systemic inflammation, BM-derived MSCs decrease both the systemic and local inflammatory responses (50). These effects did not require either lung engraftment or stem cell transdifferentiation, suggesting that humoral and physical interactions between stem cells and lung cells account for some of the beneficial effects.

Gene Delivery by MSCs

MSCs may also be used as vehicles to target gene delivery in vivo, as was demonstrated for the cystic fibrosis transmembrane conductance regulator (CFTR) gene with successful, epithelial cell-specific expression (51). Wang et al. reported MSCs in coculture with alveolar epithelial cells from ΔF508 cystic fibrosis patients to acquire expression of the wild-type CFTR protein, to adopt a columnar or epithelial shape of the human airway epithelium, and to express cytokeratin-18 (52). MSCs engineered to express vasoactive molecules and cytoprotective genes have been reported to be more effective in reducing or preventing LPS-induced lung injury in mice or monocrotaline-induced pulmonary hypertension in the rat (44,53). The therapeutic efficacy of MSCs may thus be enhanced by genetic engineering strategies to deliver and overexpress cytoprotective mediators of lung repair.

C. BPD: A Disease of Stem Cell Depletion?

Hyperoxia contributes to BPD and causes an arrest in alveolar and vascular growth in newborn rodents. Recent evidence suggests that the distal lung harbors various cells with progenitor properties. The role of these cells during lung development is unknown, but these cells seem to contribute to lung repair, because their depletion in the developing lung is associated with arrested lung development.

For example, circulating endothelial progenitor cells home to the injured lung and contribute to lung repair in experimental models of lung injury (42,54–56). Clinical reports indicate that increased circulating endothelial progenitor cells correlate with improved outcome in lung injury (57–59). In O_2-induced neonatal lung injury in newborn mice, lung resident endothelial progenitor cells (60) are decreased. Likewise, side population cells (SP, primitive multipotent progenitor cells defined by their ability to efflux the DNA dye Hoechst 33342 and to differentiate into hematopoietic, epithelial, and mesenchymal cells while lacking differentiated lineage markers) have been identified in the adult and more recently in the developing mouse lung (61). Chronic hyperoxia results in prolonged depletion of SP cells during room air recovery (61). Two weeks of chronic hyperoxic exposure of newborn rats also reduces the lung resident MSC population.

These observations suggest that chronic hyperoxia, known to result in irreversible alveolar destruction, overwhelms the repair capacity of the developing lung, resulting in destruction of resident progenitor cells and in decreased homing of putative reparative cells, and provides a rationale for exogenous supplementation of stem cells to prevent lung injury or to regenerate damaged lung.

D. Effects of MSC Therapy in Experimental BPD

Two recent observations by our groups suggest that MSCs can prevent O_2-induced lung injury in newborn rodents. In a neonatal mouse hyperoxia model, systemic delivery of BM-MSCs but not mouse lung fibroblasts ameliorated alveolar injury and prevented lung inflammation as well as lung vascular remodeling and right ventricular hypertrophy. Likewise, intratracheal delivery of MSCs in newborn rats, but not pulmonary artery smooth muscle cells (used as control cells), improved survival and exercise tolerance while attenuating alveolar and lung vascular injury and pulmonary hypertension in this model. Engrafted MSCs coexpressed SP-C. In vitro, BM-derived MSCs migrated preferentially toward O_2-damaged lung compared with undamaged normoxic lung or culture media alone. In addition, MSCs exposed to either normoxic or hyperoxic lung, but not to culture media alone or liver, developed molecular and structural characteristics of type II alveolar epithelial cells (SP-C expression and lamellar bodies). Despite the therapeutic benefit, in both studies, engraftment of MSCs was low, suggesting again that cell replacement may not be a major mechanism by which MSCs exert their beneficial effects. These studies provide proof of concept that BM-MSCs exert a therapeutic benefit in experimental chronic neonatal lung disease.

Besides the BM, another potential stem cell source is umbilical cord blood in particular with the perspective to treat diseases of the newborn. Indeed, umbilical cord blood is a currently discarded, yet easily accessible, ethically appropriate (compared to embryonic stem cells), clinically relevant source of potent stem cells (62,63). On the basis of proof of concept provided by our previous study with BM-MSCs, human cord blood–derived plastic adherent cells obtained from term deliveries were shown to prevent alveolar injury in neonatal nude rats exposed to hyperoxia similar to the administration of BM-derived MSCs.

V. Conclusion

Cell-based therapies for lung diseases hold tremendous promise. Over the last decade, numerous studies have demonstrated the ability of adult BM-derived cells to differentiate into nonhematopoietic lineages, including neural, skeletal muscle, hepatic, cardiac, and vascular lineages, and to repair these tissues. With regard to lung repair, initial reports of stem cell homing, engraftment, and lung phenotype adoption are now challenged. Nonetheless, the benefit of MSC therapy has been demonstrated in various experimental models mimicking adult and neonatal lung diseases. However, prerequisites for the potential clinical application of cell-based therapies for newborns suffering from BPD include the following: identifying the best "reparative cell(s)" and its source, determining the importance of homing-engraftment-transdifferentiation mechanisms, understanding alternate mechanisms of action beyond cell replacement, and assessing the short- and long-term efficacy and safety in rigorously well-designed preclinical studies.

References

1. Eichenwald EC, Stark AR. Management and outcomes of very low birth weight. N Engl J Med 2008; 358(16):1700–1711.
2. Kinsella JP, Greenough A, Abman SH. Bronchopulmonary dysplasia. Lancet 2006; 367(9520):1421–1431.
3. Cutz E, Chiasson D. Chronic lung disease after premature birth. N Engl J Med 2008; 358(7):743–745; author reply 745–746.
4. Wong PM, Lees AN, Louw J, et al. Emphysema in young adult survivors of moderate-to-severe bronchopulmonary dysplasia. Eur Respir J 2008; 32(2):321–328.

5. Shaffer SG, O'Neill D, Bradt SK, et al. Chronic vascular pulmonary dysplasia associated with neonatal hyperoxia exposure in the rat. Pediatr Res 1987; 21(1):14–20.
6. Korbling M, Estrov Z. Adult stem cells for tissue repair—a new therapeutic concept? N Engl J Med 2003; 349(6):570–582.
7. Blau HM, Brazelton TR, Weimann JM. The evolving concept of a stem cell: entity or function? Cell 2001; 105(7):829–841.
8. Evans MJ, Kaufman MH. Establishment in culture of pluripotential cells from mouse embryos. Nature 1981; 292(5819):154–156.
9. McLaren A. Ethical and social considerations of stem cell research. Nature 2001; 414(6859):129–131.
10. Iyer SS, Rojas M. Anti-inflammatory effects of mesenchymal stem cells: novel concept for future therapies. Expert Opin Biol Ther 2008; 8(5):569–581.
11. Ward MR, Stewart DJ, Kutryk MJ. Endothelial progenitor cell therapy for the treatment of coronary disease, acute MI, and pulmonary arterial hypertension: current perspectives. Catheter Cardiovasc Interv 2007; 70(7):983–998.
12. Slack JM. Stem cells in epithelial tissues. Science 2000; 287(5457):1431–1433.
13. Pitt BR, Ortiz LA. Stem cells in lung biology. Am J Physiol Lung Cell Mol Physiol 2004; 286(4):L621–L623.
14. Driscoll B, Buckley S, Bui KC, et al. Telomerase in alveolar epithelial development and repair. Am J Physiol Lung Cell Mol Physiol 2000; 279(6):L1191–L1198.
15. Rawlins EL, Hogan BL. Epithelial stem cells of the lung: privileged few or opportunities for many? Development 2006; 133(13):2455–2465.
16. Mason RJ, Williams MC, Moses HL, et al. Stem cells in lung development, disease, and therapy. Am J Respir Cell Mol Biol 1997; 16(4):355–363.
17. Warburton D, Wuenschell C, Flores-Delgado G, et al. Commitment and differentiation of lung cell lineages. Biochem Cell Biol 1998; 76(6):971–995.
18. Reddy R, Buckley S, Doerken M, et al. Isolation of a putative progenitor subpopulation of alveolar epithelial type 2 cells. Am J Physiol Lung Cell Mol Physiol 2004; 286(4):L658–L667.
19. Friedenstein AJ, Gorskaja JF, Kulagina NN. Fibroblast precursors in normal and irradiated mouse hematopoietic organs. Exp Hematol 1976; 4(5):267–274.
20. Pittenger MF, Mackay AM, Beck SC, et al. Multilineage potential of adult human mesenchymal stem cells. Science 1999; 284(5411):143–147.
21. Krause DS, Theise ND, Collector MI, et al. Multi-organ, multi-lineage engraftment by a single bone marrow-derived stem cell. Cell 2001; 105(3):369–377.
22. Prockop DJ. Marrow stromal cells as stem cells for nonhematopoietic tissues. Science 1997; 276(5309):71–74.
23. Petersen BE, Bowen WC, Patrene KD, et al. Bone marrow as a potential source of hepatic oval cells. Science 1999; 284(5417):1168–1170.
24. Lagasse E, Connors H, Al-Dhalimy M, et al. Purified hematopoietic stem cells can differentiate into hepatocytes in vivo. Nat Med 2000; 6(11):1229–1234.
25. Dominici M, Le Blanc K, Mueller I, et al. Minimal criteria for defining multipotent mesenchymal stromal cells. The International Society for Cellular Therapy position statement. Cytotherapy 2006; 8(4):315–317.
26. Burt RK, Loh Y, Pearce W, et al. Clinical applications of blood-derived and marrow-derived stem cells for nonmalignant diseases. JAMA 2008; 299(8):925–936.
27. Gomperts BN, Strieter RM. Stem cells and chronic lung disease. Annu Rev Med 2007; 58:285–298.
28. van Haaften T, Thebaud B. Adult bone marrow-derived stem cells for the lung: implications for pediatric lung diseases. Pediatr Res 2006; 59(4 pt 2):94R–99R.
29. Weiss DJ, Berberich MA, Borok Z, et al. Adult stem cells, lung biology, and lung disease. NHLBI/Cystic Fibrosis Foundation Workshop. Proc Am Thorac Soc 2006; 3(3):193–207.

30. Hennrick KT, Keeton AG, Nanua S, et al. Lung cells from neonates show a mesenchymal stem cell phenotype. Am J Respir Crit Care Med 2007; 175(11):1158–1164.

31. Lama VN, Smith L, Badri L, et al. Evidence for tissue-resident mesenchymal stem cells in human adult lung from studies of transplanted allografts. J Clin Invest 2007; 117(4):989–996.

32. Theise ND, Badve S, Saxena R, et al. Derivation of hepatocytes from bone marrow cells in mice after radiation-induced myeloablation. Hepatology 2000; 31(1):235–240.

33. Kotton DN, Ma BY, Cardoso WV, et al. Bone marrow-derived cells as progenitors of lung alveolar epithelium. Development 2001; 128(24):5181–5188.

34. Theise ND, Henegariu O, Grove J, et al. Radiation pneumonitis in mice: a severe injury model for pneumocyte engraftment from bone marrow. Exp Hematol 2002; 30(11): 1333–1338.

35. Abe S, Lauby G, Boyer C, et al. Transplanted BM and BM side population cells contribute progeny to the lung and liver in irradiated mice. Cytotherapy 2003; 5(6):523–533.

36. Hatch HM, Zheng D, Jorgensen ML, et al. SDF-1alpha/CXCR4: a mechanism for hepatic oval cell activation and bone marrow stem cell recruitment to the injured liver of rats. Cloning Stem Cells 2002; 4(4):339–351.

37. Wagers AJ, Sherwood RI, Christensen JL, et al. Little evidence for developmental plasticity of adult hematopoietic stem cells. Science 2002; 297(5590):2256–2259.

38. Chang JC, Summer R, Sun X, et al. Evidence that bone marrow cells do not contribute to the alveolar epithelium. Am J Respir Cell Mol Biol 2005; 33(4):335–342.

39. Herzog EL, Chai L, Krause DS. Plasticity of marrow-derived stem cells. Blood 2003; 102(10):3483–3493.

40. Kotton DN, Fabian AJ, Mulligan RC. Failure of bone marrow to reconstitute lung epithelium. Am J Respir Cell Mol Biol 2005; 33(4):328–334.

41. Zander DS, Baz MA, Cogle CR, et al. Bone marrow-derived stem-cell repopulation contributes minimally to the type II pneumocyte pool in transplanted human lungs. Transplantation 2005; 80(2):206–212.

42. Yamada M, Kubo H, Kobayashi S, et al. Bone marrow-derived progenitor cells are important for lung repair after lipopolysaccharide-induced lung injury. J Immunol 2004; 172(2): 1266–1272.

43. Gupta N, Su X, Popov B, et al. Intrapulmonary delivery of bone marrow-derived mesenchymal stem cells improves survival and attenuates endotoxin-induced acute lung injury in mice. J Immunol 2007; 179(3):1855–1863.

44. Mei SH, McCarter SD, Deng Y, et al. Prevention of LPS-induced acute lung injury in mice by mesenchymal stem cells overexpressing angiopoietin 1. PLoS Med 2007; 4(9):e269.

45. Ortiz LA, Gambelli F, McBride C, et al. Mesenchymal stem cell engraftment in lung is enhanced in response to bleomycin exposure and ameliorates its fibrotic effects. Proc Natl Acad Sci U S A 2003; 100(14):8407–8411.

46. Rojas M, Xu J, Woods CR, et al. Bone marrow-derived mesenchymal stem cells in repair of the injured lung. Am J Respir Cell Mol Biol 2005; 33(2):145–152.

47. Shigemura N, Okumura M, Mizuno S, et al. Autologous transplantation of adipose tissue-derived stromal cells ameliorates pulmonary emphysema. Am J Transplant 2006; 6(11): 2592–2600.

48. Zhen G, Liu H, Gu N, et al. Mesenchymal stem cells transplantation protects against rat pulmonary emphysema. Front Biosci 2008; 13:3415–3422.

49. Ortiz LA, Dutreil M, Fattman C, et al. Interleukin 1 receptor antagonist mediates the anti-inflammatory and antifibrotic effect of mesenchymal stem cells during lung injury. Proc Natl Acad Sci U S A 2007; 104(26):11002–11007.

50. Xu J, Woods CR, Mora AL, et al. Prevention of endotoxin-induced systemic response by bone marrow-derived mesenchymal stem cells in mice. Am J Physiol Lung Cell Mol Physiol 2007; 293(1):L131–L141.

51. Loi R, Beckett T, Goncz KK, et al. Limited restoration of cystic fibrosis lung epithelium in vivo with adult bone marrow-derived cells. Am J Respir Crit Care Med 2006; 173(2): 171–179.

52. Wang G, Bunnell BA, Painter RG, et al. Adult stem cells from bone marrow stroma differentiate into airway epithelial cells: potential therapy for cystic fibrosis. Proc Natl Acad Sci U S A 2005; 102(1):186–191.

53. Kanki-Horimoto S, Horimoto H, Mieno S, et al. Implantation of mesenchymal stem cells overexpressing endothelial nitric oxide synthase improves right ventricular impairments caused by pulmonary hypertension. Circulation 2006; 114(1 suppl):I181–I185.

54. Ishizawa K, Kubo H, Yamada M, et al. Bone marrow-derived cells contribute to lung regeneration after elastase-induced pulmonary emphysema. FEBS Lett 2004; 556(1–3):249–252.

55. Ishizawa K, Kubo H, Yamada M, et al. Hepatocyte growth factor induces angiogenesis in injured lungs through mobilizing endothelial progenitor cells. Biochem Biophys Res Commun 2004; 324(1):276–280.

56. Balasubramaniam V, Mervis C, Maxey AM, et al. Neoantal hyperoxia reduces circulating, bone marrow, and lung EPCs in neonatal mice: implications for the pathogenesis of BPD. Am J Physiol Lung Cell Mol Physiol 2007; 292(5):L1073–L1084.

57. Burnham EL, Taylor WR, Quyyumi AA, et al. Increased circulating endothelial progenitor cells are associated with survival in acute lung injury. Am J Respir Crit Care Med 2005; 172(7):854–860.

58. Yamada M, Kubo H, Ishizawa K, et al. Increased circulating endothelial progenitor cells in patients with bacterial pneumonia: evidence that bone marrow derived cells contribute to lung repair. Thorax 2005; 60(5):410–413.

59. Fadini GP, Schiavon M, Cantini M, et al. Circulating progenitor cells are reduced in patients with severe lung disease. Stem Cells 2006; 24(7):1806–1813.

60. Balasubramaniam V, Mervis CF, Maxey AM, et al. Hyperoxia reduces bone marrow, circulating, and lung endothelial progenitor cells in the developing lung: implications for the pathogenesis of bronchopulmonary dysplasia. Am J Physiol Lung Cell Mol Physiol 2007; 292(5):L1073–L1084.

61. Irwin D, Helm K, Campbell N, et al. Neonatal lung side population cells demonstrate endothelial potential and are altered in response to hyperoxia-induced lung simplification. Am J Physiol Lung Cell Mol Physiol 2007; 293(4):L941–L951.

62. Broxmeyer HE. Primitive hematopoietic stem and progenitor cells in human umbilical cord blood: an alternative source of transplantable cells. Cancer Treat Res 1996; 84:139–148.

63. Javed MJ, Mead LE, Prater D, et al. Endothelial colony forming cells and mesenchymal stem cells are enriched at different gestational ages in human umbilical cord blood. Pediatr Res 2008; 64(1):68–73.

11
Altered Growth Factor Signaling in the Pathogenesis of BPD

A. KEITH TANSWELL, SANNA PADELA, and ROBERT P. JANKOV
University of Toronto, Toronto, Ontario, Canada

I. Introduction

The majority of infants developing bronchopulmonary dysplasia (BPD) in the current era have been delivered at 23 to 28 weeks' gestation. The pathological hallmarks of BPD in this population are interstitial thickening and an arrest or inhibition of alveologenesis (1). Pulmonary hypertension is a significant adverse outcome in those most severely affected (2). As described elsewhere in this volume, inflammation may play a central role in the development of BPD. Suggested major contributors to inflammation, separately or additively, which leads to BPD are chorioamnionitis (3), hyperoxia (4,5), sepsis (6), and ventilation-induced volutrauma (7). Results from in vitro and in vivo models of lung growth, repair, and injury suggest that immaturity, oxygen concentration, sepsis, and volutrauma may all influence the expression of polypeptide growth factors in the developing lung. Whether the structural changes observed in human BPD reflect an altered pattern of secretion of polypeptide growth factors, the appearance of different factors, or both, is unknown. Available information about the role of polypeptide growth factors during the development of BPD remains sparse. This is in major part due to the limited availability of human tissue from the early stages of disease development and, until relatively recently, uncertainty as to the identity of likely mediators.

II. Reactive Oxygen Species and Cell Division

Reactive oxygen species (ROS) play important physiological roles as intra- and intercellular messengers, modulating the growth of target cells (8–11). Low concentrations of superoxide and hydrogen peroxide stimulate, and extracellular antioxidant enzymes inhibit, the in vitro growth of some cell types (9), suggesting an autocrine growth-stimulating response to cell-derived ROS. ROS production increases progressively throughout the cell cycle from G_1 to S phase, with antioxidant therapy arresting cell cycle progression at late G_1 phase, which is associated with a failure to accumulate cyclin A (12). NAD(P)H oxidase, as a source of superoxide, appears to be involved in signaling by epidermal growth factor (EGF), insulin, platelet-derived growth factor (PDGF), and transforming growth factor β_1 (TGF-β_1) (10). The primary effect that ROS use for signal transduction is reversible protein oxidation. In particular, thiol groups on molecules such as glutathione, glutaredoxin, thioredoxin, and peroxiredoxin act as redox-sensitive switches. Redox homeostasis plays a critical role in many cellular processes, including DNA synthesis, and has been the subject of recent informative reviews (10,11). Proteins with cysteine residues that undergo redox regulation include protein tyrosine phosphatases and kinases. Low concentrations of ROS stimulate the expression of the early growth-related genes, *c-fos* and *c-jun*, in various cell types (9). The subsequent binding of the Fos/Jun heterodimer to the AP-1 promoter site is also dependent on the redox state of a cysteine residue in their DNA-binding domain (13). Redox state also regulates the enhanced DNA-binding of the Fos/Jun heterodimer mediated by the nuclear protein Ref-1 (14,15), as well as that of other transcription factors (8). ROS-mediated activation of both *c-fos* and the *erg1* transcription factor genes involves modification of the serum response factor (16,17). Activation of the NF-κB is also redox dependent, but by a mechanism involving its release from an inactive cytoplasmic complex (18), which is regulated by the degree of glutathione oxidation (19).

In contrast to the growth stimulation that may be observed with low concentrations of ROS, high concentrations of ROS may inhibit or arrest cell growth. Much of our understanding of how an exposure to excessive amounts of ROS affects the lung has come from studies of the effects of hyperoxia. Newborn rats exposed to >95% O_2 for one week have arrested lung cell DNA synthesis. Upon recovery in air, lung growth is rapidly restored to allow catch-up to a near-normal alveolar number (20). This suggests that the initial growth arrest observed with >95% O_2 is, at least in part, a protective response. DNA damage caused by oxidant stress results in p53 stabilization with activation of p21, a cyclin-dependent kinase inhibitor. In addition, p21 can bind to proliferating cell nuclear antigen to inhibit its function (21). DNA breaks occur when pneumocytes from premature rat lung are exposed to 95% O_2 (22), which appear to modulate *c-fos* expression (23). There are multiple redox-sensitive cellular sites that could act as sensors to initiate protective responses (9). NAD(P)H associated with a potassium channel appears to be such a sensor in pulmonary neuroepithelial cells (24). For growth-arrested lung cells a likely candidate as a sensor is an hemoprotein, aconitase. Aconitase is a tricarboxylic acid cycle enzyme, which is extremely sensitive to superoxide (25), and is rapidly inactivated in lung tissue following exposure to 100% O_2 (26). This shuts down mitochondrial respiration, thus limiting their further production of ROS and sparing DNA and other vital cell components from further oxidative injury (27). Additional potential protective mechanisms include oxygen-responsive elements, such as those found in the 5′-flanking region of the human glutathione peroxidase gene, which allows increased transcription in response to O_2 (28). In contrast, increased catalase activity following exposure to O_2 results from increased mRNA stability (29).

Very high O_2 concentrations, as discussed in the preceding text, arrest growth of lung cells. This likely reflects an overwhelming ROS concentration. An intriguing observation has been that exposure of neonatal rats to 60% oxygen can actually stimulate secondary crest formation, under conditions in which neutrophil influx into the lung was prevented, hence limiting their considerable contribution to the ROS pool (30). At this time, one can only speculate how this effect might be mediated. In vitro studies of hyperoxic premature lung cells have demonstrated increased prostaglandin synthesis (31,32). Direct stimulation of protein kinase C (PKC) can occur in some cell types in response to *cis*-unsaturated fatty acids, including arachidonic acid (33), and in response to increased glutathione oxidation (34). Increase in certain prostaglandins can cause an increase in intracellular calcium that, in some cell types, activates protein kinases (35). Premature lung cells exposed to hyperoxia in vitro have rapidly depleted stores of reduced nonprotein thiols (22). In addition, oxidative stress can influence growth factor transduction pathways through effects on both protein tyrosine kinase and phosphatase activities (36).

III. The Influence of Lung Distension on Cell Growth

Overdistension of the lung has been recognized for many years as a mediator of ventilator-induced lung injury (37–39). High tidal volume ventilation can induce stress fractures of capillary endothelium, epithelium, and basement membranes and increase vascular filtration pressures (40). It can also stimulate proinflammatory cytokine release (41). This recognition has led to the introduction of low tidal volume ventilation (permissive hypercapnia) as a standard practice in adult intensive care, with a resultant improved survival of patients suffering from the acute adult respiratory distress syndrome (42–44) or acute lung injury (45). On the basis of this success, permissive hypercapnia has become a widely used strategy in neonatal intensive care. Targeting an arterial partial pressure of carbon dioxide ($PaCO_2$) of 45 to 55 mmHg (46) has no apparent short-term adverse consequences (47). However, multicenter trials of permissive hypercapnia in premature neonates have not, to date, demonstrated any reduction in the incidence of death or BPD (48,49). The issue of whether reduced tidal volume ventilation strategies can affect the incidence of BPD remains open, in that both the trials cited above were terminated prior to recruitment of the necessary patient numbers. Although neonatal lungs may be inherently less susceptible to ventilator-induced lung injury than adult lungs (50), the risk of ventilator-induced lung injury still requires that overdistention of functional lung units during mechanical ventilation be avoided. Premature lung tissue is structurally immature with a low tensile strength, which may contribute to ventilator-induced microvascular permeability (51). How neonatal ventilation within the usual range of tidal volumes used clinically affects growth factor expression awaits future exploration.

In vitro studies have demonstrated that excessive stretch of lung cells increases superoxide production, both from mitochondria and from NAD(P)H oxidase, with increased glutathione oxidation (52). An alternative source for superoxide when tissue is overstretched is through an increased activity of xanthine oxidoreductase (53). Exogenous sources of free radicals are from an influx of phagocytes (54) induced by ventilation-mediated release of cytokines.

As described in the preceding text, both O_2 and excessive distension share common pathways by which lung cell growth may be dysregulated. Early, and more recent, studies suggest that the effects of hyperoxia and excessive ventilation on lung injury are additive (55,56). A role for neutrophils in pulmonary oxygen toxicity appears to be firmly established, as assessed by depletion experiments (30,57,58). Barotrauma-mediated changes in airway pathology of surfactant-insufficient lungs are also phagocyte mediated (59). Although additive effects on growth factor expression have yet to be

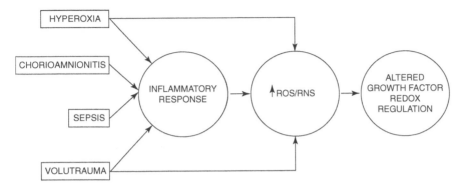

Figure 1 Schematic of how major contributors to the development of BPD (hyperoxia, chorioamnionitis, sepsis, volutrauma) may influence growth factor expression. All four insults cause inflammation with a phagocyte influx and resultant generation of ROS. Both hyperoxia and volutrauma cause additional independent ROS formation. The excess of ROS ± reactive nitrogen species (RNS) oxidize thiol groups to modify redox state and alter the expression of redox-sensitive growth factors.

explored in the laboratory, we speculate (Fig. 1) that those factors such as hyperoxia, chorioamnionitis, volutrauma, and sepsis, which are known to be positively associated with the development of BPD, all use a common pathway leading to ROS accumulation and redox regulation of growth factor expression.

IV. Specific Growth Factors and Receptors in Normal and Injured Lung

A. Epidermal Growth Factor and Transforming Growth Factor α

Both EGF and TGF-α exert their mitogenic activities through their binding to the EGF receptor (EGF-R), though they may have different ligand/receptor processing, accounting for any relative differences in potency (60). Neonatal rabbits exposed to an hyperoxia protocol that induces pulmonary fibrosis have increased TGF-α in their bronchoalveolar lavage fluid (61). A cause-and-effect relationship is suggested by the pulmonary fibrosis observed in transgenic mice overexpressing TGF-α (62). Following oxidant injury, hamster lung fibroblasts also synthesize TGF-α (63), suggesting that epithelial cells and macrophages may not be the only source following lung injury. Conditional pulmonary expression of TGF-α in late fetal life resulted in abnormal lung morphogenesis, including remodeling of the distal lung septa and arteries (64). In the immediate postnatal period, mice that overexpress TGF-α develop enlarged alveolar airspaces, pulmonary fibrosis, airway obstruction, and altered lung compliance (65). Even transient conditional overexpression of pulmonary TGF-α results in abnormal lung morphogenesis, which is carried into adult life (66). Stahlman et al. (67) described the presence of bronchiolar EGF in infants with BPD, which was not seen in unaffected infants. Strandjord et al. (68) were able to detect EGF and its receptor in all lung epithelium and TGF-α in airway epithelium of children with normal lungs, whereas children with BPD had increased EGF, EGF-R, and TGF-α in alveolar macrophages.

B. Insulin-Like Growth Factors

Insulin-like growth factor I (IGF-I) is a retinoic acid–sensitive growth factor (69), which has been implicated in air embolization-induced experimental pulmonary hypertension (70). This observation is consistent with findings that IGF-I and IGF-R1 mRNAs and proteins are increased in the lung parenchyma of adult rats exposed to 85% O_2 and that the increase in the IGF-R1 was localized to peribronchial and perivascular smooth muscle and endothelial cells (71). In a neonatal rat model of BPD, induced by a two-week exposure to 60% O_2, patchy areas of tissue thickening and active DNA synthesis had an increase in immunoreactive IGF-I and IGF-R1, whereas emphysematous areas of arrested cell growth had a reduction in immunoreactive IGF-I and IGF-R1, compared with air-exposed lungs (72). Exposure of newborn rats to 80% to 90% O_2 for four to six weeks results in a markedly increased expression of both IGF-I and IGF-II (73). IGFs have also been implicated in compensatory lung growth (74,75). Given that both surface forces and O_2 regulate IGF gene expression in experimental models, IGF-related gene products are strong candidates for contributing to the cellular changes observed in BPD. Lung tissue from patients with BPD, when compared with tissue from patients with RDS, showed increased IGF-I localized to alveolar epithelium and mesenchyme, bronchial epithelium and peribronchial myofibroblasts, and increased IGF-R1 was localized to peribronchial myofibroblasts and perialveolar mesenchyme (76). Patients with BPD have an increase in free IGF-I, i.e., IGF-I dissociated from its binding proteins, in their airway epithelial lining fluid (77).

C. Platelet-Derived Growth Factors

PDGF-A-deficient mice that survive beyond birth have a failure of alveologenesis attributed to a lack of fibroblast migration, failed differentiation into alveolar myofibroblasts, and failed elastin deposition (78). The PDGF-A gene includes a vitamin D response element (79), which, along with the observation that rachitic rats have impaired lung development (80), is consistent with vitamin D–affecting lung development through PDGF-AA. After birth in the neonatal rat, the expressions of PDGF-AA, -BB, and -αR all peak at the onset of alveologenesis (81). Treatment of rat pups with antibodies to PDGF-BB, or a truncated soluble PDGF-βR, impairs alveolarization and postnatal lung growth (81), limits pulmonary vascular smooth muscle hyperplasia secondary to 60% O_2 exposure (82), and in older pups impairs postpneumonectomy compensatory lung growth (83). Attenuation of PDGF-B function prevented pulmonary vascular remodeling associated with upregulation of PDGF-βR in fetal sheep (84). The degree of phosphorylation of the PDGF-βR following binding of PDGF-BB is redox regulated by the action of glutaredoxin on protein tyrosine phosphatases (85).

Neonatal lung injury is associated both with reduced cell proliferation and, based on the limited studies available, with downregulation of the PDGF ligands. Neonatal rats ventilated with 40% or exposed to 60% O_2 had a reduced expression of PDGF-AA (81,86), -BB, and -βR (81). Altered expression of PDGF isoforms will likely be identified as playing a role in the cellular changes of BPD, but analyses of human tissue are currently lacking.

D. Fibroblast Growth Factors

Both fibroblast growth factor 1 (FGF-1; acidic fibroblast growth factor, aFGF) and fibroblast growth factor 2 (FGF-2; basic fibroblast growth factor, bFGF) are mitogenic for type II pneumocytes (87). However, the injection of neutralizing antibodies to FGF-1 or FGF-2 had no effect on lung cell DNA synthesis in neonatal rats, though injection of a soluble receptor to FGF-R1α-IIIc did inhibit cell proliferation (88). Treatment with a soluble receptor to FGF-R1α-IIIc also impairs compensatory lung growth (89). Several members of the FGF family bind to FGF-R1α-IIIc, but it is not clear which member(s) are responsible for effects on cell proliferation, and their contribution to growth impairment in lung injury is therefore uncertain. FGF-R1α-IIIc and FGF-2, but not FGF-1, regulated physiological apoptosis in the neonatal rat lung (88).

A ligand for an FGF-R2 splice variant, FGF-R2-IIIb, is FGF-7 (keratinocyte growth factor, KGF). The FGF-R2-IIIb is not a specific receptor for FGF-7, also binding to FGF-1, -3, -7, and -10 (90–92). Late gestation fetal lung fibroblasts in vitro secrete FGF-7, which stimulates adult type II cell proliferation (90). Neonatal rats injected with antibodies to FGF-7 have arrested alveologenesis (93). FGF-18 is a vitamin A–responsive growth factor that regulates myofibroblast differentiation and elastin formation in the postnatal lung (94) and is downregulated in human and animal models of diaphragmatic hernia, in which there is impaired alveolarization (95).

Both FGF-R3 and -R4 together are required for the formation of secondary septa (96). Both are downregulated in neonatal mice exposed to hyperoxia (97). Increased levels of FGF-2 were found in tracheal aspirates from infants of less than 34 weeks' gestation destined to die or develop BPD (98). FGF-7 is known to enhance compensatory lung growth (99), and both FGF-2 and -7 are upregulated in the bleomycin- and monocrotaline-induced lung injuries of adult rats (100,101). Upregulation of FGF-7 may reflect a protective response, in that enhanced lung concentrations protected against lung injury induced by hyperoxia, ventilation, bacterial sepsis, and elastase-induced pulmonary emphysema (102–108). Neonatal rat pups show an increased expression of FGF-7 after 10 days and a decreased expression after 14 days, of exposure to 60% O_2, relative to air-exposed control animals (Fig. 2). A reduced expression of FGF-7 was also observed in neonatal mice exposed to 85% O_2 for 14 days (97). Using a soluble FGF-7 receptor, to limit FGF-7 binding to its endogenous receptor, increased sensitivity to hyperoxia (103). A high concentration of FGF-7 in the airways of premature human infants is a negative predictor for the development of BPD (109). FGF-10 has significant homology to FGF-7, is a growth factor for epithelial cells but not for cells of mesenchymal origin, and binds to the same FGF-R2-IIIb (98). Its expression is downregulated in lung tissues from infants with BPD (110).

E. Hepatocyte Growth Factor

Hepatocyte growth factor (HGF) has considerable homology with FGF-7 (111). Both HGF and its receptor, c-met, are essential for postnatal alveolar formation (112). In human infants developing BPD, the severity of their outcome has been inversely

(A)   **(B)**

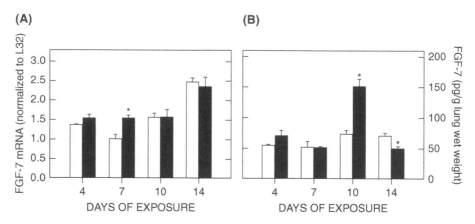

Figure 2 (A) FGF-7 mRNA content of neonatal rat pups exposed to air (*open bars*) or 60% oxygen (*solid bars*) for up to 14 days. Northern blot bands were quantified by densitometry and normalized to the housekeeping mRNA, L32. (B) FGF-7 protein content, as assessed by ELISA, of neonatal rat pups exposed to air (*open bars*) or 60% oxygen (*solid bars*) for up to 14 days; * indicates $p < 0.05$ by one-way ANOVA compared with lung FGF-7 mRNA or protein content of pups exposed to air for the same periods. Lungs from four average-sized pups in each litter of 10 to 12 pups were pooled. Values are means ± SEM for four litters in each group.

correlated with their tracheal aspirate content of HGF (113). In the neonatal rat model of BPD, induced by exposure to 60% O_2, HGF expression is upregulated (112). HGF has been reported to stimulate myofibroblast apoptosis in another lung injury (114), yet may inhibit epithelial cell apoptosis (115). This latter observation is of particular interest, in that both the neonatal rat and baboon models of BPD have been observed to have a relative increase in epithelial cells as part of the lung injury (112,116). In the neonatal rat model, preliminary data suggests that exposure to 60% O_2 causes an inhibition of physiological apoptosis (117). This may account for the observed relative increase in epithelial cells and could, in turn, be mediated by the upregulated HGF expression.

F. Transforming Growth Factor βs

Excessive signaling by TGF-β inhibits secondary septation (118,119). Increased expression of TGF-β_1 has been reported in the lungs of animals subjected to experimental asbestosis, bleomycin-induced pulmonary fibrosis, hypoxia-induced vascular injury, hypersensitivity pneumonitis, silicosis, and pulmonary O_2 toxicity (120–125). In human idiopathic pulmonary fibrosis, the intracellular form has been localized to alveolar macrophages and epithelium and to airway epithelium, whereas the extracellular form has been localized to matrix (126). The cell types contributing TGF-βs in the injured lung may vary at differing time points following the initiation of the injury process (127). In addition to the role of TGF-βs in the matrix deposition accompanying lung injury (128), they may also influence cell proliferation. In bleomycin-induced pulmonary fibrosis, there is a temporal relationship between TGF-β expression and cell proliferation (129). TGF-β-mediated fibroblast proliferation may occur either through an autocrine release of PDGF (130) or through a restoration of PDGF receptors (131). TGF-β-mediated inhibition of airway epithelial cell proliferation may be secondary to an effect on EGF-R phosphorylation (132). Overexpression of TGF-β in mice or rats (118,119) results in a BPD-like picture. Neonatal rats exposed to 100% O_2 have increased expression of TGF-β-RI and TGF-β-RII (133). Fetal sheep exposed to intra-amniotic endotoxin have increased TGF-β expression (134). Preterm lambs ventilated with O_2 have increased TGF-$β_1$ expression (135). Neonatal mice exposed to 85% O_2 have increased TGF-β, TGF-β-RII, and ALK-1 expression (119,136) and a BPD-like lung pathology. They also have altered BMP receptor expression, with downregulation of the proproliferative ALK-1 receptor and an upregulation of the antiproliferative ALK-6 receptor (136). Treatment of 85% O_2-exposed mice with a TGF-β neutralizing antibody reduced Smad 2 signaling and partially attenuated the pathological changes (137).

Very immature infants receiving supplemental O_2 have increased TGF-β levels in tracheal aspirates. A further increased in infants with BPD correlates with its severity (138–140). Autopsy tissues show increased peripheral TGF-β expression in the lungs of infants with BPD (141).

G. Connective Tissue Growth Factor

Connective tissue growth factor (CTGF) is a downstream regulator of some TGF-β-mediated effects and appears to play a critical role in lung development, in that the Ctgf-null mouse has pulmonary hypoplasia (142). CTGF is well recognized to play a role in the development of pulmonary fibrosis (143). However, exposure of neonatal rats to ≥90% O_2 results in the upregulation of CTGF expression, in association with increased collagen deposition (144,145), suggesting that it may not stimulate alveologenesis. Fetal sheep exposed to intra-amniotic endotoxin have downregulated CTGF expression, despite increased TGF-β expression (132).

H. Vascular Endothelial Growth Factor

Expression of VEGF, acting through the VEGF receptor-2 (VEGF-R2/KDR/flk-1), is necessary for alveologenesis to occur (146–149). Collectively, these observations have led to the "vascular hypothesis," in which secondary septation and alveolar formation is dependent on, and driven by, capillary formation. Exogenous VEGF also accelerates lung growth after pneumonectomy (150). VEGF expression is downregulated in neonatal rats (147,151) and rabbits (152) following exposure to hyperoxia, and in lambs following antenatal endotoxin exposure (153). This downregulation by antenatal endotoxin was further amplified in rats subsequently exposed to hyperoxia (154). Exposure to 100% O_2 has been shown to impair the synthesis of VEGF by epithelial cells (152). Neonatal mice ventilated with 40% O_2 had a reduced expression of VEGF and VEGF-R2, compared with unventilated control animals (86), as do preterm lambs ventilated with O_2 (135). In both 125-day and 140-day baboon models of BPD, expression of VEGF and the VEGF receptors, Flt-1 and Flk-1, have been reported to be decreased (155–157). The overall picture in animal models of neonatal lung injury is an initial downregulation of VEGF during the injury process, followed by an upregulation during a recovery period (158). On the basis of observations with adenovirus-mediated upregulation of VEGF, this upregulation of VEGF in a recovery phase will be associated with new lung capillary formation (147). Immature new capillaries formed in response to exogenous VEGF given during an injury process may leak and contribute to pulmonary edema (159), until the capillaries are matured with angiopoietin-1, suggesting a possible pharmacological role for combined VEGF and angiopoietin-1 therapy (147).

On the basis of the "vascular hypothesis" alluded to earlier, the inhibition of VEGF expression early in lung injury could result in, or contribute to, the impaired alveolar formation observed in BPD (160). Consistent with this hypothesis, infants who die from BPD or following brief periods of ventilation have a reduced and abnormal distal lung vasculature (146,161,162) and reduced VEGF, Flt-1, and TIE-2 expression in lung tissue (146,163,164) and tracheal fluid (165). In addition, an antiangiogenic protein, endothelial-monocyte activating protein II, is upregulated in the lung tissue of humans and baboons with BPD (166).

I. Other Factors That Influence Growth

The concentration of placental growth factor (PlGF) in cord blood in preterm infants correlates with both the development of BPD and its severity (167). The role of PlGF in lung injury requires further exploration. Another factor that may be involved in alveolar formation is the heparin-binding growth factor, midkine. This growth factor is retinoic acid sensitive and is downregulated in neonatal mice exposed to 95% O_2 (168). This review has focused on the classic group of polypeptide growth factors. However, other cytokines such as IL-1α, IL-1β, IL-6, GM-CSF, and 5-hydroxytryptamine (169–173) may have growth stimulating or inhibiting properties. Endothelin-1 is a known mitogen (174) for pulmonary vascular smooth muscle cells. That it may play a role in the pulmonary hypertension seen in BPD is suggested by intervention studies in a neonatal rat model using an endothelin receptor antagonist (175). Another reported mitogen for smooth muscle is thrombin, though this appears to be an indirect effect mediated by FGF-2 (176) or PDGFs (177,178).

The airways of infants with BPD have increased neuroendocrine cells containing gastrin-releasing peptide (mammalian bombesin), a growth regulator for airway epithelium (179). Infants who subsequently develop BPD have elevated urinary bombesin levels (180). In a baboon model of BPD, a critical role for bombesin in the inhibition of alveologenesis was demonstrated by its reversal following antibody treatment (181). Another potentially important agent is the parathyroid hormone–related protein, which inhibits proliferation of type II pneumocytes, both in vivo and in vitro (182), and may be downregulated in adult lung injury, to facilitate type II pneumocyte proliferation (183).

V. Problems of Interpretation

As our understanding of growth factor expression in neonatal lung injury increases, a very complex picture of interactions is unfolding. Many growth factors modulate the expression of other growth factors or their receptors (184–194). Complex interactions can occur between IGF and EGF receptors (195). VEGF and FGF-2 may function synergistically in angiogenesis (196). Also, different subpopulations of lung cells, in particular fibroblasts, may not be homogeneous in their secretion of, or response to, growth factors (197,198).

Growth factors may serve functions other than simply inducing DNA synthesis. It is probable that most, if not all, polypeptide growth factors will serve dual functions. Several growth factors are inhibitors of apoptosis (199), including PDGF-BB, FGF-2, VEGF, HGF, and ET-1 (200–204). Changes in growth factor expression may alter extracellular matrix composition and, as a secondary effect, alter cell growth through a variety of mechanisms. Some extracellular matrix proteins promote growth through the presence of growth factor–like domains (205). Others can affect growth by modifying cell shape (206), acting as a reservoir for some growth factors that are released by proteases to become active (207), protecting growth factors against inactivation (208) and enhancing or inhibiting growth factor presentation to a receptor on a target cell (209–211). Expression of growth factor receptors, following lung injury, may be temporally very different from that of the ligand (212,213), complicating the interpretation of any altered growth factor expression. Understanding such complex interactions in lung injury will be essential for appropriate interpretation of observations. Temporal relationships between increased cell proliferation and increased growth factor expression can only be considered a correlation, unless specific targeted interventions allow a cause and effect relationship to be confirmed.

References

1. Coalson JJ. Pathology of chronic lung disease of early infancy. In: Bland RD, Coalson JJ, eds. Chronic Lung Disease of Early Infancy. New York, NY: Marcel Dekker, 2000:85–124.
2. Thibeault DW, Truog WE, Ekekezie II. Acinar arterial changes with chronic lung disease of prematurity in the surfactant era. Pediatr Pulmonol 2003; 36:482–489.
3. Watterberg KL, Demers LM, Scott SM, et al. Chorioamnionitis and early lung inflammation in infants in whom bronchopulmonary dysplasia develops. Pediatrics 1996; 97:210–215.
4. STOP-ROP Multicenter Study Group. Supplemental therapeutic oxygen for prethreshold retinopathy of prematurity (STOP-ROP), a randomized, controlled trial. I: Primary outcomes. Pediatrics 2000; 105:295–310.
5. Askie LM, Henderson-Smart DJ, Irwig L, et al. Oxygen-saturation targets and outcomes in extremely preterm infants. N Engl J Med 2003; 349:959–967.
6. Bancalari E, Gonzales A. Clinical course and lung function abnormalities during development of neonatal chronic lung disease. In: Bland RD, Coalson JJ, eds. Chronic Lung Disease of Early Infancy. New York, NY: Marcel Dekker, 2000:41–64.
7. Albertine KH, Jones GP, Starcher BC, et al. Chronic lung injury in preterm lambs. Disordered respiratory tract development. Am J Respir Crit Care Med 1999; 159:945–958.
8. Saran M, Bors W. Oxygen radicals acting as chemical messengers: a hypothesis. Free Radic Res Commun 1989; 7:3–6.
9. Burdon RH. Superoxide and hydrogen peroxide in relation to mammalian cell proliferation. Free Radic Biol Med 1995; 18:775–794.
10. Oktyabrsky ON, Smirnova GV. Redox regulation of cellular functions. Biochemistry (Mosc) 2007; 72:132–145.
11. Chiarugi P, Fiaschi T. Redox signalling in anchorage-dependent cell growth. Cell Signal 2007; 19:672–682.
12. Havens CG, Ho A, Yoshioka N, et al. Regulation of late G_1/S phase transition and APC Cdh1 by reactive oxygen species. Mol Cell Biol 2006; 26:4701–4711.
13. Abate C, Patel L, Rauscher FJ, et al. Redox regulation of Fos and Jun DNA-binding in vitro. Science 1990; 249:1157–1161.
14. Xanthoudakis S, Curran T. Identification and characterization of Ref-1, a nuclear protein that facilitates AP-1 DNA-binding activity. EMBO J 1992; 11:653–665.

15. Xanthoudakis S, Miao G, Wang F, et al. Redox activation of Fos-Jun DNA binding activity is mediated by a DNA repair enzyme. EMBO J 1992; 11:3323–3335.

16. Datta R, Taneja N, Sukhatme VP, et al. Reactive oxygen intermediates target $CC(A/T)_6GG$ sequence to mediate activation of early growth response 1 transcription factor gene by ionising radiation. Proc Natl Acad Sci U S A 1993; 90:2419–2422.

17. Treisman RH. Identification of a protein binding site that mediates transcriptional response of the c-fos gene to serum factors. Cell 1986; 46:567–574.

18. Schreck R, Rieber P, Baeuerle PA. Reactive oxygen intermediates as apparently widely used messengers in the activation of the NF-κB transcription factor and HIV-1. EMBO J 1991; 10:2247–2258.

19. Galter D, Mihm S, Dröge W. Distinct effects of glutathione disulphide on the nuclear transcription factors κB and the activator protein-1. Eur J Biochem 1994; 221:639–648.

20. Randell SH, Mercer RR, Young SL. Postnatal growth of pulmonary acini and alveoli in normal and oxygen exposed rats studied by serial section reconstruction. Am J Anat 1989; 186:55–68.

21. Gehen SC, Vitiello PF, Bambara RA, et al. Downregulation of PCNA potentiates p21-mediated growth inhibition in response to hyperoxia. Am J Physiol 2007; 292:L716–L724.

22. Christie NA, Slutsky AS, Freeman BA, et al. A critical role for thiol, but not ATP, depletion in 95% O_2-mediated injury in preterm pneumocytes. Arch Biochem Biophys 1994; 313:131–138.

23. Amstad PA, Krupitza G, Cerutti P. Mechanism of c-fos induction by active oxygen. Cancer Res 1992; 52:3952–3960.

24. Youngson C, Nurse C, Yeger H, et al. Oxygen sensing in airway chemoreceptors. Nature 1993; 365:153–155.

25. Gardner PR, Fridovich I. Effect of glutathione on aconitase in *Escherichia coli*. Arch Biochem Biophys 1993; 301:98–102.

26. Gardner PR, Nguyen DD, White CW. Aconitase is a sensitive and critical target of oxygen poisoning in cultured mammalian cells and in rat lungs. Proc Natl Acad Sci U S A 1994; 91:12248–12252.

27. Halliwell B, Gutteridge JMC. Oxygen toxicity, oxygen radicals, transition metals and disease. Biochem J 1984; 219:1–14.

28. Cowan DB, Weisel RD, Williams WG, et al. Identification of oxygen responsive elements in the 5′-flanking region of the human glutathione peroxidase gene. J Biol Chem 1993; 36: 26904–26910.

29. Clerch LB, Massaro D. Rat lung antioxidant enzymes: differences in perinatal gene expression and regulation. Am J Physiol 1992; 263:L466–L470.

30. Yi M, Jankov RP, Belcastro R, et al. Opposing effects of 60% oxygen and neutrophil influx on alveologenesis in the neonatal rat. Am J Respir Crit Care Med 2004; 170:1188–1196.

31. Tanswell AK, Olson DM, Freeman BA. Response of fetal rat lung fibroblasts to elevated oxygen concentrations after liposome-mediated augmentation of antioxidant enzymes. Biochim Biophys Acta 1990; 1044:269–274.

32. Tanswell AK, Olson DM, Freeman BA. Liposome-mediated augmentation of antioxidant defences in fetal rat pneumocytes. Am J Physiol 1990; 258:L165–L172.

33. Dell KR, Severson DI. Effects of cis-unsaturated fatty acids on aortic protein kinase C. Biochem J 1989; 258:171–175.

34. Kass GEN, Duddy SK, Orrenius S. Activation of protein kinase C by redox-cycling quinones. Biochem J 1989; 260:499–507.

35. Suzuki A, Kozawa O, Saito H, et al. Effects of prostaglandin $F_{2\alpha}$ on Ca^{2+} influx in osteoblast-like cells: function of tyrosine kinase. J Cell Biochem 1994; 54:487–493.

36. Keyse SM, Emslie EA. Oxidative stress and heat shock induce a human gene encoding a protein tyrosine phosphatase. Nature (Lond) 1992; 359:644–647.

37. Drayfuss D, Soler P, Basset G, et al. High inflation pressure pulmonary edema. Am Rev Respir Dis 1988; 137:1159–1164.
38. Carlton DP, Cummings JJ, Scheerer RG, et al. Lung overexpansion increases pulmonary microvascular protein permeability in young lambs. J Appl Physiol 1990; 69:577–583.
39. Manning HL. Peak airway pressure: why the fuss? Chest 1994; 105:242–247.
40. Parker JC, Hernandez LA, Peevy KJ. Mechanisms of ventilator-induced lung injury. Crit Care Med 1993; 21:131–143.
41. Tremblay L, Valenza F, Ribeiro S, et al. Injurious ventilation strategies increase cytokines and c-fos mRNA expression in an isolated rat lung model. J Clin Invest 1997; 99:944–952.
42. Amato MD, Barbas CS, Medeiros DM, et al. Effects of a protective-ventilation strategy on mortality in the acute respiratory distress syndrome. N Engl J Med 1998; 338:347–354.
43. Bidani A, Tzouanakis AE, Cardenas VJ Jr, et al. Permissive hypercapnia in acute respiratory failure. JAMA 1994; 272:957–962.
44. Laffey JG, O'Coinin D, McLoughlin P, et al. Permissive hypercapnia—role in protective lung ventilatory strategies. Intensive Care Med 2004; 30:347–356.
45. Kregenow DA, Rubenfeld GD, Hudson LD, et al. Hypercapnic acidosis and mortality in acute lung injury. Crit Care Med 2006; 34:229–231.
46. Varughese M, Patole S, Shama A, et al. Permissive hypercapnia in neonates: the case of the good, the bad, and the ugly. Pediatr Pulmonol 2002; 33:56–64.
47. Mariani G, Cifuentes J, Carlo WA. Randomized trial of permissive hypercapnia in preterm infants. Pediatrics 1999; 104:1082–1088.
48. Carlo WA, Stark AR, Wright LL, et al. Minimal ventilation to prevent bronchopulmonary dysplasia in extremely-low-birth-weight infants. J Pediatr 2002; 141:370–374.
49. Thome UH, Carroll W, Wu T-J, et al. Outcome of extremely preterm infants randomized at birth to different PaCO$_2$ targets during the first seven days of life. Biol Neonate 2006; 90:218–225.
50. Kornecki A, Tsuchida S, Ondiveeran HK, et al. Lung development and susceptibility to ventilator-induced lung injury. Am J Respir Crit Care Med 2005; 171:743–752.
51. Adkins WK, Hernandez LA, Coker PJ, et al. Age affects susceptibility to pulmonary barotrauma in rabbits. Crit Care Med 1991; 19:390–393.
52. Chapman KE, Sinclair SE, Zhuang D, et al. Cyclic mechanical strain increases reactive oxygen species production in pulmonary epithelial cells. Am J Physiol 2005; 289:L834–L841.
53. Abdulnour RE, Peng X, Finigan JH, et al. Mechanical strain activates xanthine oxidoreductase through MAP kinase-dependent pathways. Am J Physiol 2006; 291:L345–L353.
54. Jobe AH, Kramer BW, Moss TJ, et al. Decreased indicators of lung injury with continuous positive expiratory pressure in preterm lambs. Pediatr Res 2002; 52:387–392.
55. Liland AE, Zapol WM, Qvist J, et al. Positive airway pressure in lambs spontaneously breathing air and oxygen. J Surg Res 1976; 20:85–92.
56. Bailey TC, Martin EL, Zhao L, et al. High oxygen concentrations predispose mouse lungs to the effects of high stretch ventilation. J Appl Physiol 2003; 94:975–982.
57. Auten RL, Whorton MH, Mason SN. Blocking neutrophil influx reduces DNA damage in hyperoxia-exposed newborn rat lung. Am J Respir Cell Mol Biol 2002; 26:391–397.
58. Auten RL, Richardson RM, White JR, et al. Nonpeptide CXCR2 antagonist prevents neutrophil accumulation in hyperoxia-exposed newborn rats. J Pharm Exp Ther 2003; 299: 90–95.
59. Kawano T, Mori S, Cybulsky M, et al. Effect of granulocyte depletion in a ventilated surfactant-depleted lung. J Appl Physiol 1987; 62:27–33.
60. Ebner R, Derynck. Epidermal growth factor and transforming growth factor-α: differential routing and processing of ligand-receptor complexes. Cell Regul 1991; 2:599–612.
61. Waheed S, D'Angio CT, Wagner CL, et al. Transforming growth factor alpha (TGFα) is increased during hyperoxia and fibrosis. Exp Lung Res 2002; 28:361–372.

62. Korfhagen TR, Swanz RJ, Wert SE, et al. Respiratory epithelial cell expression of human transforming growth factor-α induces lung fibrosis in transgenic mice. J Clin Invest 1994; 93:1691–1699.

63. Vivekananda J, Lin A, Coalson JJ, et al. Acute inflammatory injury in the lung precipitated by oxidant stress induces fibroblasts to synthesize and release transforming growth factor-α. J Biol Chem 1994; 269:25057–25061.

64. Le Cras TD, Hardie WD, Deutsch GH, et al. Transient induction of TGF-alpha disrupts lung morphogenesis, causing pulmonary disease in adulthood. Am J Physiol Lung Cell Mol Physiol 2004; 287:L718–L729.

65. Kramer EL, Deutsch GH, Sartor MA, et al. Perinatal increases in TGF-α disrupt the saccular phase of lung morphogenesis and cause remodeling: microarray analysis. Am J Physiol Lung Cell Mol Physiol 2007; 293:L314–L327.

66. Hardie WD, Bruno MD, Huelsman KM, et al. Postnatal lung function and morphology in transgenic mice expressing transforming growth factor-alpha. Am J Pathol 1997; 151: 1075–1083.

67. Stahlman MT, Orth DN, Gray ME. Immunocytochemical localization of epidermal growth factor in the developing human respiratory system and in acute and chronic lung disease in the neonate. Lab Invest 1989; 60:539–547.

68. Strandjord TP, Clark JG, Guralnick DE, et al. Immunolocalization of transforming growth factor-α, epidermal growth factor (EGF), and EGF-receptor in normal and injured developing human lung. Pediatr Res 1995; 38:851–856.

69. Liu H, Chang L, Rong Z, et al. Association of insulin-like growth factors with lung development in neonatal rats. J Huazhong Univ Sci Technolog Med Sci 2004; 24:162–165.

70. Perkett EA, Badesch DB, Roessler MK, et al. Insulin-like growth factor I and pulmonary hypertension induced by continuous air embolization in sheep. Am J Respir Cell Mol Biol 1992; 6:82–87.

71. Han RNN, Han VKM, Buch S, et al. Insulin-like growth factor-I and type I insulin-like growth factor receptor in 85% O_2-exposed rat lung. Am J Physiol 1996; 271:L139–L149.

72. Han RNN, Buch S, Tseu I, et al. Changes in structure, mechanics, and insulin-like growth factor-related gene expression in the lungs of newborn rats exposed to 60% oxygen. Pediatr Res 1996; 39:921–929.

73. Veness-Meehan KA, Moats-Staats BM, Price WA, et al. Re-emergence of a fetal pattern of insulin-like growth factor expression during hyperoxic rat lung injury. Am J Respir Cell Mol Biol 1997; 16:538–548.

74. Stiles AD, D'Ercole AJ. The insulin-like growth factors and the lung. Am J Respir Cell Mol Biol 1990; 3:93–100.

75. Nobuhara KK, DiFiore JW, Ibla JC, et al. Insulin-like growth factor-1 gene expression in three models of accelerated lung growth. J Pediatr Surg 1998; 33:1057–1060.

76. Chetty A, Andersson S, Lassus P, et al. Insulin-like growth factor-1 (IGF-1) and IGF-1 receptor (IGF-1R) expression in human lungs in RDS and BPD. Pediatr Pulmonol 2004; 37:128–136.

77. Capoluongo E, Ameglio F, Lulli P, et al. Epithelial lining fluid free IGF-I-to-PAPP-A ratio is associated with bronchopulmonary dysplasia in preterm infants. Am J Physiol Endocrinol Metab 2007; 292:E308–E313.

78. Boström H, Willetts K, Pekny M, et al. PDGF-A signaling is a critical event in lung alveolar myofibroblast development and alveogenesis. Cell 1996; 85:863–873.

79. Soriano P. The PDGFα receptor is required for neural crest cell development and for normal patterning of the somites. Development 1997; 124:2691–2700.

80. Gaultier C, Harf A, Balmain N, et al. Lung mechanics in rachitic rats. Am Rev Respir Dis 1984; 130:1108–1110.

81. Buch S, Han RNN, Cabacungan J, et al. Changes in expression of platelet-derived growth factor and its receptors in the lungs of newborn rats exposed to air or 60% O_2. Pediatr Res 2000; 48:423–433.
82. Jankov RP, Kantores C, Belcastro R, et al. A role for platelet-derived growth factor β-receptor in a newborn rat model of endothelin-mediated pulmonary vascular remodeling. Am J Physiol Lung Cell Mol Physiol 2005; 288:L1162–L1170.
83. Yuan S, Hannam V, Belcastro R, et al. A role for platelet-derived growth factor-BB in rat postpneumonectomy compensatory lung growth. Pediatr Res 2002; 52:25–33.
84. Balasubramaniam V, Le Cras TD, Ivy DD, et al. Role of platelet-derived growth factor in vascular remodeling during pulmonary hypertension in the ovine fetus. Am J Physiol Lung Cell Mol Physiol 2003; 284:L826–L833.
85. Kanda M, Ihara Y, Murata H, et al. Glutaredoxin modulates platelet-derived growth factor-dependent cell signaling by regulating the redox status of low molecular weight protein-tyrosine phosphatase. J Biol Chem 2006; 281:28518–28528.
86. Bland RD, Mokres LM, Ertsey R, et al. Mechanical ventilation with 40% oxygen reduces pulmonary expression of genes that regulate lung development and impairs alveolar septation in newborn mice. Am J Physiol 2007; 293:L1099–L1110.
87. Leslie CC, McCormick-Shannon K, Mason RJ. Heparin-binding growth factors stimulate DNA synthesis in rat alveolar type II cells. Am J Respir Cell Mol Biol 1990; 2:99–106.
88. Yi M, Belcastro R, Shek S, et al. Fibroblast growth factor-2 and receptor-1α(IIIc) regulate postnatal rat lung cell apoptosis. Am J Respir Crit Care Med 2006; 174:581–589.
89. Jankov RP, Luo X, Campbell A, et al. Fibroblast growth factor receptor-1 and compensatory neonatal lung growth after 95% oxygen exposure. Am J Respir Crit Care Med 2003; 167:1554–1561.
90. Panos RJ, Rubin JS, Csaky KG, et al. Keratinocyte growth factor and hepatocyte growth factor/scatter factor are heparin-binding growth factors for alveolar type II cells in fibroblast-conditioned medium. J Clin Invest 1993; 92:969–977.
91. Ornitz DM., Xu J, Colvin JS, et al. Receptor specificity of the fibroblast growth factor family. J Biol Chem 1996; 271:15292–15297.
92. Igarashi M, Finch PW, Aaronson SA. Characterization of recombinant human fibroblast growth factor (FGF)-10 reveals functional similarities with keratinocyte growth factor (FGF-7). J Biol Chem 1998; 273:13230–13235.
93. Padela S, Yi M, Cabacungan J, et al. A critical role for fibroblast growth factor-7 during early alveolar formation in the neonatal rat. Pediatr Res 2008; 63:232–238.
94. Gillis P, Savla U, Volpert OV, et al. Keratinocyte growth factor induces angiogenesis and protects endothelial barrier function. J Cell Sci 1989; 112:2049–2057.
95. Boucherat O, Benachi A, Barlier-Mur AM, et al. Decreased lung fibroblast growth factor 18 and elastin in human congenital diaphragmatic hernia and animal models. Am J Respir Crit Care Med 2007; 175:1066–1077.
96. Weinstein M, Xu X, Ohyama K, et al. FGFR-3 and FGFR-4 function cooperatively to direct alveologenesis in the murine lung. Development 1998; 125:3615–3623.
97. Parks MS, Rieger-Fackeldey E, Schanbacher BL, et al. Altered expressions of fibroblast growth factor receptors and alveolarization in neonatal mice exposed to 85% oxygen. Pediatr Res 2007; 62:652–657.
98. Ambalavanan N, Novak ZE. Peptide growth factors in tracheal aspirates of mechanically ventilated preterm newborns. Pediatr Res 2003; 53:240–244.
99. Kaza AK, Kron IL, Leuwerke SM, et al. Keratinocyte growth factor enhances postpneumonectomy lung growth by alveolar proliferation. Circulation 2002; 106:120–124.
100. Adamson IY, Bakowska J. Relationship of keratinocyte growth factor and hepatocyte growth factor levels in rat lung lavage fluid to epithelial cell regeneration after bleomycin. Am J Pathol 1999; 155:949–954.

101. Arcot SS, Fagerland JA, Lipke DW, et al. Basic fibroblast growth factor alterations during development of monocrotaline-induced pulmonary hypertension in rats. Growth Factors 1995; 12:121–130.
102. Frank L. Protective effects of keratinocyte growth factor against lung abnormalities associated with hyperoxia in prematurely born rats. Biol Neonate 2003; 83:263–272.
103. Barazzone C, Donati YR, Rochat AF, et al. Keratinocyte growth factor protects alveolar epithelium and endothelium from oxygen-induced injury in mice. Am J Pathol 1999; 154:1479–1487.
104. Ray P, Devaux Y, Stolz DB, et al. Inducible expression of keratinocyte growth factor (KGF) in mice inhibits lung epithelial cell death induced by hyperoxia. Proc Natl Acad Sci U S A 2003; 100:6098–6103.
105. Welsh DA, Summer WR, Dobard EP, et al. Keratinocyte growth factor prevents ventilator-induced lung injury in an *ex vivo* rat model. Am J Respir Crit Care Med 2000; 162: 1081–1086.
106. Hokuto I, Perl AK, Whitsett JA. FGF signaling is required for pulmonary homeostasis following hyperoxia. Am J Physiol 2004; 286:L580–L587.
107. Viget NB, Guery BP, Ader F, et al. Keratinocyte growth factor protects against *Pseudomonas aeruginosa*-induced lung injury. Am J Physiol 2000; 279:L1199–L1209.
108. Plantier L, Marchand-Adam S, Antico VG, et al. Keratinocyte growth factor protects against elastase-induced pulmonary emphysema in mice. Am J Physiol 2007; 293:L1230–L1239.
109. Danan C, Franco ML, Jarreau PH, et al. High concentrations of keratinocyte growth factor in airways of premature infants predicted absence of bronchopulmonary dysplasia. Am J Respir Crit Care Med 2002; 165:1384–1387.
110. Benjamin JT, Smith RJ, Halloran BA, et al. FGF-10 is decreased in bronchopulmonary dysplasia and suppressed by Toll-like receptor activation. Am J Physiol 2007; 292: L550–L558.
111. Mason RJ, Leslie CC, McCormick-Shannon K, et al. Hepatocyte growth factor is a growth factor for rat alveolar type II cells. Am J Respir Cell Mol Biol 1994; 11:561–567.
112. Padela S, Cabacungan J, Shek S, et al. Hepatocyte growth factor is required for alveologenesis in the neonatal rat. Am J Respir Crit Care Med 2005; 172:907–914.
113. Lassus P, Heikkilä P, Andersson LC, et al. Lower concentration of pulmonary hepatocyte growth factor is associated with more severe lung disease in preterm infants. J Pediatr 2003; 143:199–202.
114. Mizuno S, Matsumoto K, Li MY, et al. HGF reduces advancing lung fibrosis in mice: a potential role for MMP-dependent myofibroblast apoptosis. FASEB J 2005; 19:333–350.
115. Shigemura N, Sawa Y, Mizuno S, et al. Amelioration of pulmonary emphysema by in vivo gene transfection with hepatocyte growth factor in rats. Circulation 2005; 111: 1407–1414.
116. Maniscalco WM, Watkins RH, O'Reilly MA, et al. Increased epithelial cell proliferation in very premature baboons with chronic lung disease. Am J Physiol 2002; 283:L991–L1001.
117. Yi M, Ziino A, Johnson BH, et al. Inhibition of apoptosis in 60% oxygen-induced neonatal rat lung injury (abstr). E-PAS 2007; 61:5894.3.
118. Gauldie J, Galt T, Bonniaud P, et al. Transfer of the active form of transforming growth factor-beta-1 gene to newborn rat lung induces changes consistent with bronchopulmonary dysplasia. Am J Pathol 2003; 163:2575–2584.
119. Vincencio AG, Lee CG, Cho SJ, et al. Conditional overexpression of bioactive transforming growth factor-beta 1 in neonatal mouse lung: a new model for bronchopulmonary dysplasia? Am J Respir Cell Mol Biol 2004; 31:650–656.
120. Perdue TD, Brody AR. Distribution of transforming growth factor-β1, fibronectin, and smooth muscle actin in asbestos-induced pulmonary fibrosis in rats. J Histochem Cytochem 1994; 42:1061–1070.

121. Khalil N, O'Connor RN, Flanders KC, et al. Regulation of type II alveolar cell proliferation by TGF-β during bleomycin-induced lung injury in rats. Am J Physiol 1994; 11:498–507.
122. Kwapiszewska G, Wilhelm J, Wolff S, et al. Expression profiling of laser-microdissected intrapulmonary arteries in hypoxia-induced pulmonary hypertension. Respir Res 2005; 6:109.
123. Denis M, Ghadirian E. Transforming growth factor-β is generated in the course of hypersensitivity pneumonitis: contribution to collagen synthesis. Am J Respir Cell Mol Biol 1992; 7:156–160.
124. Williams AO, Flanders KC, Saffiotti U. Immunohistochemical localization of transforming growth factor-β1 in rats with experimental silicosis, alveolar type II hyperplasia, and lung cancer. Am J Pathol 1993; 142:1831–1840.
125. Moore AM, Buch S, Han RNN, et al. Altered expression of type I collagen, TGF-β1, and related genes in rat lung exposed to 85% O_2. Am J Physiol 1995; 268:L78–L84.
126. Khalil N, O'Connor R, Unruh H, et al. Enhanced expression and immunohistochemical distribution of transforming growth factor-β in idiopathic pulmonary fibrosis. Chest 1991; 99(3 suppl):S65–S66.
127. Ono M, Sawa Y, Matsumoto K, et al. In vivo gene transfection with hepatocyte growth factor via the pulmonary artery induces angiogenesis in the rat lung. Circulation 2002; 106:1264–1269.
128. Giri SN, Hyde DM, Hollinger MA. Effect of antibody to transforming growth factor β on bleomycin induced accumulation of lung collagen in mice. Thorax 1993; 48:959–966.
129. Raghow R, Irish P, Kang AH. Coordinate regulation of transforming growth factor β gene expression and cell proliferation in hamster lungs undergoing bleomycin-induced pulmonary fibrosis. J Clin Invest 1989; 84:1836–1842.
130. Moses HL, Coffey RJ, Leof EB, et al. Transforming growth factor β regulation of cell proliferation. J Cell Physiol 1987; 5(suppl):S1–S7.
131. Psarras S, Kletsas D, Stathakos D. Restoration of down-regulated PDGF receptors by TGF-β in human embryonic fibroblasts. FEBS Lett 1994; 339:84–88.
132. Chess PR, Ryan RM, Finkelstein JN. Tyrosine kinase activity is necessary for growth factor-stimulated rabbit type II pneumocyte proliferation. Pediatr Res 1994; 36:481–486.
133. Zhao Y, Gilmore BJ, Young SL. Expression of transforming growth factor-beta receptors during hyperoxia-induced lung injury and repair. Am J Physiol 1997; 273:L355–L362.
134. Kunzmann S, Speer CP, Jobe AH, et al. Antenatal inflammation induces TGF-β1, but suppressed CTGF in preterm lungs. Am J Physiol 2007; 292:L223–L231.
135. Bland RD, Xu L, Ertsey R, et al. Dysregulation of pulmonary elastin synthesis and assembly in preterm lambs with chronic lung disease. Am J Physiol 2007; 292:L1370–L1384.
136. Alejandre-Alcazar MA, Kwapiszewska G, Reiss I, et al. Hyperoxia modulates TGF-β/BMP signaling in a mouse model of bronchopulmonary dysplasia. Am J Physiol 2007; 292: L537–L549.
137. Nakanishi H, Sugiura T, Streisand JB, et al. TGF-β-neutralizing antibodies improve pulmonary alveologenesis and vasculogenesis in the injured newborn lung. Am J Physiol 2007; 293:L151–L161.
138. Kotecha S, Wangoo A, Silverman M, et al. Increase in the concentration of transforming growth factor beta-1 in bronchoalveolar lavage fluid before development of chronic lung disease of prematurity. J Pediatr 1996; 128:464–469.
139. Lecart C, Cayabyab R, Buckley S, et al. Bioactive transforming growth factor-beta in the lungs of extremely low birth weight neonates predicts the need for home oxygen supplementation. Biol Neonate 2000; 77:217–223.
140. Saito M, Ichiba H, Yokoi T, et al. Mitogenic activity of tracheal effluents from premature infants with chronic lung disease. Pediatr Res 2004; 55:960–965.

141. Toti P, Buoncore G, Tanganelli P, et al. Bronchopulmonary dysplasia of the premature baby: an immunohistochemical study. Pediatr Pulmonol 1997; 24:22–28.
142. Baguma-Nibasheka M, Kablar B. Pulmonary hypoplasia in the connective tissue growth factor (Ctgf) null mouse. Dev Dyn 2008; 237:485–493.
143. Pan LH, Yamauchi K, Uzuki M, et al. Type II alveolar epithelial cells and interstitial fibroblasts express connective tissue growth factor in IPF. Eur Respir J 2001; 17:1220–1227.
144. Fu JH, Xue XD. Expression and role of connective tissue growth factor mRNA in premature rats with hyperoxia-induced chronic lung disease. Zhongguo Dang Dai Er Ke Za Zhi 2007; 9:449–452.
145. Chen CM, Wang LF, Chou HC, et al. Up-regulation of connective tissue growth factor in hyperoxia-induced lung fibrosis. Pediatr Res 2007; 62:128–133.
146. McGrath-Morrow SA, Cho C, Cho C, et al. Vascular endothelial growth factor receptor-2 blockade disrupts postnatal lung development. Am J Respir Cell Mol Biol 2005; 32:420–427.
147. Thébaud B, Ladha F, Michelakis ED, et al. Vascular endothelial growth factor gene therapy increases survival, promotes lung angiogenesis, and prevents alveolar damage in hyperoxia-induced lung injury: evidence that angiogenesis participates in alveolarization. Circulation 2005; 112:2383–2385.
148. Jakkula M, Le Cras TD, Gebb S, et al. Inhibition of angiogenesis decreases alveolarization in the developing rat lung. Am J Physiol 2000; 279:L600–L607.
149. Gerber HP, Hillan KJ, Ryan AM, et al. VEGF is required for growth and survival in neonatal mice. Development 1999; 126:1149–1159.
150. Sakurai MK, Lee S, Arsenault DA, et al. Vascular endothelial growth factor accelerates compensatory lung growth after unilateral pneumonectomy. Am J Physiol 2007; 292: L742–L747.
151. Maniscalco WM, Watkins RH, Finkelstein JN, et al. Vascular endothelial growth factor mRNA increases in alveolar epithelial cells during recovery from oxygen injury. Am J Respir Cell Mol Biol 1995; 13:377–386.
152. Maniscalco WM, Watkins RH, D'Angio CT, et al. Hyperoxic injury decreases alveolar epithelial cell expression of vascular endothelial growth factor (VEGF) in neonatal rabbit lung. Am J Respir Cell Mol Biol 1997; 16:557–567.
153. Kallapur SG, Bachurski CJ, Le Cras TD, et al. Vascular changes after intra-amniotic endotoxin in preterm lamb lungs. Am J Physiol 2004; 287:L1178–L1185.
154. Wang W, Wei W, Ning Q, et al. Effect of intra-amniotic endotoxin priming plus hyperoxic exposure on the expression of vascular endothelial growth factor and its receptors in lungs of preterm newborn rats. Zhonghua Er Ke Za Zhi 2007; 45:533–538.
155. Tambunting F, Beharry KD, Waltzman J, et al. Impaired lung vascular endothelial growth factor in extremely premature baboons developing bronchopulmonary dysplasia/chronic lung injury. J Invest Med 2005; 53:253–262.
156. Maniscalco WM, Watkins RH, Roper JM, et al. Hyperoxic ventilated premature baboons have increased p53, oxidant DNA damage and decreased VEGF expression. Pediatr Res 2005; 58:549–556.
157. Asikainen TM, Waleh NS, Schneider BK, et al. Enhancement of angiogenic effectors through hypoxia-inducible factor in preterm primate lung *in vivo*. Am J Physiol 2006; 291: L588–L595.
158. D'Angio CT, Maniscalco WM. The role of vascular growth factors in hyperoxia-induced injury to the developing lung. Front Biosci 2002; 7:d1609–d1623.
159. Kunig AM, Balasubramaniam V, Markham NE, et al. Recombinant human VEGF treatment transiently increases lung edema but enhances lung structure after neonatal hyperoxia. Am J Physiol 2006; 291:L1068–L1078.
160. Thébaud B, Abman SH. Bronchopulmonary dysplasia: where have all the vessels gone? Roles of angiogenic growth factors in chronic lung disease. Am J Respir Crit Care Med 2007; 175:978–985.

161. Tomashefski JF, Oppermann HC, Vawter GF, et al. Bronchopulmonary dysplasia: a morphometric study with emphasis on the pulmonary vasculature. Pediatr Pathol 1984; 2:469–487.
162. De Paepe ME, Mao Q, Powell J, et al. Growth of pulmonary microvasculature in ventilated preterm infants. Am J Respir Crit Care Med 2006; 173:204–211.
163. Lassus P, Turanlahti M, Heikkila P, et al. Pulmonary vascular endothelial growth factor and Flt-1 in fetuses, in acute and chronic lung disease, and in persistent pulmonary hypertension of the newborn. Am J Respir Crit Care Med 2001; 15:1981–1987.
164. Bhatt AJ, Pryhuber GS, Huyck H, et al. Disrupted pulmonary vasculature and decreased vascular endothelial growth factor, Flt-1, and TIE-2 in human infants dying with bronchopulmonary dysplasia. Am J Respir Crit Care Med 2001; 164:1971–1980.
165. Lassus P, Ristamaki A, Ylikorkala O, et al. Vascular endothelial growth factor in human preterm lung. Am J Respir Crit Care Med 1999; 159:1429–1433.
166. Quintos-Alagheband ML, White CW, Schwartz MA. Potential role for antiangiogenic proteins in the evolution of bronchopulmonary dysplasia. Antioxid Redox Signal 2004; 6:137–145.
167. Tsao PN, Wei SC, Su YN, et al. Placenta growth factor elevation in the cord blood of premature neonates predicts poor pulmonary outcome. Pediatrics 2004; 113:1348–1351.
168. Matsuura O, Kadomatsua K, Takei Y, et al. Midkine expression is associated with postnatal development of the lungs. Cell Struct Funct 2002; 27:109–115.
169. Portnoy J, Pan T, Dinarello CA, et al. Alveolar type II cells inhibit fibroblast proliferation: role of IL-1alpha. Am J Physiol 2005; 290:L307–L316.
170. Bry K, Whitsett JA, Lappalainen U. IL-1 beta disrupts postnatal lung morphogenesis in the mouse. Am J Respir Cell Mol Biol 2007; 36:32–42.
171. Fries KM, Felch ME, Phipps RP. Interleukin-6 is an autocrine growth factor for murine lung fibroblast subsets. Am J Respir Cell Mol Biol 1994; 11:552–560.
172. Huffman Reed JA, Rice WR, Zsengeller ZK, et al. GM-CSF enhances lung growth and causes alveolar type II epithelial cell hyperplasia in transgenic mice. Am J Physiol 1997; 273:L715–L725.
173. Aldenborg F, Nilsson K, Jarlshammer B, et al. Mast cells and biogenic amines in radiation-induced pulmonary fibrosis. Am J Respir Cell Mol Biol 1993; 8:112–117.
174. Hassoun PM, Thappa V, Landman MJ, et al. Endothelin 1: mitogenic activity on pulmonary artery smooth muscle cells and release from hypoxic endothelial cells. Proc Soc Exp Biol Med 1992; 199:165–170.
175. Jankov RP, Luo X, Cabacungan J, et al. Endothelin-1 and O_2-mediated pulmonary hypertension in neonatal rats: a role for products of lipid peroxidation. Pediatr Res 2000; 48:289–298.
176. Weiss RH, Maduri M. The mitogenic effect of thrombin in vascular smooth muscle cells is largely due to basic fibroblast growth factor. J Biol Chem 1993; 268:5724–5727.
177. Scarpati EM, DiCorleto PE. Identification of a thrombin response element in the human platelet- derived growth factor B-chain (c-sis) promoter. J Biol Chem 1996; 271:3025–3032.
178. Stouffer GA, Sarembock IJ, McNamara CA, et al. Thrombin-induced mitogenesis of vascular SMC is partially mediated by autocrine production of PDGF-AA. Am J Physiol 1993; 265:C806–C811.
179. Sunday ME, Kaplan LM, Motoyama E, et al. Gastrin-releasing peptide (mammalian bombesin) gene expression in health and disease. Lab Invest 1988; 59:5–24.
180. Cullen A, Van Marter J, Allred EN, et al. Urine bombesin-like peptide elevation precedes clinical evidence of bronchopulmonary dysplasia. Am J Respir Crit Care Med 2002; 165:1093–1097.
181. Subramaniam M, Bausch C, Twomey A, et al. Bombesin-like peptides modulate alveolarization and angiogenesis in bronchopulmonary dysplasia. Am J Respir Crit Care Med 2007; 179:902–912.

182. Hastings RH, Summers-Torres D, Yaszay B, et al. Parathyroid hormone related protein, an autocrine growth inhibitor of alveolar type II cells. Am J Physiol 1997; 272:L394–L399.

183. Hastings RH, Berg JT, Summers-Torres D, et al. Parathyroid hormone-related protein reduces alveolar epithelial cell proliferation during lung injury in rats. Am J Physiol 2000; 279:L194–L200.

184. Fernandez-Pol JA, Klos DJ, Hamilton PD. Modulation of transforming growth factor alpha-dependent expression of epidermal growth factor receptor gene by transforming growth factor beta, triiodothyronine, and retinoic acid. J Cell Biochem 1989; 41:159–170.

185. Fernandez-Pol JA, Hamilton PD, Klos DJ. Transcriptional regulation of proto-oncogene expression by epidermal growth factor, transforming growth factor $\beta1$ and triiodothyronine in MDA-468 cells. J Biol Chem 1989; 264:4151–4156.

186. Dlogosz AA, Cheng C, Denning MF, et al. Keratinocyte growth factor receptor ligands induce transforming growth factor α expression and activate the epidermal growth factor receptor pathway in cultured epidermal keratinocytes. Cell Growth Differ 1994; 5:1283–1292.

187. Leholta L, Nistér M, Höltä E, et al. Down-regulation of cellular platelet-derived growth factor receptors induced by an activated neu receptor tyrosine kinase. Cell Regul 1991; 2:651–661.

188. Rosenthal SM, Brown EJ, Brunetti A, et al. Fibroblast growth factor inhibits insulin-like growth factor-II (IGF-II) gene expression and increases IGF-I receptor abundance in BC3H-1 muscle cells. Mol Endocrinol 1991; 5:678–684.

189. Yoshinouchi M, Baserga R. The role of the IGF-1 receptor in the stimulation of cells by short pulses of growth factors. Cell Prolif 1993; 26:139–146.

190. Barreca A, Voci A, Minuto F, et al. Effect of epidermal growth factor and insulin-like growth factor-1 (IGF-I) and IGF-binding protein synthesis by adult rat hepatocytes. Mol Cell Endocrinol 1992; 84:119–126.

191. Gohda E, Matsunaga T, Kataoka H, et al. Induction of hepatocyte growth factor in human skin fibroblasts by epidermal growth factor, platelet-derived growth factor and fibroblast growth factor. Cytokine 1994; 6:633–640.

192. Harrison P, Bradley L, Bomford A. Mechanism of regulation of HGF/SF gene expression in fibroblasts by TGF-$\beta1$. Biochem Biophys Res Commun 2000; 271:203–211.

193. Inoue T, Okada H, Kobayashi T, et al. Hepatocyte growth factor counteracts transforming growth factor-β_1, through attenuation of connective tissue growth factor induction, and prevents renal fibrogenesis in 5/6 nephrectomized mice. FASEB J 2002; 16:NIL205–NIL222.

194. Millette E, Rauch BH, Defawe O, et al. Platelet-derived growth factor-BB-induced human smooth muscle cell proliferation depends on basic FGF release and FGFR-1 activation. Circ Res 2005; 96:172–179.

195. Adams TE, McKern NM, Ward CW. Signalling by the type 1 insulin-like growth factor receptor: interplay with the epidermal growth factor receptor. Growth Factors 2004; 22:89–95.

196. Asahara T, Bauters C, Zheng LP, et al. Synergistic effect of vascular endothelial growth factor and basic fibroblast growth factor on angiogenesis in vivo. Circulation 1995; 92: SII365–SII371.

197. Kovacs EJ, Kelley J. Lymphokine regulation of macrophage-derived growth factor secretion following pulmonary injury. Am J Pathol 1985; 121:261–268.

198. Silviera MR, Sempowski GD, Phipps RP. Expression of TGFß isoforms in THY-1$^+$ and Thy-1$^-$ pulmonary fibroblast subsets: evidence for TGF β as a regulator of IL-1-dependent stimulation of IL-6. Lymphokine Cytokine Res 1994; 13:277–285.

199. Harrington EA, Bennett MR, Fanidi A, et al. c-Myc-induced apoptosis in fibroblasts is inhibited by specific cytokines. EMBO J 1994; 13:3286–3296.

200. Sano H, Ueda Y, Takakura N, et al. Blockade of platelet-derived growth factor receptor-β pathway induces apoptosis of vascular endothelial cells and disrupts glomerular capillary formation in neonatal mice. Am J Pathol 2002; 161:135–143.

201. Murphy PR, Limoges M, Dodd F, et al. Fibroblast growth factor-2 stimulates endothelial nitric oxide synthase expression and inhibits apoptosis by a nitric oxide-dependent pathway in Nb2 lymphoma cells. Endocrinology 2001; 142:81–88.

202. Kasahara Y, Tuder RM, Taraseviciene-Stewart L, et al. Inhibition of VEGF receptors causes lung cell apoptosis and emphysema. J Clin Invest 2002; 106:1311–1319.

203. Wang X, Zhou YS, Kim HP, et al. Hepatocyte growth factor protects against hypoxia/ reoxygenation-induced apoptosis in endothelial cells. J Biol Chem 2004; 279:5237–5243.

204. Jankov RP, Kantores C, Belcastro R, et al. Endothelin-1 inhibits apoptosis of pulmonary arterial smooth muscle in the neonatal rat. Pediatr Res 2006; 60:245–251.

205. Engel J. EGF-like domains in extracellular matrix proteins: localized signals for growth and differentiation? FEBBS Lett 1989; 251:1–7.

206. Ingber D. Extracellular matrix and cell shape: potential control points for inhibition of angiogenesis. J Cell Biochem 1991; 47:236–241.

207. Vlodavsky I, Fuks Z, Ishai-Michaeli R, et al. Extracellular matrix-resident basic fibroblast growth factor: implications for the control of angiogenesis. J Cell Biochem 1991; 45:167–176.

208. Murphy-Ullrich JE, Schultz-Cherry S, Höök M. Transforming growth factor-β complexes with thrombospondin. Molec Biol Cell 1992; 3:181–188.

209. Gitay-Goren H, Soker S, Vlodavsky I, et al. The binding of vascular endothelial growth factor to its receptors is dependent on cell surface-associated heparin-like molecules. J Biol Chem 1992; 267:6093–6098.

210. Roghani M, Moscatelli D. Basic fibroblast growth factor is internalized through both receptor-mediated and heparan sulfate-mediated mechanisms. J Biol Chem 1992; 267:22156–22162.

211. Raines EW, Lane TF, Iruela-Arispe ML, et al. The extracellular glycoprotein SPARC interacts with platelet-derived growth factor (PDGF)-AB and -BB and inhibits the binding of PDGF to its receptors. Proc Natl Acad Sci U S A 1992; 89:1281–1285.

212. Han RNN, Buch S, Freeman BA, et al. Platelet-derived growth factor and growth-related genes in rat lung. II. Effect of exposure to 85% O_2. Am J Physiol 1992; 262:L140–L146.

213. Buch S, Han RNN, Liu J, et al. Basic fibroblast growth factor and growth factor receptor gene expression in 85% O_2-exposed rat lung. Am J Physiol 1995; 268:L455–L464.

12
Evolving Clinical Features of the New Bronchopulmonary Dysplasia

EDUARDO BANCALARI and NELSON CLAURE

University of Miami Miller School of Medicine, Miami, Florida, U.S.A.

I. Introduction

Bronchopulmonary dysplasia (BPD) was originally described by Northway and collaborators in the late-1960s as a complication of aggressive mechanical respiratory support in preterm infants with severe respiratory distress syndrome (RDS) (1). Despite the considerable advances in the prevention and management of RDS that have occurred in the last two decades, BPD remains as one of the major complications in premature infants who require prolonged mechanical ventilation (2,3). In fact, the increasing survival of the most immature infants has produced an increase in the number of survivors with BPD (4–9).

The clinical presentation and severity of BPD varies widely, ranging from a mild form observed in small premature infants who need low levels of supplemental oxygen and mechanical ventilation for few weeks to more severe cases who remain ventilator dependent for months or years or who die during their course due to severe cardiopulmonary failure. This later form of severe BPD resembles to some degree the course that was originally described by Northway in slightly more mature infants. Northway's description of BPD included preterm infants who had severe RDS and received high inspired oxygen concentration and prolonged mechanical ventilation with very high positive airway pressures. Their clinical and radiographic course was described in four stages ending with the severe chronic lung damage, characterized by persistent respiratory failure and a chest radiograph that reveals areas of increased density due to fibrosis and collapse surrounded by areas of marked hyperinflation and emphysema. In recent years, however, with the wider use of antenatal steroids, the introduction of exogenous surfactant, and improvements in respiratory care, this form of severe BPD has become less common, but has been replaced by milder forms of chronic lung disease that are observed more frequently in the smaller preterm infants who survive after prolonged respiratory support (7,10–12). This change in presentation over the years is illustrated in Figure 1 showing a relatively constant incidence when all forms of BPD are combined, while the incidence of severe BPD decreases over time.

A large proportion of infants who develop the milder form of chronic lung damage have had no RDS or mild RDS that improves quickly after surfactant administration, and frequently require mechanical ventilation mainly because of apnea and poor respiratory effort. These infants, therefore, are not being exposed to high airway pressures or

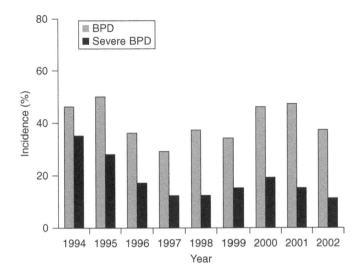

Figure 1 Incidence of BPD over time in infants born before 29 weeks of gestation, alive by 36 weeks of PMA. *Abbreviations*: BPD, bronchopulmonary dysplasia; PMA, postmenstrual age. *Source*: Data from Ref. 2.

inspired oxygen concentrations, but their hospital course is often complicated by conditions such as nosocomial infections and a prolonged patent ductus arteriosus (PDA), both of which have been identified as possible contributing pathogenic factors in the development of BPD (12).

This chapter describes the clinical characteristics and evolution of these two forms of chronic lung disease with emphasis on the new milder forms of BPD.

The reported incidence of BPD varies widely. This is due to differences in patient populations and management, but is also due to different criteria used to define BPD. (Different definitions of BPD are discussed elsewhere in chapter 14.) The incidence of BPD in infants with a birth weight ≤1500 g who survive ranges between 15% and 65% (9). This incidence increases at lower gestational age and birth weight. Most cases of BPD occur in extreme premature infants born before 28 to 30 weeks of gestation. Although BPD can occur in more mature infants, it is uncommon in infants born after 32 to 34 weeks of gestation. Figure 2 shows the incidence of BPD in infants less than 1500 g in the NICHD neonatal network (3).

II. Clinical Presentation

The diagnosis of BPD is based on the clinical and radiographic manifestations, but these are not specific. With rare exceptions, BPD occurs in premature infants and follows the use of mechanical ventilation with intermittent positive pressure during the first weeks after birth. Mechanical ventilation is usually indicated for respiratory failure resulting from RDS, but also may be required for other causes of respiratory

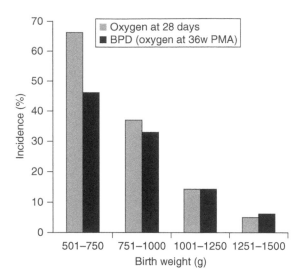

Figure 2 Incidence of BPD in infants <1500 g by birth weight strata in years 1997 to 2002 at the NICHD Neonatal Research Network. *Abbreviation*: BPD, bronchopulmonary dysplasia. *Source*: Data from Ref. 3.

failure such as pneumonia or severe apnea. The development of BPD is more likely to occur when mechanical ventilation and oxygen supplementation extend beyond 10 to 14 days. Nonetheless, definitive radiographic features do not typically develop until later in the course, usually around the third or fourth week after birth. There is a broad spectrum of clinical presentations ranging from a very mild disease where the pulmonary changes are minimal to the more severe forms, similar to those described originally by Northway et al.

III. Severe Form of BPD

The original form of BPD was common prior to the broader use of antenatal steroids and exogenous surfactant therapy, and is usually seen after severe RDS or neonatal pneumonia. Most of these infants require mechanical ventilation with high airway pressures and inspired oxygen concentration during the first week of life, and frequently their course is complicated by gas leaks and pulmonary interstitial emphysema (PIE). These complications require increased ventilator support and high inspired oxygen concentrations, which further aggravate the lung damage. Other complications such as persistent patency of a ductus arteriosus, with associated heart failure and pulmonary edema, as well as pulmonary or systemic infections frequently develop in these patients and can contribute to the progression in severity of the lung damage.

Despite all therapeutic efforts, these infants remain ventilator dependent for several weeks, and chronic radiographic changes, such as densities, linear-reticular opacities, and in some cases, cystic changes begin to appear at this stage. These infants

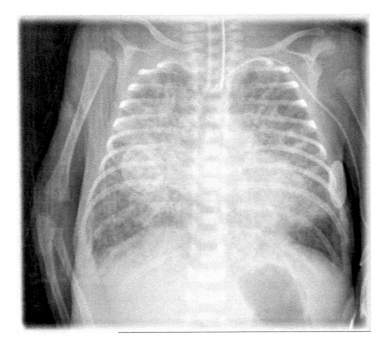

Figure 3 Chest radiograph of an infant with a severe form of BPD. *Abbreviation*: BPD, bronchopulmonary dysplasia.

usually remain oxygen dependent and display pulmonary radiographic changes that are characterized by hyperinflation and patchy atelectasis (Fig. 3). The radiographic progression of BPD through the sequence of four stages, originally described by Northway et al. (1) is now infrequent. The appearance of stage I is essentially indistinguishable from that of uncomplicated RDS. Dense parenchymal opacification, as described in stage II BPD, is commonly due to other processes such as congestive heart failure from a PDA, fluid overload, or pulmonary hemorrhage. The bubble-like pattern of stage III BPD is not always seen, and when it does occur, it does not always follow a period of parenchymal opacity. Finally, the radiographic development of the more advanced form of BPD (stage IV) may be more insidious than originally described, and it usually appears after several weeks of mechanical ventilation. The major features of stage IV BPD include hyperinflation mainly in the basal areas and nonhomogeneity of pulmonary parenchyma, with multiple fine or coarser densities extending to the periphery (Fig. 3). At this point, commonly, there is also cardiomegaly due to right ventricular hypertrophy secondary to pulmonary hypertension.

Despite surfactant administration, severe RDS sometimes can progress to this form of severe lung damage. In most instances, surfactant administration produces rapid improvement in oxygenation and lung compliance in infants with RDS (13–15). Failure to wean ventilator settings after surfactant administration may result in lung over-distention, which may lead to pneumothorax or PIE. This can further aggravate the

Table 1 The Introduction of Exogenous Surfactant and the Incidence of Severe RDS and BPD in Infants ≤1000 g Born at UM/JMMC Between 1989 and 1994

	Presurfactant (9 months, 1989–1990)	Postsurfactant (1992–1994)
	$n = 57$	$n = 243$
Severe RDS	17/57 (30%)	26/243 (11%)
Mild or no RDS	40/57 (70%)	217/243 (89%)
BPD in severe RDS	13/17 (76%)	20/26 (77%)
BPD in mild or no RDS	13/40 (32%)	76/217 (35%)
All BPD	26/47 (46%)	96/243 (39%)
BPD from severe RDS	13/26 (50%)	20/96 (21%)
BPD from mild RDS	13/26 (50%)	76/96 (79%)

Abbreviations: RDS, respiratory distress syndrome; BPD, bronchopulmonary dysplasia.

respiratory failure and require increases in the ventilator and oxygen support, thereby increasing lung damage from excessive parenchymal stretch and oxygen toxicity. Pulmonary hemorrhage is another complication associated with a PDA and exogenous surfactant therapy, which is more frequent in the more immature infants (16,17). When the hemorrhage is severe, blood enters the air spaces and inactivates surfactant, with resultant worsening of respiratory failure and increased need for ventilator support.

Other causes of initial severe respiratory failure such as pneumonia, sepsis, lung hypoplasia, and meconium aspiration are also associated with the development of BPD. Sepsis often leads to failure of multiple organ systems and respiratory failure that further prolongs the need for mechanical ventilation and supplemental oxygen. Radiographically, neonatal pneumonia cannot be distinguished from a severe RDS, but the response to surfactant replacement is usually short lived or absent, requiring aggressive ventilator support for prolonged periods. Frequently, pneumonia is complicated by air leaks, shock, and persistent pulmonary hypertension. These infants may succumb early from cardiorespiratory failure, and among those who survive, particularly those who are extremely premature, a substantial number develop BPD.

With the wider use of antenatal steroids and surfactant replacement combined with improvements in ventilator management, the incidence of the severe form of BPD has decreased considerably. Table 1 shows the impact of the introduction of surfactant treatment in the incidence of severe RDS and BPD in our institution. The incidence of severe initial respiratory failure decreased from 30% to 11%, and consequently, the proportion of infants with BPD and who initially presented with severe RDS declined considerably from 50% to 21%. Currently, this pattern of disease progression accounts for less than one-fifth of all the infants who develop BPD in our institution.

Severe forms of RDS are more common in males and Caucasians, and are inversely related to the gestational age of the infant (18–20). Each of these characteristics has also been shown to be an important risk factor for the development of BPD. The main factors that increase the risk for severe lung injury are the exposure to excessive positive airway pressures and high inspired oxygen concentration in an infant with an immature lung. The role of each of these variables in the development of lung injury is discussed in detail in other sections of this book.

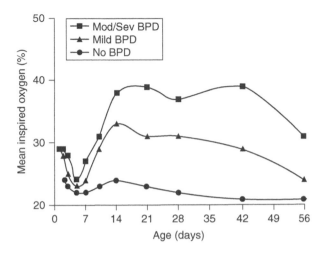

Figure 4 Evolution of oxygen requirement in the two forms of BPD. Infants born at University of Miami/Jackson Memorial Medical Center years 1996 to 2002, birth weight 500 to 1000 g, alive at 36 weeks of PMA. *Abbreviations*: BPD, bronchopulmonary dysplasia; PMA, postmenstrual age.

IV. Evolution of Severe BPD

As a result of the severe lung damage, these infants present signs of chronic respiratory failure, such as tachypnea, chest retractions, and frequent episodes of hypoxemia, especially with agitation and nursing procedures. Figure 4 illustrates the typical pattern of the oxygen requirement of these infants during the first month of life. Oxygen need is high during the severe initial respiratory failure, and then remains moderately elevated over time, usually for several weeks. Pulmonary edema frequently develops in these infants, complicating their respiratory course. This can be associated with reopening of the ductus arteriosus or it may be a manifestation of the lung damage, with associated capillary leak and increased lung fluid. These patients frequently have crackles on auscultation, and the chest radiograph reveals lung opacities. Fluid restriction, diuretics, and prompt intervention to close the PDA usually improve this condition. During the evolution of severe BPD, blood gas measurements usually reveal chronic CO_2 retention accompanied by metabolic alkalosis.

Severe BPD is also characterized by airway damage and increased smooth muscle with increased airway resistance (21–23). This manifests clinically with distress, wheezing with scattered or diffuse rhonchi on auscultation, overexpansion of the lungs on the chest radiograph, and hypercapnia. The cause of the increased airway resistance is multifactorial, including airway inflammation with hyperplasia and metaplasia of bronchial epithelium, increased mucus production from glandular hyperplasia, mucosal edema, localized infections, and increased airway smooth muscle with bronchial hyperreactivity. These infants may also develop large airway damage with bronchomalacia that can lead to dynamic expiratory airway obstruction, especially during episodes of agitation and increased intrathoracic pressure (23,24). Most infants with severe BPD have lobar or segmental atelectasis resulting from retained secretions and airway obstruction.

Acute pulmonary infection, either bacterial or viral, frequently complicates the course of the disease, sometimes resulting in severe respiratory failure and even death in infants with severe lung damage (25).

Infants with severe BPD frequently display signs of right heart failure secondary to pulmonary hypertension, with cardiomegaly, hepatomegaly, and fluid retention (26,27). The electrocardiogram shows signs of right ventricular hypertrophy, which is confirmed by echocardiography. In some infants, anastomoses develop between the systemic and pulmonary circulations, which may further aggravate pulmonary hypertension. Pulmonary hypertension with cor pulmonale is frequently the main cause of heart and respiratory failure. As it becomes resistant to treatment, it is one of the leading causes of death in infants with severe BPD (28). Infants with severe BPD can also display left ventricular dysfunction that can contribute to the pulmonary hypertension and pulmonary edema (29).

V. Outcome of Severe BPD

Once lung damage has developed, these infants require mechanical ventilation and increased inspired oxygen concentration for many weeks, months, or years in the most severe cases. Infants with more severe lung damage may die of progressive respiratory failure, cor pulmonale, or acute complications, especially intercurrent infections. Mortality rates of around 30% to 40% have been reported in infants with severe BPD, and most of them occur during the first year of life secondary to respiratory failure, sepsis, or intractable cor pulmonale (27,28).

Most survivors show slow but steady improvement in their lung function (22) and radiographic pictures, and after variable periods of time, they can be weaned from the ventilator and oxygen therapy but some may remain on supplemental oxygen after discharge. After extubation, most infants continue to have marked distress with chest wall retractions and tachypnea, and they frequently have rales and bronchial sounds on auscultation.

Because of the respiratory failure, most infants with severe BPD take oral feedings with difficulty and frequently require nasogastric or orogastric feeding. Although weight gain is usually below that expected for their age, children who receive adequate oxygen supplementation and appropriate nutritional support may achieve consistent rates of growth (30,31). The lower weight gain is multifactorial, and among the mechanisms that may limit growth are a higher energy expenditure required by the increased work of breathing, increased oxygen consumption, inadequate caloric intake, and chronic hypoxemia (32–34). Adequate nutrition is important for lung growth and repair, and nutritional deficits may impair recovery and adversely affect the outcome of these infants (35). With adequate nutrition, oxygen therapy, and control of infections and heart failure, gradual improvement in pulmonary function may be accompanied by resolution of cor pulmonale and radiographic evidence of healing.

Among the survivors with severe BPD, lower respiratory tract infections are common during the first two years of life (36). Frequently they require hospitalization for prolonged periods, and no specific organisms are isolated, suggesting a viral etiology. Episodes of wheezing and airway obstruction are also common during the first years of life, and infection with influenza or respiratory syncytial virus can be life-threatening (25). Acute hyperinflation may be difficult to appreciate in infants with severe BPD because their baseline radiograph often shows lung overexpansion. Such acute episodes of airway obstruction are frequently accompanied by radiographic evidence of focal segmental or lobar atelectasis.

Pulmonary function in infants with severe BPD may remain abnormal for many years, even though the infants may be asymptomatic (37). They present a high incidence of obstructive airway disease that can persist into adulthood (38,39).

Infants with severe BPD also have more neurodevelopmental sequelae when compared with control groups, and they exhibit impaired growth curves (40–44). It is apparent that neurodevelopmental prognosis depends on the severity of the BPD and on the presence of other risk factors for developmental delays that occur frequently in infants with severe BPD, such as intracranial hemorrhage, hearing impairment, and retinopathy of prematurity (see chaps. 22 and 23).

VI. "New" Or Mild Form of BPD

As a result of the wider use of antenatal steroids and postnatal surfactant, a large portion of small premature infants who develop BPD at present have a mild initial respiratory course and require prolonged respiratory support for management of apnea and poor respiratory effort (12,45,46). These infants represent more than 80% of all infants diagnosed with BPD in our institution. In contrast to infants with severe BPD, these infants commonly require mechanical ventilation with low ventilator rates and peak airway pressures and low inspired oxygen concentration, and therefore are not exposed to the same degree of barotrauma and oxygen toxicity. The typical oxygen requirement for these infants is illustrated in Figure 4. These infants require low or moderate initial concentrations of oxygen for the treatment of mild RDS that usually responds favorably to exogenous surfactant. This is often followed by a few days with minimal or no supplemental oxygen need ("honeymoon"). After this, many of these infants, however, have a progressive deterioration in their lung function that persists over time, wherein their ventilator and oxygen requirements increase, accompanied by signs of respiratory failure (tachypnea, retractions, etc). This deterioration is frequently triggered by pulmonary or systemic bacterial or viral infections or heart failure and pulmonary edema secondary to a PDA. In these patients, the functional and radiographic lung changes are usually mild, sometimes showing only diffuse haziness that persists over time, without the more coarse changes of nonuniform inflation and cystic nature that is often observed in the original classic severe form of BPD (Fig. 5). Chest CT in these infants can still show hyperlucent areas, linear opacities, and triangular subpleural opacities, but in contrast with severe BPD, these infants do not show bronchial involvement (47).

Epidemiological studies to identify the main risk factors that predispose these infants to BPD revealed that besides prematurity, severe RDS, presence of episodes of symptomatic PDA, and systemic infections were associated with a significantly higher risk for the development of BPD (12,48), as shown in Figure 6. Furthermore, when both complications (PDA and infection) occurred at the same time, they produced a synergistic interaction, further increasing their impact on the development of BPD (49). This is likely a consequence of the left-to-right shunting through the ductus with increased pulmonary blood flow and lung fluid that negatively affect lung function and gas exchange, thereby increasing the risk for BPD (50–52).

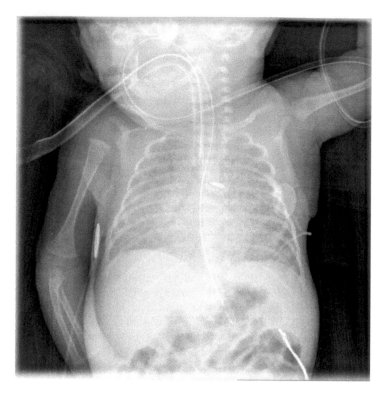

Figure 5 Chest radiograph of an infant with mild or new form of BPD. *Abbreviation*: BPD, bronchopulmonary dysplasia.

There is also compelling evidence that support the role of antenatal and postnatal infection and inflammation in the pathogenesis of BPD (53,54). Prolonged neutrophil influx and increased cytokine activity in bronchoalveolar lavage fluid have been associated with an increased likelihood of BPD in ventilator-dependent premature infants (55,56). Antenatal exposure to infection and colonization with specific microorganisms such as *Cytomegalovirus* and *Ureaplasma urealyticum* also have been associated with increased risk of BPD (57–62).

The presence of infections in the premature infant adversely affects permanent closure of the ductus, often inducing late ductal opening and failure to respond to medical treatment with prostaglandin inhibitors (63). One possible mechanism for this interaction is the elevated serum level of prostaglandins and tumor necrosis factor observed in infants with infections. In addition, infants with infections frequently have complications that delay or impede the treatment of the PDA. As a result, the ductus remains open for prolonged periods, maintaining an increased pulmonary blood flow, high capillary pressure, and pulmonary edema. The epidemiological data linking the persistence of a PDA with an increased risk of BPD has been recently supported by the results of studies in preterm baboons. In this animal model, the persistence of a PDA was

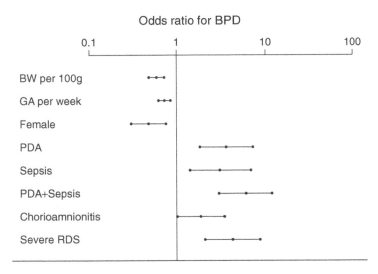

Figure 6 Perinatal and postnatal risk factors for BPD (≥28 days of oxygen) among premature infants born at University of Miami/Jackson Memorial Medical Center years 1995 to 2000, birth weight 500 to 1000 g, gestational age (GA), 23 to 32 weeks, alive at day 28. *Source*: Data from Ref. 49.

associated with a significant reduction in formation of alveolar septae and capillaries and a reduced alveolar surface area (64). Early pharmacological closure of the ductus decreased lung water and improved lung mechanics with a decreased need for mechanical ventilation, leading to improved alveolarization (65). The reduction in formation of alveolar septae and capillaries is one of the hallmarks of the new milder form of BPD.

VII. Evolution of Mild BPD

As in infants with severe BPD, but to a lesser degree, infants with mild BPD also show signs of chronic respiratory failure, such as tachypnea, chest wall retractions, and frequent episodes of hypoxemia, especially with agitation, and mild hypercapnia. As observed in Figure 4, the initial oxygen dependence of these infants is modest. Chronic pulmonary edema occurs frequently and is manifested by rales on auscultation and a chest radiograph revealing diffuse lung opacification. These infants also may have signs of increased airway resistance (retraction, wheezing, with scattered or diffuse rhonchi on auscultation, overexpanded lungs in the chest radiograph, and hypercapnia), but this is usually not as pronounced as in the infants with severe BPD. Some infants with mild BPD also may have lobar or segmental atelectasis, resulting from retained secretions and airway obstruction. Signs of right heart failure secondary to pulmonary hypertension are less common in this milder form of BPD. Acute pulmonary infections, either bacterial or viral, also may complicate the course of these infants, but when they occur they are better tolerated with less lung dysfunction.

VIII. Outcome of Mild BPD

Because of their extreme prematurity, these infants may also require respiratory support and elevated inspired oxygen concentration for prolonged periods, usually several weeks or months. Occasionally they may progress to more severe lung damage and die of progressive respiratory failure or acute complications, especially intercurrent infections. However, most of these infants survive and show slow but steady improvement in their lung function and radiographic changes and, after variable periods, can be weaned from respiratory support and oxygen therapy.

Infants with this form of BPD may also be difficult to feed, tolerate fluids poorly, and their growth may be below the expected rate for infants of similar gestational ages. However, with adequate nutrition, oxygen supplementation, and control of infections and heart failure, gradual improvement in pulmonary function is accompanied by radiographic evidence of healing. Lower respiratory tract infections are common during the first two years of life, and these infants may also require hospitalizations for episodes of acute airway obstruction and respiratory failure. There is limited follow-up data of pulmonary function in these infants, but the abnormalities are less pronounced and tend to improve during the first years of life (22) (see chaps. 21 and 22).

IX. Differential Diagnosis of BPD

The diagnosis of BPD is based on the clinical and radiographic course described earlier, but these signs are not specific. Although the pathogenesis of BPD is not conclusively established, it is accepted that in most cases the lung damage results from the interaction of a variety of factors, among which the most important are prematurity, mechanical ventilation with high airway pressures and increased inspired oxygen concentrations, PDA, and infections. Other factors that may lead to chronic lung damage and must be investigated before concluding that the infant has BPD are specific viral, fungal, or bacterial perinatal infections, congenital heart diseases such as total anomalous pulmonary venous drainage, pulmonary lymphangiectasia, sequestration, chemical pneumonitis resulting from recurrent aspiration, cystic fibrosis, and idiopathic pulmonary fibrosis.

Of all differential diagnostic possibilities, Wilson–Mikity syndrome has probably engendered the greatest confusion with BPD, especially with the new milder forms of BPD (66). It is likely that the cases described originally by Wilson and Mikity correspond to the milder form of BPD seen today in the smaller infants. The radiographic and clinical similarities between the two conditions have caused some investigators to associate these two entities. Like in the new BPD, patients with Wilson–Mikity syndrome generally had an initially benign course, with an insidious onset of respiratory failure and radiographic abnormalities. In contrast, patients with the severe form of BPD have a greater degree of acute respiratory failure from the beginning and greater need for high inspired oxygen concentrations and respiratory support. In recent years, there has been a notable decline in the reporting of this syndrome, which is rarely diagnosed today.

X. Prediction of BPD

A number of studies have been performed to develop scores that may predict the risk of BPD in ventilated preterm infants (67–71). Most of these scores include the state of maturity of the infant and factors that reflect the severity of the initial respiratory failure, and therefore are more useful to identify the severe forms of BPD than the more common milder forms observed today. It is clear that the risk for developing BPD is related to low gestational age and the severity of the initial respiratory failure. For this reason, a number of investigators have attempted to develop predictive models for BPD by relating the severity of the respiratory failure during the first days of life with the risk for BPD. These studies have identified factors such as low birth weight and gestational age, low Apgar score, male gender, white race, and outborn status as characteristics that increase the risk for BPD (5,68–70). Oxygen requirement at 14 days is also a strong predictor of BPD and the risk increases at higher inspired oxygen concentrations (71). Prolonged oxygen treatment is also associated with worse long-term pulmonary function (72). These scores are helpful to identify patients for clinical trials to prevent BPD and may become more useful in the future as more effective preventive therapies become available.

References

1. Northway WH, Rosan RC, Porter DY. Pulmonary disease following respiratory therapy of hyaline membrane disease. Bronchopulmonary dysplasia. N Engl J Med 1967; 276:357–336.
2. Smith VC, Zupancic JAF, McCormick MC, et al. Trends in severe bronchopulmonary dysplasia rates between 1994 and 2002. J Pediatr 2005; 146:469–473.
3. Fanaroff AA, Stoll BJ, Wright LL, et al. Trends in neonatal morbidity and mortality for very low birthweight infants. Am J Obstet Gynecol 2007; 106:147.e1–147.e8.
4. Avery ME, Tooley WH, Keller JB, et al. Is chronic lung disease in low birth weight infants preventable? A survey of eight centers. Pediatrics 1987; 79:26–30.
5. Palta M, Gabbert D, Weinstein MR, et al. Multivariate assessment of traditional risk factors for chronic lung disease in very low birth weight neonates. J Pediatr 1991; 119:285–292.
6. Van Marter LJ, Gabbert D, Weinstein MR, et al. Rate of bronchopulmonary dysplasia as a function of neonatal intensive care practices. J Pediatr 1992; 120:938–946.
7. Parker RA, Pagano M, Allred EN. Improved survival accounts for most, but not all, of the increase in bronchopulmonary dysplasia. Pediatrics 1992; 90:663–668.
8. Horbar JD, McAuliffe TL, Adler SM, et al. Variability in 28-day outcomes for very low birth weight infants: an analysis of 11 neonatal intensive care units. Pediatrics 1988; 82:554–559.
9. Walsh MC, Yao Q, Gettner P, et al. Impact of a physiological definition on bronchopulmonary dysplasia rates. Pediatrics 2004; 114(5):1305–1311.
10. Wung JT, Koons AH, Driscoll JM, et al. Changing incidence of bronchopulmonary dysplasia. J Pediatr 1979; 95:845–847.
11. Heneghan MA, Sosulski R, Baquero JM. Persistent pulmonary abnormalities in newborns: the changing picture of bronchopulmonary dysplasia. Pediatr Radiol 1986; 16:180–184.
12. Rojas MA, Gonzalez A, Bancalari E, et al. Changing trends in the epidemiology and pathogenesis of neonatal chronic lung disease. J Pediatr 1995; 126:605–610.
13. Davis JM, Veness-Meehan K, Notter RH, et al. Changes in pulmonary mechanics after the administration of surfactant to infants with respiratory distress syndrome. N Engl J Med 1988; 319:476–479.
14. Goldsmith LS, Greenspan JS, Rubenstein SD, et al. Immediate improvement in lung volume after exogenous surfactant: alveolar recruitment versus increased distension. J Pediatr 1991; 119: 750–755.
15. Bhutani VK, Abbasi S, Long W, et al. Pulmonary mechanics and energetics in preterm infants who had respiratory distress syndrome treated with synthetic surfactant. J Pediatr 1992; 120:S18–S24.

16. Raju TNK, Langenber P. Pulmonary hemorrhage and exogenous surfactant therapy: a meta-analysis. J Pediatr 1993; 123:603–610.
17. Pappin A, Shenker N, Hack M. Extensive intraalveolar pulmonary hemorrhage in infants dying after surfactant therapy. J Pediatr 1994; 124:621–626.
18. Miller HC, Futrakul P. Birth weight, gestational age, and sex as determining factors in the incidence of respiratory distress syndrome of prematurely born infants. J Pediatr 1968; 72: 628–635.
19. Farrell PM, Avery ME. Hyaline membrane disease. Am Rev Respir Dis 1975; 111:657–687.
20. Perelman RH, Palta M, Kirby R, et al. Discordance between male and female deaths due to the respiratory distress syndrome. Pediatrics 1986; 78:238–244.
21. Goldman SL, Gerhardt T, Sonni R, et al. Early prediction of chronic lung disease by pulmonary function testing. J Pediatr 1983; 102:613–617.
22. Gerhardt T, Hehre D, Feller R, et al. Serial determination of pulmonary function in infants with chronic lung disease. J Pediatr 1987; 110:448–456.
23. Miller RW, Woo P, Kellman RK, et al. Tracheobronchial abnormalities in infants with bronchopulmonary dysplasia. J Pediatr 1987; 111:779–782.
24. McCubbin M, Frey EE, Wagener JS, et al. Large airway collapse in bronchopulmonary dysplasia. J Pediatr 1989; 114:304–307.
25. Groothuis JR, Gutierrez KM, Lauer BA. Respiratory syncytial virus infection in children with bronchopulmonary dysplasia. Pediatrics 1988; 82:199–203.
26. Goodman G, Perkin RM, Anas NG, et al. Pulmonary hypertension in infants with bronchopulmonary dysplasia. J Pediatr 1988; 112:67–72.
27. Khemani E, McElhinney DB, Rhein L, et al. Pulmonary artery hypertension in formerly premature infants with bronchopulmonary dysplasia: clinical features and outcomes in the surfactant era. Pediatrics 2007; 120(6):1260–1269.
28. Shankaran S, Szego E, Eizert D, et al. Severe BPD: predictors of survival and outcome. Chest 1984; 88:607–610.
29. Mourani PM, Ivy DD, Rosenberg AA, et al. Left ventricular diastolic dysfunction in bronchopulmonary dysplasia. J Pediatr 2008; 152:291–293.
30. Abman SH, Accurso FJ, Koops BL. Experience with home oxygen in the management of infants with BPD. Clin Pediatr 1984; 23:471–476.
31. Groothuis JR, Rosenberg AA. Home oxygen promotes weight gain in infants with BPD. Pediatrics 1988; 82:199–203.
32. Kurzner SI, Garg M, Batista M, et al. Growth failure in BPD: elevated metabolic rates and pulmonary mechanics. J Pediatr 1988; 112:73–80.
33. Weinstein MR, Oh W. Oxygen consumption in infants with BPD. J Pediatr 1981; 99: 958–961.
34. Koops BL, Abman SH, Accurso FJ. Outpatient management and follow-up of BPD. Clin Perinat 1984; 11:101–122.
35. Sosenko IRS, Frank L. Nutritional influences on lung development and protection against chronic lung disease. Seminars in Perinatology 1991; 15:462–168.
36. Cunningham CK, McMillan JA, Gross SJ. Rehospitalization for respiratory illness in infants less than 32 weeks gestation. Pediatrics 1991; 88:527–533.
37. Blayney M, Kerem E, Whyte H, et al. BPD: improvement in lung function between 7 and 10 years of age. J Pediatr 1991; 118:201–206.
38. Smyth JA, Tabachnik E, Duncan WJ, et al. Pulmonary function and bronchial hyper-reactivity in long-term survivors of bronchopulmonary dysplasia. Pediatrics 1981; 68:336–340.
39. Northway WH, Moss RB, Carlisle KB, et al. Late pulmonary sequelae of bronchopulmonary dysplasia. N Engl J Med 1990; 323:1793–1799.
40. Vohr BR, Bell EF, Oh W. Infants with bronchopulmonary dysplasia: growth pattern and neurologic and developmental outcome. Am J Dis Child 1982; 136:443–447.

41. Markestad T, Fitzhardinge PM. Growth and development in children recovering from bronchopulmonary dysplasia. J Pediatr 1981; 98:597–602.
42. Meisels SJ, Rivers A, Hack M. Growth and development of preterm infants with respiratory distress syndrome and bronchopulmonary dysplasia. Pediatrics 1986; 77:345–352.
43. Bozynski MEA, Brown ER, Neff RK, et al. Bronchopulmonary dysplasia and postnatal growth in extremely premature black infants. Early Hum Dev 1990; 21:83–92.
44. Skidmore MD, Rivers A, Hack M. Increased risk of cerebral palsy among very low-birthweight infants with chronic lung disease. Dev Med Child Neurolo 1990; 32:325–332.
45. Charafedine L, D'Angio CT, Phelps D. Atypical chronic lung disease patterns in neonates. Pediatrics 1999; 103(4):759–765.
46. Streubel AH, Donohue PK, Aucott SW. The epidemiology of atypical chronic lung disease in extremely low birth weight infants. J Perinatol 2008; 28:141–148.
47. Mahut B, De Blic J, Emond S, et al. Chest computed tomography findings in broncho-pulmonary dysplasia and correlation with lung function. Arch Dis Child Fetal Neonatal Ed 2007; 92:F459–F464.
48. Marshall DD, Kotelchuck M, Young TE, et al. Risk factors for chronic lung disease in the surfactant era: a North Carolina population-based study of very low birth weight infants. Pediatrics 1999; 104(6):1345–1350.
49. Bancalari E, Claure N, Sosenko I. Bronchopulmonary dysplasia: changes in pathogenesis, epidemiology and definition. Semin Neonatol 2003; 8(1):63–67.
50. Gerhardt T, Bancalari E. Lung compliance in newborns with patent ductus arteriosus before and after surgical ligation. Biol Neonate 1980; 38:96–105.
51. Stefano JL, Abbasi S, Pearlman SA, et al. Closure of the ductus arteriosus with indomethacin in ventilated neonates with respiratory distress syndrome. Effects on pulmonary compliance and ventilation. Am Rev Respir Dis 1991; 143:236–239.
52. Brown ER. Increased risk of bronchopulmonary dysplasia in infant with patent ductus arteriosus. J Pediatr 1979; 95:865–866.
53. Pierce MR, Bancalari E. The role of inflammation in the pathogenesis of bronchopulmonary dysplasia. Pediatr Pulmonol 1995; 19:371–378.
54. Young K, del Moral T, Claure N, et al. The association between early tracheal colonization and bronchopulmonary dysplasia. J Perinatol 2005; 25:403–407.
55. Ogden BE, Murphy S, Saunders GC, et al. Lung lavage of newborns with respiratory distress syndrome: prolonged neutrophil influx is associated with bronchopulmonary dysplasia. Chest 1983; 83:31S–33S.
56. Bagghi A, Viscardi RM, Taciak V, et al. Increased activity of interleukin-6 but not tumor necrosis factor-α in lung lavage of premature infants is associated with the development of bronchopulmonary dysplasia. Pediatr Res 1994; 36:244–252.
57. Sawyer MH, Edwards DK, Spector SA. Cytomegalovirus infection and bronchopulmonary dysplasia in premature infants. Am J Dis Child 1987; 141:303–305.
58. Cassell GH, Crouse DT, Cannup KC, et al. Association of Ureaplasma urealyticum infection of the lower respiratory tract with chronic lung disease and death in very low birth weight infants. Lancet 1988; 2:240–244.
59. Wang EEL, Ohlsson A, Kellner JD. Association of ureaplasma urealyticum colonization with chronic lung disease of prematurity: results of a meta-analysis. J Pediatr 1995; 127:640–644.
60. Colayzy TT, Morris CD, Lapidus J, et al. Detection of ureaplasma DNA in endotracheal samples is associated with bronchopulmonary dysplasia after adjustment for multiple risk factors. Pediatr Res 2007; 61:578–583.
61. Van Marter LJ, Dammann O, Allred EN, et al. Chorioamnionitis, mechanical ventilation, and postnatal sepsis as modulators of chronic lung disease in preterm infants. J Pediatr 2002; 140(2): 171–176.

62. Schelonka RL, Waites KB. Ureaplasma infection and neonatal lung disease. Semin Perinatol 2008; 31:2–9.
63. Gonzalez A, Sosenko IRS, Chandar J, et al. Influence of infection on patent ductus arteriosus and chronic lung disease in premature infants ≤ 1000 g. J Pediatr 1996; 128:470–478.
64. Chang LY, McCurnin D, Yoder B, et al. Ductus arteriosus ligation and alveolar growth in preterm baboons with a patent ductus arteriosus. Pediatr Res 2008; 63(3):299–302.
65. McCurnin D, Seidner S, Chang LY, et al. Ibuprofen-induced patent ductus arteriousus closure: physiologic, histologic, and biochemical effects on the premature lung. Pediatrics 2008; 121: 945–956.
66. Wilson MG, Mikity VG. A new form of respiratory disease in premature infants. Am J Dis Child 1960; 99:489–499.
67. Shennan AT, Dunn MS, Ohlsson A, et al. Abnormal pulmonary outcomes in premature infants: prediction from oxygen requirements in the neonatal period. Pediatrics 1988; 82:527–532.
68. Sinkin RA, Cox C, Phelps DL. Predicting risk for bronchopulmonary dysplasia: selection criteria for clinical trials. Pediatrics 1990; 86:728–736.
69. Ryan SW, Wild NJ, Arthur RJ, et al. Prediction of chronic neonatal lung disease in very low birthweight neonates using clinical and radiological variables. Arch Dis Child 1994; 71:F36–F39.
70. Ambavalanan N, Van Meurs KP, Perritt R, et al. Predictors of death or bronchopulmonary dysplasia in preterm infants with respiratory failure. J Perinatol 2008; 28(6):420–426.
71. Groves AM, Briggs KA, Kuschel CA, et al. Predictors of chronic lung disease in the 'CPAP era'. J Paediatr Child Health 2004; 40:290–294.
72. Halvorsen T, Skadberg BT, Eide GE, et al. Better care of immature infants; has it influenced long-term pulmonary outcome? Acta Paediatr 2006; 95:547–554.

13

Epidemiology of Bronchopulmonary Dysplasia

LINDA J. VAN MARTER
Harvard Medical School, Boston, Massachusetts, U.S.A.

I. Introduction

First described in 1967 by Northway and colleagues (1), bronchopulmonary dysplasia (BPD) remains the most prevalent and one of the most serious of the long-term sequelae of preterm birth. Improvements in neonatal intensive care that have reduced mortality among even the most preterm infants have not been accompanied by diminished occurrence of BPD. This chronic lung disease of prematurity primarily, but not exclusively, affects infants who have been treated with mechanical ventilation for surfactant deficiency or structural lung immaturity and its prevalence is highest among extremely preterm and very low birth weight infants. With an average BPD rate of 23% among infants whose birth weights are below 1500 g (2), at the current U.S. annual birth rate of approximately 4.1 million, 1.49% of whom are born below 1500 g (3), greater than 14,000 infants born each year in the United States are destined to develop BPD.

Impairments of health, neurodevelopment, and quality of life frequently accompany BPD. Indeed, for some survivors of preterm birth, BPD leads to lifelong health compromise. Infants with BPD are at increased risk of death following discharge (4–7) as well as during their initial newborn intensive care unit (NICU) hospitalizations. Pulmonary impairments associated with BPD (8–10) include asthma (11,12) and emphysema (13), and these conditions can persist into young adulthood (13–15). Their pulmonary vulnerability leads infants with BPD to experience significantly higher rates of rehospitalization, especially during the early years of life (16,17), for respiratory infection (18–21) or airway reactivity (12,22,23), compared with their gestational age equivalent peers without BPD. Infants with BPD are at substantially increased risk of other major health and neurodevelopment impairments (24) including pulmonary hypertension (25–28) or other cardiovascular compromise (29,30), undernutrition (31,32), and growth failure (24,33). Associated neurodevelopmental disabilities are common and BPD severity (34–36) and duration of mechanical ventilation (37) influence the extent (6,10) of cognitive deficits (38–40), cerebral palsy (41–43), and global neurodevelopmental impairment (44). Recent work by Wilkinson et al. (45,46) suggests that the neurological basis of the functional impairments that occur among infants with BPD are explained, in part, by inadequate brainstem myelination and synaptic function. Of the serious comorbidities associated with BPD, only neurosensory impairments have shown a trend toward improvement over time and with advances in neonatal intensive care (37).

II. The "New" Bronchopulmonary Dysplasia

In their landmark report, published in 1967 (1), Northway and colleagues described 32 preterm infants who developed chronic lung disease and characteristic clinical, radiographic, and pathological features following mechanical ventilation for respiratory distress syndrome (RDS). The histology of the classical BPD described by Northway (1) featured prominent interstitial fibrosis, alveolar overdistention alternating with regions of atelectasis, and airway abnormalities, including squamous metaplasia and excessive muscularization. In the four decades since the first description of BPD, very preterm infants have been surviving in progressively greater numbers, and this trend has been accompanied by changes in the epidemiology and pathological features of a new BPD.

What new BPD shares with the disorder described by Northway is a substantial prevalence among preterm infants, most of whom have been treated with mechanical ventilation, and an association with prolonged need for supplemental oxygen. New BPD differs from the classical description of BPD in the demographics of the population of affected preterm infants and the pulmonary pathological features accompanying the disorder. In the current era, the infants at greatest risk of BPD are survivors of extremely preterm birth: infants born at 22 to 26 weeks' gestation whose lungs exhibit profound structural underdevelopment. These infants are born at the intersection of the canalicular and saccular phases of lung development that substantially precedes alveolarization (Fig. 1).

Disruptions in alveolarization (47) and microvascularization (48) were observed as sequelae of BPD as early as 1982. New BPD, first identified in autopsy specimens by Hussain et al. (49), is characterized by a histological pattern consistent with developmental arrest and impaired alveolar development: alveolar numbers are reduced and the alveoli are larger than normal in diameter; fibrosis, squamous metaplasia, and excessive airway muscularization are absent. In new BPD, there is a failure of the normal pattern of microvascular proliferation in late gestation that typically is associated with elevated levels of vascular endothelial growth factor (VEGF) (50). Vascular and airway growth are impaired in new BPD, as evidenced by decreased levels of VEGF and angiogenic receptors, Flt-1 and Tie-2, noted among infants who died following development of BPD (51).

Features analogous to human pathological changes of BPD are evident in baboon and lamb models. Two baboon models have been developed by Jacqueline Coalson's research group at the University of Texas, San Antonio: the 140-day gestation (75% of the normal 185-day gestation) baboon model of classical BPD (52–54) and the 125-day gestation extremely preterm baboon model of 'new' BPD, (approximately equivalent to 27-week human gestation) (55,56) (Fig. 2). The 125-day extremely preterm baboon model has provided important information regarding the combined effects of moderate oxygen and mechanical ventilation on the extremely preterm lung (Fig. 3). In the preterm lamb model developed by Bland and colleagues (57–59), the histological features analogous to the disrupted lung development of new BPD appear to result from insufficient or aberrant microvascularization that interferes with alveolar crest formation and,

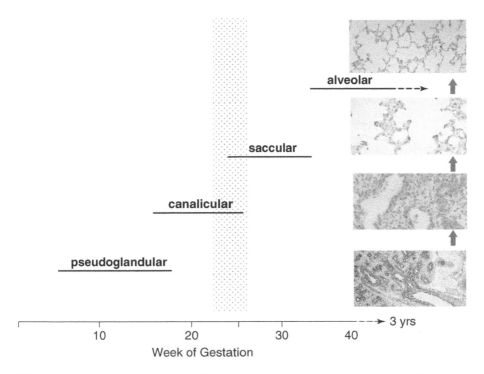

Figure 1 Stages of lung development. The human embryo and fetus progress through four stages of lung development: pseudoglandular, canalicular, saccular, and alveolar. Infants at greatest risk of "new" BPD are those born at 22 to 26 weeks' gestation, the intersection of the canalicular and saccular stages of development. Alveolarization begins at approximately 36 weeks of gestation.

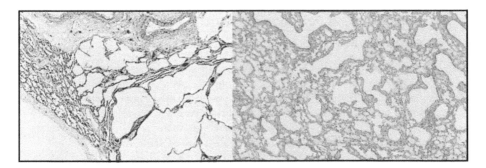

Figure 2 Classical and new BPD—baboon model. Images from two baboon models of BPD depicting the histological features of classical and new BPD. On the left, lung injury in the 140-day-gestation baboon, born at three-quarters of the normal 185 day gestation, shows the changes of classical BPD: marked interstitial fibrosis, areas of alveolar destruction and emphysematous change alternating with atelectasis, and increased airway muscularization. The image on the right, of the 125-day-gestation baboon model of BPD, approximately equivalent to an infant at 27 weeks' human gestation, reveals histology similar to new BPD: alveolar oversimplification with blunting and deficiency of alveolar secondary crests; inflammatory infiltrate is also evident. *Source*: Images courtesy of Steven Seidner, MD

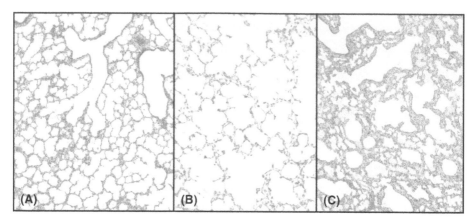

Figure 3 Effects of mechanical ventilation on the immature lung—baboon model. A series of three images of the 125-day-gestation baboon model of BPD contrasting the progression of the normal fetal lung at 125 days of gestation (*panel A*) and its maturation during an additional two weeks of fetal development (*panel B*) versus the effects of two weeks of mechanical ventilation (*panel C*). *Source*: Images courtesy of Steven Seidner, MD

thus, impairs the normal process of alveolarization (57) (Fig. 4). The likelihood that inhibition of microvascular growth is an important factor in the impaired alveolar septation, a key component of new BPD, is supported by detection of reduced angiogenic factors and microvascular growth in the immature sheep and baboon models of BPD (57,60,61).

III.   Incidence and Definition of Bronchpulmonary Dysplasia

A.   BPD Incidence

BPD rates vary with gestational age distribution and other characteristics of the study population, by the definition applied (62), and among medical centers. Northway (63) found, among infants born before 32 weeks' gestation in a single center (Stanford University) over more than 20 years of the pre–surfactant era, a consistent rate of ∼30% stage IV BPD. During this period, however, there was increased survival of progressively more immature infants who had very high rates of BPD, which obscured the falling BPD rates among infants born at more advanced gestation. A similar trend was observed at Vanderbilt University Medical Center (64) among infants born below 1500 g during three time periods over the years 1979 to 1990: mortality fell from 26.4% to 18.3% to 15.9% and BPD increased from 10.6% to 21.7% to 32.9%, in parallel.

Following its introduction in 1991, surfactant treatment became widespread and some centers reported a modest decline in BPD rates soon thereafter (65). Despite availability of surfactant and introduction of other technological advances in neonatal respiratory management, adoption of a new definition of BPD referencing the need for supplemental oxygen at 36 weeks' postmenstrual age (PMA) was accompanied by BPD rates that subsequently remained stable or increased. Data from the Eunice Kennedy

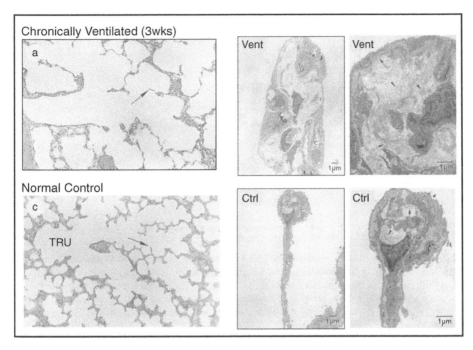

Figure 4 Chronic ventilation and disrupted alveolarization—lamb model. Left (*upper and lower*): Lung histology illustrating the effect of prolonged mechanical ventilation on the loss of alveoli and alveolar secondary crests in terminal respiratory units (trichrome stain). The panels are the same magnification. (*a*) Chronically ventilated preterm lamb that was managed at 20 breaths/ minute for three weeks and (*c*) control term lamb <1-day old and matched for developmental age. Middle (*upper and lower*): Transmission electron micrographs illustrating the effect of prolonged mechanical ventilation on alveolar secondary crest structure. Both panels are the same magnification. (*Top*) Chronically ventilated preterm lamb that was managed at 20 breaths/minute for three weeks. (*Bottom*) Control term lamb <1-day old and matched for developmental age. The alveolar secondary crest of the chronically ventilated preterm lamb is thicker and lacks capillaries (*c*) at its tip when compared with the alveolar secondary crest of the control term lamb. Right (*upper and lower*): Transmission electron micrographs illustrating the effect of prolonged mechanical ventilation on alveolar secondary crest structure. Both panels are the same magnification. (*Top*) Chronically ventilated preterm lamb that was managed at 20 breaths/minute for three weeks. (*Bottom*) Control term lamb <1-day old and matched for developmental age. The alveolar secondary crest of the chronically ventilated preterm lamb is thicker and lacks capillaries (*c*) at its tip when compared with the alveolar secondary crest of the control term lamb. *Source*: Ref. 57.

Shriver National Institutes of Child Health and Human Development Neonatal Research Network (NICHD Neonatal Network) suggest that increasing BPD rates are closely linked with progressively improving survival of infants born at or below 1000 g (Fig. 5) or, as others report (66), before 26 weeks of gestation. The highest BPD rates occur among infants of the lowest birth weight and most immature gestational age groups. Summarizing outcomes among infants 501 to 1500 g birth weight, Fanaroff et al. (2)

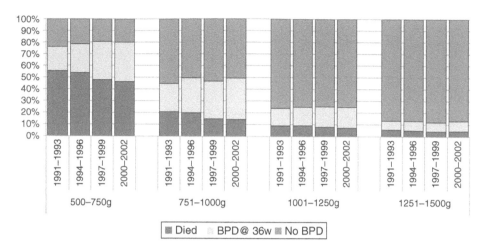

Figure 5 BPD and neonatal mortality. Progression over time in rates of BPD and death among infants at NICHD Neonatal Network centers. The data are shown, in 250 g increments from 500 to 1250 g birth weight, in two-year increments from 1997 to 2002. A trend is evident, among infants born at or below 1000 g birth weight, in the direction of increasing BPD accompanying lower mortality rates. *Source*: Data are provided by and shown with permission of the NICHD Neonatal Research Network.

reported that BPD rates among NICHD Neonatal Network sites during the period from 1997 to 2002 were 23%, overall: 57% at 501 to 750 g, 32% at 751 to 1000 g, 14% at 1001 to 1250 g, and 6% at 1251 to 1500 g birth weight.

Avery et al. (67) noted intercenter variability in BPD rates among infants born at eight major academic medical centers, suggesting that population characteristics and/or specific care practices might be important determinants of BPD risk. In their study of infants with birth weights 700 to 1500 g born at eight centers, Avery et al. (67) discovered a range in rates of BPD (i.e., receipt of supplemental oxygen at postnatal age 28 days) of 6% to 33%. Other early estimates of BPD prevalence (68–70) placed BPD rates among infants ventilated for surfactant deficiency at 4% to 40%. Using the most frequently applied contemporary definition of BPD, oxygen requirement at 36 weeks' PMA, the two largest neonatal networks in the United States, the Vermont Oxford Network and the NICHD Neonatal Network, also have detected intercenter variation in overall and birth weight–specific rates of BPD. Data from the Vermont Oxford Network suggest that intercenter differences persist and are not eradicated by efforts to decrease BPD rates: among infants born at 501 to 1500 g, the average BPD rate among Vermont Oxford Network sites was 29% and rates at individual sites varied from 13.4% to 66% in 2001 and from 4% to 58.3% in 2003, following a quality improvement initiative (71,72). Intercenter variability in BPD rates also is observed internationally: among 494,463 infants born in 2003 at 24 to 31 weeks' gestation at centers in 10 European regions, the rate of BPD (oxygen requirement at 36 weeks' PMA) recently was reported to vary from 10.5% to 21.5% (73). The proportion of the intercenter variations attributable to population characteristics versus to modifiable care practices remains controversial.

The Vermont Oxford Network (71,72) demonstrated that a package of pre-specified potentially better practices lowered BPD rates in initially underperforming centers. Such a benefit, however, did not result from a cluster randomized trial among NICHD Neonatal Network centers (74) in which 14 underperforming NICUs were cluster randomized to adopt best clinical practices of the three centers with the lowest BPD rates.

B. Progress in the Definition of BPD

The diagnosis of BPD has been made on the basis of pathological (1,75–77), clinical (67,68,78), and conventional radiographic (1,68,79) criteria. Northway described four stages of BPD, defined by clinical characteristics and radiographic findings: stage I (2–3 days) RDS; stage II (4–10 days) regeneration; stage III (11–20 days) transition to chronic disease; stage IV (>1 month) chronic disease. Bancalari et al. (68) subsequently defined BPD as a disorder occurring among infants receiving mechanical ventilation for at least three days in the first postnatal week who also had respiratory signs, such as the need for supplemental oxygen at 28 postnatal days, as well as characteristic radiographic findings. Among neonatologists, growing recognition that infants who did not receive mechanical ventilation also are at risk of chronic lung disease (80) led to a definition of BPD that was simplified to simply receipt of supplemental oxygen at 28 days' postnatal age (67). Shennan et al. (78) identified oxygen requirement at 36 weeks' PMA as a more accurate predictor of later pulmonary outcome and proposed this improved definition that still appears to predict pulmonary outcomes among infants with new BPD (81) and, in contemporary practice, remains the most commonly applied definition of BPD. Although not incorporated as a standard diagnostic procedure in current care of infants with BPD, chest CT images appear to offer greater detail (82,83) and to better predict later pulmonary outcomes (84) than do conventional chest radiographs, raising the possibility that chest imaging by CT scan or magnetic resonance imaging might become an important component of future BPD diagnostic techniques.

A definition of BPD that relies solely on receipt of supplemental oxygen is a crude measure of pulmonary disease and is at risk of being influenced, not only by the infant's inherent lung disease and genuine need for supplemental oxygen, but also caregivers' practice styles and oxygenation targets. In an effort to develop a consensus definition that would provide an estimate of disease severity as well as the presence or absence of BPD, participants in an NICHD-NHLBI workshop (85) convened to define mild, moderate, and severe BPD. Applying clinical criteria from both 28 days' and 36 weeks' PMA, workshop participants defined mild BPD as the need for supplemental oxygen at or beyond 28 days but not at 36 weeks' PMA; moderate BPD was defined as the need for supplemental oxygen at 28 days, in addition to supplemental oxygen at F_iO_2 at or below 0.30 at 36 weeks' PMA; and criteria for severe BPD included the need for supplemental oxygen at 28 days and, at 36 weeks' PMA, the need for mechanical ventilation and/or $F_iO_2 > 0.30$. In a validation study, the NICHD consensus definitions correlated well with pulmonary outcomes, including rates of treatment with pulmonary medications and rehospitalization for pulmonary causes (86).

Walsh et al. (87) took the concept of diagnostic accuracy of BPD a step further in proposing a physiological test for BPD (oxygen requirement) at 36 weeks' PMA to establish the need for supplemental oxygen by objective criteria. In the algorithm developed by Walsh et al. (87), infants receiving mechanical support or $F_iO_2 > 0.30$ are designated as having BPD and infants receiving $F_iO_2 \leq 0.30$ undergo an oxygen challenge test that determines their diagnostic categorization (87). In a study of 1598 preterm infants born at 501 to 1249 g, Walsh et al. (88) found approximately 30% of infants diagnosed with BPD by conventional criteria could safely and successfully pass an oxygen challenge test during which they maintained normal oxygen saturation when supplemental oxygen was tapered incrementally to room air and the application of a physiological definition of BPD resulted in a lower overall incidence of BPD (35–25%) and diminished variability in BPD rates among centers (15–66% vs. 9–57%). The average center-specific difference in BPD rates by clinical versus physiological definition was 10% with a range of 0% to 44%. Of 17 participating centers, 16 showed decreased BPD rates with use of the physiological definition of BPD. Failure to pass the oxygen challenge test correlated with duration of hospitalization and discharge on supplemental oxygen.

IV. Epidemiology: Northway to New BPD

Pulmonary immaturity is the primary risk factor for BPD and manifests as incomplete structural development and inadequacy of biochemical components or protectants such as surfactant, antioxidants, and proteinase inhibitors (89,90). Northway and colleagues speculated that oxygen toxicity and barotrauma were responsible for the lung injury leading to BPD and epidemiological studies supported this hypothesis. Early reports of the antecedents of classical BPD by Northway and colleagues and others focused on contributing neonatal clinical factors, many of which reflected inherent risk of or association with surfactant deficiency.

A. Demographic and Perinatal Risk Factors

Descriptive epidemiological studies of BPD identified many factors that modify BPD risk. Endogenous factors linked with BPD include gestational immaturity (91–96), lower birth weight (67,91,93,94), male sex (67,91,93–96), White or non-Black race (67,96), a family history of asthma (97), and being small for gestational age (98,99). Perinatal risk factors for BPD include absence of maternal glucocorticoid treatment (100,101), lower Apgar scores (96), perinatal asphyxia (93,94), and RDS (93,94).

B. Neonatal Antecedents

Many factors relating to neonatal health and pulmonary status, as well as respiratory support and other medical interventions, have been associated with BPD risk. Markers indicating greater severity of initial pulmonary disease (91), including pneumothorax (102), pulmonary interstitial emphysema (103), and more severe atelectasis (95), are associated with increased risk of BPD. Greater BPD risk also has been linked with a host of other early neonatal influences, including patent ductus arteriosus (80,96,104), pulmonary edema (105), higher weight-adjusted fluid intake (96,106), earlier use of parenteral lipids (107), light-exposed parenteral nutrition (108,109), and duration of oxygen therapy (110). Among at-risk infants, the duration (92,111) and/or features of mechanical ventilation, including high inspired oxygen (91,96,112), high peak inspiratory pressure (96,112–114), lower positive end expiratory pressure (115), and higher ventilation rate (95), also are associated with BPD, relationships that could be causal or might simply reflect confounding by severity of acute respiratory disease. Kraybill and colleagues' detection of increased BPD risk associated with hypocarbia, indicated by highest $PCO_2 <$ 40 at 48 or 96 hours, however, suggests that aggressive ventilation directly contributes to lung injury leading to BPD (95,96). Colonization or infection with Ureaplasma urealyticum (116,117) and postnatal sepsis (112) also appear to predispose to BPD.

Epidemiological studies of BPD yielded a number of predictive models (113,118–120). Although none currently is routinely applied in caring for infants at risk of BPD, such models might serve as valuable risk adjustment tools for therapeutic trials and other clinical research studies.

C. Experimental Evidence and the Epidemiology of New BPD

Preterm infants are especially susceptible to injury due to mechanical, oxidant, and inflammatory forces because of the extreme structural and biochemical immaturity of the preterm lung (121). Laboratory studies of the developing lung have identified three major causes of lung injury: oxidant stress, mechanical injury, and inflammation. Volutrauma, inflammation, and genetic contributions are recognized as especially important factors in the development of new BPD.

The effort to minimize mechanical injury to the lung of the extremely preterm infant at risk of new BPD is an extraordinary challenge. The total lung capacities of the most immature infants in the NICU are miniscule in comparison with those of adults making it difficult to provide mechanical support that achieves the delicate ventilation balance that will maintain the preterm lung in the optimal zone that avoids both alveolar overdistention and atelectasis (122,123) (Fig. 6). Mechanical ventilation of the structurally underdeveloped and surfactant-deficient lung often requires (as positive pressure) an increase

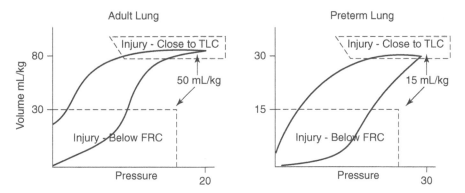

Figure 6 Optimal zone of ventilation. Hypothetical pressure-volume curves for adult and preterm lungs. Injury occurs if the lung is ventilated from below functional residual capacity (FRC) or to volumes close to total lung capacity (TLC). When the graphs are scaled such that the 80 mL/kg TLC of the adult lung is shown to be similar to the 30 mL/kg TLC for the preterm lung, the large difference in the lung volume available for ventilation is not apparent. As indicated, this volume is about 50 mL/kg in the adult and about 15 mL/kg in the preterm infant who has respiratory distress syndrome. Also note that higher pressures are required to recruit volume for the preterm than for the adult lung. *Source*: From Ref. 122.

of fivefold or more in the pressure exerted (as negative pressure) during normal respiration of the structurally mature surfactant-replete lung. Although pressure-induced injury (barotrauma) might play a role in the injury leading to new BPD, alveolar overdistention (volutrauma) currently is believed to be a more important contributing factor (124–126).

Injury to the preterm lung does not require prolonged or sustained volutrauma. In a study of the preterm lamb, Bjorklund and colleagues (127) found that just six overdistended breaths disrupted surfactant function. Even pretreatment with exogenous surfactant did not completely protect the immature lung from volutrauma (128). Atelectasis also contributes to BPD: ventilation of the atelectatic lung leads to pulmonary parenchymal injury through the shear stress of repeatedly opening atelectatic alveoli (129,130). These are important considerations in providing respiratory support to preterm infants, not only because they demonstrate the need for meticulous attention to potential volutrauma during mechanical ventilation in the NICU, but also because they heighten awareness of potential lung injury during neonatal resuscitation. In a study of infants 23 to 28 weeks' gestation, 26% had $PaCO_2$ levels below 30 torr during delivery room resuscitation and 38% had PaO_2 levels above 100 torr (131). Use of 100% oxygen during resuscitation has been associated with lower Apgar scores and longer time to the first breath, factors that increase the likelihood that a preterm infant will require intubation and mechanical ventilation, beginning in the delivery room (132).

Groneck and Speer (133) were among the first to appreciate the importance of inflammation in BPD pathogenesis. Infection is not the only neonatal stimulus provoking inflammation: inflammatory mediators are released in response to direct pulmonary toxins, including oxidant stress and release of free radicals, hypoxia, infection, volutrauma, or alveolar shear stress resulting from ventilating atelectatic alveoli. One of the early events in the injury process appears to involve sequestration of neutrophils in the lung, accompanied by reduced numbers of circulating neutrophils (134). Subsequent physiological events leading to BPD are mediated directly or through downstream effects of proinflammatory cytokines, chemokines, and proteinases (135–140).

Evidence that a systemic inflammatory response of extrapulmonary origin might contribute to BPD pathogenesis (141) led investigators to explore the contributions of antenatal (142), perinatal, and postnatal inflammation to lung injury. Observational studies of biomarkers of chorioamnionitis by Watterberg and colleagues (143) established the association between amniotic fluid markers of chorioamnionitis and BPD. The link between chorioamnionitis and BPD was confirmed by additional studies of amniotic fluid markers (144) and placental and umbilical cord pathology (145–147), showing an association between chorioamnionitis, pulmonary inflammation, and BPD (148). The combined effects of antenatal infection or inflammation and clinical factors might contribute to the occurrence of BPD via a number of mechanisms: direct injury of pulmonary parenchyma, disruption of the developmental milieu, impaired angiogenesis (57,149), or activation (priming) of immune cells in the lung, thus provoking an exaggerated inflammatory injury in response to a variety of prenatal, perinatal, and postnatal insults (150). In a case-control study of 386 infants born at or below 1500 g, after adjusting for other BPD risk factors, Van Marter and colleagues found that chorioamnionitis alone appeared to be associated with reduced risk of BPD but chorioamnionitis followed by seven days of mechanical ventilation or postnatal sepsis had a synergistic effect that substantially increased the risk of BPD over the independent effect of either factor. These data suggest that chorioamnionitis might make the lung more

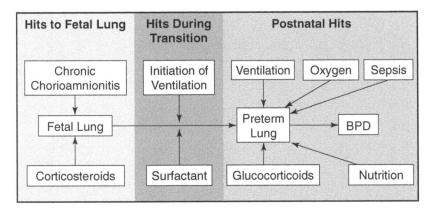

Figure 7 Antenatal, transitional, and postnatal contributions to BPD. The progression in pulmonary insults from fetal life to perinatal transition and the early neonatal experience culminates in BPD. This appears to be the result of a series of events and interventions, or "hits," that initially prime the lung for accelerated injury by later insults and, thus, alter the course of development. *Source*: From Ref. 142.

vulnerable to later insults (151), supporting Jobe's hypothesis that BPD is the product of a "multiple hit" sequential process in which prenatal lung injury represents one factor that primes the lung for accelerated injury by later insults (Fig. 7) (142).

Genetic predisposition is likely to be an important regulator of structural and functional lung development as well as the response of the preterm lung to physiological stressors. Laboratory work in the mouse already has shown pulmonary morphology similar to new BPD in association with a specific genetic polymorphism (152). Although the role of genetic factors in protecting from or predisposing to BPD is still largely unexplored, Lavoie et al. reported results of a study of 318 twins of known zygosity that suggested as much as 82% of the observed variance in BPD susceptibility could be explained by genetic effects (153). Advanced genetic technologies and analytic approaches (154) offer the potential to explore the role of genetic polymorphisms in modifying BPD risk among preterm infants. Although there are few published studies of BPD genetics, a number of genetic polymorphisms have been linked with BPD, including surfactant protein B (SP-B intron 4 deletion variant) (155), glutathione-*S*-transferase (GST P1 val105ile isoform) (156), dystroglycan (NH494H homozygous genotype) (157), angiotension converting enzyme (deletion allele) (158), tumor necrosis factor-α (adenine allele of TNF-α-238) (159), and vascular endothelial growth factor (VEGF -460T>C) (160).

V. Prevention of Bronchopulmonary Dysplasia

Marked variation, among medical centers, in risk adjusted BPD rates (88) and demonstrated success in reducing BPD rates within individual institutions through quality improvement efforts such as the Vermont Oxford Network "breathsavers" quality improvement initiative (71,72) suggest that specific care practices (Table 1) modify BPD occurrence. Quality improvement interventions, however, have not proven

Table 1 Cochrane Systematic Reviews. This table summarizes the results of systematic reviews, by the Cochrane Collaboration, of clinical trials of potential preventive therapies for bronchopulmonary dysplasia. Original reports are cited and updates for many are available at the Cochrane Collaborative website. Full text of these reviews can be viewed online at: http://www.cochrane.org/reviews/.

Therapeutic comparison	Cochrane author(s), (yr)	Trials, N (36-wk PMA outcomes)	Subjects in 36-wk PMA analyses, N	BPD at 36 wk PMA risk ratio (95% CI)	BPD or death at 36 wk PMA risk ratio (95% CI)
Biochemical/Hormonal Treatments					
α-1 Proteinase inhibitor vs. placebo	Shah and Ohlsson, 2001 (287)	2 (2)	151	0.64 (0.35,1.18)	0.84 (0.53, 1.34)
Superoxide dismutase vs. placebo	Suresh et al., 2001 (291)	1 (1)	33	1.0 (0.10, 9.86)	NR
Prophylactic vs. selective surfactant	Soll and Morley, 2001 (292)	8 (0)	0	NR	NR
Early surfactant with brief ventilation then CPAP vs. selective surfactant and continued ventilation	Stevens et al., 2007 (207)	6 (0)	0	NR[a]	NR
Thyrotropin-releasing hormone and steroids vs. placebo	Crowther et al., 2004 (293)	13 (0)	0	NR	NR
Glucocorticoids					
Early inhaled corticosteroid vs. placebo	Shah et al., 2007 (271)	7 (5)	429	0.97 (0.62, 1.52)	0.86 (0.63, 1.17)
Inhaled vs. systemic corticosteroids	Shah et al., 2007 (294)	1 (1)	292	1.10 (0.82, 1.47)	1.00 (0.90, 1.12)
Early (<8 days) corticosteroids vs. placebo	Halliday et al., 2003 (274)	27 (21)	3286	0.79 (0.79, 0.88)	0.89 (0.84, 0.95)
Moderately early (7–14 days) postnatal corticosteroids vs. placebo	Halliday et al., 2003 (295)	6 (5)	247	0.62 (0.47, 0.82)	0.63 (0.51, 0.78)
Late (>7days) postnatal corticosteroids vs. placebo	Halliday et al., 2003 (296)	16 (8)	471	0.72 (0.61, 0.85)	0.72 (0.63, 0.82)
Nutritional Treatments					
Inositol vs. placebo	Howlett and Ohlsson, 2003 (297)	3 (0)	0	NR	NR[a]
Vitamin A (IM) vs. placebo	Darlow and Graham, 2007 (161)	8 (2)	847	0.84 (0.73 0.97)	0.89 (0.79, 0.99)

234

Respiratory Technologies

Intervention	Study				
CPAP (prophylactic) vs. placebo	Subramaniam et al., 2005 (298)	2 (1)	230	2.0 (0.18, 21.75)	NR
NCPAP (after extubation) vs. placebo	Davis and Henderson-Smart, 2003 (299)	9 (0)	0	NR	NR
NIPPV vs. CPAP (after extubation)	Davis et al., 2001 (211)	3 (2)	118	0.73 (0.49, 1.07)	NR
Synchronized IMV vs. CMV	Greenough et al., 2008 (300)	14 (2)	1310	0.90 (0.75, 1.08)	NR
HFJV (elective) vs. CMV	Bhuta and Henderson-Smart, 1998 (301)	3 (2)	170	0.58 (0.34, 0.98)	NR
HFOV (all elective) vs. CMV	Henderson-Smart et al., 2007 (221)	15 (13)	2820	0.98 (0.83, 1.14)	0.93 (0.86, 1.00)
iNO vs. placebo	Barrington and Finer, 2007 (302)	11 (10)	2488	< 3d: 0.89 (0.76, 1.05) >3 days: 0.89 (0.78, 1.02) Routine use: 0.96 (0.85, 1.08)	< 3d: 0.95 (0.88, 1.02) >3 days: 0.90 (0.80, 1.02) Routine use: 0.91 (0.84, 0.99)

Respiratory Management

Permissive hypercapnia	Woodgate and Davies, 2001 (215)	2 (2)	269	1.05 (0.16, 6.77)	0.94 (0.78, 1.15)

Other Treatments

Bronchodilators vs. placebo	Ng et al., 2001 (303)	1 (0)	173	NR[b]	NR
Erythromycin vs. placebo (infants at risk for or colonized with ureaplasma urealyticum)	Mabanta et al., 2003 (304)	2 (0)	0	NR[b]	NR[b]

[a] Improved outcome(s) at 28 days.

[b] No difference in outcome(s) at 28 days.

Abbreviations: CPAP, continuous positive airway pressure; CMV, conventional mechanical ventilation; IM, intramuscular injection; iNO, inhaled nitric oxide; HFJV, high frequency jet ventilation; HFOV, high-frequency oscillatory ventilation; nCPAP, nasal continuous positive airway pressure; NIPPV, nasal intermittent positive pressure ventilation; NR, not reported.

uniformly successful (74) and efforts to identify the "silver bullet," a single modifiable care practice most likely to prove useful in preventing BPD, have proven unsuccessful.

A. Evidence-Based Preventive Treatment for BPD: Vitamin A

Vitamin A

Vitamin A is a safe and effective preventive therapy for BPD with a modest treatment effect (161). The biological benefits conferred by vitamin A and it metabolites include improved epithelial integrity and response to infection or injury. Vitamin A is necessary for normal lung development, and the immature lung appears to require a constant supply to compensate for its inability to recycle retinol (162). The pulmonary developmental effects of vitamin A vary by species. Normal alveolarization in the mouse (163) and ongoing alveolarization after dexamethasone exposure in the rat (164) are retinoic acid dependent. In the preterm baboon, however, retinoids do not enhance angiogenesis or alveolar development (165). In the preterm lamb, proliferation of pulmonary elastin in response to injury is antagonized by retinoic acid treatment (166).

Shenai et al. (167) discovered that infants who progressed to BPD differed from a comparison group of infants without serious pulmonary disease in having lower levels of vitamin A that declined in the first postnatal month. Among infants born at or below 1000 g, intramuscular vitamin A supplementation is associated with a modest reduction in BPD-free survival without observed increases in other neonatal morbidities (161,168). In the masked clinical trial by Tyson et al. of 807 infants below 1000 g birth weight born at centers in the NICHD Neonatal Network, the group randomized to receive intramuscular vitamin A at 5000 IU or sham treatment three times per week for one month were at reduced risk of death or BPD at 36 weeks' PMA (7% reduction in BPD; RR 0.89; 95% CI 0.79, 0.99) (168). No differences in neurodevelopmental impairment were noted between treatment groups at 18 to 22 months (169). A dosing schedule of intramuscular injection of vitamin A 5000 IU three times per week achieves superior retinol levels than 15,000 IU once-weekly dose and similar levels to 10,000 IU given three times per week (170). Vitamin A administered orally appears to offer no protection from BPD (171).

B. Potentially Beneficial Respiratory Therapies That Require Further Study: Inhaled Nitric Oxide, Noninvasive Respiratory Support, Permissive Hypercapnia, and High-Frequency Ventilation

Inhaled Nitric Oxide

Of the potential new therapies for BPD prevention, inhaled nitric oxide (iNO) is considered one of the most promising. Nitric oxide isoforms are detectable in the airways and vascular tree early in human lung development (172), and its physiological effects of make iNO a logical candidate in the search for an ideal therapy for prevention of new BPD. In animal models of pulmonary immaturity and mechanically induced lung injury, nitric oxide reduces neutrophil accumulation and pulmonary edema (173,174), diminishes inflammatory markers of lung injury (175,176) and fibrin deposition (175), alleviates hyperoxia suppressed phosphotidylcholine synthesis (177), enhances lung growth (178),

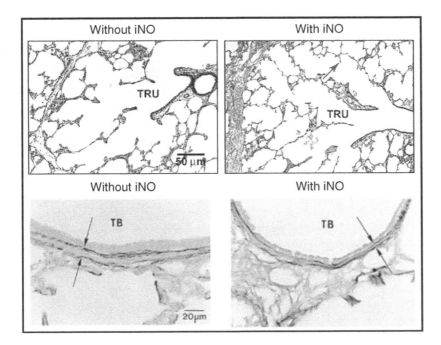

Figure 8 iNO effects and the preterm lung—lamb model. (*Top*) Lung tissue images illustrating differences in radial alveolar counts for preterm lambs that were mechanically ventilated for three weeks without iNO (*left*) or with iNO (*right*). Radial alveolar counts averaged 1.5 ± 0.3 alveoli/terminal bronchiole in lambs that did not receive iNO and 3.6 ± 1.5 alveoli/terminal bronchiole in lambs that received iNO. The *arrow* points to a secondary crest (alveolar septa). TRU the terminal respiratory unit, which is the landmark for measuring radial alveolar counts. (*Bottom*) Representative photomicrographs showing smooth muscle wall thickness between the internal and external elastic laminae (*arrows*; Hart's elastin stain) of terminal bronchioles (TB) in lungs of preterm lambs that were mechanically ventilated for 3 weeks either without iNO (control, *left*) or with iNO (5–15 ppm, *right*). *Source*: From Ref. 182.

and decreases apoptosis of endothelial cells following inhibition of VEGF (179). In experimental models of lung injury, nitric oxide treatment has been shown to improve lung growth (180), morphology, volume and compliance (181), and normalize airway smooth muscle and alveolar development (Fig. 8) (182). Administration of nitric oxide to eNOS-deficient mice during the recovery period was shown by Balasubramaniam et al. to rescue oxygen-exposed animals from the usual patterns of disrupted structure and impaired lung growth (183). In vitro studies suggest that such iNO-induced improvements in lung growth and structure might be attributable to the proangiogenic effects of nitric oxide that promote associated alveolarization (184).

Six masked randomized clinical trials have investigated the potential of inhaled iNOs as a preventive treatment for BPD (Table 2). Each of the studies enrolled and randomized to iNO versus placebo very low birth weight infants receiving mechanical ventilation who, therefore, were at substantial risk of developing BPD; four (185–188) were large multicenter double-masked randomized clinical trials. Schreiber et al. (187)

Table 2 Inhaled Nitric Oxide and BPD Prevention. This table provides an overview of key details of the both masked and unmasked trials of iNO for prevention of BPD among preterm infants

Author	Year	Study population	Age at randomization	iNO/placebo, N/N	BPD at 36 wk: %iNO vs. placebo (RR; 95% CI) (p)	Death or BPD at 36 wk, % (RR; 95% CI) (p)	IVH (Gr 3–4) or PVL, % (RR; 95% CI) (P)	Neuro-developmental outcomes, % iNO vs. placebo (RR; 95% CI) (p)	Comment
Unmasked Trials									
Subhedar (305,306)	1997	GA < 32 wk	96 hr	10/11 (additional 21 randomized to dexa-methasone with or without iNO)	NR	NR	NR	At 30 mo: ND delay 57 vs. 64 (0.89; 0.37–1.75) Severe Disability 0 vs. 35 (p = 0.12) Cerebral Palsy 0 vs. 14 (p = 0.53)	Factorial design also evaluating 6 days of high-dose dexamethasone. Death or CLD (defined by prediction score) no different between study groups.
Franco Belgium (307)	1999	GA <33wk: OI 12.5–30 GA ≥33wk: OI 15–40	<7 days	97 (45 <33 wk)/ 95 (40 <33 wk)	Among GA <33 wk 24 vs. 29 (0.95; 0.44–2.04)	NR	Among GA <33 wk 32 vs. 27 (0.82; 0.38–1.76)	NR	
Srisuparp (308)	2002	BW 500–2000 g	72 hr	16/18	NR	NR	IVH (Gr 3–4) 25 vs. 28 (p = 1.0)	NR	

Study	Year	Inclusion	Age	N					Comments
Hascoet et al. (309)	2005	GA < 32wk	at birth	49/45	NR	NR	NR	NR	28-day outcomes: no difference in mortality, CLD, respiratory failure, any grade IVH, or PDA
Field (INNOVO) (310,311)	2005	<34 wk; <28 days	<28 days	55/53	On O$_2$ at expected date of delivery: 16 vs. 12	71 vs. 85 (0.98; 0.87–1.12)	NR	NR	At 12 mo: death or severe NDI 67 vs. 68 (0.99; 0.76–1.29) At 4–5 yr: death or severe disability 62 vs. 70 (0.89; 0.67–1.16) ($p > 0.59$)	
Dani et al. (312)	2006	GA < 30 wk	<7 days	20/20	30 vs. 60 ($p = 0.067$)	50 vs. 90 ($p = 0.016$)	10 vs. 15 ($p = $ ND)	ND	BW <750 g predicted failure of iNO
Masked Trials									
Kinsella et al. (313)	1999	GA ≤ 34 wk; severe respiratory failure with ≥50% predicted mortality	<48 hr	48/32	60 vs. 80 (0.75; 0.5–1.13) ($p = 0.30$)	77 vs. 91 (0.85; 0.7–1.03) ($p = 0.14$)	Gr 3–4 IVH: 37 vs. 40 ($p = 0.92$)	NR	Survival at discharge was no difference between groups: 52% iNO vs. 47% placebo

(Continued)

239

Table 2 Inhaled Nitric Oxide and BPD Prevention. This table provides an overview of key details of the both masked and unmasked trials of iNO for prevention of BPD among preterm infants (*Continued*)

Author	Year	Study population	Age at randomization	iNO/placebo, N/N	BPD at 36 wk: %iNO vs. placebo (RR; 95% CI) (p)	Death or BPD at 36 wk, % (RR; 95% CI) (p)	IVH (Gr 3–4) or PVL, % (RR; 95% CI) (P)	Neuro-developmental outcomes, % iNO vs. placebo (RR; 95% CI) (p)	Comment
Schreiber (187,191)	2003	GA <34 wk; BW <2000 g	<72 hr	105/102	39 vs. 53 (0.74; 0.53–1.03) (p = 0.07)	49 vs. 64 (0.76; 0.60–0.97) (p = 0.03)	12 vs. 24 (0.53; 0.28–0.98) (p = 0.04)	At 24 mo: NDI (CP, bilateral blindness, bilateral hearing loss, one BSID II score < 70) 24 vs. 46 (0.53; 0.33–0.87) (p = 0.01)	Benefit of iNO was greatest among infants with initial OI < 6.94. 24 mo outcomes primarily reflected iNO treated infants' better Bayley MDI scores.
Van Meurs (188,192)	2005	GA < 34 wk; BW 401–1500 g	24–48 hr	210/210	60 vs. 68 (0.90; 0.75–1.08) (p = 0.26)	80 vs. 82 (0.97; 0.86–1.06) (p = 0.52) BW > 1000 g: 50 vs. 69 (0.72; 0.54–0.96) (p = 0.03)	39 vs. 32 (1.25; 0.95–1.66) (p = 0.11)	At 18–22 mo: Death or NDI 78 vs. 73 (1.07; 0.95–1.19) (p = 0.32)	iNO treated infants at BW ≤ 1000 g BW had increased rate of BPD or death. 18–22 mo: iNO treated infants had an increase in adjusted risk of moderate to severe CP and iNO treated at BW ≤ 1000 g had increased rate of death or CP.

Study	Year	Inclusion criteria	Timing	N			IVH	Outcome	Comments
Ballard (185,314,315)	2006	GA < 32 wk; BW 500–1250 g	7–21 days	294/288	51 vs. 57	56 vs. 63 (0.81; 0.66–0.99) (p = 0.04)	IVH, Gr 3 or 4: 12 vs. 16 (p = 0.13)	Preliminary 24 mo outcomes: no difference	Benefits of iNO occurred among those randomized at 7–14 days; but not 15–21 days. At 12 mo: iNO treated received fewer outpatient respiratory medications.
Kinsella et al. (186,316)	2006	GA < 34 wk	<48 hr	398/395	65 vs. 68 (0.96; 0.86–1.09)	72 vs. 75 (0.79; 0.61–1.03) (p = 0.24) BW > 1000 g: 39 vs. 64 (0.60; 0.42–0.86)	IVH Gr 3 or 4, PVL or ventriculomegaly: 18 vs. 24 (0.73; 0.55–0.98) (p = 0.03)	Preliminary 24 mo outcomes: no difference	Benefit in primary outcome (death or BPD) detected among iNO treated who were of BW >1000 g
Van Meurs et al. (317)	2007	BW > 1500 g and GA < 34 wk; 2 OI strata	24–48 hr	14/15	30 vs. 45 (0.66; 0.21–2.08) (p = 0.66)	50 vs. 60 (0.83; 0.43–1.62) (p = 0.87)	IVH Gr 3 or 4, PVL: 0 vs. 22 (p = 0.47)	At 18 mo: no differences	Study terminated due to Gr 3–4 IVH or PVL among iNO treated

Abbreviations: BSID II, Bayley Scales of Infant Development II; BW, birth weight; Gr, grade; Hrs, hours; INO, inhaled nitric oxide; IVH, intraventricular hemorrhage; MDI, mental development index; N, number(s); ND, neurodevelopmental; NDI, neurodevelopmental impairment; NR, not reported; OI, oxygenation index (%inspired oxygen × mean airway pressure/partial pressure of oxygen); P, probability; PVL, periventricular leukomalacia.

randomized 207 preterm infants born before 34 weeks' gestation to iNO versus placebo and found a benefit of iNO initiated before 72 hours of age in the primary outcome, death or BPD (48.6% vs. 63.7%) (RR 0.76; 95% CI 0.60–0.97), as well as in severe intraventricular hemorrhage (IVH) or periventricular leukomalacia (12.4% vs. 23.5%) (RR 0.53; 95% CI 0.28–0.98). In post hoc analyses, the benefit in primary outcome (death or BPD) was found to be greatest among the group of infants whose oxygenation index at study entry was below 6.94; no effect of type of ventilation was observed. A benefit of iNO treatment in promoting BPD-free survival to 36 weeks (43.9% vs. 36.8%) (RR 1.23; 95% CI 1.01–1.51) also was observed by Ballard et al. (185) in their randomized clinical trial of 582 infants with birth weights at or below 1250 g who required ventilatory assistance and were randomized between 7 and 21 days of age. This study showed no differences between study groups in airway inflammatory markers (189) or adverse effects of iNO on surfactant composition and function (190). Two additional studies found improvement in the primary outcome, death or BPD, only among iNO treated infants born at or greater than 1000 g birth weight. (186,188). Van Meurs et al. (188) randomized 420 infants with respiratory distress who were born before 34 weeks' gestation and between 401 and 1500 g birth weight to receive iNO or placebo, beginning before 48 hours of age, and observed no overall benefit in death or BPD (80% vs. 82%) (RR 0.97; 95% CI 0.86–1.06). Post hoc analyses revealed a reduction in the primary outcome among infants whose birth weights were above 1000 g (50% vs. 69%) (RR 0.72; 95% CI 0.54–0.96) offset by increased risk of severe IVH or PVL among nitric oxide–treated infants born below 1000 g (43% vs. 33%) (RR 1.40; 95% CI 1.03–1.88). The high rates of BPD or death might have been attributable to greater than average severity of illness among the Van Meurs' study population. In the trial by Kinsella et al. (186), 793 preterm infants born at or below 34 weeks' gestation were randomized to iNO or placebo before 48 hours of age. No benefit was observed in the overall study population with respect to the primary outcome, death or BPD (71.6% vs. 75.3%) (RR 0.95 (0.87–1.03). Post hoc analyses, however, revealed, among infants 1000 to 1250 g, a benefit of iNO treatment in reducing death or BPD (38.5% vs. 64.1%) (RR 0.60; 95% CI 0.42–0.86). Further, iNO treatment was associated with reduction in significant ultrasonographic abnormalities (i.e., grade 3–4 IVH, ventriculomegaly or PVL) among the entire study population (17.5% vs. 23.9%) (RR 0.73; 95% CI 0.55–0.98).

Neurodevelopmental and other health outcomes are important considerations in assessment of the risks and benefits of iNO treatment of preterm infants. At 24-month evaluations of infants enrolled in the study by Schreiber et al. (187), Mestan et al. (191) found reduced risk of neurodevelopmental disability (cerebral palsy, bilateral blindness, bilateral hearing loss, or one score < 70 on Bayley II) among infants who had been randomized to receive iNO (24% vs. 46%) (RR 0.53; 95% CI 0.33–0.87). This effect was primarily explained by a 47% reduction among iNO-treated infants in low MDI on the Bayley II examination. Hintz et al. (192) conducted follow-up evaluations of infants enrolled in Van Meurs and colleagues' trial (188) and found no difference between study groups in the outcome death or neurdevelopmental impairment (78% vs. 73%) (RR 1.07; 95% CI 0.95–1.19); however, a greater adjusted risk of moderate to severe cerebral palsy among iNO-treated infants (20% vs. 11%) (RR 2.41; 95% CI 1.01–5.75). Twenty-four-month outcomes are awaited for the Ballard and Kinsella studies, and these data are needed to establish long-term safety of inhaled nitric oxide for BPD prevention.

Noninvasive Respiratory Support: Continuous Positive Airway Pressure and Nasal Intermittent Positive Pressure Ventilation

Nasal Continuous Positive Airway Pressure

Nasal continuous positive airway pressure (nCPAP) offers the theoretical pulmonary benefit of gentle noninvasive support that can be accomplished without an endotracheal tube and mechanical ventilation, thus minimizing the risk of infection, volutrauma, and barotrauma. In a study of the baboon model of BPD that compared surfactant treatment followed by early (24 hours) versus later (5 days) extubation to nCPAP, Thomson et al. provide compelling evidence in support of this approach, noting substantial reductions in proinflammatory biomarkers and pathological indicators of BPD as well as normal pressure-volume relationship after 28 days among preterm baboons randomized to early extubation to nCPAP (Fig. 9) (193).

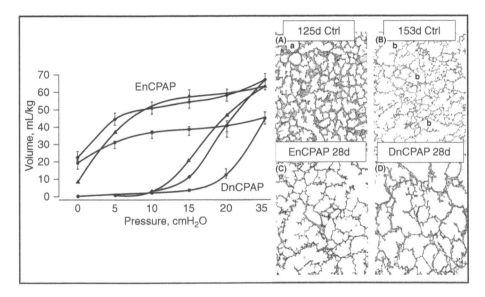

Figure 9 Early and delayed extubation to nasal continuous positive airway pressure. On the left, pressure-volume curves at necropsy of lungs of animals early extubated to CPAP (EnCPAP) (at 24 hours) achieved significantly higher volumes at maximum pressure ($p = 0.0253$). Median and 25th to 75th interquartile ranges are depicted. Pressure-volume curve for the term animals are included for reference only. p 0.0253. (*Upper left*) the 125-day gestational control. Bronchioles and rounded saccular spaces with thickened walls can be seen. Bulges or protuberances from walls into air spaces are progenitor secondary crests. (*Upper right*) 153-day-gestational control. Air spaces larger than 125-day control and thinned saccular walls have abundant secondary crests and alveolar structures. (*Lower left*) EnCPAP 28-day specimen. Air spaces well expanded and thinned saccular walls show increase in alveolar complexity (i.e., elongated branching walls with secondary crests and alveolar formation). (*Lower right*) Delayed extubation to nCPAP 28-day specimen. Walls of thinned saccular structures may be slightly more cellular than EnCPAP, but ongoing alveolar formation is present. Hematoxylin and eosin: original magnification, 10×. *Source*: From Ref. 193.

In the delivery room, rapid initiation of CPAP following a sustained inflation reduces the likelihood of the preterm infant requiring delivery room intubation (194). Although only a minority of extremely preterm infants in whom CPAP is initiated in the delivery room will avoid the need for intubation within 72 hours of birth (194,195), a gestational age–matched case-control analysis by te Pas et al. (196) found that delivery room initiation of respiratory support with CPAP, compared with immediate intubation, diminished the likelihood of an infant later developing BPD (4% vs. 35%; $p < 0.004$) without increasing neonatal mortality or risks of other significant neonatal morbidities. Large randomized clinical trials of nCPAP are few and other observational studies have yielded conflicting results (197–199) regarding the potential of nCPAP to reduce BPD occurrence.

The "CPAP or Intubation" (COIN) study (200), an international multicenter clinical trial, randomized 610 infants born at 25 to 28 weeks' gestation to nCPAP or ventilation at five minutes after birth. There was no significant benefit of nCPAP over mechanical ventilation in the primary outcome: death or BPD at 36 weeks' PMA (33.9% vs. 38.9%) (RR 0.80; 95% CI 0.58–1.12). The group randomized to nCPAP, however, had lower rates of intubation and surfactant use and, among those who required mechanical ventilation, shorter durations of ventilation. The rate of pneumothorax was increased among infants randomized to nCPAP (9% vs. 3%; $p < 0.001$). Inadequate treatment of surfactant deficiency might have contributed to the failure of the COIN trial (200) to detect a benefit of nCPAP for respiratory distress: 77% of infants in the ventilated group received surfactant; however infants in the nCPAP group received surfactant only if they required intubation (38%) ($p < 0.001$).

The potential benefit of surfactant treatment immediately followed by extubation to nCPAP, advocated by Blennow (201), was shown by Verder et al. (202) to reduce the need for mechanical ventilation with surfactant pretreatment compared with nCPAP alone. Several clinical trials of relatively modest size studied moderately (203,204) and very preterm (205) infants who were randomized to receive a single dose of surfactant then extubation to nCPAP versus ongoing mechanical ventilation. Each of these studies of surfactant followed by extubation to nCPAP (203–205) detected, among infants randomized to nCPAP, reductions in days of oxygen, mechanical ventilation, and/or hospitalization, without concurrent reduction in rates of BPD. A larger study by the Texas Neonatal Research Group (206) randomized, at one hour of age, 132 infants born at or above 1250 g and at or below 36 weeks' gestational age to intubation, surfactant, and expedited extubation to nCPAP versus expectant management and found only that surfactant-treated infants were less likely to require intubation and mechanical ventilation for worsening respiratory distress (26% vs. 43%) (RR 0.60; 95% CI 0.37–0.99). Meta-analysis of these, as well as published and unpublished data from a number of studies that were either terminated early or published only in abstract form, showed no differences in rates of neonatal mortality or oxygen requirement at 28 postnatal days (RR 0.51; 95% CI 0.26–0.99) but insufficient data to assess outcomes at 36 weeks' PMA (207). A large multicenter clinical trial of surfactant and nCPAP currently being conducted by the Vermont Oxford Network will contribute important knowledge regarding the potential benefits of surfactant treatment followed by immediate extubation to nCPAP among preterm infants requiring respiratory support.

Nasal Intermittent Positive Pressure Ventilation

A noninvasive alternative to nCPAP, nasal intermittent positive pressure ventilation (NIPPV) appears to enhance success of extubation from mechanical ventilation when compared with nCPAP (208–210). These findings are summarized in a Cochrane Collaborative systematic review that cites a benefit of NIPPV compared with nCPAP in reducing need for reintubation (RR 0.21; 95% CI 0.10, 0.45) (211) without an apparent excess in adverse effects such as abdominal distention or disrupted feeding. No benefit of NIPPV was detected with respect to BPD (i.e., receipt of supplemental oxygen at 36 weeks' PMA) (RR 0.73; 95% CI 0.49, 1.07) (211). Synchronization might enhance the effectiveness of NIPPV. A randomized clinical trial of 41 infants born at 600 to 1250 g birth weight who required mechanical ventilation found a benefit of early extubation to synchronized SNIPPV compared with continued conventional ventilation for the outcome BPD or death at 36 weeks' PMA (212) (52% vs. 20%; $p = 0.03$). Before NIPPV or SNIPPV can be considered for broader use, short- and long-term safety and efficacy must be established through larger-scale randomized clinical trials and safe, reliable equipment for delivery of SNIPPV must be commercially available.

Permissive Hypercapnia

Permissive hypercapnia was proposed as a surrogate that would lead to reduced pulmonary barotrauma and volutrauma among intubated infants and, thus, reduce lung injury leading to BPD. Kraybill et al. (95) provided support for this approach, noting that infants who had a $PaCO_2$ above 50 at 48 or 96 hours were at reduced risk of BPD, and suggested that less aggressive ventilation and/or higher levels of carbon dioxide might offer some protection to the preterm lung. The potential beneficial effects of permissive hypercapnia were further supported by intriguing data from the lamb model of BPD, suggesting that high $PaCO_2$ might have a direct effect in ameliorating pulmonary injury (213).

An early-randomized controlled clinical trial of permissive hypercapnia by Mariani et al. (214,215) compared the effects of 96 hours of relative hypercapnia ($PaCO_2$ between 45 and 55 mmHg and pH > 7.20) versus normocapnea ($PaCO_2$ 35 to 45 mmHg and pH >7.25) among 49 infants 601 to 1250 g birth weight with RDS at <24 hours of age and found no differences in respiratory or other clinical outcomes. The largest published study of permissive hypercapnia among preterm newborns was reported by Carlo et al. (216). This 2×2 factorial design, in which both minimal ventilation and early postnatal corticosteroid treatment were studied, randomized 220 infants 501 to 1000 g birth weight requiring mechanical ventilation at <12 hours of age (751–1000 g birth weight infants were also required to receive $F_iO_2 \geq 0.30$) to dexamethasone versus placebo and minimal ventilation ($PaCO_2 > 52$ mmHg) versus routine ventilation ($PaCO_2 < 48$ mmHg) for 10 days or until extubation with a primary study outcome of death or BPD at 36 weeks' PMA. The study was terminated at approximately half of the projected enrollment due to complications attributed to glucocorticoid treatment. In analyses focused on the limited study sample, no benefit of permissive hypercapnia in BPD prevention was appreciated: the relative risk for death or BPD at 36 weeks' PMA was 0.93 (95% CI 0.77–1.12). Ventilator support, however, was significantly reduced at 36 weeks among infants randomized to receive permissive hypercapnia (1% vs. 16%; $p < 0.01$).

High-Frequency Ventilation

High-Frequency Oscillatory Ventilation

Multicenter randomized clinical trials by Courtney et al. (217), Johnson et al. (218), Moriette et al. (219), and Van Reempts et al. (220) provide conflicting results regarding the potential effectiveness of elective high-frequency oscillatory ventilation (HFOV) compared with conventional mechanical ventilation (CMV) in BPD prevention. Courtney et al. (217) reported the results of a multicenter randomized clinical trial of 500 infants born at 601 to 1200 g who were hospitalized at 1 of 26 tertiary neonatal care units in the United States in which randomization to HFOV before four hours of age was associated with a modest improvement in survival without the need for supplemental oxygen at 36 weeks' PMA (56% in the HFOV group compared with 47% among the infants who received conventional ventilation; $p = 0.046$). On the other hand, no improvement in the composite outcome death or BPD at 36 weeks' PMA was observed in a study conducted by Johnson et al. (218) of 797 preterm infants born at 23 to 28 weeks' gestation who were hospitalized at 1 of 25 centers in the United Kingdom, Australia, and Singapore, or in two other large trials: a multicenter study of 292 infants 24 to 29 weeks' gestation with evidence of RDS (219) and a single-center Belgian study of 300 infants born before 32 weeks of completed gestation (220). Systematic review of these four and nine additional heterogeneous studies (221) by Henderson-Smart revealed a benefit of borderline statistical significance in 36-week PMA outcomes: BPD (OR 0.89; 95% CI 0.81–0.99) and the composite outcome death or BPD (OR 0.93; 95% CI 0.86–1.0).

High-Frequency Jet Ventilation

Two clinical trials evaluated 36-week BPD outcomes among preterm infants randomized early elective use of high-frequency jet ventilation (HFJV) versus conventional mechanical ventilation (222,223). A multicenter trial by Keszler et al. (222) randomized 166 infants born at or below 750 g birth weight who were at or below 7 days of age to HFJV versus CMV found a reduction in receipt of supplemental oxygen at 36 weeks' PMA among infants randomized to HFJV. Wiswell and colleagues (223) randomized 73 infants born before 33 weeks' gestation who were above 500 g birth weight to HFJV versus CMV before 24 hours of age and, on average, used lower HFJV mean airway pressures to provide respiratory support. The study revealed no benefit in oxygen requirement at 36 weeks' PMA and increased risk of periventricular leukomalacia among infants randomized to HFJV. Meta-analysis of these two studies shows a benefit in BPD reduction of borderline statistical significance (RR 0.59; 95% CI 0.35–0.99). Although HFJV might offer pulmonary benefit, its routine use for BPD prevention cannot be recommended until clinical trials are conducted that fully establish efficacy and safety with respect to both pulmonary and neurological outcomes.

C. Potentially Beneficial Medications That Require Further Study: Caffeine and Low-Dose Glucocorticoids

Caffeine

Caffeine enhances respiratory drive and improves the likelihood of successful extubation from mechanical ventilation. Post hoc analyses of the largest published randomized trial of caffeine therapy for apnea of prematurity (224) showed reduction in BPD among infants randomized to caffeine therapy, an effect that persisted after adjustment for other risk factors. In a multicenter placebo-controlled randomized trial of caffeine treatment for apnea of prematurity among 963 infants born at 500 to 1250 g, conducted by Schmidt et al. (224), the caffeine-treated group exhibited pulmonary benefits. Infants randomized to receive caffeine were more of younger corrected gestational age at their last exposure to an endotracheal tube (median PMA 29.1 vs. 30.0 weeks; $p < 0.001$), last receipt of positive airway pressure (median PMA 31.0 vs. 32.0 weeks; $p < 0.001$), and last use of supplemental oxygen (median PMA 33.6 vs. 35.1 weeks; $p < 0.001$). There were no differences between study groups with respect to other short-term adverse outcomes, including mortality, ultrasonographic signs of brain injury, and necrotizing enterocolitis (224) or neurodevelopmental disability at 18 to 21 months (225). Role of caffeine in enhancing extubation success might explain the reduced rate of supplemental oxygen use at 36 weeks' PMA, possibly most benefiting the infants at greatest risk of developing BPD: those who require intubation and mechanical ventilation. Alternatively, caffeine might exert an anti-inflammatory or other salutary effect.

Low-Dose Glucocorticoids

Endogenous corticosteroids are necessary for many vital physiological functions including the stress response and modulation of inflammation. Because of their powerful anti-inflammatory properties, glucocorticoids modulate the pulmonary inflammation that is an integral component of BPD pathogenesis. Furthermore, preterm infants are at risk of cortisol deficiency (226), prenatal inflammation contributes to this deficiency (227), and cortisol deficiency is associated with greater risk of poor respiratory outcome, possibly including BPD (228,229). Following a promising pilot study of early low-dose prophylactic hydrocortisone treatment in BPD prevention (230), a multicenter randomized clinical trial was launched. The study was terminated at approximately half the intended enrollment due to higher rates of spontaneous gastrointestinal perforation among infants randomized to receive hydrocortisone (231). Among the 360 mechanically ventilated infants with birth weights between 500 and 999 g enrolled in this randomized masked placebo-controlled multicenter trial of low-dose hydrocortisone, there was no observed effect of hydrocortisone on BPD rate at 36 weeks' PMA. There was, however, a significant benefit of hydrocortisone treatment in BPD-free survival to 36 weeks' PMA observed among the 149 infants who were born in the context of chorioamnionitis (38% vs. 24%) (OR 2.84; 95% CI 1.21–6.67). Among 252 survivors evaluated at 18 to 22 months, there was no difference between study groups in the rate of neurodevelopment impairment (39% in hydrocortisone treated vs. 44% among those in the placebo group) (232). These findings are consistent with results of an observational study of 226 infants born at or below 32 weeks' gestation that found, although initially smaller and sicker, the 62 infants treated with low-dose hydrocortisone for BPD (starting dose 5 mg/kg/day; median duration 27.5 days) had no greater likelihood of having cerebral palsy, abnormal developmental testing, or MRI abnormalities than their untreated counterparts (233).

A multicenter clinical trial by Doyle et al. (234), intended to evaluate low-dose dexamethasone, was abandoned due to slow enrollment. The final study population consisted of 70 infants born before 28 weeks' gestation or below 1000 g birth weight,

10% of the intended sample size. No differences were observed between the study groups in neonatal mortality or oxygen requirement at 36 weeks' PMA. However, among the group randomized to low-dose dexamethasone, a greater proportion of dexamethasone-treated infants were extubated by 10 days of treatment (60% vs. 12%) (OR 11.2; 95% CI 3.2–39.0). There was no difference between study groups in the primary outcome, death or severe BPD (234) or in neurodevelopmental outcomes at age 2 (235); however, limited study power might have obscured other positive or negative effects of low-dose dexamethasone.

D. Effective Therapy with Substantial Risk: Early High-Dose Glucocorticoids

High-Dose Glucocorticoids

Among infants at risk of BPD, early or moderately early use of high-dose dex- amethasone leads to improved survival and pulmonary benefits, including reductions in pulmonary inflammation (236), duration of mechanical ventilation (237–244), and oxygen requirement at 28 days (242,244) and 36 weeks' PMA (242,245–247) or more (248). There is some evidence that dexamethasone-mediated pulmonary benefits are enhanced by surfactant treatment (248) and are achieved only at higher doses (249). The pulmonary benefits are substantially counterbalanced by increased risk of other serious morbidities including cerebral palsy (250,251) and intestinal perforation (247,252). In randomized clinical trials by Yeh et al. (244) and Kothadia et al. (239), treatment assignment to high-dose dexamethasone was linked with greater risk of cerebral palsy at age two (250) and neurodevelopmental disability at two years (253) and school age (251), possibly reflecting impaired regional or overall brain growth and development (254). Differences between study groups in later neurodevelopmental outcomes might be less pronounced: follow-up of infants enrolled in the study by O'Shea et al. (255) at 4 to 11 years revealed rates of death or major neurodevelopmental impairment that were similar between the treatment groups (47% and 41%) (OR 1.3; 95% CI 0.6–2.7). Other adverse effects of early high-dose dexamethsone administration include impaired growth (244,256), hypertension (244,256–259), hypertrophic cardiomyopathy (260–265), hyperglycemia (244,256–258,266), intestinal hemorrhage (256,258), adrenal suppression (267,268), and systemic infection (240,257,269). Inhaled steroids are associated with fewer adverse systemic effects; however none have proven useful in preventing BPD (266,270,271).

Although some investigators have noted increased risk of BPD in the era in which steroid treatment has declined (272), the risk-benefit ratio for glucocorticoids currently does not favor routine use of early high-dose glucocorticoids BPD prevention (273,274). Evidence-based concerns are substantial, yet corticosteroids might prove lifesaving for selected infants. Doyle et al. demonstrated that the effect of postnatal corticosteroids on the combined outcome of death or cerebral palsy varies with the level of BPD risk and estimated that the risk-to-benefit ratio tips in favor of glucocorticoid treatment when the risk of BPD exceeds approximately 65% (275). Clinical guidelines recommend reserving glucocorticoid treatment for critically ill infants who fail alternative therapies and, when needed, steroids are used at the lowest effective dose and for the briefest possible duration (275–278).

E. Additional Proposed Preventive Treatments: Antioxidants, Antiproteinases, and Indomethacin

Antioxidants

The lung of the preterm infant is deficient in endogenous antioxidants (279,280) and therefore is vulnerable to oxidative stress produced by a host of provocative stimuli, including inspired oxygen, infection, inflammation, consumption of iron, and therapies such as inhaled nitric oxide and parenteral nutrition (281). Several antioxidant therapies have been evaluated for their potential in preventing or ameliorating lung injury leading to BPD. Rosenfeld et al. (282) studied the use of subcutaneous bovine superoxide dismutase (SOD) versus saline placebo in mechanically ventilated preterm infants with RDS and found fewer radiographic abnormalities and signs of asthma among the survivors who received SOD; no specific clinical criteria for BPD were evaluated. Ahola et al. (283) randomized mechanically ventilated infants (birth weights 500–999 g) to intravenous antioxidant therapy with *N*-acetylcysteine (a glutathione substrate) or placebo and showed no significant reduction in mortality or requirement for supplemental oxygen at 28 days or 36 weeks' PMA. In a multicenter clinical trial, Davis et al. (284) randomized 102 infants 600 to 1200 g birth weight who received surfactant for respiratory distress to intratracheal recombinant human Copper Zinc Superoxide Dismutase (r-h CuZn SOD) or normal saline placebo, administering the study drug every 48 hours for up to one month among intubated and ventilated extremely preterm infants, and found no difference in mortality or 36-week oxygen dependence between the two study groups (36% vs. 37%; $p = 0.51$). However, at one year of age, the r-h CuZn SOD–treated infants had lower rates of hospitalization (30% vs. 54%; $p = 0.05$), emergency room visits (19%. vs. 42%; $p = 0.01$), and treatment with asthma medications (19% vs. 42%; $p = 0.01$) (284).

Antiproteinases

Proteolytic enzyme–induced lung injury accompanies pulmonary inflammation and unopposed antioxidant stress and disruption of the proteinase: antiproteinase balance is thought to produce lung injury that results in BPD. Rigorously conducted studies of α-1-proteinase inhibitor (α1PI), using two different treatment regimens (285,286) failed to show a benefit of α1PI in mortality or oxygen requirement at 36 weeks' PMA, independently or in a meta-analysis of the total 195 subjects (287). Larger-scale multicenter clinical trials of α1PI or other antiproteinase therapies are needed to evaluate their potential effectiveness in BPD prevention.

Indomethacin

Indomethacin exerts anti-inflammatory effects and facilitates closure of the ductus arteriosus, two physiological responses that might benefit infants at risk of BPD. In the baboon model of BPD (288), ibuprofen-induced patent ductus arteriosus closure improved pulmonary mechanics, increased epithelial sodium channel expression, decreased total lung water, and was associated with improved alveolarization. The benefits of indomethacin on the human preterm lung, however, have not yet been demonstrated.

Post hoc analyses of the 999 infants born at 500 to 999 g who were enrolled in Schmidt and colleagues' (289) Trial of Indomethacin Prophylaxis in Preterms (TIPP) study, a multicenter randomized masked clinical trial of indomethacin prophylaxis for patent ductus arteriosus showed no benefit of prophylactic indomethacin in BPD prevention, an effect that was consistent in both crude analyses [BPD rates: 45% (indomethacin) vs. 43% (placebo); $p = 0.41$] and those stratified by the presence or absence of PDA. BPD rates in the subgroup of infants with PDA were 52% after indomethacin prophylaxis and 56% after placebo. In contrast, among the subgroup of infants without a PDA, BPD rates were 43% after indomethacin prophylaxis and 30% after placebo [p (interaction) $= 0.05$]. The reasons underlying the failure to observe a benefit of indomethacin in BPD prevention are unclear. Possible explanations for TIPP study results include (*i*) the presence of a PDA does not contribute to new BPD, (*ii*) the treatment dose and/or schedule offer inadequate anti-inflammatory effects, or (*iii*) indomethacin exerts direct toxicity to the immature lung. Results of an observational study showing an increased incidence of BPD following antenatal administration of indomethacin for preterm labor do not exclude the possibility that indomethacin might exert a direct toxic effect on the neonatal lung (290).

VI. Summary

Four decades after its discovery, Bronchopulmonary dysplasia has evolved pathologically and epidemiologically yet remains the most prevalent and one of the most serious of the adverse sequelae of prematurity. BPD is no longer predominantly the disease of lung destruction and fibrosis described by Northway et al. (1): the new BPD is characterized by aberrant pulmonary development that features impaired angiogenesis and fewer and larger alveoli. From the outset, Northway et al. recognized pulmonary immaturity, oxygen toxicity, and ventilator-induced lung injury as important antecedents of BPD. These factors remain central to BPD pathogenesis, interacting with and being modulated by a host of more recently identified risks, including genetic predisposition and exposures, such as chorioamnionitis, that begin during prenatal life. The study of BPD has enjoyed strong collaborative and interactive relationships between the laboratory and clinical research communities. Studies of the epidemiology of BPD and newer translational approaches to BPD prevention have benefited from the wealth of information gleaned from laboratory work, including the significant contributions of the baboon (52–56) and lamb (57–59) models of BPD. Although the silver bullet for BPD remains elusive, several current therapeutic interventions—vitamin A, caffeine, noninvasive respiratory support, and inhaled nitric oxide, among the most promising—appear to modulate BPD occurrence. Ultimately, eradication of BPD will occur as a consequence of prevention of preterm birth as well as improved pulmonary therapies that enable normal lung growth and development among preterm infants.

Acknowledgments

The author thanks Steven Abman, MD, for the providing opportunity to contribute this chapter to his outstanding book. She also thanks Steven Seidner, MD, for sharing images of the baboon model of BPD, generated from his work in collaboration with Jacqueline Coalson, MD, of the University of Texas, San Antonio; as well as Rosemary Higgins, MD and the Eunice Kennedy Shriver National Institutes of Child Health and Human Development Neonatal Research Network for generously providing Network data on trends in birth weight–specific mortality and BPD. In addition, the author thanks Sarah Gately for her leadership in coordinating all clerical components of manuscript preparation and Katherine Scarpelli and Katherine Juhasz for clerical support. Finally, Dr. Van Marter wishes to thank Alison Clapp for assistance in retrieval of selected references and for demystifying EndNote.

References

1. Northway WH Jr, Rosan RC, Porter DY. Pulmonary disease following respirator therapy of hyaline-membrane disease. Bronchopulmonary dysplasia. N Engl J Med 1967; 276: 357–368.
2. Fanaroff AA, Stoll BJ, Wright LL, et al. Trends in neonatal morbidity and mortality for very low birthweight infants. Am J Obstet Gynecol 2007; 196:147 e1–e8.
3. Martin J, Hamilton B, Sutton P, et al. Births: final data for 2006. Natl Vital Stat Rep 2009; 57:1–102.
4. Cunningham CK, McMillan JA, Gross SJ. Rehospitalization for respiratory illness in infants of less than 32 weeks' gestation. Pediatrics 1991; 88:527–532.
5. Sauve RS, Singhal N. Long-term morbidity of infants with bronchopulmonary dysplasia. Pediatrics 1985; 76:725–733.
6. Schmidt B, Asztalos EV, Roberts RS, et al. Impact of bronchopulmonary dysplasia, brain injury, and severe retinopathy on the outcome of extremely low-birth-weight infants at 18 months: results from the trial of indomethacin prophylaxis in preterms. JAMA 2003; 289:1124–1129.
7. Werthammer J, Brown ER, Neff RK, et al. Sudden infant death syndrome in infants with bronchopulmonary dysplasia. Pediatrics 1982; 69:301–304.
8. Gross SJ, Iannuzzi DM, Kveselis DA, et al. Effect of preterm birth on pulmonary function at school age: a prospective controlled study. J Pediatr 1998; 133:188–192.
9. Hennessy EM, Bracewell MA, Wood N, et al. Respiratory health in pre-school and school age children following extremely preterm birth. Arch Dis Child 2008; 93:1037–1043.
10. Vohr BR, Bell EF, Oh W. Infants with bronchopulmonary dysplasia. Growth pattern and neurologic and developmental outcome. Am J Dis Child 1982; 136:443–447.
11. Gibson RL, Jackson JC, Twiggs GA, et al. Bronchopulmonary dysplasia. Survival after prolonged mechanical ventilation. Am J Dis Child 1988; 142:721–725.
12. Greenough A. Long-term pulmonary outcome in the preterm infant. Neonatology 2008; 93:324–327.
13. Wong PM, Lees AN, Louw J, et al. Emphysema in young adult survivors of moderate-to-severe bronchopulmonary dysplasia. Eur Respir J 2008; 32:321–328.
14. Doyle LW, Faber B, Callanan C, et al. Bronchopulmonary dysplasia in very low birth weight subjects and lung function in late adolescence. Pediatrics 2006; 118:108–113.
15. Northway WH Jr., Moss RB, Carlisle KB, et al. Late pulmonary sequelae of bronchopulmonary dysplasia. N Engl J Med 1990; 323:1793–1799.
16. Jeng SF, Hsu CH, Tsao PN, et al. Bronchopulmonary dysplasia predicts adverse developmental and clinical outcomes in very-low-birthweight infants. Dev Med Child Neurol 2008; 50:51–57.
17. Smith VC, Zupancic JA, McCormick MC, et al. Rehospitalization in the first year of life among infants with bronchopulmonary dysplasia. J Pediatr 2004; 144:799–803.

18. Greenough A. Bronchopulmonary dysplasia—long term follow up. Paediatr Respir Rev 2006; 7(suppl 1):S189–S191.

19. Gregoire MC, Lefebvre F, Glorieux J. Health and developmental outcomes at 18 months in very preterm infants with bronchopulmonary dysplasia. Pediatrics 1998; 101:856–860.

20. Groothuis JR, Gutierrez KM, Lauer BA. Respiratory syncytial virus infection in children with bronchopulmonary dysplasia. Pediatrics 1988; 82:199–203.

21. Truog WE, Jackson JC, Badura RJ, et al. Bronchopulmonary dysplasia and pulmonary insufficiency of prematurity. Lack of correlation of outcome with gas exchange abnormalities at 1 month of age. Am J Dis Child 1985; 139:351–354.

22. Motoyama EK, Fort MD, Klesh KW, et al. Early onset of airway reactivity in premature infants with bronchopulmonary dysplasia. Am Rev Respir Dis 1987; 136:50–57.

23. Smyth JA, Tabachnik E, Duncan WJ, et al. Pulmonary function and bronchial hyperreactivity in long-term survivors of bronchopulmonary dysplasia. Pediatrics 1981; 68: 336–340.

24. Vohr BR, Coll CG, Lobato D, et al. Neurodevelopmental and medical status of low-birthweight survivors of bronchopulmonary dysplasia at 10 to 12 years of age. Dev Med Child Neurol 1991; 33:690–697.

25. Berman W Jr., Yabek SM, Dillon T, et al. Evaluation of infants with bronchopulmonary dysplasia using cardiac catheterization. Pediatrics 1982; 70:708–712.

26. Bush A, Busst CM, Knight WB, et al. Changes in pulmonary circulation in severe bronchopulmonary dysplasia. Arch Dis Child 1990; 65:739–745.

27. Goodman G, Perkin RM, Anas NG, et al. Pulmonary hypertension in infants with bronchopulmonary dysplasia. J Pediatr 1988; 112:67–72.

28. Khemani E, McElhinney DB, Rhein L, et al. Pulmonary artery hypertension in formerly premature infants with bronchopulmonary dysplasia: clinical features and outcomes in the surfactant era. Pediatrics 2007; 120:1260–1209.

29. de Sa D. Myocardial changes in immature infants requiring prolonged ventilation. Arch Dis Child 1977; 52:138–147.

30. Mourani PM, Ivy DD, Rosenberg AA, et al. Left ventricular diastolic dysfunction in bronchopulmonary dysplasia. J Pediatr 2008; 152:291–293.

31. Bott L, Beghin L, Devos P, et al. Nutritional status at 2 years in former infants with bronchopulmonary dysplasia influences nutrition and pulmonary outcomes during childhood. Pediatr Res 2006; 60:340–344.

32. Kurzner SI, Garg M, Bautista DB, et al. Growth failure in infants with bronchopulmonary dysplasia: nutrition and elevated resting metabolic expenditure. Pediatrics 1988; 81: 379–384.

33. Korhonen P, Hyodynmaa E, Lenko HL, et al. Growth and adrenal androgen status at 7 years in very low birth weight survivors with and without bronchopulmonary dysplasia. Arch Dis Child 2004; 89:320–324.

34. Moon NM, Mohay HA, Gray PH. Developmental patterns from 1 to 4 years of extremely preterm infants who required home oxygen therapy. Early Hum Dev 2007; 83:209–216.

35. Shankaran S, Szego E, Eizert D, et al. Severe bronchopulmonary dysplasia. Predictors of survival and outcome. Chest 1984; 86:607–610.

36. Short EJ, Kirchner HL, Asaad GR, et al. Developmental sequelae in preterm infants having a diagnosis of bronchopulmonary dysplasia: analysis using a severity-based classification system. Arch Pediatr Adolesc Med 2007; 161:1082–1087.

37. Kobaly K, Schluchter M, Minich N, et al. Outcomes of extremely low birth weight (<1 kg) and extremely low gestational age (<28 weeks) infants with bronchopulmonary dysplasia: effects of practice changes in 2000 to 2003. Pediatrics 2008; 121:73–81.

38. Hughes CA, O'Gorman LA, Shyr Y, et al. Cognitive performance at school age of very low birth weight infants with bronchopulmonary dysplasia. J Dev Behav Pediatr 1999; 20:1–8.

39. O'Shea TM, Goldstein DJ, deRegnier RA, et al. Outcome at 4 to 5 years of age in children recovered from neonatal chronic lung disease. Dev Med Child Neurol 1996; 38:830–839.
40. Singer L, Yamashita T, Lilien L, et al. A longitudinal study of developmental outcome of infants with bronchopulmonary dysplasia and very low birth weight. Pediatrics 1997; 100:987–993.
41. Majnemer A, Riley P, Shevell M, et al. Severe bronchopulmonary dysplasia increases risk for later neurological and motor sequelae in preterm survivors. Dev Med Child Neurol 2000; 42:53–60.
42. Skidmore MD, Rivers A, Hack M. Increased risk of cerebral palsy among very low-birthweight infants with chronic lung disease. Dev Med Child Neurol 1990; 32:325–332.
43. Walsh MC, Morris BH, Wrage LA, et al. Extremely low birthweight neonates with protracted ventilation: mortality and 18-month neurodevelopmental outcomes. J Pediatr 2005; 146:798–804.
44. Anderson PJ, Doyle LW. Neurodevelopmental outcome of bronchopulmonary dysplasia. Semin Perinatol 2006; 30:227–232.
45. Jiang ZD, Brosi DM, Wilkinson AR. Brain-stem auditory function in very preterm infants with chronic lung disease: delayed neural conduction. Clin Neurophysiol 2006; 117:1551–1559.
46. Wilkinson AR, Brosi DM, Jiang ZD. Functional impairment of the brainstem in infants with bronchopulmonary dysplasia. Pediatrics 2007; 120:362–371.
47. Sobonya RE, Logvinoff MM, Taussig LM, et al. Morphometric analysis of the lung in prolonged bronchopulmonary dysplasia. Pediatr Res 1982; 16:969–972.
48. Tomashefski JF Jr, Oppermann HC, Vawter GF, et al. Bronchopulmonary dysplasia: a morphometric study with emphasis on the pulmonary vasculature. Pediatr Pathol 1984; 2:469–487.
49. Hussain NA, Siddiqui NH, Stocker JR. Pathology of arrested acinar development in post surfactant bronchopulmonary dysplasia. Human Pathol 1998; 29:710–717.
50. Albertine KH, Sun J, Dahl MJ, et al. Lung abundance of vascular endothelial growth factor and it's receptor, fetal liver kinase-1, proteins coincides with perinatal changes of pulmonary capillary surface density in sheep. Pediatr Res 2002; 51:63A.
51. Bhatt AJ, Amin SB, Chess PR, et al. Expression of vascular endothelial growth factor and Flk-1 in developing and glucocorticoid-treated mouse lung. Pediatr Res 2000; 47:606–613.
52. Coalson JJ, Kuehl TJ, Escobedo MB, et al. A baboon model of bronchopulmonary dysplasia. II. Pathologic features. Exp Mol Pathol 1982; 37:335–350.
53. Coalson JJ, Winter V, deLemos RA. Decreased alveolarization in baboon survivors with bronchopulmonary dysplasia. Am J Resp Crit Care Med 1995; 152:640–646.
54. Escobedo MB, Hilliard JL, Smith F, et al. A baboon model of bronchopulmonary dysplasia. I. Clinical features. Exp Mol Pathol 1982; 37:323–334.
55. Seidner S, McCurnin D, Coalson J, et al. A new model of chronic lung injury in surfactant-treated preterm baboons delivered at very early gestations. Pediatr Res 1993; 33:344A.
56. Seidner SR, Jobe AH, Coalson JJ, et al. Abnormal surfactant metabolism and function in preterm ventilated baboons. Am J Respir Crit Care Med 1998; 158:1982–1989.
57. Albertine KH, Jones GP, Starcher BC, et al. Chronic lung injury in preterm lambs. Disordered respiratory tract development. Am J Respir Crit Care Med 1999; 159:945–958.
58. Bland RD, Kullama L, Day RW, et al. Nitric oxide inhalation decreases pulmonary vascular resistance in preterm lambs with evolving chronic lung disease. Pediatr Res 1997; 41:247A.
59. Pierce RA, Albertine KH, Starcher BC, et al. Chronic lung injury in preterm lambs: disordered pulmonary elastin deposition. Am J Physiol 1997; 272:L452–L460.
60. Coalson JJ, Winter V, Yodar B. Decreased alveoli and surface area in premature baboons with long-term bronchopulmonary dysplasia. Am J Resp Crit Care Med 1998; 157:A373.
61. Maniscalco WM, Watkins RH, Pryhuber GS, et al. Angiogenic factors and alveolar vasculature: development and alterations by injury in very premature baboons. Am J Physiol Lung Cell Mol Physiol 2002; 282:L811–L823.

62. Bancalari E, Claure N, Sosenko IR. Bronchopulmonary dysplasia: changes in pathogenesis, epidemiology and definition. Semin Neonatol 2003; 8:63–71.
63. Northway WH Jr. Bronchopulmonary dysplasia: then and now. Arch Dis Child 1990; 65:1076–1081.
64. Parker RA, Lindstrom DP, Cotton RB. Improved survival accounts for most, but not all, of the increase in bronchopulmonary dysplasia. Pediatrics 1992; 90:663–668.
65. Byrne BJ, Mellen BG, Lindstrom DP, et al. Is the BPD epidemic diminishing? Semin Perinatol 2002; 26:461–466.
66. de Kleine MJ, den Ouden AL, Kollee LA, et al. Lower mortality but higher neonatal morbidity over a decade in very preterm infants. Paediatr Perinat Epidemiol 2007; 21:15–25.
67. Avery ME, Tooley WH, Keller JB, et al. Is chronic lung disease in low birth weight infants preventable? A survey of eight centers. Pediatrics 1987; 79:26–30.
68. Bancalari E, Abdenour GE, Feller R, et al. Bronchopulmonary dysplasia: clinical presentation. J Pediatr 1979; 95:819–823.
69. Greenough A, Roberton NR. Morbidity and survival in neonates ventilated for the respiratory distress syndrome. Br Med J (Clin Res Ed) 1985; 290:597–600.
70. Reynolds EO, Taghizadeh A. Improved prognosis of infants mechanically ventilated for hyaline membrane disease. Arch Dis Child 1974; 49:505–515.
71. Payne NR, LaCorte M, Karna P, et al. Reduction of bronchopulmonary dysplasia after participation in the Breathsavers Group of the Vermont Oxford Network Neonatal Intensive Care Quality Improvement Collaborative. Pediatrics 2006; 118(suppl 2):S73–S77.
72. Payne NR, LaCorte M, Sun S, et al. Evaluation and development of potentially better practices to reduce bronchopulmonary dysplasia in very low birth weight infants. Pediatrics 2006; 118(suppl 2):S65–S72.
73. Zeitlin J, Draper ES, Kollee L, et al. Differences in rates and short-term outcome of live births before 32 weeks of gestation in Europe in 2003: results from the MOSAIC cohort. Pediatrics 2008; 121:e936–e944.
74. Walsh M, Laptook A, Kazzi SN, et al. A cluster-randomized trial of benchmarking and multimodal quality improvement to improve rates of survival free of bronchopulmonary dysplasia for infants with birth weights of less than 1250 grams. Pediatrics 2007; 119:876–890.
75. Edwards DK, Colby TV, Northway WH Jr. Radiographic-pathologic correlation in bronchopulmonary dysplasia. J Pediatr 1979; 95:834–836.
76. Lee RM, O'Brodovich H. Airway epithelial damage in premature infants with respiratory failure. Am Rev Respir Dis 1988; 137:450–457.
77. O'Brodovich HM, Mellins RB. Bronchopulmonary dysplasia. Unresolved neonatal acute lung injury. Am Rev Resp Dis 1985; 132:694–709.
78. Shennan AT, Dunn MS, Ohlsson A, et al. Abnormal pulmonary outcomes in premature infants: prediction from oxygen requirement in the neonatal period. Pediatrics 1988; 82:527–532.
79. Edwards DK. Radiographic aspects of bronchopulmonary dysplasia. J Pediatr 1979; 95:823–829.
80. Rojas MA, Gonzalez A, Bancalari E, et al. Changing trends in the epidemiology and pathogenesis of neonatal chronic lung disease. J Pediatr 1995; 126:605–610.
81. Davis PG, Thorpe K, Roberts R, et al. Evaluating "old" definitions for the "new" bronchopulmonary dysplasia. J Pediatr 2002; 140:555–560.
82. Aukland SM, Halvorsen T, Fosse KR, et al. High-resolution CT of the chest in children and young adults who were born prematurely: findings in a population-based study. Am J Roentgenol 2006; 187:1012–1018.
83. Mahut B, De Blic J, Emond S, et al. Chest computed tomography findings in bronchopulmonary dysplasia and correlation with lung function. Arch Dis Child Fetal Neonatal Ed 2007; 92:F459–F464.

84. Ochiai M, Hikino S, Yabuuchi H, et al. A new scoring system for computed tomography of the chest for assessing the clinical status of bronchopulmonary dysplasia. J Pediatr 2008; 152:90–95, 95.e1–3.
85. Jobe AH, Bancalari E. Bronchopulmonary dysplasia. Am J Respir Crit Care Med 2001; 163:1723–1729.
86. Ehrenkranz RA, Walsh MC, Vohr BR, et al. Validation of the National Institutes of Health consensus definition of bronchopulmonary dysplasia. Pediatrics 2005; 116:1353–1360.
87. Walsh MC, Wilson-Costello D, Zadell A, et al. Safety, reliability, and validity of a physiologic definition of bronchopulmonary dysplasia. J Perinatol 2003; 23:451–456.
88. Walsh MC, Yao Q, Gettner P, et al. Impact of a physiologic definition on bronchopulmonary dysplasia rates. Pediatrics 2004; 114:1305–1311.
89. Randell SH, Young SL. Unique features of the immature lung that make it vulnerable to injury. In: Bland RD, Coalson JJ, eds. Chronic Lung Disease in Early Infancy. New York: Marcel Dekker Inc., 2000:377–403.
90. Speer CP. Inflammation and bronchopulmonary dysplasia: a continuing story. Semin Fetal Neonatal Med 2006; 11:354–362.
91. Ambalavanan N, Van Meurs KP, Perritt R, et al. Predictors of death or bronchopulmonary dysplasia in preterm infants with respiratory failure. J Perinatol 2008; 28:420–426.
92. Antonucci R, Contu P, Porcella A, et al. Intrauterine smoke exposure: a new risk factor for bronchopulmonary dysplasia? J Perinat Med 2004; 32:272–277.
93. Darlow BA, Horwood LJ. Chronic lung disease in very low birthweight infants: a prospective population-based study. J Paediatr Child Health 1992; 28:301–305.
94. Hakulinen A, Heinonen K, Jokela V, et al. Occurrence, predictive factors and associated morbidity of bronchopulmonary dysplasia in a preterm birth cohort. J Perinat Med 1988; 16:437–446.
95. Kraybill EN, Runyan DK, Bose CL, et al. Risk factors for chronic lung disease in infants with birth weights of 751 to 1000 grams. J Pediatr 1989; 115:115–120.
96. Palta M, Gabbert D, Weinstein MR, et al. Multivariate assessment of traditional risk factors for chronic lung disease in very low birth weight neonates. The Newborn Lung Project. J Pediatr 1991; 119:285–292.
97. Nickerson BG, Taussig LM. Family history of asthma in infants with bronchopulmonary dysplasia. Pediatrics 1980; 65:1140–1144.
98. Egreteau L, Pauchard J, Semama D, et al. Chronic oxygen dependency in infants born at less than 32 weeks' gestation: incidence and risk factors. Pediatrics 2001; 108:E26.
99. Reiss I, Landmann E, Heckmann M, et al. Increased risk of bronchopulmonary dysplasia and increased mortality in very preterm infants being small for gestational age. Arch Gynecol Obstet 2003; 269:40–44.
100. Doyle L, Kitchen W, Ford G. Effects of antenatal steroid therapy on mortality and morbidity in very low birth weight infants. J Pediatr 1986; 108:287–292.
101. Van Marter LJ, Leviton A, Kuban KC, et al. Maternal glucocorticoid therapy and reduced risk of bronchopulmonary dysplasia. Pediatrics 1990; 86:331–336.
102. Yu VY, Orgill AA, Lim SB, et al. Bronchopulmonary dysplasia in very low birthweight infants. Aust Paediatr J 1983; 19:233–236.
103. Moylan FM, Walker AM, Kramer SS, et al. Alveolar rupture as an independent predictor of bronchopulmonary dysplasia. Crit Care Med 1978; 6:10–13.
104. Brown ER. Increased risk of bronchopulmonary dysplasia in infants with patent ductus arteriosus. J Pediatr 1979; 95:865–866.
105. Brown ER, Stark A, Sosenko I, et al. Bronchopulmonary dysplasia: possible relationship to pulmonary edema. J Pediatr 1978; 92:982–984.
106. Van Marter LJ, Leviton A, Allred EN, et al. Hydration during the first days of life and the risk of bronchopulmonary dysplasia in low birth weight infants. J Pediatr 1990; 116:942–949.

107. Cooke RW. Factors associated with chronic lung disease in preterm infants. Arch Dis Child 1991; 66:776–779.
108. Brown LA, Gauthier TW. Highlight commentary on "influence of lung oxidant and anti-oxidant status on alveolarization: role of light-exposed total parenteral nutrition". Free Radic Biol Med 2008; 45:570–571.
109. Chessex P, Harrison A, Khashu M, et al. In preterm neonates, is the risk of developing bronchopulmonary dysplasia influenced by the failure to protect total parenteral nutrition from exposure to ambient light? J Pediatr 2007; 151:213–214.
110. Edwards DK, Dyer WM, Northway WH Jr. Twelve years' experience with broncho-pulmonary dysplasia. Pediatrics 1977; 59:839–846.
111. Young TE, Kruyer LS, Marshall DD, et al. Population-based study of chronic lung disease in very low birth weight infants in North Carolina in 1994 with comparisons with 1984. The North Carolina Neonatologists Association. Pediatrics 1999; 104:e17.
112. Van Marter LJ, Allred EN, Pagano M, et al. Do clinical markers of barotrauma and oxygen toxicity explain interhospital variation in rates of chronic lung disease? Pediatrics 2000; 105:1194–1201.
113. Sinkin RA, Cox C, Phelps DL. Predicting risk for bronchopulmonary dysplasia: selection criteria for clinical trials. Pediatrics 1990; 86:728–736.
114. Taghizadeh A, Reynolds EO. Pathogenesis of bronchopulmonary dysplasia following hyaline membrane disease. Am J Pathol 1976; 82:241–264.
115. Van Marter LJ, Pagano M, Allred EN, et al. Rate of bronchopulmonary dysplasia as a function of neonatal intensive care practices. J Pediatr 1992; 120:938–946.
116. Goldenberg RL, Andrews WW, Goepfert AR, et al. The alabama preterm birth study: umbilical cord blood Ureaplasma urealyticum and Mycoplasma hominis cultures in very preterm newborn infants. Am J Obstet Gynecol 2008; 198:43.e1–43.e5.
117. Oue S, Hiroi M, Ogawa S, et al. Association of gastric fluid microbes at birth with severe bronchopulmonary dysplasia. Arch Dis Child Fetal Neonatal Ed 2009; 94:F17–F22.
118. Bhering CA, Mochdece CC, Moreira ME, et al. Bronchopulmonary dysplasia prediction model for 7-day-old infants. J Pediatr (Rio J) 2007; 83:163–170.
119. Ryan SW, Nycyk J, Shaw BN. Prediction of chronic neonatal lung disease on day 4 of life. Eur J Pediatr 1996; 155:668–671.
120. Ryan SW, Wild NJ, Arthur RJ, et al. Prediction of chronic neonatal lung disease in very low birthweight neonates using clinical and radiological variables. Arch Dis Child Fetal Neo-natal Ed 1994; 71:F36–F39.
121. Auten RL Jr. Mechanisms of neonatal lung injury. In: Polin RA, Fox WW, Abman S, eds. Fetal and Neonatal Physiology. 3rd ed. Philadelphia: Saunders, 2004:934–941.
122. Jobe A. The new BPD. NeoReviews 2006; 7:531–545.
123. Vilstrup CT, Bjorklund LJ, Werner O, et al. Lung volumes and pressure-volume relations of the respiratory system in small ventilated neonates with severe respiratory distress syn-drome. Pediatr Res 1996; 39:127–133.
124. Auten RL, Vozzelli M, Clark RH. Volutrauma. What is it, and how do we avoid it? Clin Perinatol 2001; 28:505–515.
125. Dreyfuss D, Saumon G. Ventilator-induced lung injury: lessons from experimental studies. Am J Respir Crit Care Med 1998; 157:294–323.
126. Parker JC, Hernandez LA, Peevy KJ. Mechanisms of ventilator-induced lung injury. Crit Care Med 1993; 21:131–143.
127. Bjorklund LJ, Ingimarsson J, Curstedt T, et al. Manual ventilation with a few large breaths at birth compromises the therapeutic effect of subsequent surfactant replacement in immature lambs. Pediatr Res 1997; 42:348–355.
128. Ingimarsson J, Bjorklund LJ, Curstedt T, et al. Incomplete protection by prophylactic surfactant against the adverse effects of large lung inflations at birth in immature lambs. Intensive Care Med 2004; 30:1446–1453.

129. Muscedere JG, Mullen JB, Gan K, et al. Tidal ventilation at low airway pressures can augment lung injury. Am J Respir Crit Care Med 1994; 149:1327–1334.
130. Taskar V, John J, Evander E, et al. Surfactant dysfunction makes lungs vulnerable to repetitive collapse and reexpansion. Am J Respir Crit Care Med 1997; 155:313–320.
131. Tracy M, Downe L, Holberton J. How safe is intermittent positive pressure ventilation in preterm babies ventilated from delivery to newborn intensive care unit? Arch Dis Child Fetal Neonatal Ed 2004; 89:F84–F87.
132. Saugstad OD, Rootwelt T, Aalen O. Resuscitation of asphyxiated newborn infants with room air or oxygen: an international controlled trial: the Resair 2 study. Pediatrics 1998; 102:e1.
133. Groneck P, Speer CP. Inflammatory mediators and bronchopulmonary dysplasia. Arch Dis Child Fetal Neonatal Ed 1995; 73:F1–F3.
134. Ferreira PJ, Bunch TJ, Albertine KH, et al. Circulating neutrophil concentration and respiratory distress in premature infants. J Pediatr 2000; 136:466–472.
135. Baier RJ, Majid A, Parupia H, et al. CC chemokine concentrations increase in respiratory distress syndrome and correlate with development of bronchopulmonary dysplasia. Pediatr Pulmonol 2004; 37:137–148.
136. Beresford MW, Shaw NJ. Detectable IL-8 and IL-10 in bronchoalveolar lavage fluid from preterm infants ventilated for respiratory distress syndrome. Pediatr Res 2002; 52:973–978.
137. Kotecha S. Cytokines in chronic lung disease of prematurity. Eur J Pediatr 1996; 155(suppl 2):S14–S17.
138. Kotecha S, Wilson L, Wangoo A, et al. Increase in interleukin (IL)-1 beta and IL-6 in bronchoalveolar lavage fluid obtained from infants with chronic lung disease of prematurity. Pediatr Res 1996; 40:250–256.
139. Munshi UK, Niu JO, Siddiq MM, et al. Elevation of interleukin-8 and interleukin-6 precedes the influx of neutrophils in tracheal aspirates from preterm infants who develop bronchopulmonary dysplasia. Pediatr Pulmonol 1997; 24:331–336.
140. Speer CP. New insights into the pathogenesis of pulmonary inflammation in preterm infants. Biol Neonate 2001; 79:205–209.
141. Romero R, Chaiworapongsa T, Espinoza J. Micronutrients and intrauterine infection, preterm birth and the fetal inflammatory response syndrome. J Nutr 2003; 133:1668S–1673S.
142. Jobe AH. Antenatal associations with lung maturation and infection. J Perinatol 2005; 25 (suppl 2):S31–S35.
143. Watterberg KL, Demers LM, Scott SM, et al. Chorioamnionitis and early lung inflammation in infants in whom bronchopulmonary dysplasia develops. Pediatrics 1996; 97: 210–215.
144. Yoon BH, Romero R, Jun JK, et al. Amniotic fluid cytokines (interleukin-6, tumor necrosis factor – alpha, interleukin-1 beta, and interleukin-8) and the risk for the development of bronchopulmonary dysplasia. Am J Obstet Gynecol 1997; 177:825–830.
145. Kim CJ, Yoon BH, Park SS, et al. Acute funisitis of preterm but not term placentas is associated with severe fetal inflammatory response. Hum Pathol 2001; 32:623–629.
146. Matsuda T, Nakajima T, Hattori S, et al. Necrotizing funisitis: clinical significance and association with chronic lung disease in premature infants. Am J Obstet Gynecol 1997; 177:1402–1407.
147. Viscardi RM, Muhumuza CK, Rodriguez A, et al. Inflammatory markers in intrauterine and fetal blood and cerebrospinal fluid compartments are associated with adverse pulmonary and neurologic outcomes in preterm infants. Pediatr Res 2004; 55:1009–1017.
148. Schmidt B, Cao L, Mackensen-Haen S, et al. Chorioamnionitis and inflammation of the fetal lung. Am J Obstet Gynecol 2001; 185:173–177.
149. Kallapur SG, Jobe AH, Ikegami M, et al. Increased IP-10 and MIG expression after intra-amniotic endotoxin in preterm lamb lung. Am J Respir Crit Care Med 2003; 167: 779–786.

150. Ikegami M, Kallapur SG, Jobe AH. Initial responses to ventilation of premature lambs exposed to intra-amniotic endotoxin 4 days before delivery. Am J Physiol Lung Cell Mol Physiol 2004; 286:L573–L579.

151. Van Marter LJ, Dammann O, Allred EN, et al. Chorioamnionitis, mechanical ventilation, and postnatal sepsis as modulators of chronic lung disease in preterm infants. J Pediatr 2002; 140:171–176.

152. Purevdorj E, Zscheppang K, Hoymann HG, et al. ErbB4 deletion leads to changes in lung function and structure similar to bronchopulmonary dysplasia. Am J Physiol Lung Cell Mol Physiol 2008; 294:L516–L522.

153. Lavoie PM, Pham C, Jang KL. Heritability of bronchopulmonary dysplasia, defined according to the consensus statement of the national institutes of health. Pediatrics 2008; 122:479–485.

154. Meng H, Gruen JR. Genetic approaches to complications of prematurity. Front Biosci 2007; 12:2344–2351.

155. Hallman M, Haataja R. Surfactant protein polymorphisms and neonatal lung disease. Semin Perinatol 2006; 30:350–361.

156. Manar MH, Brown MR, Gauthier TW, et al. Association of glutathione-S-transferase-P1 (GST-P1) polymorphisms with bronchopulmonary dysplasia. J Perinatol 2004; 24:30–35.

157. Concolino P, Capoluongo E, Santonocito C, et al. Genetic analysis of the dystroglycan gene in bronchopulmonary dysplasia affected premature newborns. Clin Chim Acta 2007; 378:164–167.

158. Kazzi SN, Quasney MW. Deletion allele of angiotensin-converting enzyme is associated with increased risk and severity of bronchopulmonary dysplasia. J Pediatr 2005; 147:818–822.

159. Kazzi SN, Kim UO, Quasney MW, et al. Polymorphism of tumor necrosis factor-alpha and risk and severity of bronchopulmonary dysplasia among very low birth weight infants. Pediatrics 2004; 114:e243–e248.

160. Kwinta P, Bik-Multanowski M, Mitkowska Z, et al. Genetic risk factors of broncho-pulmonary dysplasia. Pediatr Res 2008; 64:682–688.

161. Darlow BA, Graham PJ. Vitamin A supplementation to prevent mortality and short and long-term morbidity in very low birthweight infants. Cochrane Database Syst Rev 2007; (4):CD000501.

162. Blomhoff R, Green MH, Norum KR. Vitamin A: physiological and biochemical processing. Annu Rev Nutr 1992; 12:37–57.

163. McGowan S, Jackson SK, Jenkins-Moore M, et al. Mice bearing deletions of retinoic acid receptors demonstrate reduced lung elastin and alveolar numbers. Am J Respir Cell Mol Biol 2000; 23:162–167.

164. Massaro GD, Massaro D. Postnatal treatment with retinoic acid increases the number of pulmonary alveoli in rats. Am J Physiol 1996; 270:L305–L310.

165. Pierce RA, Joyce B, Officer S, et al. Retinoids increase lung elastin expression but fail to alter morphology or angiogenesis genes in premature ventilated baboons. Pediatr Res 2007; 61:703–709.

166. Bland RD, Albertine KH, Pierce RA, et al. Impaired alveolar development and abnormal lung elastin in preterm lambs with chronic lung injury: potential benefits of retinol treatment. Biol Neonate 2003; 84:101–102.

167. Shenai JP, Chytil F, Stahlman M. Vitamin A status of neonates with bronchopulmonary dysplasia. Pediatr Res 1985; 19:185–189.

168. Tyson JE, Wright LL, Oh W, et al. Vitamin A supplementation for extremely-low-birth-weight infants. National Institute of Child Health and Human Development Neonatal Research Network. N Engl J Med 1999; 340:1962–1968.

169. Ambalavanan N, Tyson JE, Kennedy KA, et al. Vitamin A supplementation for extremely low birth weight infants: outcome at 18 to 22 months. Pediatrics 2005; 115:e249–e254.

170. Ambalavanan N, Wu TJ, Tyson JE, et al. A comparison of three vitamin A dosing regimens in extremely-low-birth-weight infants. J Pediatr 2003; 142:656–661.
171. Wardle SP, Hughes A, Chen S, et al. Randomised controlled trial of oral vitamin A supplementation in preterm infants to prevent chronic lung disease. Arch Dis Child Fetal Neonatal Ed 2001; 84:F9–F13.
172. Sheffield M, Mabry S, Thibeault DW, et al. Pulmonary nitric oxide synthases and nitrotyrosine: findings during lung development and in chronic lung disease of prematurity. Pediatrics 2006; 118:1056–1064.
173. Hu X, Guo C, Sun B. Inhaled nitric oxide attenuates hyperoxic and inflammatory injury without alteration of phosphatidylcholine synthesis in rat lungs. Pulm Pharmacol Ther 2007; 20:75–84.
174. Kinsella JP, Parker TA, Galan H, et al. Effects of inhaled nitric oxide on pulmonary edema and lung neutrophil accumulation in severe experimental hyaline membrane disease. Pediatr Res 1997; 41:457–463.
175. ter Horst SA, Walther FJ, Poorthuis BJ, et al. Inhaled nitric oxide attenuates pulmonary inflammation and fibrin deposition and prolongs survival in neonatal hyperoxic lung injury. Am J Physiol Lung Cell Mol Physiol 2007; 293:L35–L44.
176. Zhu Y, Guo C, Cao L, et al. Different effects of surfactant and inhaled nitric oxide in modulation of inflammatory injury in ventilated piglet lungs. Pulm Pharmacol Ther 2005; 18:303–313.
177. Gong X, Guo C, Huang S, et al. Inhaled nitric oxide alleviates hyperoxia suppressed phosphatidylcholine synthesis in endotoxin-induced injury in mature rat lungs. Respir Res 2006; 7:5.
178. Tang JR, Markham NE, Lin YJ, et al. Inhaled nitric oxide attenuates pulmonary hypertension and improves lung growth in infant rats after neonatal treatment with a VEGF receptor inhibitor. Am J Physiol Lung Cell Mol Physiol 2004; 287:L344–L351.
179. Tang JR, Seedorf G, Balasubramaniam V, et al. Early inhaled nitric oxide treatment decreases apoptosis of endothelial cells in neonatal rat lungs after vascular endothelial growth factor inhibition. Am J Physiol Lung Cell Mol Physiol 2007; 293:L1271–L1280.
180. Lin YJ, Markham NE, Balasubramaniam V, et al. Inhaled nitric oxide enhances distal lung growth after exposure to hyperoxia in neonatal rats. Pediatr Res 2005; 58:22–29.
181. McCurnin DC, Pierce RA, Chang LY, et al. Inhaled NO improves early pulmonary function and modifies lung growth and elastin deposition in a baboon model of neonatal chronic lung disease. Am J Physiol Lung Cell Mol Physiol 2005; 288:L450–L459.
182. Bland RD, Albertine KH, Carlton DP, et al. Inhaled nitric oxide effects on lung structure and function in chronically ventilated preterm lambs. Am J Respir Crit Care Med 2005; 172:899–906.
183. Balasubramaniam V, Maxey AM, Morgan DB, et al. Inhaled NO restores lung structure in eNOS-deficient mice recovering from neonatal hypoxia. Am J Physiol Lung Cell Mol Physiol 2006; 291:L119–L127.
184. Balasubramaniam V, Maxey AM, Fouty BW, et al. Nitric oxide augments fetal pulmonary artery endothelial cell angiogenesis in vitro. Am J Physiol Lung Cell Mol Physiol 2006; 290:L1111–L1116.
185. Ballard RA, Truog WE, Cnaan A, et al. Inhaled nitric oxide in preterm infants undergoing mechanical ventilation. N Engl J Med 2006; 355:343–353.
186. Kinsella JP, Cutter GR, Walsh WF, et al. Early inhaled nitric oxide therapy in premature newborns with respiratory failure. N Engl J Med 2006; 355:354–364.
187. Schreiber MD, Gin-Mestan K, Marks JD, et al. Inhaled nitric oxide in premature infants with the respiratory distress syndrome. N Engl J Med 2003; 349:2099–2107.
188. Van Meurs KP, Wright LL, Ehrenkranz RA, et al. Inhaled nitric oxide for premature infants with severe respiratory failure. N Engl J Med 2005; 353:13–22.

189. Truog WE, Ballard PL, Norberg M, et al. Inflammatory markers and mediators in tracheal fluid of premature infants treated with inhaled nitric oxide. Pediatrics 2007; 119:670–678.
190. Ballard PL, Merrill JD, Truog WE, et al. Surfactant function and composition in premature infants treated with inhaled nitric oxide. Pediatrics 2007; 120:346–353.
191. Mestan KK, Marks JD, Hecox K, et al. Neurodevelopmental outcomes of premature infants treated with inhaled nitric oxide. N Engl J Med 2005; 353:23–32.
192. Hintz SR, Van Meurs KP, Perritt R, et al. Neurodevelopmental outcomes of premature infants with severe respiratory failure enrolled in a randomized controlled trial of inhaled nitric oxide. J Pediatr 2007; 151:16–22, e1–e3.
193. Thomson MA, Yoder BA, Winter VT, et al. Delayed extubation to nasal continuous positive airway pressure in the immature baboon model of bronchopulmonary dysplasia: lung clinical and pathological findings. Pediatrics 2006; 118:2038–2050.
194. te Pas AB, Walther FJ. A randomized, controlled trial of delivery-room respiratory management in very preterm infants. Pediatrics 2007; 120:322–329.
195. Finer NN, Carlo WA, Duara S, et al. Delivery room continuous positive airway pressure/positive end-expiratory pressure in extremely low birth weight infants: a feasibility trial. Pediatrics 2004; 114:651–657.
196. te Pas AB, Lopriore E, Engbers MJ, et al. Early respiratory management of respiratory distress syndrome in very preterm infants and bronchopulmonary dysplasia: a case-control study. PLoS ONE 2007; 2:e192.
197. Ammari A, Suri M, Milisavljevic V, et al. Variables associated with the early failure of nasal CPAP in very low birth weight infants. J Pediatr 2005; 147:341–347.
198. De Klerk AM, De Klerk RK. Nasal continuous positive airway pressure and outcomes of preterm infants. J Paediatr Child Health 2001; 37:161–167.
199. Narendran V, Donovan EF, Hoath SB, et al. Early bubble CPAP and outcomes in ELBW preterm infants. J Perinatol 2003; 23:195–199.
200. Morley CJ, Davis PG, Doyle LW, et al. Nasal CPAP or intubation at birth for very preterm infants. N Engl J Med 2008; 358:700–708.
201. Blennow M, Jonsson B, Dahlstrom A, et al. [Lung function in premature infants can be improved. Surfactant therapy and CPAP reduce the need of respiratory support]. Lakartidningen 1999; 96:1571–1576.
202. Verder H, Robertson B, Greisen G, et al. Surfactant therapy and nasal continuous positive airway pressure for newborns with respiratory distress syndrome. Danish-Swedish Multicenter Study Group. N Engl J Med 1994; 331:1051–1055.
203. Dani C, Bertini G, Pezzati M, et al. Early extubation and nasal continuous positive airway pressure after surfactant treatment for respiratory distress syndrome among preterm infants <30 weeks' gestation. Pediatrics 2004; 113:e560–e563.
204. Reininger A, Khalak R, Kendig JW, et al. Surfactant administration by transient intubation in infants 29 to 35 weeks' gestation with respiratory distress syndrome decreases the likelihood of later mechanical ventilation: a randomized controlled trial. J Perinatol 2005; 25:703–708.
205. Tooley J, Dyke M. Randomized study of nasal continuous positive airway pressure in the preterm infant with respiratory distress syndrome. Acta Paediatr 2003; 92:1170–1174.
206. Texas Neonatal Research Group. Early surfactant for neonates with mild to moderate respiratory distress syndrome: a multicenter, randomized trial. J Pediatr 2004; 144:804–808.
207. Stevens TP, Harrington EW, Blennow M, et al. Early surfactant administration with brief ventilation vs. selective surfactant and continued mechanical ventilation for preterm infants with or at risk for respiratory distress syndrome. Cochrane Database Syst Rev 2007:CD003063.
208. Barrington KJ, Bull D, Finer NN. Randomized trial of nasal synchronized intermittent mandatory ventilation compared with continuous positive airway pressure after extubation of very low birth weight infants. Pediatrics 2001; 107:638–641.

209. Friedlich P, Lecart C, Posen R, et al. A randomized trial of nasopharyngeal-synchronized intermittent mandatory ventilation versus nasopharyngeal continuous positive airway pressure in very low birth weight infants after extubation. J Perinatol 1999; 19:413–418.

210. Khalaf MN, Brodsky N, Hurley J, et al. A prospective randomized, controlled trial comparing synchronized nasal intermittent positive pressure ventilation versus nasal continuous positive airway pressure as modes of extubation. Pediatrics 2001; 108:13–17.

211. Davis PG, Lemyre B, de Paoli AG. Nasal intermittent positive pressure ventilation (NIPPV) versus nasal continuous positive airway pressure (NCPAP) for preterm neonates after extubation. CochraneDatabase Syst Rev 2001:CD003212.

212. Bhandari V, Gavino RG, Nedrelow JH, et al. A randomized controlled trial of synchronized nasal intermittent positive pressure ventilation in RDS. J Perinatol 2007; 27:697–703.

213. Strand M, Ikegami M, Jobe AH. Effects of high PCO2 on ventilated preterm lamb lungs. Pediatr Res 2003; 53:468–472.

214. Mariani G, Cifuentes J, Carlo WA. Randomized trial of permissive hypercapnia in preterm infants. Pediatrics 1999; 104:1082–1088.

215. Woodgate PG, Davies MW. Permissive hypercapnia for the prevention of morbidity and mortality in mechanically ventilated newborn infants. Cochrane Database Syst Rev 2001: CD002061.

216. Carlo WA, Stark AR, Wright LL, et al. Minimal ventilation to prevent bronchopulmonary dysplasia in extremely-low-birth-weight infants. J Pediatr 2002; 141:370–374.

217. Courtney SE, Durand DJ, Asselin JM, et al. High-frequency oscillatory ventilation versus conventional mechanical ventilation for very-low-birth-weight infants. N Engl J Med 2002; 347:643–652.

218. Johnson AH, Peacock JL, Greenough A, et al. High-frequency oscillatory ventilation for the prevention of chronic lung disease of prematurity. N Engl J Med 2002; 347:633–642.

219. Moriette G, Paris-Llado J, Walti H, et al. Prospective randomized multicenter comparison of high-frequency oscillatory ventilation and conventional ventilation in preterm infants of less than 30 weeks with respiratory distress syndrome. Pediatrics 2001; 107:363–372.

220. Van Reempts P, Borstlap C, Laroche S, et al. Early use of high frequency ventilation in the premature neonate. Eur J Pediatr 2003; 162:219–226.

221. Henderson-Smart DJ, Cools F, Bhuta T, et al. Elective high frequency oscillatory ventilation versus conventional ventilation for acute pulmonary dysfunction in preterm infants. Cochrane Database Syst Rev 2007:CD000104.

222. Keszler M, Modanlou HD, Brudno DS, et al. Multicenter controlled clinical trial of high-frequency jet ventilation in preterm infants with uncomplicated respiratory distress syndrome. Pediatrics 1997; 100:593–599.

223. Wiswell TE, Graziani LJ, Kornhauser MS, et al. High-frequency jet ventilation in the early management of respiratory distress syndrome is associated with a greater risk for adverse outcomes. Pediatrics 1996; 98:1035–1043.

224. Schmidt B, Roberts RS, Davis P, et al. Caffeine therapy for apnea of prematurity. N Engl J Med 2006; 354:2112–2121.

225. Schmidt B, Roberts RS, Davis P, et al. Long-term effects of caffeine therapy for apnea of prematurity. N Engl J Med 2007; 357:1893–1902.

226. Nykanen P, Anttila E, Heinonen K, et al. Early hypoadrenalism in premature infants at risk for bronchopulmonary dysplasia or death. Acta Paediatr 2007; 96:1600–1605.

227. Watterberg KL, Scott SM, Naeye RL. Chorioamnionitis, cortisol, and acute lung disease in very low birth weight infants. Pediatrics 1997; 99:E6.

228. Banks BA, Stouffer N, Cnaan A, et al. Association of plasma cortisol and chronic lung disease in preterm infants. Pediatrics 2001; 107:494–498.

229. Watterberg KL, Scott SM, Backstrom C, et al. Links between early adrenal function and respiratory outcome in preterm infants: airway inflammation and patent ductus arteriosus. Pediatrics 2000; 105:320–324.

230. Watterberg KL, Gerdes JS, Gifford KL, et al. Prophylaxis against early adrenal insufficiency to prevent chronic lung disease in premature infants. Pediatrics 1999; 104: 1258–1263.
231. Watterberg KL, Gerdes JS, Cole CH, et al. Prophylaxis of early adrenal insufficiency to prevent bronchopulmonary dysplasia: a multicenter trial. Pediatrics 2004; 114:1649–1657.
232. Watterberg KL, Shaffer ML, Mishefske MJ, et al. Growth and neurodevelopmental outcomes after early low-dose hydrocortisone treatment in extremely low birth weight infants. Pediatrics 2007; 120:40–48.
233. Rademaker KJ, Uiterwaal CS, Groenendaal F, et al. Neonatal hydrocortisone treatment: neurodevelopmental outcome and MRI at school age in preterm-born children. J Pediatr 2007; 150:351–357.
234. Doyle LW, Davis PG, Morley CJ, et al. Low-dose dexamethasone facilitates extubation among chronically ventilator-dependent infants: a multicenter, international, randomized, controlled trial. Pediatrics 2006; 117:75–83.
235. Doyle LW, Davis PG, Morley CJ, et al. Outcome at 2 years of age of infants from the DART study: a multicenter, international, randomized, controlled trial of low-dose dexamethasone. Pediatrics 2007; 119:716–21.
236. Yoder MC Jr., Chua R, Tepper R. Effect of dexamethasone on pulmonary inflammation and pulmonary function of ventilator-dependent infants with bronchopulmonary dysplasia. Am Rev Respir Dis 1991; 143:1044–1048.
237. Avery GB, Fletcher AB, Kaplan M, et al. Controlled trial of dexamethasone in respirator-dependent infants with bronchopulmonary dysplasia. Pediatrics 1985; 75:106–111.
238. Cummings JJ, D'Eugenio DB, Gross SJ. A controlled trial of dexamethasone in preterm infants at high risk for bronchopulmonary dysplasia. N Engl J Med 1989; 320:1505–1510.
239. Kothadia JM, O'Shea TM, Roberts D, et al. Randomized placebo-controlled trial of a 42-day tapering course of dexamethasone to reduce the duration of ventilator dependency in very low birth weight infants. Pediatrics 1999; 104:22–27.
240. Mammel MC, Green TP, Johnson DE, et al. Controlled trial of dexamethasone therapy in infants with bronchopulmonary dysplasia. Lancet 1983; 1:1356–1358.
241. Ohlsson A, Calvert SA, Hosking M, et al. Randomized controlled trial of dexamethasone treatment in very-low-birth-weight infants with ventilator-dependent chronic lung disease. Acta Paediatr 1992; 81:751–756.
242. Rastogi A, Akintorin SM, Bez ML, et al. A controlled trial of dexamethasone to prevent bronchopulmonary dysplasia in surfactant-treated infants. Pediatrics 1996; 98:204–210.
243. Sinkin RA, Dweck HS, Horgan MJ, et al. Early dexamethasone-attempting to prevent chronic lung disease. Pediatrics 2000; 105:542–548.
244. Yeh TF, Lin YJ, Hsieh WS, et al. Early postnatal dexamethasone therapy for the prevention of chronic lung disease in preterm infants with respiratory distress syndrome: a multicenter clinical trial. Pediatrics 1997; 100:E3.
245. Bhuta T, Ohlsson A. Systematic review and meta-analysis of early postnatal dexamethasone for prevention of chronic lung disease. Arch Dis Child Fetal Neonatal Ed 1998; 79: F26–F33.
246. Durand M, Sardesai S, McEvoy C. Effects of early dexamethasone therapy on pulmonary mechanics and chronic lung disease in very low birth weight infants: a randomized, controlled trial. Pediatrics 1995; 95:584–590.
247. Garland JS, Alex CP, Pauly TH, et al. A three-day course of dexamethasone therapy to prevent chronic lung disease in ventilated neonates: a randomized trial. Pediatrics 1999; 104:91–99.
248. Kari MA, Hallman M, Eronen M, et al. Prenatal dexamethasone treatment in conjunction with rescue therapy of human surfactant: a randomized placebo-controlled multicenter study. Pediatrics 1994; 93:730–736.

249. Onland W, De Jaegere AP, Offringa M, et al. Effects of higher versus lower dexamethasone doses on pulmonary and neurodevelopmental sequelae in preterm infants at risk for chronic lung disease: a meta-analysis. Pediatrics 2008; 122:92–101.

250. O'Shea TM, Kothadia JM, Klinepeter KL, et al. Randomized placebo-controlled trial of a 42-day tapering course of dexamethasone to reduce the duration of ventilator dependency in very low birth weight infants: outcome of study participants at 1-year adjusted age. Pediatrics 1999; 104:15–21.

251. Yeh TF, Lin YJ, Lin HC, et al. Outcomes at school age after postnatal dexamethasone therapy for lung disease of prematurity. N Engl J Med 2004; 350:1304–1313.

252. Stark AR, Carlo WA, Tyson JE, et al. Adverse effects of early dexamethasone in extremely-low-birth-weight infants. National Institute of Child Health and Human Development Neonatal Research Network. N Engl J Med 2001; 344:95–101.

253. Yeh TF, Lin YJ, Huang CC, et al. Early dexamethasone therapy in preterm infants: a follow-up study. Pediatrics 1998; 101:E7.

254. Parikh NA, Lasky RE, Kennedy KA, et al. Postnatal dexamethasone therapy and cerebral tissue volumes in extremely low birth weight infants. Pediatrics 2007; 119:265–272.

255. O'Shea TM, Washburn LK, Nixon PA, et al. Follow-up of a randomized, placebo-controlled trial of dexamethasone to decrease the duration of ventilator dependency in very low birth weight infants: neurodevelopmental outcomes at 4 to 11 years of age. Pediatrics 2007; 120:594–602.

256. Vermont Oxford Study Group. Early postnatal dexamethasone therapy for the prevention of chronic lung disease. Pediatrics 2001; 108:741–748.

257. Papile LA, Tyson JE, Stoll BJ, et al. A multicenter trial of two dexamethasone regimens in ventilator-dependent premature infants. N Engl J Med 1998; 338:1112–1118.

258. Shinwell ES, Karplus M, Zmora E, et al. Failure of early postnatal dexamethasone to prevent chronic lung disease in infants with respiratory distress syndrome. Arch Dis Child Fetal Neonatal Ed 1996; 74:F33–F37.

259. Smets K, Vanhaesebrouck P. Dexamethasone associated systemic hypertension in low birth weight babies with chronic lung disease. Eur J Pediatr 1996; 155:573–575.

260. Bensky AS, Kothadia JM, Covitz W. Cardiac effects of dexamethasone in very low birth weight infants. Pediatrics 1996; 97:818–821.

261. Brand PL, van Lingen RA, Brus F, et al. Hypertrophic obstructive cardiomyopathy as a side effect of dexamethasone treatment for bronchopulmonary dysplasia. Acta Paediatr 1993; 82:614–617.

262. Evans N. Cardiovascular effects of dexamethasone in the preterm infant. Arch Dis Child Fetal Neonatal Ed 1994; 70:F25–F30.

263. Haney I, Lachance C, van Doesburg NH, et al. Reversible steroid-induced hypertrophic cardiomyopathy with left ventricular outflow tract obstruction in two newborns. Am J Perinatol 1995; 12:271–274.

264. Israel BA, Sherman FS, Guthrie RD. Hypertrophic cardiomyopathy associated with dexamethasone therapy for chronic lung disease in preterm infants. Am J Perinatol 1993; 10:307–310.

265. Skelton R, Gill AB, Parsons JM. Cardiac effects of short course dexamethasone in preterm infants. Arch Dis Child Fetal Neonatal Ed 1998; 78:F133–F137.

266. Halliday HL, Patterson CC, Halahakoon CW, Behalf of the European Multicenter Steroid Study G. A multicenter, randomized open study of early corticosteroid treatment (OSECT) in preterm infants with respiratory illness: comparison of early and late treatment and of dexamethasone and inhaled budesonide. Pediatrics 2001; 107:232–240.

267. Arnold JD, Leslie GI, Williams G, et al. Adrenocortical responsiveness in neonates weaned from the ventilator with dexamethasone. Aust Paediatr J 1987; 23:227–229.

268. Ford LR, Willi SM, Hollis BW, et al. Suppression and recovery of the neonatal hypothalamic-pituitary-adrenal axis after prolonged dexamethasone therapy. J Pediatr 1997; 131:722–726.

269. Stoll BJ, Temprosa M, Tyson JE, et al. Dexamethasone therapy increases infection in very low birth weight infants. Pediatrics 1999; 104:e63.

270. Cole CH, Colton T, Shah BL, et al. Early inhaled glucocorticoid therapy to prevent bronchopulmonary dysplasia. N Engl J Med 1999; 340:1005–1010.

271. Shah V, Ohlsson A, Halliday HL, et al. Early administration of inhaled corticosteroids for preventing chronic lung disease in ventilated very low birth weight preterm neonates. Cochrane Database Syst Rev 2007:CD001969.

272. Shinwell ES, Lerner-Geva L, Lusky A, et al. Less postnatal steroids, more broncho-pulmonary dysplasia: a population-based study in very low birthweight infants. Arch Dis Child Fetal Neonatal Ed 2007; 92:F30–F33.

273. Banks BA. Postnatal dexamethasone for bronchopulmonary dysplasia. NeoReviews 2004; 3:e24–e34.

274. Halliday HL, Ehrenkranz RA, Doyle LW. Early postnatal (<96 hours) corticosteroids for preventing chronic lung disease in preterm infants. Cochrane Database Syst Rev 2003: CD001146.

275. Doyle LW, Halliday HL, Ehrenkranz RA, et al. Impact of postnatal systemic corticosteroids on mortality and cerebral palsy in preterm infants: effect modification by risk for chronic lung disease. Pediatrics 2005; 115:655–661.

276. AAP Committee on Fetus and Newborn. CPS Fetus and Newborn Committee. Postnatal Corticosteroids to treat or prevent chronic lung disease in preterm infants. Pediatrics 2002; 109:330–340.

277. Eichenwald E, Stark A. Are postnatal steroids ever justified to treat severe broncho-pulmonary dysplasia? Arch Dis Child 2007; 92:F334–F337.

278. Grier DG, Halliday HL. Management of bronchopulmonary dysplasia in infants: guidelines for corticosteroid use. Drugs 2005; 65:15–29.

279. Collard KJ, Godeck S, Holley JE, et al. Pulmonary antioxidant concentrations and oxidative damage in ventilated premature babies. Arch Dis Child Fetal Neonatal Ed 2004; 89: F412–F416.

280. Kaarteenaho-Wiik R, Kinnula VL. Distribution of antioxidant enzymes in developing human lung, respiratory distress syndrome, and bronchopulmonary dysplasia. J Histochem Cytochem 2004; 52:1231–1240.

281. Zoban P, Cerny M. Immature lung and acute lung injury. Physiol Res 2003; 52:507–516.

282. Rosenfeld W, Evans H, Concepcion L, et al. Prevention of bronchopulmonary dysplasia by administration of bovine superoxide dismutase in preterm infants with respiratory distress syndrome. J Pediatr 1984; 105:781–785.

283. Ahola T, Lapatto R, Raivio KO, et al. N-acetylcysteine does not prevent bronchopulmonary dysplasia in immature infants: a randomized controlled trial. J Pediatr 2003; 143:713–719.

284. Davis JM, Parad RB, Michele T, et al. Pulmonary outcome at 1 year corrected age in premature infants treated at birth with recombinant human CuZn superoxide dismutase. Pediatrics 2003; 111:469–476.

285. Dunn M, Stiskal J, O'Brien K, et al. A1 proteinase inhibitor (A1P1) therapy for the pre-vention of chronic lung disease of prematurity (CLD)—a dose ranging study and meta analysis with previous randomized clinical trial (RTC). Pediatr Res 2000:397A.

286. Stiskal JA, Dunn MS, Shennan AT, et al. alpha1-Proteinase inhibitor therapy for the pre-vention of chronic lung disease of prematurity: a randomized, controlled trial. Pediatrics 1998; 101:89–94.

287. Shah P, Ohlsson A. Alpha-1 proteinase inhibitor (a1PI) for preventing chronic lung disease in preterm infants. Cochrane Database Syst Rev 2001:CD002775.

288. McCurnin D, Seidner S, Chang LY, et al. Ibuprofen-induced patent ductus arteriosus closure: physiologic, histologic, and biochemical effects on the premature lung. Pediatrics 2008; 121:945–956.
289. Schmidt B, Roberts RS, Fanaroff A, et al. Indomethacin prophylaxis, patent ductus arteriosus, and the risk of bronchopulmonary dysplasia: further analyses from the Trial of Indomethacin Prophylaxis in Preterms (TIPP). J Pediatr 2006; 148:730–734.
290. Eronen M, Pesonen E, Kurki T, et al. Increased incidence of bronchopulmonary dysplasia after antenatal administration of indomethacin to prevent preterm labor. J Pediatr 1994; 124:782–788.
291. Suresh GK, Davis JM, Soll RF. Superoxide dismutase for preventing chronic lung disease in mechanically ventilated preterm infants. Cochrane Database Syst Rev 2001:CD001968.
292. Soll RF, Morley CJ. Prophylactic versus selective use of surfactant in preventing morbidity and mortality in preterm infants. Cochrane Database Syst Rev 2001:CD000510.
293. Crowther CA, Alfirevic Z, Haslam RR. Thyrotropin-releasing hormone added to corticosteroids for women at risk of preterm birth for preventing neonatal respiratory disease. Cochrane Database Syst Rev 2004:CD000019.
294. Shah SS, Ohlsson A, Halliday H, et al. Inhaled versus systemic corticosteroids for the treatment of chronic lung disease in ventilated very low birth weight preterm infants. Cochrane Database Syst Rev 2007:CD002057.
295. Halliday HL, Ehrenkranz RA, Doyle LW. Moderately early (7–14 days) postnatal corticosteroids for preventing chronic lung disease in preterm infants. Cochrane Database Syst Rev 2003:CD001144.
296. Halliday HL, Ehrenkranz RA, Doyle LW. Delayed (>3 weeks) postnatal corticosteroids for chronic lung disease in preterm infants. Cochrane Database Syst Rev 2003:CD001145.
297. Howlett A, Ohlsson A. Inositol for respiratory distress syndrome in preterm infants. Cochrane Database Syst Rev 2003:CD000366.
298. Subramaniam P, Henderson-Smart DJ, Davis PG. Prophylactic nasal continuous positive airways pressure for preventing morbidity and mortality in very preterm infants. Cochrane Database Syst Rev 2005:CD001243.
299. Davis PG, Henderson-Smart DJ. Nasal continuous positive airways pressure immediately after extubation for preventing morbidity in preterm infants. Cochrane Database Syst Rev 2003:CD000143.
300. Greenough A, Dimitriou G, Prendergast M, et al. Synchronized mechanical ventilation for respiratory support in newborn infants. Cochrane Database Syst Rev 2008:CD000456.
301. Bhuta T, Henderson-Smart D. Elective high frequency jet ventilation versus conventional ventilation for respiratory distress syndrome in preterm infants. Cochrane Database Syst Rev 1998:CD000328.
302. Barrington KJ, Finer NN. Inhaled nitric oxide for respiratory failure in preterm infants. Cochrane Database Syst Rev 2007:CD000509.
303. Ng GY, da S, Ohlsson A. Bronchodilators for the prevention and treatment of chronic lung disease in preterm infants. Cochrane Database Syst Rev 2001:CD003214.
304. Mabanta CG, Pryhuber GS, Weinberg GA, et al. Erythromycin for the prevention of chronic lung disease in intubated preterm infants at risk for, or colonized or infected with Ureaplasma urealyticum. Cochrane Database Syst Rev 2003:CD003744.
305. Bennett AJ, Shaw NJ, Gregg JE, et al. Neurodevelopmental outcome in high-risk preterm infants treated with inhaled nitric oxide. Acta Paediatr 2001; 90:573–576.
306. Subhedar NV, Ryan SW, Shaw NJ. Open randomised controlled trial of inhaled nitric oxide and early dexamethasone in high risk preterm infants. Arch Dis Child Fetal Neonatal Ed 1997; 77:F185–F190.
307. Franco Belgium Collaborative NO Trial Group. Early compared with delayed inhaled nitric oxide in moderately hypoxaemic neonates with respiratory failure: a randomised controlled trial. Lancet 1999; 354:1066–1071.

308. Srisuparp P, Heitschmidt M, Schreiber MD. Inhaled nitric oxide therapy in premature infants with mild to moderate respiratory distress syndrome. J Med Assoc Thai 2002; 85 (suppl 2):S469–S478.

309. Hascoet JM, Fresson J, Claris O, et al. The safety and efficacy of nitric oxide therapy in premature infants. J Pediatr 2005; 146:318–323.

310. Field D, Elbourne D, Truesdale A, et al. Neonatal ventilation with inhaled nitric oxide versus ventilatory support without inhaled nitric oxide for preterm infants with severe respiratory failure: the INNOVO multicentre randomised controlled trial (ISRCTN 17821339). Pediatrics 2005; 115:926–936.

311. Huddy CL, Bennett CC, Hardy P, et al. The INNOVO multicentre randomised controlled trial: neonatal ventilation with inhaled nitric oxide versus ventilatory support without nitric oxide for severe respiratory failure in preterm infants: follow up at 4–5 years. Arch Dis Child Fetal Neonatal Ed 2008; 93:F430–F435.

312. Dani C, Bertini G, Pezzati M, et al. Inhaled nitric oxide in very preterm infants with severe respiratory distress syndrome. Acta Paediatr 2006; 95:1116–1123.

313. Kinsella JP, Walsh WF, Bose CL, et al. Inhaled nitric oxide in premature neonates with severe hypoxaemic respiratory failure: a randomised controlled trial. Lancet 1999; 354:1061–1065.

314. Hibbs AM, Walsh MC, Martin RJ, et al. One-year respiratory outcomes of preterm infants enrolled in the Nitric Oxide (to prevent) Chronic Lung Disease trial. J Pediatr 2008; 153:525–529.

315. Walsh M, Hibbs A, Martin R, et al. Neurodevelopmental outcomes at 24 months for extremely low birth weight neonates in the NO CLD trial of inhaled nitric oxide (iNO) to prevent bronchopulmonary dysplasia (BPD). Pediatric Academic Societies. Honolulu, Hawaii; 2008.

316. Kinsella J, Cutter G, Walsh W, et al. Outcomes of premature infants enrolled in the early inhaled nitric oxide for the prevention of chronic lung disease trial. Pediatric Academic Societies. Baltimore, Maryland; 2009.

317. Van Meurs KP, Hintz SR, Ehrenkranz RA, et al. Inhaled nitric oxide in infants >1500 g and <34 weeks gestation with severe respiratory failure. J Perinatol 2007; 27:347–352.

14
Definitions of Bronchopulmonary Dysplasia and the Use of Benchmarking to Compare Outcomes

MICHELE C. WALSH

Rainbow Babies and Children's Hospital, Case Western Reserve University School of Medicine, Cleveland, Ohio, U.S.A.

I. Introduction

Improved treatments of smaller and sicker infants with mechanical ventilation in the 1960s led to increasing survival. Soon thereafter, pulmonary sequelae were described by Northway and colleagues who introduced the term bronchopulmonary dysplasia (BPD) (1). Both the terms bronchopulmonary dysplasia (BPD) and chronic lung disease (CLD) have been used interchangeably. At a 2001 National Institutes of Health, participants recommended that the term BPD be used to describe the pulmonary sequelae of respiratory distress syndrome (RDS) and prematurity because BPD emphasized the involvement of all of the tissues of the lung, and was a term reserved solely to survivors of preterm birth (2). Since the original description by Northway, the natural history of BPD has evolved and newer definitions have been proposed. Original definitions were dichotomous based on exposure to oxygen supplementation at various time points. However, increasingly it has been recognized that dichotomous outcomes fail to adequately describe the long-term pulmonary outcomes of these fragile infants. These definitions attempt to improve the specificity of the diagnosis of BPD as an outcome measure of clinical care and research trials. This chapter discusses the definitions of BPD and the use of benchmarking techniques to compare BPD outcomes.

II. Definition of Northway

All infants originally described by Northway and colleagues had severe RDS, received prolonged mechanical ventilation, and were exposed to high concentrations of inspired oxygen (1). Northway described a progression of disease through four stages that ended with severe chronic changes, characterized by persistent respiratory failure, hypoxemia, and hypercapnia. Radiographs of infants with stage IV disease showed areas of increased density due to fibrosis alternating with areas of hyperinflation. Late follow-up of these infants at age 7 to 11 years demonstrated persistent and significant pulmonary morbidity (3). By the late 1970s, there was increasing recognition that damage from large tidal volume ventilation strategies contributed to BPD. Modifications of these strategies decreased the incidence of the classic stages described by Northway. Therefore, investigators proposed definitions based on clinical and radiographic characteristics.

III.   Definitions Based on Oxygen Utilization

Bancalari and colleagues were among the first to propose a definition based on clinical characteristics including the need for oxygen on 28 of the first 28 days, together with a compatible chest radiograph (4). Subsequently, Tooley (5) and O'Brodovich and Mellins (6) provided additional support for this definition. Palta et al. explored the utility and predictive validity of various definitions of BPD in the Newborn Lung Project in the late 1980s (7). Her group found that clinical characteristics combined with chest radiograph were predictive of later pulmonary morbidity. These early definitions focused on outcomes at the first month of life. However, as smaller and more immature neonates were resuscitated, treated for RDS, and survived, the significance of a continued oxygen requirement at 28 days was questioned: Could the continued oxygen requirement represent pulmonary immaturity rather than true pulmonary injury? By the late 1970s, authors noted that the radiographic abnormalities in ELBW differed from those described by Northway (8). Fletcher and colleagues compared different definitions of BPD and found that radiographs did not improve either the sensitivity or the specificity of the diagnosis (9).

In 1988, Shennan and coworkers compared the ability of continued treatment with oxygen at 28 days of age and 36 weeks of postmenstrual age (PMA) in neonates less than 1500 g birth weight (10). The authors defined abnormal pulmonary outcomes as one or more of the following in the first two years of life: death in the first two years of life, oxygen at 40 weeks' PMA, surgical procedure involving respiratory tract, two or more hospitalizations for respiratory cause, wheezing requiring drug treatment, and persistent radiographic changes at one year of age. The study cohort had a mean birth weight of 1132 g in those with a normal outcome ($n = 486$) and 992 g in those with an abnormal outcome ($n = 119$); 74 of the 119 (62%) with abnormal outcome were ventilated. The 28-day definition did correctly identify neonates less than 30 weeks' gestation who went on to have an abnormal pulmonary outcome; however, it performed less well for older infants. A requirement for oxygen at 28 days had a positive predictive value of only 38% for later abnormal pulmonary function. In contrast, oxygen requirement at 36 weeks' PMA increased the positive predictive value to 63% and the sensitivity from 79% to 83%.

In another study, Davis and colleagues evaluated the utility of defining BPD at different PMA cutoff points. They compared serial time points from 28 days postnatal to 2-week intervals between 32 and 40 weeks' PMA (11). The investigators found that while 36 weeks' PMA was the most accurate time point for prediction of later sequelae, continued oxygen use at 40 weeks' PMA was a better predictor of long-term neuro-sensory outcomes (Table 1).

Since the original work by Shennan, many studies have validated the utility of the diagnosis of clinical BPD at 36 weeks' PMA as a significant risk factor for future pulmonary and neurodevelopmental impairment (12–17). Even after the adjustment for gestational age and initial severity of illness, BPD is among the most significant predictors of future neurodevelopmental impairment in infancy, early childhood, and adolescence. In a longitudinal study by Short and coworkers evaluating survivors at eight years of age, neonates with BPD (54%) were more likely to be enrolled in special

Table 1 Duration After Which Oxygen Therapy Stopped and Prediction of Pulmonary and Neurological Outcomes

	Postmenstrual age (wk)			
	34	36	38	40
Pulmonary outcomes				
Positive predictive value	68	75	82	90
Negative predictive value	57	57	56	55
Accuracy	62	63	62	62
Neurological outcomes				
Positive predictive value	42	45	51	53
Negative predictive value	73	72	72	71
Accuracy	59	63	67	68

education classes (54%) compared with a matched very low birth weight (VLBW) cohort (37%) or with term children (25%) (17). In addition, more BPD children (20%) achieved full-scale IQ scores <70 in the mental retardation range, compared with either VLBW (11%) or term (3%) children. Only recently, the pulmonary outcomes of these infants have been studied (18). The findings are sobering with higher rates of asthma, and diminished pulmonary function into adolescence. The longer-term impact on the development of chronic obstructive pulmonary disease in the presence and absence of tobacco exposure is not known, nor is the impact on longevity.

IV. Definitions Based on Continuous Measures

While moving the definition of BPD to a time point at 36 weeks improved the specificity and positive predictive value of the BPD definition, many remained concerned that neonates who might have suffered significant pulmonary injury were lost in the 36-week definition. In addition, neonates >32 weeks were not well classified by the 36-week definition, as it was possible for a 2-week-old, 34-week gestational age neonate who remained in oxygen to be classified as BPD at 36 weeks' PMA but to have resolved lung injury and weaned to room air at 38 weeks' PMA (28 days postdelivery).

The NIH Consensus definition addressed these competing needs (2). The definition increased the information contained in it to include a range of severity of outcomes from no BPD to mild, moderate, or severe BPD (Table 3). Neonates are assessed for the BPD outcome at different time points to account for different gestational trajectories. Those born at <32 weeks' gestation are assessed at 36 weeks' PMA or discharge home, whichever comes first. Those born at ≥32 weeks' PMA are assessed at >28 days, but <56 days, or discharge home, whichever comes first. The severity of the lung injury is assessed by a combination of early support and the degree of support needed at the assessment endpoint. In every case, the definition requires support on 28 of the first 28 days of life plus continued support at the assessment endpoint (Table 2). The definition was constructed by consensus from a panel of neonatal experts. While the definition had high face validity with neonatologists and pediatric pulmonologists, it was not derived from a body of evidence.

Table 2 NIH Consensus Definition of Bronchopulmonary Dysplasia

Gestational age	<32 wk	≥32 wk
Time point of assessment	36 wk PMA or discharge to home, whichever comes first	>28 day but <56 day postnatal age or discharge to home, whichever comes first
	Treatment with oxygen >21% for at least 28 day plus	
Mild BPD	Breathing room air at 36 wk PMA or discharge, whichever comes first	Breathing room air by 56 day postnatal age or discharge, whichever comes first
Moderate BPD	Need[a] for <30% oxygen at 36 wk PMA or discharge, whichever comes first	Need[a] for <30% oxygen at 56 day postnatal age or discharge, whichever comes first
Severe BPD	Need[a] for ≥30% oxygen and/or positive pressure (PPV or NCPAP) at 36 wk PMA or discharge, whichever comes first	Need[a] for ≥30% oxygen and/or positive pressure (PPV or NCPAP) at 56 day postnatal age or discharge, whichever comes first

[a]As defined by a physiological test developed by Walsh and colleagues (22). Infants treated with oxygen >21% and/or positive pressure for nonrespiratory disease (e.g., central apnea or diaphragmatic paralysis) do not have BPD unless they also develop parenchymal lung disease and exhibit clinical features of respiratory distress. A day of treatment with oxygen >21% means that the infant received oxygen >21% for more than 12 hours on that day. Treatment with oxygen >21% and/or positive pressure at 36-week PMA, or at 56 days postnatal age or discharge, should not reflect an "acute" event, but should rather reflect the infant's usual daily therapy for several days preceding and following 36 weeks' PMA, 56 days postnatal age, or discharge.
Abbreviations: BPD, bronchopulmonary dysplasia; NCPAP, nasal continuous positive airway pressure; PMA, postmenstrual age; PPV, positive-pressure ventilation.
Source: Adapted from Ref. 2.

Table 3 BPD Definitions and Selected Pulmonary Outcomes at 18 to 22 Months' Corrected Age[a]

Consensus BPD definition	NICU infants n (%); N = 4866	Infants at 18–22 mo n (%); N = 3848	Pulmonary medications (%)[a]	Rehospitalized for pulmonary cause (%)[a]	RSV prophylaxis (%)[a]
None	1124 (23.1)	876 (22.8)	27.2	23.9	12.5
Mild	1473 (30.3)	1186 (30.8)	29.7	26.7	16.6
Moderate	1471 (30.2)	1143 (29.7)	40.8	33.5	19.2
Severe	798 (16.4)	643 (16.7)	46.6[b]	39.4[b]	28.4[b]

[a]Percent among cohort of infants who were seen at 18 to 22 months' corrected age.
[b]$p < 0.001$, Mantel–Haenszel χ^2 for linear association across the categories of the consensus definition (none to severe).
Abbreviations: BPD, bronchopulmonary dysplasia; NICU, newborn intensive care units; RSV, respiratory syncitial virus.
Source: Modified from Ref. 19.

To validate the consensus definition, Ehrenkranz et al. applied the NIH Consensus definition in the large NICHD Neonatal Research Network (NRN) database (19). Use of the consensus definition increased the number of infants diagnosed with BPD by adding a group termed mild BPD, who were on oxygen at 28 days of age, but in room air at 36 weeks' PMA. The overall rate of BPD was increased from 46% to 77%. The assessment of severity of BPD adds richness to the outcome measure and identifies a spectrum of adverse pulmonary and neurodevelopmental outcomes. As the severity of BPD increases, the incidence of adverse pulmonary and neurological events also increases (Table 3). Subsequent work has replicated the validity in an independent cohort (20).

V. Physiological Definition

All of the earlier definitions are based on the use of oxygen at varying time points. The need for oxygen is determined by individual physicians, rather than on the basis of a physiological assessment. Implicit in the definition is the assumption that the criteria on which the decision to administer oxygen is uniform and applied similarly across institutions; however, such an assumption is erroneous. Because there is no consensus in the literature, neonatologists have widely divergent practices regarding oxygen saturation targets (21). Indeed, published literature cites acceptable saturation ranges from 84% to 98%. Thus, we developed a definition of BPD at 36 weeks' PMA based on a timed challenge in room air in selected infants receiving <30% effective oxygen (22,23). Infants in room air were assumed to have no BPD. Infants receiving >30% effective oxygen, support on a ventilator or continuous positive airway pressure (CPAP), were defined as BPD without a challenge. The physiological definition identified infants treated with oxygen that were able to maintain saturations exceeding 90% in room air. Overall, the physiological definition resulted in a 6% reduction in the number of infants diagnosed as having BPD compared with the clinical definition of BPD by oxygen use alone from 31% to 25% (Fig. 1). Out of 227 infants, 101 passed the challenge of a reduction of oxygen to room air. The magnitude of the impact did differ by center with the largest impact being a reduction in the BPD rate from 60% to 16% (Fig. 2). It became apparent through this study that large numbers of infants were receiving oxygen for reasons other than compromised pulmonary function. Such reasons included treatment of retinopathy of prematurity and apnea of prematurity. The main utility of this definition will be in the context of clinical trials; however, the room air challenge may also be useful clinically in identifying infants who are candidates for trials of room air. Many of these infants receive oxygen by nasal cannulae, which may make it difficult to determine the true amounts of oxygen delivered and may lead to days of treatment with low amounts of oxygen that are not needed (24).

In a similar approach to the physiological definition, Quine and colleagues studied 21 preterm infants who remained in oxygen supplementation at 36 weeks' PMA. The authors varied delivered oxygen in steps to manipulate the saturation between 86% and 94%. They demonstrated that the oxygen dissociation curve was shifted to the right in all patients. They verified that such an oxygen challenge could aid in quantifying the severity of BPD (25).

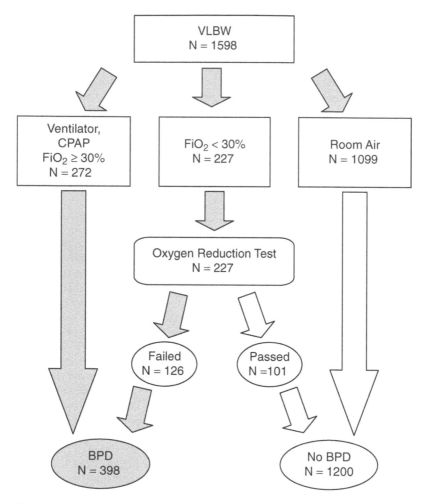

Figure 1 Impact of the physiological definition on the diagnosis of BPD. *Abbreviations*: BPD, bronchopulmonary dysplasia; CPAP, continuous positive airway pressure; VLBW, very low birth weight. *Source*: Modified from Ref. 23.

VI. An Embarrassment of Riches: Are Too Many Definitions a Bad Thing?

While studies of the optimal definition of BPD have added more objectivity and generalizability to the definition of BPD, during this transition phase, there has been considerable confusion and ambiguity for both investigators and clinicians. How many definitions of BPD are needed or helpful? Which definition is optimal for a randomized clinical trial, for patient care? For the purposes of clinical trials design and for comparing outcomes between centers, the use of an objective oxygen challenge based test,

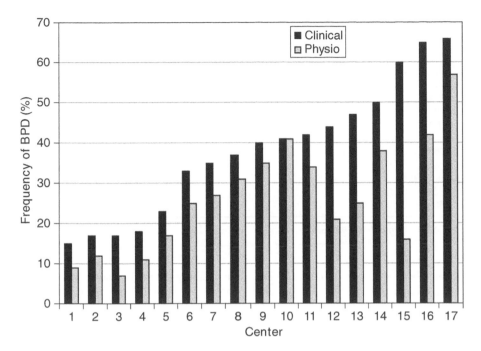

Figure 2 Variation in the impact of the physiological definition on rates of bronchopulmonary dysplasia by center. *Source*: Modified from Ref. 23.

such as the physiological definition, combined with criteria that grade BPD severity as suggested by the NIH Consensus definitions may be optimal. One approach to combine these definitions is shown in the Figure 1.

An additional twist, which remains to be adequately addressed, is the optimal approach to evaluating infants in centers at altitude. Because of the relative hypoxia in high-altitude environments, recovering neonates are exposed to oxygen longer than at centers at sea level. One possible approach to this dilemma is to utilize the alveolar gas equation to calculate the FiO_2 at the centers altitude, which corresponds to room air at sea level. In this way, infants who have been weaned to this threshold can be assigned to the mild BPD group, allowing comparisons to centers at sea level. A study to test this approach is in progress.

VII. Clinical Scores to Predict BPD

It is clear that the outcome of BPD occurs late in the neonatal course. However, increasing evidence from basic science studies and meta-analyses suggests that markers of inflammation can be identified in the first days of life that differentiate those neonates that will resolve their RDS from those who will progress to BPD. In addition, data suggests that the optimal time to intervene and potentially modify the illness is early in

Table 4 Scores to Predict Risk of Bronchopulmonary Dysplasia at Early Assessment

Study	Assessment time point	Outcome time point	Sensitivity	Specificity	ROC
Toce, 84	21 day	30 day	Correlation	Na	Na
Palta, 90 ($n = 42$)	First days of life		Correlation	Na	Na
Sinkin, 90 (validation $n = 160$)	12 hr, day 10	28 day	57%	96	Na
Corcoran, 93	Not stated	28 day	65	88	Na
Ryan, 96 ($n = 204$, <32 wk)	4 day	36 wk	88	90	0.85
Romagnoli, 98 ($n = 228$, <1250 g)	3 day, 5 day	28 day	93	97	0.96

Source: Adapted from Refs. 29 to 33.

the course between 7 and 21 days (26–28). Thus, waiting for the diagnosis of BPD at 36 weeks' PMA is not useful. Another earlier marker for those at high risk for BPD is needed. In the clinical arena, biochemical markers of airway inflammation are not yet available. Thus, there has been increasing interest in developing scores that identify infants at high predicted risk of BPD. A number of different risk scores have been proposed (29–34) (Table 4). The score developed by Ryan appears to have a desirable combination of both sensitivity and specificity with a high value for the receiver operating curve. The elements included in the Ryan risk score include birth weight, peak inspiratory pressure, and the need for ventilation on day 4 of life (33). Using a cut point of 0.4 for the score leads to sensitivity and specificity as shown in the table. The Romagnoli score requires similar information and includes clinical data up to and including day 5 of life: birth weight, gestational age, concentration of inspired oxygen, and peak inspiratory pressure (34). Both of these scores are also attractive as they do not require knowledge of the partial pressure of oxygen for their calculation. An alternative score, the oxygenation index, has been validated as a predictor of mortality in preterm infants with respiratory failure, but it has not been validated as a predictor of BPD (35). It has the disadvantage of requiring knowledge of the arterial partial pressure of oxygen, which may not be available in every patient. None of these scores has been validated in an independent cohort.

VIII. Benchmarking Outcomes in Neonatology

In neonatology today, as in healthcare in general, there is a desire to compare outcomes across institutions. The goals of these comparisons are diverse and range from a desire to reduce costs of care to improving patient outcomes. A newer goal of these comparisons is to reward institutions with practices that emphasize patient safety such as the efforts launched by the Leapfrog Foundation and recently by the Center for Medicare and Medicaid Services. Numerous studies have documented rampant variation in different aspects of neonatal care at well-respected NICUs (newborn intensive care units)

(36–38). Some of this practice variation is driven by uncertainty, which is the lack of sound evidence for any specific course of treatment.

Horbar and others have proposed a theoretical framework to explain variation in practice. In this model, as the strength of evidence increases, agreement on standard practice increases and the expected variation in a practice should decrease, and in fact any variation may be considered inappropriate. Conversely, when the evidence is weak, variation is expected to increase. Horbar together with the Vermont Oxford Network have, however, shown that differences do exist in the frequency of use of even practices that have been shown to be highly effective, such as the administration of antenatal corticosteroids and the early administration of surfactant. As predicted by the model, other less well-studied practices in neonatology vary widely between institutions. Differences have been shown to exist in rates of CLD, methods of treating persistent pulmonary hypertension, use of inotropes, pain medication, analgesic agents, and blood transfusions (36–39). This inherent variation in practice constitutes a natural experiment and allows us to explore the impact of different practices on outcomes. One tool that is useful in exploiting this variation is termed benchmarking.

Benchmarking, a technique developed in the business world in the 1980s, is the process of comparing outcomes and processes together. In benchmarking, one identifies an institution as the leader and then emulates its practices with the goal of improving one's own outcomes. For example, a business in the hospitality industry that wished to improve the treatment of its customers might study the practices of industry leaders such as the Ritz Carlton Hotel or Disney World. The practices that employees in those outstanding industries utilized are called "best practices," and these practices would then be adopted in the industry that wished to improve. The terminology of "best practices" elicits a strong negative reaction in some physicians. They argue that such terminology within health care implies that the practices have been exhaustively researched and proven to be superior. Further they argue that the practice of benchmarking runs counter to the movement that seeks sound evidence for medical practices. In fact, benchmarking is a tool that complements evidence-based medicine. Evidence-based medical practices are based on a rigorous scientific tradition. Unfortunately, most practices in neonatology have not been rigorously studied, and evidence of effectiveness does not exist. Proponents of benchmarking argue that application of benchmarking together with quality improvement methodologies that incorporate rapid cycles of change can improve care faster than change instituted through randomized clinical trials. Opponents of benchmarking argue that it is unlikely that teams can interact with a benchmark institution over a brief time period, and reliably extract the few care practice differences out of the hundreds that are applied to a given patient on a given day. These skeptics argue that any improvements seen are likely due to a Hawthorn effect, that is, observation of a phenomenon inherently changes the process observed. This worry is heightened when the outcome measure can be influenced by the caregivers conducting the observation: a classic example is BPD. If one wished to lower BPD rate, one unscrupulous method would be to encourage more aggressive oxygen weaning and not check saturations during the brief period of time needed to declare the infant BPD-free! Clinicians would not choose this approach explicitly, but may be influenced in subtle ways by the pressure from administrators and external reviewers to shade outcomes.

In neonatology, there have been two large experiences with benchmarking to reduce BPD (40). As part of their ongoing quality collaboratives, Vermont Oxford

Network sponsored a group of 16 centers with the specific goal to reduce BPD by 10% without increasing mortality using pre-post comparison. There was no control group. The group collectively reduced BPD by 27%. Specific practices changed in the collaborative were decreased use of mechanical ventilation, increased use of nasal continuous airway pressure, and lower oxygen saturation targets. The group also showed significant reductions in other adverse outcomes during their follow-up epoch. One criticism has been the lack of use of a definition that included an oxygen challenge. Thus, the BPD outcome could be subject to manipulation. However, the investigators viewed this as unlikely, given the improvements in other more objective endpoints.

In a study sponsored by NICHD in the Neonatal Research Network, the ability of benchmarking to accelerate change was explicitly tested in 14 centers with 7 centers randomized to intervention and 7 randomized to control (41). BPD was assessed by the physiological definition described previously. Use of the definition led to a 10% reduction in the average rates of BPD compared with rates calculated using oxygen at 36 weeks' PMA. In a three-year collaborative, centers randomized to intervention changed practices. Both intervention and control centers decreased the time of delivery of the first surfactant dose; with intervention centers decreased from a median of 51 to 31 minutes and control centers from a median of 41 to 21 minutes. The intervention group significantly increased the use of continuous positive pressure on the first day of life (year 1 16.9% to year 3 24.2%), but despite the 7.3% increase usage was still below the rate of CPAP use in the control centers in both study year 1 (26.5%) and 3 (28.2%). Intervention centers also decreased the duration of mechanical ventilation in the first week of life from 4.0 to 3.5 days, whereas the control centers did not change significantly, 3.5 to 3.4 days. Despite having persistently higher rates of intubation on day 1 of life than the control centers between study year 1 and study year 3, intervention centers decreased total duration of respiratory support by 5.3 days while the control group decreased by 4.1 days.

Thus, while steadily improving their practices, by chance the centers randomized to control already were practicing closer to the benchmark centers. Although practices improved, survival free of BPD rates remained stable in both the intervention and control groups (intervention pre-rate 63.3%, intervention post-rate 62.2%; control pre-rate 62.7%, and control post-rate 62.8%). The benchmark centers rate of survival free of BPD was 73.3%. In post hoc analyses, it appeared that centers that focused on interventions that reduced pressure exposure through lower ventilating pressure and through enhanced use of CPAP were more likely to decrease BPD rates than those that focused on oxygen saturation reductions.

It is perplexing why one group would show reductions in BPD, while the other would show no difference than the control centers. Key elements of the design of the trials were very different. The NRN trial was a randomized trial while Vermont Oxford trial included self-selected participants with no control group. The NRN trial used the physiological definition in both the intervention and the control groups that showed a 10% decrement in rates of BPD; thus, an intervention that focused attention on oxygen delivery occurred in both groups. This may have minimized the impact of additional changes in care.

Centers that use benchmarking must be very careful to adhere to the principles on which it is based. Benchmarking begins with an assumption that patient populations are similar and that the outcomes studied are clearly defined and identical between institutions. A common but incorrect methodology that is labeled benchmarking seeks to use the shortcut of claims data such as the Medicare database, or information drawn from hospital charge data, to compare outcomes between institutions. Such efforts are not true benchmarking in that they look at outcomes only and do not provide detailed data on the processes of this care. They are also fraught with errors because inherently different patient populations are compared. Neonatologists must beware of the potential pitfalls that exist in comparing such charge-based data and must insist on rigorous definitions and adjustment for severity of illness.

IX. Conclusion

The ideal definition of BPD would be both sensitive and specific, easy to apply, highly reliable across time periods and institutions, and highly predictive of future pulmonary and neurodevelopmental impairment, although while having high face validity among neonatologists. In the future, the definition may include pulmonary function testing or another biomarker. Until that time, we are left with the imprecise markers described in this chapter as the best definitions available.

References

1. Northway WH Jr., Rosan RC, Porter DY. Pulmonary disease following respirator therapy of hyaline-membrane disease: bronchopulmonary dysplasia. N Engl J Med 1967; 276:357–368.
2. Jobe A, Bancalari E. NICHD/NHLBI/ORD workshop summary—bronchopulmonary dysplasia. Am J Respir Crit Care Med 2001; 163:1723–1729.
3. Northway WM Jr., Rosan RC, Carlisle KB, et al. Late pulmonary sequelae of broncho-pulmonary dysplasia. N Engl J Med 1990; 323:1793–1799.
4. Bancalari E, Abdenour GE, Feller R, et al. Bronchopulmonary dysplasia: clinical presentation. J Pediatr 1979; 85:819–823.
5. Tooley WH. Epidemiology of bronchopulmonary dysplasia. J Pediatr 1979; 85:851–855.
6. O'Brodovich HM, Mellins RB. Bronchopulmonary dysplasia: unresolved neonatal acute lung injury. Am Rev Respir Dis 1958; 132:694–709.
7. Palta M, Gabbert D, Weinstein MR, et al. Multivariate assessment of traditional risk factors for chronic lung disease in VLBW neonates. J Pediatr 1991; 119:285–292.
8. Heneghan MA, Sosulski R, Baquero JM. Persistent pulmonary abnormalities in newborns: the changing picture of bronchopulmonary dysplasia. Pediatr Radiol 1986; 16:180–184.
9. Fletcher BD, Wright LL, Oh W, et al. Evaluation of radiographic (CXR) scoring system for predicting outcomes of very low birthweight (VLBW) infants with BPD. Pediatr Res 1993; 33:326A.
10. Shennan AT, Dunn MS, Ohlsson A, et al. Abnormal pulmonary outcomes in premature infants: prediction from oxygen requirements in the neonatal period. Pediatrics 1988; 82:527–532.
11. Davis PG, Thorpe K, Roberts R, et al.; and the Trial of Indomethacin Prophylaxid in Preterms (TIPP) Investigators. Evaluating old definitions for the new BPD. J Pediatr 2002; 140: 555–560.
12. Hack M, Taylor HG, Klein N, et al. Functional limitations and special health care needs of 10- to 14-year-old children weighing <750 grams at birth. Pediatrics 2000; 106:554–600.
13. Hack M, Wilson-Costello D, Friedman H, et al. Neurodevelopment and predictors of outcomes of children with birthweights of less than 1000 g: 1992-1995. Arch Pediatr Adolesc Med 2000; 154:725–731.

14. Vohr BR, Wright LL, Dusick AM, et al. Neurodevelopmental and functional outcomes of extremely low birth weight infants in the National Institute of Child Health and Human Development Neonatal Research Network, 1993-1994. Pediatrics 2000; 105:1216–1226.

15. Vohr BR, Wright LL, Poole WK, et al. Neurodevelopmental outcomes of extremely low birthweight infants <32-33wks gestation between 1993-1998. Pediatrics 2005; 116:635–643.

16. Singer L, Yamashita T, Lilien L, et al. A longitudinal study of developmental outcome of infants with bronchopulmonary dysplasia and very low birth weight. Pediatrics 1997; 100: 987–993.

17. Short EJ, Klein NK, Lewis BA, et al. Cognitive and academic consequences of bronchopulmonary dysplasia and very low birth weight: 8-year-old outcomes. Pediatrics 2003; 112:e359.

18. Baraldi E, Bonetto G, Zacchello F, et al. Low exhaled nitric oxide in school-age children with bronchopulmonary dysplasia and airflow limitation. Am J Respir Crit Care Med 2005; 171:68–72.

19. Ehrenkranz RA, Walsh MC, Vohr BR, et al. Validation of the National Institutes of Health consensus definition of bronchopulmonary dysplasia. Pediatrics 2005; 116:1353–1360.

20. Sahni R, Ammari A, Suir MD, et al. Is the new definition of bronchopulmonary dysplasia more useful? J Perinatology 2005; 25:41–46.

21. Ellsbury DL, Acarregui M, McGuinness G, et al. Variability in the use of supplemental oxygen for bronchopulmonary dysplasia. J Pediatr 2002; 140:247–249.

22. Walsh MC, Wilson-Costello D, Zadell A, et al. Safety, reliability, and validity of a physiologic definition of bronchopulmonary dysplasia. J Perinatol 2003; 23:451–456.

23. Walsh MC, Yao Q, Gettner P, et al. Impact of a physiologic definition on bronchopulmonary dysplasia rates. Pediatrics 2004; 114:1305–1311.

24. Walsh MC, Engle W, Laptook A, et al. Oxygen delivery by nasal cannula to preterm infants: can practice be improved? Pediatrics 2005; 116(4):857–861.

25. Quine D, Wong CM, Boyle EM, et al. Non-invasive measurement of reduced ventilation: perfusion ratio and shunt in infants with bronchopulmonary dysplasia: a physiological definition of the disease. Arch Dis Child Fetal Neonatal Ed 2006; 91:F409–F414.

26. Halliday HL, Ehrenkrantz RA, Doyle LW. Early postnatal (<96 hours) corticosteroids for preventing chronic lung disease in preterm infants. Cochrane Database Syst Rev 2003; (1): CD001146.

27. Halliday HL, Ehrenkrantz RA, Doyle LW. Moderately early (7–14 days) postnatal corticosteroids for chronic lung disease in preterm infants. Cochrane Database Syst Rev 2003; (1): CD001144.

28. Halliday HL, Ehrenkrantz RA, Doyle LW. Delayed (>3 weeks) postnatal corticosteroids for chronic lung disease in preterm infants. Cochrane Database Syst Rev 2003; (1):CD001145.

29. Toce SS, Farrell PM, Leavitt LA, et al. Clinical and roentgenographic scoring systems for assessing bronchopulmonary dysplasia. Am J Dis Child 1984; 138:581–585.

30. Palta M, Gabbert D, Fryback D, et al. Development and validation of an index for scoring baseline respiratory disease in the very low birth weight neonate. Severity Index Development and Validation Panels and Newborn Lung Project. Pediatrics 1990; 86:714–721.

31. Sinkin RA, Cox C, Phelps DL. Predicting risk for bronchopulmonary dysplasia: selection criteria for clinical trials. Pediatrics 1990; 86:728–736.

32. Corcoran JD, Patterson CC, Thomas PS, et al. Reduction in the risk of BPD from 1980–1990: results of a multivariate logistic regression analysis. Eur J Pediatr 1993; 152:677–681.

33. Ryan SW, Nycyk J, Shaw BNJ. Prediction of chronic neonatal lung disease on day 4 of life. Eur J Pediatr 1996; 155:668–671.

34. Romagnoli C, Zecca E, Tortorolo L, et al. A scoring system to predict the evolution of respiratory distress syndrome into chronic lung disease in preterm infants. Intensive Care Med 1998; 24:476–480.

35. Subhedar NV, Tan AT, Sweeney EM, et al. A comparison of indices of respiratory failure in ventilated preterm infants. Arch Dis Child Fetal Neonatal Ed 2000; 83:F97–F100.
36. Walsh-Sukys MC, Tyson J, Wright LL, et al. Persistent pulmonary hypertension of the newborn in the era before nitric oxide: practice variations and outcomes. Pediatrics 2000; 105:14–20.
37. Ringer SA, Richardson DK, Sacher RA, et al. Variations in transfusion practice in neonatal intensive care. Pediatrics 1998; 101:194–200.
38. Kahn DJ, Richardson DK, Gray JE, et al. Variation in the neonatal intensive care units in narcotic administration. Arch Pediatr Adolesc Med 1998; 152:844–851.
39. Horbar JD. Hospital and patient characteristics associated with variation in 28 day mortality rates for VLBW infants. Pediatrics 1997; 99:149–156.
40. Payne NR, LaCorte M, Karna P, et al., on behalf of the Breath Savers Group. Reduction of BPD after participation in the breathsavers group of the Vermont Oxford NICU quality improvement collaborative. Pediatrics 2006; 118:S73–S77.
41. Walsh MC, Laptook A, Kazzi N, et al.; for the NICHD Neonatal Research Network. A cluster randomized trial of benchmarking and multi-modal quality improvement to improve rates of survival free of BPD for infants with birthweights less than 1250 g. Pediatrics 2007; 119: 876–890.

15

Genetics of Bronchopulmonary Dysplasia

VINEET BHANDARI

Yale University School of Medicine, New Haven, Connecticut, U.S.A.

I. Introduction

Bronchopulmonary dysplasia (BPD), the most common respiratory disease in infants, is a devastating disease in the developmental program of the immature lung, secondary to preterm birth (1). The incidence of BPD in infants with birth weights of <1000 g is 43% (2). The incidence of preterm birth, specifically of low birth weight (LBW) infants, has increased by 11% from 1994 to 2004 and is expected to continue to rise, leading one to anticipate an increase in the burden of BPD. Babies of <1500 g birth weight [very low birth weight (VLBW)] infants comprise ~10 to 15 per 1000 live births; their survival rates now exceed 80% (3,4). BPD has been described in ~40% of VLBW survivors, and the rate rises as the birth weight falls. The prevalence of VLBW survivors with BPD reaching adulthood is approaching 3 to 4 per 1000, a prevalence greater than that for many childhood diseases known to affect the respiratory system, such as cystic fibrosis (4). There is currently no specific or effective prevention or treatment of this condition. BPD can no longer be considered a pediatric disease, as it has far-reaching consequences into adolescence and adulthood (1).

II. Pathogenesis of BPD

BPD is a complex disorder with multiple factors involved in the pathogenesis of the lung phenotype characterized by a dysmorphic microvascular network and fewer, larger simplified alveoli (1,2,5,6). Figure 1 illustrates the possible pathophysiologic mechanisms underlying BPD. An imbalance in the release of pro- and anti-inflammatory cytokines, secondary to the impact of environmental factors (chorioamnionitis, ventilation, hyperoxia, pulmonary edema, and/or sepsis), damages the immature lung. This is followed by either healing (resolution of injury) or repair of the lung (BPD). Cytokine release and the responses of the immature lung are determined by allelic differences of genes that create genetic susceptibility. Differential interactions between genetic susceptibility and environmental factors would create intermediate phenotypes that would modify the degree of the final clinical outcome, as mild, moderate, or severe BPD.

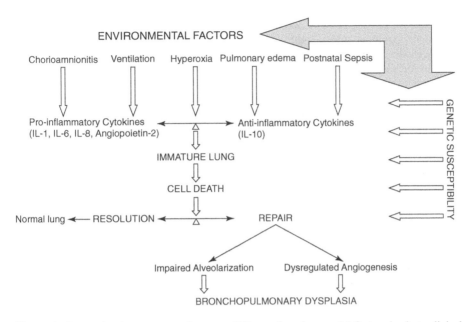

Figure 1 Interaction between genetic susceptibility and environmental factors leads to clinical phenotypes that modify the final outcome of BPD.

III. Definitions of BPD

Mild BPD is defined as a need for supplemental oxygen (O_2) for $\geq$ 28 days but not at 36 weeks' postmenstrual age (PMA) or discharge. Moderate BPD is O_2 for $\geq$ 28 days in addition to treatment with <30% O_2 at 36 weeks' PMA. Severe BPD is O_2 for $\geq$28 days in addition to $\geq$30% O_2 and/or positive pressure at 36 weeks' PMA (7,8). In some of the studies discussed below, the older definitions of need for supplemental O_2 for $\geq$28 days or at 36 weeks' PMA are used.

IV. Multiple Births and BPD

Studies of multiple births suggested a link between genetic susceptibility and risk for BPD (9–11). In a study of VLBW twins ($n = 108$), after adjusting for birth weight, gestational age, gender, respiratory distress syndrome (RDS), pneumothorax, and patent ductus arteriosus, BPD status in one twin was a highly significant predictor of BPD in the other twin (adjusted OR 12.3, $p < 0.001$), irrespective of birth order, Apgar scores, and other factors (12).

Mixed effects logistic regression probit models were used to assess the relationship between covariates and outcome for BPD within twin pairs born at $\leq$32 weeks of gestation. The study population consisted 450 twin pairs from 4 institutions with an overall BPD incidence of 21.3%. Mixed effects logistic regression analyses showed that male gender, birth weight, RDS, and treating institution (all $p < 0.001$) were significant independent variables. After controlling for the effects of the other significant risk factors, genetic modeling of twin data showed that 65.2% ($p < 0.001$, 95%CI: 52.6–78.9%) of the variance in liability for BPD could be accounted for by a combination of shared genetic plus environmental factors (6).

To isolate the contribution due to genetic factors alone, a subgroup of the cohort with zygosity data was analyzed further. Since monozygotic (MZ) twins share 100% of their genome and on average dizygotic (DZ) twins share about 50%, studies that compare concordance can quantify heritability. Sixty-three MZ and 189 DZ twin pairs were compared. While there were more DZ than MZ twins, demographic data for birth weight, gestational age, and other variables were comparable. MZ twins, however, had more BPD ($p = 0.04$) and a longer duration of hospitalization ($p = 0.03$). BPD occurred in either one or both of the twins in 18 of 63 (29%) pairs of MZ twins and in 43 of 189 (23%) pairs of DZ twins. The ratio between the observed to the expected concordance was significantly higher ($p < 0.0001$) in the MZ compared with the DZ group. After controlling for covariates such as birth weight, gestational age, gender, RDS, Apgar scores, duration of ventilation, and birth order, genetic factors accounted for 53% ($p = 0.004$, 95% CI: 16–89%) of the variance in liability for BPD (6).

V. Candidate Genes and BPD

Lung injury and healing is regulated by a variety of genes and the balance between inflammatory factors, oxygen toxicity, cell injury and death, tissue repair, and infection. Genetic association studies of BPD have attempted to identify specific candidate genes that are known to be involved in the biologic pathways governing the processes mentioned above. These studies, however, involve small sample sizes, and a majority of them have not been replicated in additional cohorts. Regardless, they represent a shift in the way physicians and scientists have traditionally thought about BPD, from a disease that is exclusively developmental to one that is the consequence of interaction between genetic and environmental factors (Fig. 1).

The following text will summarize the data regarding various candidate gene association studies with BPD. These have been arbitrarily classified into five groups: adhesion molecules, antioxidant systems, inflammatory mediators, surfactant proteins, and miscellaneous.

VI. Adhesion Molecules

A. Dystroglycan

Dystroglycan is an extracellular matrix receptor that serves as an adhesion molecule and stabilizes the plasma membrane. In a study linking abnormalities in the gene DAG1 to BPD, the N494H homozygous genotype was found more often in patients with BPD ($n = 11$, defined as O_2 requirement at 36 weeks' PMA), compared with those without BPD ($n = 22$) (13). No correction was done for differences in gestational age, birth weight, or known environmental factors.

Table 1 Candidate Genes for BPD: Adhesion Molecules

Marker	Polymorphism	N	BPD susceptibility	Reference no.
DAG1	N449H	33	Increased in homozygotes	13
L-Selectin	pro213ser	125	Increased	14

Abbreviation: BPD, bronchopulmonary dysplasia.

B. L-Selectin

Selectins are lectin-binding proteins that mediate rolling and capture of leukocytes to endothelial cells. In the adhesion cascade, this first step eventually results in the movement of leukocytes to areas of inflammation (14). L-Selectin is expressed on leukocytes. The pro213ser polymorphism causes an amino acid alteration in the short consensus repeat domain-1 of L-Selectin and could potentially alter leukocyte-endothelial interactions (14). In a cross-sectional analysis of 24 LBW infants with BPD (28 day definition) compared with 101 LBW infants without BPD, greater risk was conferred by the 213ser allele (OR 2.45, 95% CI 1.01–5.05, $p = 0.04$) (14).

These have been summarized in Table 1.

VII. Antioxidant Systems

A. Glutathione-*S*-transferase

Glutathione-*S*-transferases (GSTs) provide an important line of cellular defense against reactive oxygen species (ROS). GST polymorphisms can alter the detoxification of oxidizing agents. The GST P1 gene, which encodes the human class GST π, has a single nucleotide polymorphism (SNP) at nucleotide 313 that causes a valine to isoleucine change at amino acid 105. The valine isoform is better at reducing oxidative toxins (15). After controlling for race and gender, BPD cases ($n = 35$; controls $= 98$) were less likely to be homozygous for the valine/valine isoform (OR 0.21, CI 0.045–0.95, $p = 0.04$) and more likely to possess the less-efficient isoleucine isoform (OR 4.5, CI 1.0–20.7, $p = 0.05$) (16).

B. Microsomal Epoxide Hydrolases

These microsomal enzymes metabolize ROS by catalyzing the hydrolysis of various epoxides and reactive epoxide intermediates. The alteration in the 113tyr isoform to histidine leads to slower catalysis of reduction of ROS metabolites. BPD cases had an approximate sixfold increase (not statistically significant) in 113His homozygotes (16).

These have been summarized in Table 2.

Table 2 Candidate Genes for BPD: Antioxidant Systems

Marker	Polymorphism	N	BPD susceptibility	Reference no.
GST	Valine/isoleucine	35	Increased (ile) Decreased (val)	16
mEPHx	Tyr113His	35	None	16

Abbreviations: BPD, bronchopulmonary dysplasia; GST, glutathione-*S*-transferase; mEPHx, microsomal epoxide hydrolases.

VIII. Inflammatory Mediators

A. Interleukin 4

Interleukin 4 (IL-4) is a potent anti-inflammatory cytokine, capable of inhibiting monocyte and macrophage production of pro-inflammatory cytokines and chemokines. Since it downregulates many of the inflammatory mediators that are elevated in tracheal aspirates (TA) from infants with BPD, it may have a protective effect. In a case-control study of IL-4 polymorphisms in 224 Taiwanese infants (<30 weeks) with RDS requiring ventilation, there were no significant differences in allelic frequencies of the IL-4 intron 3 or IL-4 promoter polymorphisms between infants who developed BPD and those who did not (17).

B. Interleukin 10

IL-10 inhibits mononuclear cell synthesis of a variety of pro-inflammatory cytokines including tumor necrosis factor (TNF), IL-1α, IL-1β, IL-6, IL-8, IFN-γ, IL-12, IL-18, and chemokines. Its main mode of action is by inhibiting synthesis and promoting degradation of pro-inflammatory cytokines. These actions may help to diminish the inflammation, cell injury, and cell death seen in BPD. IL-10 expression is affected by a G to A SNP at position 1082. The A allele is associated with lower IL-10 production (18). The frequency of the 1082 SNP in ventilated VLBW infants ($n = 294$) had no significant effect on mortality or the development of BPD (28-day or 36 weeks' PMA definitions) (19).

C. Interferon γ

Interferon-γ (IFN-γ) is considered a Th1 cytokine. The functions of IFN include host defense against viral and parasitic infections, regulation of cell growth and differentiation, activation of monocytes/macrophages, and cytotoxic T and natural killer cells. Carriers of the IFN-γ +874T allele in LBW infants ($n = 153$) were found to be protective of BPD ($p = 0.049$), compared with those with IFN-γ +874 AA genotype (20).

D. Mannose-Binding Lectin 2

Mannose-binding lectin (MBL) is a collectin molecule found in serum and produced by the liver. MBL activates the complement system in an antibody-independent manner on binding and enhances phagocytosis; it is also said to be an acute-phase reactant (21). The MBL protein is encoded by the MBL2 gene. Low serum levels of MBL and MBL2 genetic variants have been associated with infection in premature newborns; however, genotypic MBL concentrations correlations may not always be true in individuals (21). In a study of premature infants ($n = 75$), the R52C mutation was associated with an increased risk of BPD (36 weeks' PMA definition), corrected for gestational age and birth weight (21).

E. Monocyte Chemoattractant Protein 1

Chemokines form the largest subgroup of the family of cytokines and have chemotactic, homing, and activating effects on leukocytes. Monocyte chemoattractant protein 1

(MCP-1) levels were increased in the bronchoalveolar lavage (BAL) fluid of ventilated preterm infants ($n = 56$) who developed BPD (22). In contrast, the A/G polymorphism at MCP-1-2518 was not associated with BPD in ventilated VLBW infants ($n = 178$) or differences in MCP-1 concentration in TA (23).

F. Transforming Growth Factor β

TGF-β is a growth inhibitor for most epithelial cell types and leukocytes, but it generally stimulates the proliferation of fibroblasts and smooth muscle cells. It also has a strong anti-inflammatory effect. Overexpression of TGF-β1 in a neonatal mouse model has been reported to mimic BPD (24). However, in ventilated VLBW infants ($n = 178$), the TGF-β1 +915 noncoding C to G polymorphism, which is associated with decreased production of TGF-β1 in vitro (C allele), had no effect on the development of BPD (23).

G. Tumor Necrosis Factor

TNF is one of the principal mediators of the inflammatory cascade response. This cascade may play a role in the inflammation seen in BPD as evidenced by elevated levels of TNF-α (TNF-α) in the BAL fluid of ventilated preterm infants who develop BPD (25,26). High levels of TNF-α may promote chronic inflammation by overwhelming counter-regulatory mechanisms, while low levels may decrease the risk and severity of BPD (27).

The expression of both TNF-α and TNF-β are regulated at the transcriptional level, and various SNPs have been identified in their respective promoter sequences that could modulate expression. A to G substitutions at positions 308 and 238 for TNF-α and position 250 for TNF-β have been studied. The A alleles of TNF-α-308 and TNF-β-250 have been associated with increased levels of TNF-α, whereas the A allele of TNF-α-238 produces lower levels after stimulation. The inverse is true for the G allele.

No difference in allele frequencies were found in ventilated VLBW infants ($n = 178$) genotyped for the TNF-α-308 A to G allele in those who developed BPD versus those who did not (23). In another study, the allele frequencies of TNF-α-308 and TNF-β-250 were comparable in BPD cases ($n = 51$; 36 weeks' PMA definition) and controls ($n = 69$) (27). While the authors suggest that the A allele in TNF-α-238 genotype is protective for BPD (BPD: AA = 0/51, 0%, GA = 10/51, 14%, $p = 0.026$), the number of subjects are small, and the p value is relatively weak (27). In contrast, other investigators have reported no association for the following TNF-α SNPs: -1031, -863, -857, -308, -238 and severity of BPD (28).

These have been summarized in Table 3.

IX. Surfactant Proteins

Pulmonary surfactant stabilizes alveoli, lowers surface tension, and diminishes lung injury due to atelectasis and barotrauma. Surfactant contains 90% phospholipids and 10% proteins [surfactant proteins (SP)-A, -B, -C, and -D]. The SP-A 6A[6] allele appears to be overrepresented in infants with BPD (29).

More than 27 loss of function mutations have been identified in the SP-B gene resulting in lethal neonatal respiratory failure. Of the several known common variants,

Table 3 Candidate Genes for BPD: Inflammatory Mediators

Marker	Polymorphism	N	BPD susceptibility	Reference no.
IL-4	Intron 3	224	None	17
IL-4	590 Promoter	224	None	17
IL-10	1082 Adenine/guanine	294	None	19
IFN-γ	+874T	153	Decreased	20
MBL2	R52C	75	Increased	21
MCP-1	2518 Adenine/guanine	178	None	23
TGF-β	915 Guanine/cytosine	178	None	23
TNF-α 238	Adenine/guanine	100	Decreased	27
TNF-α 238	Adenine/guanine	105	None	28
TNF-α 308	Adenine/guanine	100	None	27
TNF-α 308	Adenine/guanine	178	None	23
TNF-α 308	Adenine/guanine	105	None	28
TNF-α 857	Cytosine/thymidine	105	None	28
TNF-α 863	Cytosine/adenine	105	None	28
TNF-α 1031	Thymidine/cytosine	105	None	28
TNF-β 250	Adenine/guanine	100	None	27

Abbreviation: BPD, bronchopulmonary dysplasia.

the most common is the frameshift in exon 4 (121ins2) accounting for 60% to 70% of mutations. One study evaluated SP-B intron 4 polymorphisms to identify a possible genetic predisposition to BPD (30). In this study, group 1 ($n = 111$, with the intron 4 wild type) and group 2 ($n = 29$, with intron 4 variations) were compared. Both groups were well matched for gestational age, gender distribution, and birth weight. The incidence of BPD (28-day definition, 21.6% vs. 48.3%, $p < 0.01$) was higher in infants in group 2. Using the 36 weeks definition resulted in loss of that association (30). In a study from Finland, the frequency of the SP-B intron 4 deletion variant allele was increased in infants with BPD ($n = 67$) compared with controls ($n = 178$; OR 2.0, 95% CI 1.2–3.4, $p = 0.008$). However, in addition to the small number of cases the p value is not compelling—as reflected by the wide confidence interval—and in any event would disintegrate with most corrections for multiple testing (31).

In a family-based association study, in the SP-B gene, allele B-18_C was associated with susceptibility to BPD (36 weeks' PMA definition; $n = 19$) and the microsatellite marker AAGG_6 was associated with susceptibility to BPD (28-day definition, $n = 52$ and at 36 weeks' PMA; $n = 19$) (32). Haplotype analysis showed 10 susceptibility, 1 protective haplotypes for SP-B, while 2 protective haplotypes were revealed for SP-A-SP-D (32). These have been summarized in Table 4.

X. Miscellaneous

A. Angiotensin-Converting Enzyme

Renin, secreted exclusively by the kidneys into the circulation, splits the decapeptide angiotensin I (AG I) from the amino terminal end of angiotensinogen. Angiotensin-converting enzyme (ACE) converts the physiologically inactive AG I to the active

Table 4 Candidate Genes for BPD: Surfactant Proteins

Marker	Polymorphism	N	BPD susceptibility	Reference no.
SP-A	SPA1-6A6	46	Increased	29
SP-B	Intron 4	140	None	30
SP-B	Allele_6 AAGG	71	Increased	32
SP-B	B-18 (A/C)	71	Increased with allele C	32

Abbreviation: BPD, bronchopulmonary dysplasia.

AG II. Conversion to AG II mostly occurs in endothelial cells in the lung. AG II is a direct vasoconstrictor and stimulates the adrenal cortex to produce aldosterone. Aldosterone causes sodium and hence water absorption in the distal collecting tubules of the kidneys. The extra cellular fluid retention via aldosterone resulting from ACE polymorphisms that increase AGII may increase the predisposition to BPD. Thus, it is speculated that increased activity of ACE leads to an increased risk for BPD. The ACE gene contains a polymorphism consisting of either the presence (insertion, I) or absence (deletion, D) of a 287-bp alu repeat in intron 16. The D allele is associated with increased ACE activity in both tissue and plasma. ACE I and D alleles were genotyped in mechanically ventilated infants ($n = 245$) with birth weights <1250 g and their outcomes (death and/or development of BPD) compared (33); 88 (35.9%) infants were homozygous DD, 107 (43.7%) were heterozygous ID, and 50 (20.4%) were homozygous II. There were no significant differences between genotype groups with respect to ethnic origin, birth weight, gestation, or gender. There was no effect of the ACE ID polymorphism on mortality or development of BPD, using either the 28-day or 36-week definitions (33). In another study comparing infants with BPD ($n = 51$) with controls ($n = 60$), it was reported that VLBW infants with DD or ID genotypes of ACE were more likely to have BPD than infants with the II genotype (47% vs. 22%, $p = 0.025$). However, more infants with DD or ID genotypes did not have BPD (51/97 = 53%) compared with those that did (46/97 = 47%), and the real difference in this study were the 23 infants with II, with the I allele not being "causative." The authors further noted that the number of D alleles correlated with severity, but they had a small number of infants in the mild (16/62) and moderate (46/62) categories of BPD (34).

B. Factor VII

The factor VII-323 del/ins (323 A1/A2) promoter polymorphism has been shown to result in ~20% decrease in factor VII coagulant activity (35). This polymorphism was found to be a potential protective factor against BPD (8.3% in carriers vs. 14.6% in noncarriers, $p = 0.011$; $n = 1004$) (35). The biochemical explanation for such an effect remains unknown.

C. Human Leukocyte Antigen-A2

Preterm infants ($n = 77$) weighing $\leq$ 1500 g were human leukocyte antigen (HLA) genotyped in one of the earliest prospective blinded studies associating genes to BPD

(36). Their HLA phenotype was correlated with their clinical course. All infants with BPD (defined by chest X ray) had HLA-A2 antigens (36).

D. Insulin-Like Growth Factor 1 and Insulin-Like Growth Factor 1 Receptor

Insulin-like growth factor 1 (IGF-1), with most effects mediated through insulin-like growth factor 1 receptor (IGF-1R), is involved in both prenatal and postnatal lung growth. Low serum IGF levels were associated with BPD in VLBW subjects ($n = 22$) (37). In contrast, IGF-1 and IGF-1R immunocytochemistry in human lung tissue obtained at autopsy was found to be low during fetal development ($n = 6$), acutely upregulated in RDS ($n = 5$), and further upregulated in BPD ($n = 4$) (38). No association between an IGF-1R noncoding G to A SNP at +3174 and development of BPD was noted in a study of LBW infants ($n = 132$) (39). In that study, the SNP in the IGF-1R was used as a proxy for IGF-1 plasma levels. However, the ability of this SNP to predict IGF-1 levels is at best tenuous with very wide standard errors (GG:2.95 ± 2.61, AG:2.34 ± 2.41, AA:1.94 ± 2.17) (40), casting concern as to the utility of the assay and the results of the above BPD study (39).

E. Transporter Associated with Antigen Processing

Together transporter associated with antigen processing 1 (TAP1) and TAP2 proteins translocate peptides from the cytosol to MHC class I molecules in the endoplasmic reticulum. TAP1 polymorphisms may play a role in inflammation, specifically affecting IFN-γ responsiveness and activation of adhesion molecules. In a study of ventilated infants ($n = 224$; <30 weeks) in the Taiwanese population, no association was noted with BPD and the DpnII polymorphism (41).

F. Urokinase

Urokinase is an enzyme that catalyzes the conversion of plasminogen to plasmin, thus stimulating fibrinolysis and degradation of major basement membrane glycoproteins such as fibronectin and laminin (42). In a study of ventilated preterm infants ($n = 204$) from Taiwan, the urokinase 3'-UTR polymorphism did not differ significantly between those who developed or did not develop BPD (43).

These have been summarized in Table 5.

Table 5 Candidate Genes for BPD: Miscellaneous

Marker	Polymorphism	N	BPD susceptibility	Reference no.
ACE	Insertion/deletion	245	None	33
ACE	Deletion	111	Increased	34
Factor VII	323 Deletion/insertion	1004	Decreased	35
HLA	A2	77	Increased	36
IGF-1R	IGF-1R G+3174	132	None	39
TAP1	DpnII adenine/guanine	224	None	41
Urokinase	3' UTR	204	None	43

Abbreviation: BPD, bronchopulmonary dysplasia.

XI. Conclusions

Twin studies have shown a familial tendency for BPD, with the zygosity analyses confirming a strong genetic component. The pathogenesis of BPD is complex, likely involving multiple genetic-environmental interactions.

The studies described in Tables 1 to 5 interrogated variations of candidate genes in a wide distribution of sample sizes. Eleven studies have reported an increased or decreased risk. It is striking to note that only two have been replicated: TNF-α-238 and ACE insertion/deletion polymorphisms. Both these associations with BPD have not held up in studies with larger cohorts. This is not surprising. The frequency that genetic association is replicated in follow-up studies has been looked at in a meta-analyses (44). About half of initial genetic association studies, even those with strong effects (OR > 2.0) or with low p values (<0.001), are not replicated. The reasons include population admixture (unmatched cases and controls), phenotypic heterogeneity (inclusion of both genetic and nongenetic cases), and commonly, underpowered studies (not enough subjects). It is therefore likely that subsequent studies with larger cohorts will diminish the initial reports of association with BPD done with smaller sample sizes.

It is critical, therefore, to undertake studies with sample sizes that would be adequately powered for robust genetic associations with BPD. This is especially important with the subcategorization of BPD into mild, moderate, and severe grades, using the consensus definition (7).

Finally, it is also important to remember that identification of molecular determinants associated with BPD in such genetic studies does not necessarily mean that they are amenable to specific therapeutic targeting. Once identified, the next logical step would involve their validation using developmentally appropriate animal models of BPD, before confirmation in human neonates. Significant improvements in the outcome of premature neonates at risk for BPD will likely depend on our ability to identify these genetic components and to specify therapeutic targets.

Acknowledgments

V.B. was supported by grants from NHLBI K08 HL 074195, AHA 0755843T, ATS 07-005.

References

1. Baraldi E, Filippone M. Chronic lung disease after premature birth. N Engl J Med 2007; 357 (19):1946–1955.
2. Bhandari A, Bhandari V. Bronchopulmonary dysplasia: an update. Indian J Pediatr 2007; 74 (1):73–77.
3. Fanaroff AA, Hack M, Walsh MC. The NICHD neonatal research network: changes in practice and outcomes during the first 15 years. Semin Perinatol 2003; 27(4):281–287.
4. Doyle LW, Faber B, Callanan C, et al. Bronchopulmonary dysplasia in very low birth weight subjects and lung function in late adolescence. Pediatrics 2006; 118(1):108–113.
5. Bhandari A, Bhandari V. Pathogenesis, pathology and pathophysiology of pulmonary sequelae of bronchopulmonary dysplasia in premature infants. Front Biosci 2003; 8:e370–e380.

6. Bhandari V, Bizzarro MJ, Shetty A, et al. Familial and genetic susceptibility to major neonatal morbidities in preterm twins. Pediatrics 2006; 117(6):1901–1906.
7. Jobe AH, Bancalari E. Bronchopulmonary dysplasia. Am J Respir Crit Care Med 2001; 163 (7):1723–1729.
8. Ehrenkranz RA, Walsh MC, Vohr BR, et al. Validation of the National Institutes of Health consensus definition of bronchopulmonary dysplasia. Pediatrics 2005; 116(6):1353–1360.
9. Chen SJ, Vohr BR, Oh W. Effects of birth order, gender, and intrauterine growth retardation on the outcome of very low birth weight in twins. J Pediatr 1993; 123(1):132–136.
10. Nielsen HC, Harvey-Wilkes K, MacKinnon B, et al. Neonatal outcome of very premature infants from multiple and singleton gestations. Am J Obstet Gynecol 1997; 177(3):653–659.
11. Shinwell ES, Blickstein I, Lusky A, et al. Effect of birth order on neonatal morbidity and mortality among very low birthweight twins: a population based study. Arch Dis Child Fetal Neonatal Ed 2004; 89(2):F145–F148.
12. Parker RA, Lindstrom DP, Cotton RB. Evidence from twin study implies possible genetic susceptibility to bronchopulmonary dysplasia. Semin Perinatol 1996; 20(3):206–209.
13. Concolino P, Capoluongo E, Santonocito C, et al. Genetic analysis of the dystroglycan gene in bronchopulmonary dysplasia affected premature newborns. Clin Chim Acta 2007; 378(1–2): 164–167.
14. Derzbach L, Bokodi G, Treszl A, et al. Selectin polymorphisms and perinatal morbidity in low-birthweight infants. Acta Paediatr 2006; 95(10):1213–1217.
15. Hayes JD, Strange RC. Glutathione S-transferase polymorphisms and their biological consequences. Pharmacology 2000; 61(3):154–166.
16. Manar MH, Brown MR, Gauthier TW, et al. Association of glutathione-S-transferase-P1 (GST-P1) polymorphisms with bronchopulmonary dysplasia. J Perinatol 2004; 24(1):30–35.
17. Lin HC, Su BH, Chang JS, et al. Nonassociation of interleukin 4 intron 3 and 590 promoter polymorphisms with bronchopulmonary dysplasia for ventilated preterm infants. Biol Neonate 2005; 87(3):181–186.
18. Turner DM, Williams DM, Sankaran D, et al. An investigation of polymorphism in the interleukin-10 gene promoter. Eur J Immunogenet 1997; 24(1):1–8.
19. Yanamandra K, Boggs P, Loggins J, et al. Interleukin-10 -1082 G/A polymorphism and risk of death or bronchopulmonary dysplasia in ventilated very low birth weight infants. Pediatr Pulmonol 2005; 39(5):426–432.
20. Bokodi G, Derzbach L, Banyasz I, et al. Association of interferon gamma T+874A and interleukin 12 p40 promoter CTCTAA/GC polymorphism with the need for respiratory support and perinatal complications in low birthweight neonates. Arch Dis Child Fetal Neonatal Ed 2007; 92(1):F25–F29.
21. Capoluongo E, Vento G, Rocchetti S, et al. Mannose-binding lectin polymorphisms and pulmonary outcome in premature neonates: a pilot study. Intensive Care Med 2007; 33(10): 1787–1794.
22. Baier RJ, Majid A, Parupia H, et al. CC chemokine concentrations increase in respiratory distress syndrome and correlate with development of bronchopulmonary dysplasia. Pediatr Pulmonol 2004; 37(2):137–148.
23. Adcock K, Hedberg C, Loggins J, et al. The TNF-alpha -308, MCP-1 -2518 and TGF-beta1 +915 polymorphisms are not associated with the development of chronic lung disease in very low birth weight infants. Genes Immun 2003; 4(6):420–426.
24. Vicencio AG, Lee CG, Cho SJ, et al. Conditional overexpression of bioactive transforming growth factor-beta1 in neonatal mouse lung: a new model for bronchopulmonary dysplasia? Am J Respir Cell Mol Biol 2004; 31(6):650–656.
25. Jonsson B, Tullus K, Brauner A, et al. Early increase of TNF alpha and IL-6 in tracheobronchial aspirate fluid indicator of subsequent chronic lung disease in preterm infants. Arch Dis Child Fetal Neonatal Ed 1997; 77(3):F198–F201.

26. Tullus K, Noack GW, Burman LG, et al. Elevated cytokine levels in tracheobronchial aspirate fluids from ventilator treated neonates with bronchopulmonary dysplasia. Eur J Pediatr 1996; 155(2):112–116.
27. Kazzi SN, Kim UO, Quasney MW, et al. Polymorphism of tumor necrosis factor-alpha and risk and severity of bronchopulmonary dysplasia among very low birth weight infants. Pediatrics 2004; 114(2):e243–e248.
28. Strassberg SS, Cristea IA, Qian D, et al. Single nucleotide polymorphisms of tumor necrosis factor-alpha and the susceptibility to bronchopulmonary dysplasia. Pediatr Pulmonol 2007; 42(1):29–36.
29. Weber B, Borkhardt A, Stoll-Becker S, et al. Polymorphisms of surfactant protein A genes and the risk of bronchopulmonary dysplasia in preterm infants. Turk J Pediatr 2000; 42(3): 181–185.
30. Makri V, Hospes B, Stoll-Becker S, et al. Polymorphisms of surfactant protein B encoding gene: modifiers of the course of neonatal respiratory distress syndrome? Eur J Pediatr 2002; 161(11):604–608.
31. Rova M, Haataja R, Marttila R, et al. Data mining and multiparameter analysis of lung surfactant protein genes in bronchopulmonary dysplasia. Hum Mol Genet 2004; 13(11): 1095–1104.
32. Pavlovic J, Papagaroufalis C, Xanthou M, et al. Genetic variants of surfactant proteins A, B, C, and D in bronchopulmonary dysplasia. Dis Markers 2006; 22(5–6):277–291.
33. Yanamandra K, Loggins J, Baier RJ. The angiotensin converting enzyme insertion/deletion polymorphism is not associated with an increased risk of death or bronchopulmonary dysplasia in ventilated very low birth weight infants. BMC Pediatr 2004; 4(1):26.
34. Kazzi SN, Quasney MW. Deletion allele of angiotensin-converting enzyme is associated with increased risk and severity of bronchopulmonary dysplasia. J Pediatr 2005; 147(6):818–822.
35. Hartel C, Konig I, Koster S, et al. Genetic polymorphisms of hemostasis genes and primary outcome of very low birth weight infants. Pediatrics 2006; 118(2):683–689.
36. Clark DA, Pincus LG, Oliphant M, et al. HLA-A2 and chronic lung disease in neonates. JAMA 1982; 248(15):1868–1869.
37. Hellstrom A, Engstrom E, Hard AL, et al. Postnatal serum insulin-like growth factor I deficiency is associated with retinopathy of prematurity and other complications of premature birth. Pediatrics 2003; 112(5):1016–1020.
38. Chetty A, Andersson S, Lassus P, et al. Insulin-like growth factor-1 (IGF-1) and IGF-1 receptor (IGF-1R) expression in human lung in RDS and BPD. Pediatr Pulmonol 2004; 37(2): 128–136.
39. Balogh A, Treszl A, Vannay A, et al. A prevalent functional polymorphism of insulin-like growth factor system is not associated with perinatal complications in preterm infants. Pediatrics 2006; 117(2):591–592.
40. Bonafe M, Barbieri M, Marchegiani F, et al. Polymorphic variants of insulin-like growth factor I (IGF-I) receptor and phosphoinositide 3-kinase genes affect IGF-I plasma levels and human longevity: cues for an evolutionarily conserved mechanism of life span control. J Clin Endocrinol Metab 2003; 88(7):3299–3304.
41. Lin HC, Su BH, Hsu CM, et al. No association between TAP1 DpnII polymorphism and bronchopulmonary dysplasia. Acta Paediatr Taiwan 2005; 46(6):341–345.
42. Wu HC, Chang CH, Chen WC, et al. Urokinase gene 3'-UTR T/C polymorphism is not associated with bladder cancer. Genet Mol Biol 2004; 27:15–16.
43. Lin HC, Su BH, Lin TW, et al. No association of urokinase gene 3'-UTR polymorphism with bronchopulmonary dysplasia for ventilated preterm infants. Acta Paediatr Taiwan 2004; 45(6): 315–319.
44. Trikalinos TA, Ntzani EE, Contopoulos-Ioannidis DG, et al. Establishment of genetic associations for complex diseases is independent of early study findings. Eur J Hum Genet 2004; 12(9):762–769.

16

Role of Management in the Delivery Room and Beyond in the Evolution of Bronchopulmonary Dysplasia

MAXIMO VENTO
Hospital Universitario Materno Infantil La Fe, Valencia, Spain

OLA DIDRIK SAUGSTAD
University of Oslo, Oslo, Norway

I. Introduction

Evolution of modern neonatology has dramatically increased the number of survivors of extremely low birth weight (ELBW) infants (birth weight < 1000 g) and extremely low gestational age (ELGA) neonates (postconceptional age < 28 weeks) (1–3). Of interest is that most recently, emerging reports for ELBW and ELGA neonates suggest improving neurodevelopmental outcomes in developed countries, including declining rates of cerebral palsy at the turn of the century (4–6). An examination of which factors may have contributed to the improved outcome include common use of antenatal corticosteroids and surfactant therapy, drastic reduction in the use of postnatal corticosteroids, less time on ventilator, minimizing nosocomial infections, and regionalization to tertiary care centers with high level and volume of care (7,8). Although the rates of mortality have declined, the incidence of bronchopulmonary dysplasia (BPD) has remained almost unchanged, affecting approximately 22% to 23% of ELBW infants, and around 50% in the group of the most premature infants. The improved survival rates of ELBW infants, particularly those weighing less than 1000 g, may explain, in part, the consistent rate of BPD (1). Transient episodes of oxygen desaturation followed by hyperoxic peaks during mechanical ventilation or on continuous positive airway pressure (CPAP), high rates of nosocomial sepsis, poor growth and nutrition, and separation from the mother associated with prolonged hospitalization, altogether may be important factors contributing to unfavorable outcome in these babies (8). In addition, more babies of the smallest gestational age (<25 weeks) may survive and contribute to poorer outcome in total of this group of babies.

Because the outcomes of children with BPD are suboptimal regardless of the recent therapeutic progress, it will be important to focus attention on strategies that specifically prevent the development of this condition. Retrospective cohort and experimental studies suggest that the initial ventilation strategy may play an important role in the development of BPD (9,10). In this regard, it has been reported very recently that reduction of BPD incidence from single centers after introduction of early management changes (11,12).

This chapter reviews some of the factors in the delivery room and the early period of life that may influence development of BPD.

II. Fetal to Neonatal Transition

Fetal to neonatal transition is characterized by an abrupt increase in the availability of oxygen to the tissue (13). As a consequence, there is a burst of reactive oxygen species (ROS), some of which act as oxygen free radicals (14). Free radicals are highly reactive molecules capable of attacking almost any biological compound such as DNA, RNA, lipids, or proteins. The most abundant ROS are superoxide anion, hydrogen peroxide, and hydroxyl radical (14). In addition, nitric oxide (NO) can act as a pro- or antioxidant, and the combination of NO with other reactive species produces reactive nitrogen species (RNS). NO may establish an equimolecular combination with the superoxide anion generating peroxynitrite. Its relative stability, high reactivity, and ability to act and release superoxide or a superoxide-like ROS, at sites distant from its generation, make it a potentially very damaging molecule (15). To counteract the deleterious effects of ROS and RNS, an array of biological antioxidants is available (16). Antioxidants may be broadly classified as enzymatic and nonenzymatic. The most representative of the former group are manganese, copper, zinc, and their extracellular superoxide dismutases (MnSOD, CuZnSOD, and ECSOD, respectively); catalases (CAT); and glutathione and thioredoxin peroxidases (GPx and TPx, respectively) and their associated glutathione and thioredoxin reductases (GR and TR, respectively) (Fig. 1) (17). The most relevant natural nonenzymatic antioxidants are reduced glutathione (GSH), thioredoxin (TRx), heme oxygenases, and other smaller molecules such as vitamins C and E, β-carotene, and transition metal chelators such as transferrin or ceruloplasmin (14–17). GSH is a tripeptide composed of L-cysteine, glutamic acid, and glycine, which is primarily located in the cytoplasm, although it may also be found in the mitochondria, nucleus, and endoplasmic reticulum (Fig. 1) (18). Glutathione is a powerful antioxidant that controls the intracellular redox status of the cell because its reduced form has a high capacity to neutralize free radicals and to easily recover accepting electrons from NADPH in a redox reaction catalyzed by GR (18). The antioxidant capacity of glutathione depends on its ability to capture highly energized electrons from oxidized molecules, especially superoxide anions. GPx is the specific enzyme that catalyzes this reaction promoting the binding of two molecules of GSH through a disulphide bond of L-cysteine to form oxidized glutathione (GSSG) (19–21). In addition, GSH has an important role in the synthesis of nuclear DNA, telomerase activity, and cell proliferation (22,23).

Antioxidant enzymes (AOEs) as well as glutathione synthesis–regulating enzymes are not fully expressed until late in gestation. Thus, they parallel the synthesis of alveolar lining surfactant as if in preparation for birth into oxygen-enriched atmosphere (24–31). Therefore, it is not until near term that the expression of AOEs of neonates is fully developed to face increased oxidative and nitrosative stress associated to fetal-neonatal transition (27–29). However, it has been shown that response to a hyperoxic challenge differs between animal species and also among different age groups within the same species (17). In some animal species, a rapid increase in the AOE activity when challenged with hyperoxia is exhibited, with apparently a relative tolerance to hyperoxia is developed; others do not have this capability (24–26). In respect to the human neonate, both types of responses have been found, although most of the recent work indicates that extremely premature infants are unable to upregulate the expression of AOE activity as

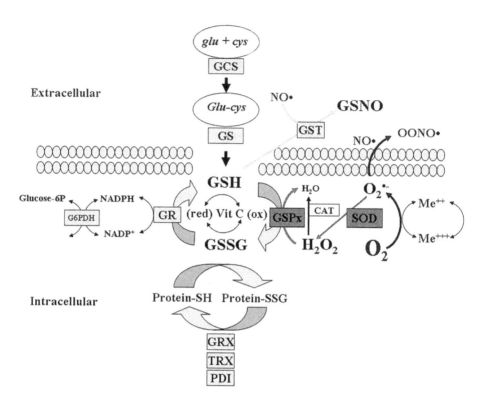

Figure 1 Enzymatic and nonenzymatic antioxidant metabolism. Glutathione metabolism and its interrelationship with pro- and antixoxidant metabolism in cells. *Abbreviations:* CAT, catalase; GSH, reduced glutathione; GSSG, oxidized glutathione; GCS, γ-glutamyl-cystein-synthase; G6PD, glucose-6-phosphate dehydrogenase; GPx, glutathione peroxidase; GR, glutathione reductase; GRX, glutaredoxin; GS, glutathione synthase; GSNO, *S*-nitroso-glutathione; GST, glutathione-*S*-transferase; Me, transition metal; SOD, superoxide dismutases; PDI, protein disulfide isomerases; TRx, thioredoxin.

well as the synthesis of GSH (17,30). Studies in preterm neonates have shown that glutathione is insufficiently synthesized before 33 weeks of gestation in spite they are able to adequately express γ-glutamyl-cysteine synthase (EC 6.3.2.2), a key regulating enzyme of glutathione synthesis in the second trimester of gestation as shown in studies performed in fetal and neonatal human liver (27–29). The low rate of GSH synthesis is dependent on the low expression of γ-cystathionase (EC 4.4.1.1), the limiting enzyme for the synthesis of L-cysteine (an essential component of GSH). This enzyme is not fully expressed in immature animals, therefore limiting the ability to synthesize glutathione (31).

The immature lung therefore seems neither to be adequately prepared to initiate respiration of a gas admixture with severalfolds higher oxygen content than during fetal life nor able to adjust to a hyperoxic stress by upregulation of protective enzyme systems. A subsequent oxidative stress therefore may have greater impact on a preterm than a term subject. Of note is that both the administration of prenatal corticosteroids and the induction of prenatal inflammation increase the activity of the AOE, as shown in the preterm lamb (32,33) However, in a prospective clinical study, a lower AOE activity and total reduced to oxidized glutathione ratios in blood were found in extremely premature infants (<28 weeks postconceptional age) compared to term babies (Fig. 2) (34). Although administration of a full course of prenatal corticosteroids substantially improved AOE activity and GSH/GSSG ratio, improvement was not sufficient as to

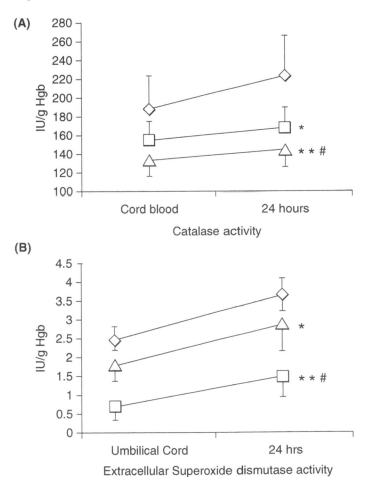

Figure 2 Enzymatic antioxidant activity in premature infants with or without prenatal corticosteroids. Antioxidant enzyme activity, (**A**) catalase and (**B**) extracellular superoxide dismutase, in extremely preterm babies (<28 weeks of gestation) treated or not with prenatal corticosteroids at birth and 24 hours thereafter. ◇, Control term newly born infants; □, preterm infants treated with prenatal corticosteroids; △, preterm infants not treated with prenatal corticosteroids. *Source*: From Ref. 124.

attain values found in term newborn (34). Under these circumstances, extremely premature infants are at risk of oxidative stress in spite of receiving prenatal corticosteroids. In fact, several studies have shown that preterm infants who develop BPD have elevated products both from lipid and from protein peroxidation at very early postnatal stages (35–37).

A. Respiratory Adaptation of the ELBW Infant Immediately After Birth

ELBW infants are born at the end of the canalicular and beginning of the saccular stage of lung development. Sacculi are characterized by the lack of secondary septation, thus having a reduced gas exchange surface. In addition, alveolar type II cells are scarcely represented and with limited capacity for surfactant production. This increases surface tension, facilitates alveolar collapse during expiration, and increases work of breathing during inspiration. Moreover, mesenchymal tissue contains low elastin and collagen, therefore having limited elastic properties (38–40). Finally, the thoracic cage of extremely premature infants is highly compliant, therefore having the tendency to collapse during forced inspiratory movements. Taken together, these factors make it difficult to establish a functional residual capacity (FRC), and favor expiratory alveolar collapse (atelectasis) (41,42). For all these reasons, most ELBW infants will need positive inspiratory pressure to allow lung expansion and positive end expiratory pressure to adequately establish an FRC immediately after birth. In fact, a recent report from the United States indicates that 60% to 70% of the babies born at 26 to 28 weeks of gestation and everyone born at less than 25 weeks are intubated in the delivery room (DR) almost immediately after birth (43). Morley et al. recently reported similar effectiveness of using nasal CPAP shortly after birth in ELBW infants of 25 to 28 weeks of gestation, compared with the intubation group, unfortunately without any reduction in BPD (44).

Using tidal volumes that would be considered adequate for a normal lung to initiate ventilation may cause lung injury secondary to overstretching in an immature lung (45,46). Indeed, administration of a few supraphysiological tidal volumes to immature lambs inhibited the positive effect on lung mechanics of subsequently administered surfactant (47). However, disruption of lung mechanics was not accompanied by alterations in oxygen exchange, and PaO_2 increased significantly in these animals (47). A similar phenomenon was encountered in human infants when late rescue treatment of surfactant was given for respiratory distress syndrome (RDS), in which there was no correlation between early improvement in oxygenation and lung volume changes (48). Although no explanation has yet been found for this apparent paradox, it may be related to changes in ventilation-perfusion matching within the lung.

Newborn lungs with adequate surfactant content can be ventilated at high pressures (consequently large tidal volumes) at least for short periods (10 minutes), with no untoward effect, as the alveoli expand synchronously and the inspired gas is distributed uniformly in the parenchyma (49). By contrast, ventilation with high tidal volumes of very immature lungs at the end stage of the canalicular and beginning of the saccular phase will lead to an uneven distribution of gas. Therefore, some alveoli will alternatively overstretch (volutrauma) and collapse, whereas others will remain unexpanded (atelectotrauma). This result could be anticipated because the unventilated immature lung with a high fluid content would not have time to recruit a sufficient number of alveoli to approach the maximal lung volume (50). Increased shear forces may also contribute to a need for higher pressures and tidal volumes contributing to early disruption of the epithelial lining and overstretching of alveoli (50).

It is known that one of the most relevant features defining BPD is the reduction of secondary septation of the saccules, thus reducing the exchange surface and elastic recoil (38,39). As a consequence, gas exchange is impaired and tendency to alveolar collapse during expiration enhanced. Elastic fibers' synthesis and assembly implies an extremely complex series of events. For instance, tropoelastin is secreted from lung myofibroblasts onto microfibril scaffolds that attach to the cell through the interaction of fibrillins, microfibril-associated glycoproteins, and integrin receptors on the cell membrane. Through the action of specific enzymes, microfibrils are stabilized in the form of elastin and collagen, thus providing resilience and distensibility to the lung's respiratory units and blood vessels (51). The cyclic stretching due to the action of mechanical ventilation increases the secretion of tropoelastin but it is not corresponded with an adequate production of matrix proteins regulating elastin assembly. The consequences are a defective elastin assembly, increased production of poorly organized elastic fibers, and abnormal lung structure characteristic of BPD (51,52). Ventilation with a too high or too low tidal volume triggers cytokine production in the lung (see sect. II.B).

B. Inflammatory Response of the Immature Lung

A body of evidence accumulated in the last two decades also suggests that subclinical infection/inflammation of the amnion/chorion/decidua is implicated in the pathogenesis of premature rupture of membranes and preterm labor, as well as long-term pulmonary inflammation (53–58). Most infants delivered before 30 weeks of gestation seem to have been exposed in utero to inflammatory processes frequently caused by intrauterine bacterial colonization of the fetal membranes (for review, see Ref. 58). In addition, physical injury in the form of high-stretch ventilation in the delivery room using high tidal volume and high oxygen concentrations will trigger release of proinflammatory cytokines and recruitment of inflammatory cells into the alveolar space (45–48,58–60). These processes have been associated with white matter injury in the brain (61) and chronic lung disease (62).

Although the use of prenatal corticosteroids has become the standard practice for preventing RDS in preterm infants, its anti-inflammatory effect on prenatal lung inflammation and, moreover, on postnatal proinflammatory interventions such as oxygen, lung stretching, or infection has still to be deciphered. It has been therefore emphasized that premature infants should be reoxygenated with as low inspiratory fractions of oxygen (FiO_2) and optimal tidal volumes as possible (63). However, recent surfactant trials have promoted the use of intubation and administration of surfactant directly into the lungs while in the DR as a protective strategy to avoid overstretching and triggering inflammatory responses (64,65). Therefore, evaluating the consequences of resuscitation maneuvers as a second inflammatory hit to the lung has become a matter of interest in the recent years.

The relation between BPD and fetal inflammation seems to be well established (56–59,62). Thus, experimental (66–73) and clinical studies (35,58,74–78) have shown that early increase of macrophages in tracheal aspirate in infants and elevation of proinflammatory cytokines in the first days of life correlate with later development of

BPD. Among inflammatory mediators, tumor necrosis factor (TNF)-1α, which mediates CXC chemokine expression in models of lung inflammation, has received special attention. However, its role in the development of BPD remains controversial (68–70). Despite the strong evidence that TNF-1α is able to influence the progression of pulmonary edema by altering the function of epithelial and endothelial cells, the predicted net effects of TNF-1α on pulmonary edema formation are conflicting in the literature (71). Thus, TNF-1α may either promote pulmonary edema by increasing epithelial and endothelial permeability or oppose edema formation by enhancing fluid reabsorption (72). These apparently opposed effects depend on the differential signaling of TNF receptors, specifically p55 and p75. Both of these TNF receptors can signal through different intracellular pathways and may induce different cellular responses. For example, activation of p55 receptor favors high-stretch edema formation, whereas p75 receptor activation may play an opposing role (72). TNF signaling through the p55 receptor, in promoting high-stretch-induced pulmonary edema is independent from its effects on neutrophil recruitment. If confirmed, these findings could imply a novel therapeutic approach for high-stretch lung damage in the coming future by modulating the TNF signaling pathway.

Inflammatory processes triggered in the early postnatal events may aggravate this and also contribute separately to the development of BPD.

Genetic studies have shown that cyclic stretching of distal airways and primitive saccules upregulates cysteine-rich 61 gene (cyr61/CCN1) as well as connective tissue growth factor (CTGF/CCN2) and early growth response gene (EGR1) (73). In addition, there is an increased expression of different interleukins (IL-1β, IL-6, IL-8) immediately after the initiation of mechanical ventilation, and these remain overexpressed for several hours after cessation of the aggression. Activation of the above-mentioned genes will cause negative effects on the lung such as hypercellularity, capillary dysplasia, inflammation, and abnormal extracellular matrix deposition and fibrosis (73). Mechanical ventilation always induces structural and functional changes.

Lambs ventilated with increased tidal volume exhibited an increased number of inflammatory cells and proteins in bronchoalveolar lavage fluid, heat shock protein-70 immunostaining, IL-1β, IL-6, IL-8, monocyte chemotactic protein-1, serum amyloid A-3. Toll-like receptor (TLR)-2 and TLR-4 mRNA in the lungs were also increased compared with control animals. Thus, the injurious process triggered by lung stretching with high tidal volumes elicits a pulmonary and also a hepatic acute-phase response (50).

C. Clinical Interventions Meant to Reduce High-Stretch Damage to the Lung

Until a clear understanding of the intrinsic molecular mechanisms implicated in the development of inflammatory lung damage is achieved, clinicians facing the necessity of ventilating ELBW infants have pursued the use of less aggressive and equally effective ventilation modalities.

CPAP is a distending pressure applied at a pressure of a few centimeter H_2O to the airways usually through the nose (nCPAP), and was developed for infants with RDS (79). However, since the introduction of surfactant and more efficient mechanical ventilation devices, the use of CPAP as primary therapy for RDS in preterm infants declined. CPAP has been recently pointed out as the first choice therapy for neonatal RDS (80).

CPAP has a series of beneficial effects derived from splinting the airways, enhancing lung expansion and the release of surfactant and aiding to maintain the surfactant present on the alveolar surface. CPAP also stabilizes the chest wall and dilates the airways; hence, it reduces inspiratory resistance, increases lung compliance, counteracts paradoxical movements, and reduces thoracoabdominal asynchrony of the chest wall. Consequently, CPAP makes it possible to reduce the work of breathing using lower peak pressures and FiO_2 to attain adequate tidal volumes (V_t) and adequate oxygenation. Finally, evidence has shown that the administration of nCPAP may reduce the rate of intubation and the need of reintubation after extubation in very preterm infants (for review, see Refs. 81–89).

However, there are still some problems associated with the use of CPAP. Trauma involving the nasal septum and *alae nasi* is seen with all the interfaces and injuries ranging from mild inflammation to laceration having been associated with increased risk of gram-negative sepsis (90,91). In addition, an increased rate of air leak in the thoracic cavity (pneumothorax, pneumomediastinum, and pneumopericardium) has been described especially when CPAP pressures are applied at 8 cm H_2O or higher as shown in the CPAP or Intubation (COIN) trial (45) and reported recently in a Cochrane Review (92).

Numerous observational studies have confirmed the feasibility of using early CPAP in the DR in ELBW infants (for review, see Refs. 81,86–89). Already in 1999, Lindner et al. (10) were able to resuscitate ELBW infants in the DR using CPAP with no increase in neonatal mortality or morbidity. Aly et al. concluded that an individualized approach and progressive ability acquisition by the resuscitation team could diminish significantly the number of intubations, especially in infants above 25 weeks of gestation (9). Ammari et al. successfully managed 50% of their infants of less than 750 g and 76% of those below 1250 g with the early use of "bubble" CPAP (93). More recently, again Lindner and Pohlandt published a prospective observational study regarding oxygenation and ventilation in spontaneous breathing very preterm infants with nCPAP in the DR (94). After an initial lung recruitment maneuver consisting of sustained pressure-controlled inflation that was repeated as necessary based on heart rate response, a substantial number of infants (67%) did not need intubation and mechanical ventilation in the DR. Moreover, initial FiO_2 could be substantially reduced short after birth to avoid hyperoxemia (94).

An observational clinical trial compared a gentle ventilatory strategy in the DR as performed in Stockholm, Sweden, with a more aggressive approach (frequent use of intubation and conventional mechanical ventilation) used in Boston, United States (95). Although no difference in BPD was observed between these NICUs, at 40 weeks, fewer infants in Stockholm were on supplementary oxygen (95). Very recently, Gearly et al. (12) performed a historical cohort study comparing the clinical impact of three early management changes for infant's ≤ 1000 g in two different periods (2001–2002 vs. 2004–2005). Babies recruited in the second period received surfactant early in the DR and were immediately switched to nCPAP whereas those in the first period were on mechanical ventilation. In addition, in the second period, target SpO_2 was substantially lowered, and babies received supplementary amino acids in the parenteral nutrition. The authors reported a substantial decrease in the incidence and severity of BPD in the second period (12) that correlated with receiving CPAP in the first 24 to 48 hours.

Only few randomized trials have compared DR use of CPAP or conventional approach. Finer et al. (43) recruited 104 ELBW infants, and demonstrated the feasibility of the use of nCPAP in the DR; however, this study was not designed for outcomes such as efficacy or safety. Recently, te Pas and Walther published a randomized trial comparing conventional approach in the DR (early intubation plus surfactant) with early nCPAP with sustained inflation to nonaggressively recruit the lung in ELBW infants (11). The number of intubations at 72 hours after birth and the number of doses of surfactant given were significantly reduced with less BPD developed in those ELBW infants treated with early CPAP compared with those with the conventional approach (11). Finally, the COIN trial has to date been the largest randomized multicenter trial (610 babies recruited) comparing nCPAP in the DR with conventional intubation and ventilation early after birth in babies between 25 and 28 weeks of postconceptional age (45). The rate of death or BPD at 36th week of gestation did not differ between the groups, although patients in the CPAP group needed less oxygen at 28 days after birth and had fewer days of ventilation. However, the use of early nCPAP was associated with a greater incidence of pneumothorax, compared with those in the intubation group (45).

The incidence of BPD reported in centers which introduced INSURE (intubation–surfactant treatment–extubation) was lower when compared with centers using mechanical ventilation with surfactant supplementation (96,97). However, although noninvasive ventilation in the DR especially in spontaneously breathing very preterm neonates is becoming more popular, there have not so far been sufficiently powered evidence-based studies supporting its systematic use in the DR for prevention of BPD. Although in a country like Denmark, which pioneered the use of early CPAP, the incidence of BPD that was relatively low has increased in the latter years, probably due to the survival of ELGA neonates (80). Increased rates of pneumothorax in infants not receiving surfactant without endotracheal intubation should be a concern (87). Taken into consideration the apparent advantages of using early nCPAP, the question still remains whether it is beneficial to use it in the DR for recovering ELBW infants in an attempt to reduce acute complications associated with intubation, as well as long-term respiratory consequences of various types of trauma to the lung caused by mechanical ventilation.

There is unfortunately no clear evidence that early nCPAP reduces the incidence of BPD. Obviously, more randomized trials are required in this field.

III. Oxygenation in the Delivery Room and Beyond

Oxygen transfer across the placenta is probably flow limited, and the driving force for net oxygen exchange is the partial pressure difference for the gas between maternal intervillous space and fetal capillary (98). The partial pressure of oxygen (PaO_2) in utero in blood taken in large umbilical vessels in the second and third trimesters ranges between 4.0 and 7.0 kPa (99–102). The values for PaO_2, PCO_2, and base excess have correlation with gestational age (101,102). Fetal oximetry ($FSpO_2$) has been studied by using reflectance pulse oximetry (103,104). $FSpO_2$ is an accurate measurement to determine fetal oxygen saturation during labor. Excellent correlation between oxygen saturation simultaneously measured in blood and oxygen saturation measured by $FSpO_2$ was shown in sheep (for review, see Ref. 104). Consistent $FSpO_2$ values of 43% to 45% in healthy fetal neonates have been reported, and values >30% are considered sufficient (105,106). Moreover, in human fetuses with abnormal non-reassuring fetal heart rate, administration of supplemental oxygen to the mother significantly increased $FSpO_2$

especially in those fetuses with the lowest initial oxygen saturation (107). Aerobic metabolism in the fetus is dependent on its capacity to adequately deliver oxygen to the different tissue. The total oxygen content of the blood is related to the oxygen saturation and hemoglobin content of arterial blood. However, although the oxygen content is linearly related to saturation, the relation between partial pressure of oxygen and saturation is nonlinear. Diffusion to the tissue depends on the oxygen tension gradient and the diffusion distance, which is related to the capillary density (108,109). These factors vary with gestational age of the fetus (110,111).

Hemoglobin is the oxygen-carrying molecule in the blood, and its concentration will affect the oxygen content of blood. Particularly, the hemoglobin concentration, which is very sensitive to PaO_2, will increase when fetal hypoxia is present over a prolonged period. Because of the oxygen-carrying capacity of hemoglobin, the oxygen tension in the blood can be lowered. Hemoglobin therefore seems to be a major factor to reduce oxidative stress. Erythropoietin, a glycoprotein which specifically is produced in the liver in the early gestation and thereafter also in the kidney, acting as a cytokine promotes bone marrow red cell production (112). Fetuses are growing and developing in a relatively hypoxic environment. To overcome such a disadvantageous condition, fetal hemoglobin (HbF), which has a high affinity toward oxygen, is produced. Because of its peculiar characteristics, HbF can easily pick up oxygen molecules from the maternal venous side (approximately 70% saturation), and deliver it to the target organs/tissues. The left shifting of oxygen dissociation curve of HbF indicates the increased binding between HbF and oxygen. This may be related to the decreased binding of 2,3-diphosphoglycerate by HbF (γ-chains). It has been shown that the in vivo effect of 2,3-diphosphoglycerate on the oxygen affinity of HbF is approximately 40% of that of adult hemoglobin (HbA) (113). The oxygen affinity of fetal blood decreases during gestation and depends on the relative proportions of HbA and HbF and on the level of red cell 2,3-diphosphoglycerate. However, it also has been shown that gestational age had no effect on 2,3-diphosphoglycerate levels and ΔpH between plasma and red cell (114). It has been therefore concluded that the decrease in fetal oxygen affinity as gestation progresses is related mainly to the increase in the amount of HbA. The levels of 2,3-diphosphoglycerate or ΔpH between plasma and red cells are not a function of gestational age. The presence of HbF with its higher affinity to oxygen therefore may be protective to the premature infant because a lower FiO_2 is needed to oxygenate the tissues compared with later in life.

A. Arterial Oxygen Saturation Changes in the Fetal to Neonatal Transition

With the lung expansion and initiation of aerial respiration, alveolar oxygen tension (PaO_2) will abruptly raise and will provide the driving pressure for oxygen diffusion into the pulmonary capillary bed (115). A series of studies have reported evolution in oxygen saturation during the first minutes of life in the DR determined by pulse oximetry (SpO_2) under different conditions [(117–122); for review, see Ref. 116)] (Fig. 3). Thus, House et al. (117) evaluated a total of one hundred newborn infants ranging from 850 to 5230 g, delivered vaginally or by C-section. Preductal readings showed an average SpO_2 of 59% at 1 minute, 68% at 2 minutes, 82% at 5 minutes, and 90% at 15 minutes (117). Dimich et al. performed a study that included pre- and postductal SpO_2 at 1, 5, 10 minutes, and 24 hours (118). They found significant differences at 1 and 5 minutes between pre- and

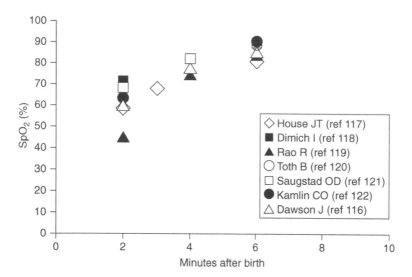

Figure 3 Arterial oxygen saturation in the first minutes of life. Saturation of oxyhemoglobin (SpO_2) in the first minutes of life as measured by pulse oximetry in the delivery room. Ref. 119 reflects SpO_2 in asphyxiated term babies, and Ref. 116 reflects SpO_2 in extremely premature babies of <30 weeks of gestation. *Source*: Modified from Ref. 123.

postductal readings. Differences disappeared almost at 10 minutes, and completely at 24 hours (118). From these and other studies, it may be concluded that it is possible to read reliable saturations in the delivery room as early as 1.2 minutes after birth. There is a gradual increase in preductal SpO_2 during the first 10 minutes of life; SpO_2 in babies born vaginally are consistently higher than in those born by C-section, the latter ones needing almost two more minutes to reach plateau SpO_2 of 90%, and that initial SpO_2 can be in normal babies as low as 53% (lower interquartile range at 1 minute of age), not reflecting a hypoxic situation but rather fetal oxygen saturation (123).

ELBW infants having an unstressed fetal to neonatal transition and who received mask or CPAP ventilation needed an average of 5 minutes to achieve an SpO_2 of 70% to 75%, and 10 to 15 minutes to reach SpO_2 of 80% to 85% (124,125). From these studies, it may be deduced that fetal to neonatal transition is a relatively slow process taking minutes. Hence, the time needed to achieve extrauterine SpO_2 values of approximately 85% inversely correlates with gestational age; thus, extremely premature infants with gestational ages around 24 to 25 weeks of gestation will need 10 or more minutes to reach a plateau SpO_2 of 80% to 85%.

B.   Lowering Inspiratory Fraction of Oxygen in the Delivery Room

The sudden increase in tissue oxygen content at transition from intra- to extrauterine life leads to oxidative stress (125–129). However, under normal circumstances, birth-associated oxidative stress is moderate, and will have beneficial effects on the term fetus favoring expression of enzymes that are essential for postnatal adaptation (26–31). Conversely, in adverse situations, such as extreme immaturity, compromised antioxidative capacity of the system may predispose to oxidative stress–induced injury capable of damaging cellular structures (14). As mentioned, the antioxidant defense system matures late in gestation, paralleling the maturation of the surfactant system (17,24–36). Therefore, extremely low gestational neonates are at special risk of developing conditions associated with oxidative stress–derived damage. In 1998, Saugstad coined the term "oxygen radical disease in neonatology," thus unifying the role of ROS in the pathogenesis of a wide range of morbidities; the implication being that they are different manifestations of the same condition (130,131). Neonatal morbidities in which oxidant stress has been hypothesized to play a crucial role include BPD (35–37,60), retinopathy of prematurity (132–135), necrotizing enterocolitis (136–138), intraventricular hemorrhage, and periventricular leukomalacia (139–141; for review, see Refs. 142 and 143).

Although extremely low gestational neonates have an immature antioxidant defense system and are therefore highly susceptible to oxidative stress and damage, a connection between high oxygen concentrations during resuscitation and development of BPD has not been yet established. Experimental studies indicate that the use of high oxygen concentrations triggers oxidative stress and causes damage in term babies (124,129,144–153). It is known that markers of oxidative stress are increased after a few days in infants who later develop BPD; thus, there is an association between early oxidative stress and BPD (35,74–78). Whether oxidative stress in utero or immediately after birth or a combination of both triggers the development of BPD is not known. Of interest is that there are data that establish a link between high oxygen concentration during resuscitation of ELGA and non-cyclooxygenase-dependent by-products derived from arachidonic acid oxidation (154); however, these are only partial results from a pilot study that need further confirmation.

Treatment Strategies

Possible strategies to avoid lung injury caused by overstretching or underventilation, oxidative stress, or inflammation would be as follows: (*i*) optimize ventilation from the first breaths of life; (*ii*) use inflammatory modulators: among these could be nutrients as polyunsaturated free fatty acids provided via the nutrition of the pregnant woman or given directly to the immature infant (for review, see Refs. 155,156), other nutritional approaches with early amino acids, shielding of vitamins for light, etc. may also be important measures to prevent BPD; (*iii*) increase the antioxidant capacity providing external antioxidants, blocking the negative consequences of free radicals (e.g., blocking the proapoptotic or proinflammatory pathways); and (*iv*) avoid the production of oxygen free radicals by reducing the amount of oxygen given during resuscitation.

Up to date, in the experimental but also in the clinical setting, ample arrays of therapeutic strategies have been proven. Thus, administration of extracellular SOD (157–159), inhaled NO (160–166), stabilization of HIF-1α (167–169), vitamin A (170–173), etc. have shown various degrees of success.

The use of lowest possible oxygen supplementation during resuscitation or adaptation maneuvers applied to the very premature infants in the DR would at least theoretically offer the advantage of decreasing the amount of oxygen free radicals generated upon reoxygenation. It has been shown in the experimental setting that the generation of superoxide anion as well as of hydrogen peroxide relates directly to the availability of oxygen on reoxygenation (144). Moreover, the use of high oxygen concentrations causes increased damage and inflammation in lung, brain, liver, platelet function, or reactivity of the pulmonary vessels (145–151). A growing body of clinical evidence has substantiated the negative effects of the use of 100% oxygen in the resuscitation of the asphyctic term newly born infant. Seemingly, the use of pure oxygen increases mortality, the risk of brain injury, and damage to heart and kidney (148,149). However, little information has been collected in relation to the resuscitation of preterm infants. In the last recommendations of the International Liaison Committee on Resuscitation (63) as well as a recent review (174), no specific initial inspiratory fraction of oxygen is indicated, although a special concern regarding the use of oxygen in preterm babies is made.

Up to date only two randomized trials investigating the feasibility of resuscitating ELGA neonates with FiO_2 lower than 100% have been published (175,176). In the first of the trials by Escrig et al. (175), researchers pursued to achieve a preestablished targeted SpO_2 of 85% at 10 minutes after birth in extremely low gestational neonates (<28 weeks of postconceptional age). Babies were randomly assigned to an initial FiO_2 of 30% or 90% respectively, which was adjusted sequentially (every 60 seconds) according to SpO_2 readings, heart rate, and patient's responsivity. No differences in SpO_2 between both groups were detected at the different time points. Moreover, no differences in the mortality rates in the early neonatal period (<7 days) were found between both groups. However, the oxygen load was significantly higher for the group starting with the high FiO_2; in fact, this group received almost 50% more oxygen as expressed in milliliters of pure oxygen per kilogram of the body weight as the group starting with lower initial FiO_2 (Fig. 4). The second published study was also a prospective, randomized controlled trial performed by Wang et al. (176) in two referral

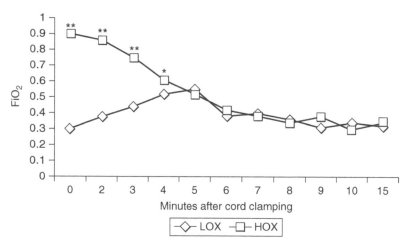

Figure 4 Resuscitation of preterm infants with higher or lower oxygen inspiratory fraction. Inspiratory fraction of oxygen (FiO_2) received by extremely low gestational age neonates randomly assigned to receive 90% (□, Hox group) or 30% (◇, Lox group) oxygen as initial gas admixture to initiate resuscitation after birth and attain a target SpO_2 of 85% at 10 minutes after birth while keeping heart rate above 100 beats/min. *Source*: Data to draw this figure have been obtained from Ref. 175.

centers. Babies enrolled who had gestational ages between 23 and 32 weeks and required resuscitation in the DR were randomly assigned to initial FiO_2 of 100% (oxygen group) or 21% (room air group). These researchers found that all their babies in the room air group needed increments of supplemental oxygen, some of them were directly switched to 100% oxygen and others reached this concentration by gradual increments of FiO_2. No differences in secondary outcomes as BPD were found. Thus, they concluded that it was not feasible to reach a targeted SpO_2 at three minutes of life when initiating resuscitation with room air.

Both of these studies were performed in very premature infants who required some type of active resuscitation maneuver. However, it would be desirable to obtain normative data of the temporal profile of the oxygenation in blood.

IV. Conclusions

The immature newborn infant is susceptible to develop BPD due to a number of risk factors. A lowered antioxidant defense makes these newborns less prepared to be born into an oxygen-enriched atmosphere. Inflammations both intrauterine and postnatally may add to the oxidative stress and injury. Overstretching and hypoventilation of the lung further adds to the inflammation through cytokine release.

Hemoglobin, especially HbF, may protect against oxidative stress because its high affinity for oxygen makes it possible to oxygenate with a lower FiO_2. In the future, new and more optimal ventilatory strategies may reduce incidence of BPD. An improved nutrition both intrauterine and postnatally may contribute to this. Antioxidant agents may come into use. However, most important today is to avoid hyperoxia including hyperoxic peaks. This strategy should be combined with a careful ventilation of the lungs. Together with inflammation control, these strategies probably make it possible to reduce severity and incidence of BPD substantially.

References

1. Fanaroff AA, Stoll BJ, Wright LL, et al. and NICHD Neonatal Research Network. Trends in neonatal morbidity and mortality for very low birth weight infants. Am J Obstet Gynecol 2007; 196:147c1–c8.
2. Field DJ, Dorling JS, Manktelow BN, et al. Survival of extremely premature babies in a geographically defined population: prospective cohort study of 1994-9 compared with 2000-5. BMJ 2008; 336(7655):1221–1223.
3. Landmann E, Misselwitz B, Steiss JO, et al. Mortality and morbidity of neonates born at <26 weeks gestation (1998-2003). A population based study. J Perinat Med 2008; 36(2): 168–174.
4. Himmelmann K, Hagberg G, Beckung E, et al. The changing panorama of cerebral palsy in Sweden. IX. Prevalence and origin in the birth year 1995-1998. Acta Paediatr 2005; 94:287–294.
5. Wilson-Costello D, Friedman H, Minich N, et al. Improved neurodevelopmental outcomes for extremely low birth weight infants in 2000-2002. Pediatrics 2007; 119:37–45.
6. Platt MJ, Cans C, Johnson A, et al. Trends in cerebral palsy among infants of very low birth-weight (<1500 g) or born prematurely (<32 weeks) in 16 European centres. Lancet 2007; 369:43–50.

7. Wilson-Costello D. Is there evidence that long-term outcomes have improved with intensive care? Semin Fetal Neonatal Med 2007; 12:344–354.

8. Phibbs CS, Baker LC, Caughey AB, et al. Level and volume of neonatal intensive care and mortality in very-low-birth-weight infants. N Engl J Med 2007; 356:2165–2175.

9. Aly H, Massaro AN, Patel K, et al. Is it safer to intubate premature infants in the delivery room? Pediatrics 2005; 115:1660–1665.

10. Lindner W, Vossbeck S, Hummler H, et al. Delivery room management of extremely low birth weight infants: spontaneous breathing or intubation? Pediatrics 1999; 103:961–967.

11. te Pas AB, Walther FJ. A randomized, controlled trial of delivery-room respiratory management in very preterm infants. Pediatrics 2007; 120:322–329.

12. Gearly C, Caskey M, Fonseca R, et al. Decreased incidence of bronchopulmonary dysplasia after early management changes, including surfactant and nasal continuous positive airway pressure treatment at delivery, lowered oxygen saturation goals, and early amino acid administration: a historical cohort study. Pediatrics 2008; 121:89–96.

13. Teitel D, Rudolph AM. Perinatal oxygen delivery and cardiac function. Adv Pediatr 1985; 32:321–347.

14. Jankov RP, Negus A, Keith Tanswell A. Antioxidants therapy in the newborn: some words of caution. Pediatr Res 2001; 50:681–687.

15. Droge W. Free radicals in the physiological control of cell function. Physiol Rev 2002; 82:47–95.

16. Terada LS. Specificity in reactive oxidant signaling: think globally, act locally. J Cell Biol 2006; 174:615–623.

17. Asikainen TM, White CW. Antioxidant defenses in the preterm lung: role for hypoxia inducible factors in BPD? Tox Appl Pharmacol 2005; 203:177–188.

18. Viña J, ed. Glutathione Metabolism and Physiological Function. Boston: CRC Press, 1990.

19. Wu G, Fang YZ, Yang S, et al. Glutathione metabolism and its implications for health. J Nutr 2004; 134:489–492.

20. Fang YZ, Yang S, Wu G. Free radicals, antioxidants, and nutrition. Nutrition 2002; 18: 872–879.

21. Lei XG. In vivo antioxidant role of glutathione peroxidase: evidence from knockout mice. Methods Enzymol 2002; 347:213–225.

22. Markovic J, Borras C, Ortega A, et al. Glutathione is recruited into the nucleus in early phases of cell proliferation. J Biol Chem 2007; 282:20416–20424.

23. Borras C, Esteve JM, Viña JR, et al. Glutathione regulates telomerase activity in 3T3 fibroblasts. J Biol Chem 2004; 279:34332–34335.

24. Frank L, Sosenko IR. Prenatal development of lung antioxidant enzymes in four species. J Pediatr 1987; 110:106–110.

25. Sosenko IR, Frank L. Thyroid inhibition and developmental increases in fetal rat lung antioxidant enzymes. Am J Physiol 1989; 257:L94–L99.

26. Chen Y, Sosenko IR, Frank L. Premature rats treated with propyl-thio-uracil show enhanced pulmonary antioxidant enzyme gene expression and improved survival during prolonged exposure to hyperoxia. Pediatr Res 1995; 38:292–297.

27. Viña J, Vento M, García-Sala F, et al. L-cysteine and glutathione metabolism are impaired in premature infants due to cistathionase deficiency. Am J Clin Nutr 1995; 61:1067–1069.

28. Levonen AL, Lapatto R, Saksela M, et al. Expression of gamma-glutamylcysteine synthase during development. Pediatr Res 2000; 278:C118–C125.

29. Levonen AL, Lapatto R, Saksela M, et al. Human cistathionine gamma-lyase developmental and in vitro expression of two isoforms. Biochem J 2000; 347(pt 1):291–295.

30. Jain A, Mehta T, Auld PA, et al. Glutathione metabolism in newborns: evidence for glutathione deficiency in plasma, bronchoalveolar lavage fluid, and lymphocytes in prematures. Pediatr Pulmonol 1995; 20:160–166.

31. Martin JA, Pereda J, Martínez-López I, et al. Oxidative stress as a signal to up-regulate gamma-cystathionase in the fetal to neonatal transition in rats. Cell Mol Biol (Noisy-le-grand) 2007; 53(suppl):OL1010–OL1017.
32. Walther FJ, Jobe AH, Ikegami M. Repetitive prenatal glucocorticoid therapy reduces oxidative stress in the lungs of preterm lambs. J Appl Physiol 1998; 85:273–278.
33. Sosenko IR, Jobe AH. Intraamniotic endotoxin increases lung antioxidant enzyme activity in preterm lambs. Pediatr Res 2003; 53:679–683.
34. Vento M, Escrig R, Saénz P, et al. Prenatal corticosteroids enhance the antioxidant defense system in extremely premature infants. E-PAS 2006; 59:2861.222.
35. Ahola T, Fellman V, Kjellmer I, et al. Plasma 8 isoprostane is increased in preterm infants who develop bronchopulmonary dysplasia or periventricular leukomalacia. Pediatr Res 2004; 56:88–93.
36. Collard KJ, Godeck S, Holley JE, et al. Pulmonary antioxidant concentrations and oxidative damage in ventilated premature babies. Arch Dis Child Fetal Neonatal Ed 2004; 89: F412–F416.
37. Saugstad OD. Oxidative stress in the newborn- a 30-year perspective. Biol Neonate 2005; 88:228–236.
38. Thebaud B. Angiogenesis and lung development. Neonatology 2007; 91:291–297.
39. Stenmark KR, Abman SH. Lung vascular development: implications for the pathogenesis of bronchopulmonary dysplasia. Annu Rev Physiol 2005; 67:623–661.
40. Bland RD. Neonatal chronic lung disease in the post-surfactant era. Lessons learned from the authentic animal models. Biol Neonate 2005; 88:181–191.
41. Gerhardt T, Bancalari E. Chestwall compliance in full-term and premature infants. Acta Paediatr Scand 1980; 69:359–364.
42. Heldt GP, McIlroy MB. Dynamics of chest wall in preterm infants. J Appl Physiol 1987; 62:170–174.
43. Finer NN, Carlo WA, Duara S, et al. for the National Institute of Child Health and Human Development Neonatal Research Network. Delivery room continuous positive airway pressure/positive end-expiratory pressure in extremely low birth weight infants: a feasibility trial. Pediatrics 2004; 114:651–657.
44. Morley CJ, Davis PG, Doyle LW, et al. Nasal CPAP or intubation at birth of very preterm infants. N Engl J Med 2008; 358:700–708.
45. Jobe AH, Ikegami M. Mechanisms' initiating lung injury in the preterm. Early Hum Dev 1998; 53:81–94.
46. Wada K, Jobe AH, Ikegami M. Tidal volume effects on surfactant treatment responses with the initiation of ventilation in preterm lambs. J Appl Physiol 1997; 83:1054–1061.
47. Björklund LJ, Ingemarson J, Curstedt T, et al. Manual ventilation with a few large breaths at birth compromises the therapeutic effect of subsequent surfactant replacement in premature lambs. Pediatr Res 1997; 42:348–355.
48. Kendig JW, Notter RH, Cox C, et al. A comparison of surfactant as immediate prophylaxis and as a rescue therapy in newborns of less than 30 wk gestation. N Engl J Med 1991; 324:865–871.
49. Grossmann G, Nilsson R, Robertson B. Scanning electron microscopy of epithelial lesions induced by artificial ventilation of the immature neonatal lung; the prophylactic effect of surfactant replacement. Eur J Pediatr 1986; 145:361–367.
50. Hillman NH, Moss TJM, Kallapur SH, et al. Brief, large tidal volume ventilation initiates lung injury and a systemic response in fetal sheep. Am J Respir Crit Care Med 2007; 176:575–581.
51. Bland RD, Xu L, Ertsey R, et al. Dysregulationof pulmonary elastin synthesis and assembly in preterm lambs with chronic lung disease. Am J Physiol Lung Cell Mol Physiol 2007; 292:L1370–L1384.

52. Bland RD, Ertsey R, Mokres LM, et al. Mechanical ventilation uncouples synthesis and assembly of elastin and increases apoptosis in lungs of newborn mice. Prelude to defective alveolar septation during lung development? Am J Physiol Lung Cell Mol Physiol 2008; 294: L3–L14.

53. Goldenberg RL, Culhane JF, Iams JD, et al. Epidemiology and causes of preterm birth. Lancet 2008; 371:75–84.

54. Goldenberg RL, Hauth JC, Andrews WW. Intrauterine infection and preterm delivery. N Engl J Med 2000; 342:1500–1507.

55. Romero R, Espinoza J, Chaiworapongsa T, et al. Infection and prematurity and the role of preventive strategies. Semin Neonatol 2002; 7:259–274.

56. Miralles R, Hodge R, McParland PC, et al. Relationship between antenatal inflammation and antenatal infection identified by detection of microbial genes by polymerase chain reaction. Pediatr Res 2005; 57:570–577.

57. Steel JH, Malatos S, Kennea N. Bacteria and inflammatory cells in fetal membranes do not always cause preterm labor. Pediatr Res 2005; 57:404–411.

58. Kallapur SG, Jobe AH. Contribution of inflammation to lung injury and development. Arch Dis Child Fetal Neonatal Ed 2006; 91:F132–F135.

59. Wilson MR, Choudhury S, Goddard ME, et al. High tidal volumes upregulates intrapulmonary cytokines in an in vivo mouse model of ventilatory-induced lung injury. J Appl Physiol 2003; 95:1385–1393.

60. Saugstad OD. Chronic lung disease: the role of oxidative stress. Biol Neonatol 1998; 74 (suppl 1):21–28.

61. Leviton A, Paneth N, Reuss ML, et al. Maternal infection, fetal inflammatory response and brain damage in very low birth weight infants. Developmental Epidemiology Network Investigators. Pediatr Res 1999; 46:566–575.

62. Jobe AH, Ikegami M. Antenatal infection/inflammation and postnatal lung maturation and injury. Respir Res 2001; 2:27–32.

63. The International Liaison Committee on Resuscitation (ILCOR) consensus on science with treatment recommendation for pediatric and neonatal patients: neonatal resuscitation. Pediatrics 2006; 117:978–988.

64. Horbar JD, Carpenter JH, Buzas J, et al. Vermont Oxford Network. Timing of initial surfactant treatment for infants 23 to 29 weeks' gestation: is routine practice evidence based? Pediatrics 2004; 113:1593–1602.

65. Horbar JD, Carpenter JH, Buzas J, et al. Collaborative quality improvement to promote evidence based surfactant or preterm infants: a cluster randomised trial. BMJ 2004; 329:1004.

66. Belperio JA, Keane MP, Burdick MD, et al. Critical role for CXCR2 and CXCR2 ligands during the pathogenesis of ventilator-induced lung injury. J Clin Invest 2002; 110:1703–1716.

67. Tremblay L, Valenza F, Ribeiro SP, et al. Injurious ventilatory strategies increase cytokines and c-fos m-RNA expression in an isolated rat lung model. J Clin Invest 1997; 99:944–952.

68. Tremblay LN, Miatto D, Hamid Q, et al. Injurious ventilation induces widespread pulmonary epithelial expression of tumor necrosis factor-alpha and interleukin-6 messenger RNA. Crit Care Med 2002; 30:1693–1700.

69. Nwariaku FE, Rothenbach P, Liu Z, et al. Rho inhibition decreases TNF-induced endothelial MAPK activation and monolayer permeability. J Appl Physiol 2003; 95:1889–1895.

70. Petrache I, Birukova A, Ramirez SI, et al. The role of the microtubules in tumor necrosis factor-alpha-induced endothelial cell permeability. Am J Respir Cell Mol Biol 2003; 28:574–581.

71. Braun C, Hamacher J, Morel DR, et al. Dichotomal role of TNF in experimental pulmonary edema reabsorption. J Immunol 2005; 175:3402–3408.

72. Wilson MR, Goddard ME, O'Dea KP, et al. Differential roles of p55 and p75 tumor necrosis factor receptors on stretch-induced pulmonary edema in mice. Am J Physiol Lung Cell Mol Physiol 2007; 293:L60–L68.

73. Sozo F, Wallace MJ, Zara VA, et al. Gene expression profiling during increased fetal lung expansion identifies genes to regulate the development of the distal airways. Physiol Genomics 2006; 24:105–113.

74. Speer CP. Pre- and postnatal inflammatory mechanisms in chronic lung disease of preterm infants. Paediatr Respir Rev 2003; 83(suppl 2):S255–S258.

75. Ogihara T, Hirano K, Morinobu T, et al. Raised concentrations of aldehyde lipid peroxidation products in premature infants with chronic lung disease. Arch Dis Child Fetal Neonatal Ed 1999; 80:F21–F25.

76. Schock BC, Sweet DG, Halliday HL, et al. Oxidative stress in lavage fluid of preterm infants at risk of chronic lung disease. Am J Physiol Lung Cell Mol Physiol 2001; 281: L1386–L139.

77. Ahola T, Lapatto R, Raivio KO, et al. N-acetylcysteine does not prevent bronchopulmonary dysplasia in immature infants: a randomized controlled trial. J Pediatr 2003; 143:713–719.

78. Speer CP. Pulmonary inflammation and bronchopulmonary dysplasia. J Perinatol 2006; 26(suppl 1):S57–S62.

79. Gregory GA, Kitterman JA, Phibbs RH, et al. Treatment of the ideopathic respiratory distress system with continuous positive airway pressure. N Engl J Med 1971; 284: 1333–1340.

80. Verder H. Nasal CPAP has become an indispensable part of the primary treatment of newborns with respiratory distress syndrome. Acta Paediatr 2007; 96:482–484.

81. Halamek LP, Morley C. Continuous positive airway pressure during neonatal resuscitation. Clin Perinatol 2006; 33:83–89.

82. Gittermann MK, Fusch C, Gittermann AR, et al. Early nasal continuous positive airway pressure treatment reduces the need for intubation in very low birth weight infants. Eur J Pediatr 1997; 156:384–388.

83. Davis P, Jankov R, Doyle L, et al. Randomised controlled trial of nasal continuous positive airway pressure in the extubation of infants weighing 600 to 1250 g. Arch Dis Child Fetal Neonatal Ed 1998; 78:F1–F4.

84. Jacobsen T, Gronvall J, Petersen S, et al. "Minitouch" treatment of very low-birth-weight infants. Acta Paediatr 1993; 82:934–938.

85. Lundstrom K, Griesen G. Early treatment with nasal CPAP. Acta Paediatr 1993; 82: 856–862.

86. Polin RA, Sahni R. Newer experience with CPAP. Semin Neonatol 2002; 7:379–389.

87. Ambalavanalan N, Carlo WA. Ventilatory strategies in the prevention and management of bronchopulmonary dysplasia. Semin Perinatol 2006; 30:192–199.

88. Morley CJ, Davis PG. Continuous positive airway pressure: scientific and clinical rational. Curr Opin Pediatr 2008; 20:119–124.

89. Bohlin K, Jonsson B, Gustafsson AS, et al. Continuous positive airway pressure and surfactant. Neonatology 2008; 93:309–315.

90. Shanmugananda K, Rawal J. Nasal trauma due to nasal continuous positive airway pressure in newborns. Arch Dis Child Fetal Neonatal Ed 2007; 92:F18.

91. Aly H, Herson V. Nasal continuous positive airway pressure and gram-negative sepsis in low-birthweight infants. Pediatr Infect Dis J 2006; 25:663–664.

92. Ho JJ, Subramaniam P, Henderson-Smart DJ, et al. Continuous distending pressure for respiratory distress syndrome in preterm infants. Cochrane Database Syst Rev 2002; 2: CD002271.

93. Ammari A, Suri M, Milisavljevic V, et al. Variables associated with the early failure of nasal CPAP in very low birth weight infants. J Pediatr 2005; 147:341–347.

94. Lindner W, Pohlandt F. Oxygenation and ventilation in spontaneously breathing very preterm infants with nasopharyngeal CPAP in the delivery room. Acta Paediatr 2007; 96:17–22.

95. Vanpée M, Walfridsson-Schultz U, Katz-Salomon M, et al. Resuscitation and ventilation strategies for extremely preterm infants: a comparison study between two neonatal centers in Boston and Stockholm. Acta Paediatr 2007; 96:10–16.

96. Halliday HL, Tarnow-Mordi WO, Cocoran JD, et al. Multicentre randomised trial comparing high and low dose surfactant regimens for the treatment of respiratory distress syndrome (the Curosurf 4 trial). Arch Dis Child 1993; 69:276–280.

97. The Osiris Collaborative Group. Early versus delayed neonatal administration of a synthetic surfactant—the judgment of Osiris. Lancet 1992; 340:1363–1369.

98. Sibley CP, Boyd RDH. Mechanisms of transfer across the human placenta. In: Polin RA, Fox WW, Abman SH, eds. Fetal and Neonatal Physiology. 4th ed. Philadelphia: Saunders-Elsevier, 2004:111–122.

99. Soothill PW, Nicolaides KH, Rodeck CH, et al. Blood gases and acid base status of the human second-trimester fetus. Obstet Gynecol 1986; 68:173–176.

100. Nicolaides KH, Soothill PW, Rodeck CH, et al. Ultrasound-guided sampling of umbilical cord and placental blood to assess fetal wellbeing. Lancet 1986; 1:1065–1067.

101. Lazarevic B, Ljubic A, Stevic R, et al. Respiratory gases and acid base parameter of the fetus during second and third trimester. Clin Exp Obstet Gynecol 1991; 18:81–84.

102. Bon C, Raudrant D, Poloce F, et al. Acid base equilibrium and oxygenation in the human fetus. Study of 73 samples obtained by cordocentesis. Ann Biol Clin (Paris) 1997; 55: 455–459.

103. Stiller R, von Mering R, König V, et al. How well does reflectance pulse oximetry reflect intrapartum fetal acidosis? Am J Obstet Gynecol 2002; 186:1351–1357.

104. East CE, Colditz PB. Intrapartum oximetry on the fetus. Anesth Analg 2007; 105:S59–S65.

105. Seelbach-Gobel B, Heupel M, Kuhnert M, et al. The prediction of fetal acidosis by means of intrapartum fetal pulse oximetry. Am J Obstet Gynecol 1996; 175:682–687.

106. Dildy GA, Thorp JA, Yeast JD, et al. The relationship between oxygen saturation and pH in umbilical blood: implications for intrapartum fetal oxygen saturation monitoring. Am J Obstet Gynecol 1996; 175:682–687.

107. Haydon ML, Gorenberg DM, Nageotte MP, et al. The effect of maternal oxygen administration on fetal pulse oximetry during labor in fetuses with non-reassuring fetal heart rate patterns. Am J Obstet Gynecol 2006; 195:735–738.

108. Leach RM, Treacher DF. Oxygen transport-2. Tissue hypoxia. BMJ 1998; 317:1370–1373.

109. Consensus conference on tissue hypoxia. Am J Respir Crit Care Med 1996; 154:1573–1578.

110. Kirschbaum TH. Variability of magnitude of the Bohr effect in human fetal blood. J Appl Physiol 1963; 18:729–733.

111. Nijland R, Jongsma HW, Nijhuis JG, et al. Arterial oxygen saturation in relation to metabolic acidosis in fetal lambs. Am J Obstet Gynecol 1995; 172:810–819.

112. Fisher JW. Erythropoietin: physiology and pharmacology update. Exp Biol Med 2003; 228:1–14.

113. Bard H, Teasdale F. Red cell oxygen affinity, hemoglobin type, 2,3-di-phospho-glycerate, and pH as a function of fetal development. Pediatrics 1979; 64:483–487.

114. Orzalesi MM, Hay WW. The regulation of oxygen affinity of fetal blood. I. In vitro experiments and results in normal infants. Pediatrics 1971; 48:857–864.

115. Treacher DF, Leach RM. Oxygen transport-1. Basic principles. BMJ 1999; 317:1320–1326.

116. Dawson JA, Davis PG, O'Donnell CP, et al. Pulse oximetry for monitoring infants in the delivery room: a review. Arch Dis Child Fetal Neonatal Ed 2007; 92:F4–F7.

117. House JT, Schultetus RR, Gravenstein N. Continuous neonatal evaluation in the delivery room by pulse oximetry. J Clin Monit 1987; 3:96–100.

118. Dimich I, Singh PP, Adell A, et al. Evaluation of oxygen saturation monitoring by pulse oximetry in neonates in the delivery system. Can J Anaesth 1991; 38:985–988.
119. Rao R, Ramji S. Pulse oximetry in asphyxiated newborns in the delivery room. Indian Pediatr 2001; 38:967–972.
120. Toth B, Becker A, Seelbach-Gobel B. Oxygen saturation in healthy newborn infants immediately after birth measured by pulse oximetry. Arch Gynecol Obstet 2002; 266:105–107.
121. Saugstad OD, Ramji S, Rootwelt T, et al. Response to resuscitation of the newborn: early prognostic variables. Acta Paediatr 2005; 94:890–895.
122. Kamlin CO, O'Donnell CPF, Davis PG, et al. Oxygen saturation in healthy infants immediately after birth. J Pediatr 2006; 148:585–589.
123. Saugstad OD. Oxygen saturations immediately after birth. J Pediatr 2006; 148:569–570.
124. Escrig R, Izquierdo I, Saénz P, et al. Glutathione redox status at birth predicts oxygen needs in the extremely preterm infant. Eur J Pediatr 2006; 165(suppl 1):65.
125. Vento M, Asensi M, Sastre J, et al. Oxidative stress in asphyxiated term infants resuscitated with 100% oxygen. J Pediatr 2003; 142:240–246.
126. Blackburn S. Alterations of the respiratory system in the neonate: implications for clinical practice. J Perinat Neonatal Nurs 1992; 6:46–58.
127. Pallardo FV, Sastre J, Asensi M, et al. Physiological changes in glutathione metabolism in foetal and newborn rat live. Biochem J 1991; 274:891–893.
128. Sastre J, Asensi M, Rodrigo F, et al. Antioxidant administration to the mother prevents oxidative stress associated with birth in neonatal rat. Life Sci 1994; 54:2055–2059.
129. Vento M, Asensi M, Sastre J, et al. Resuscitation with room air instead of 100% oxygen prevents oxidative stress in moderately asphyxiated term neonates. Pediatrics 2001; 107:642–647.
130. Saugstad OD. Hypoxanthine as an indicator of hypoxia: its role in health and disease through free radical production. Pediatr Res 1988; 23:143–150.
131. Saugstad OD. Oxygen radical disease in neonatology. Semin Neonatol 1998; 3:229–238.
132. Tin W, Milligan DW, Pennefather P, et al. Pulse oximetry, severe retinopathy, and outcome at one year in babies of less than 28 weeks gestation. Arch Dis Child Fetal Neonatal Ed 2001; 84:F106–F110.
133. Chow LC, Wright KW, Sola A, CSMC Oxygen Administration Study Group. Can changes in clinical practice decrease the incidence of severe retinopathy of prematurity in very low birth weight infants? Pediatrics 2003; 111:339–345.
134. Askie LM, Henderson-Smart DJ, Irwig L, et al. Oxygen-saturation targets and outcomes in extremely preterm infants. N Engl J Med 2003; 349:959–967.
135. Vanderveen DK, Mansfield TA, Eichenwald EC. Lower oxygen saturation alarm limits decrease the severity of retinopathy of prematurity. J AAPOS 2006; 10:445–448.
136. Haase E, Bigam DL, Nakonechny QB, et al. Resuscitation with 100% oxygen causes intestinal glutathione oxidation and reoxygenation injury in asphyxiated newborn piglets. Ann Surg 2004; 240:364–373.
137. Zhou Y, Wang Q, Mark Evers BM, et al. Oxidative stress-induced intestinal epithelial cell apoptosis is mediated by p38 MAPK. Biochem Biophys Res Commun 2006; 350:860–865.
138. Song J, Li J, Lulla A, et al. Protein kinase D protects against oxidative stress-induced intestinal epithelial cell injury via Rho/ROK/PKC-delta pathway activation. Am J Physiol Cell Physiol 2006; 290:C1469–C1476.
139. Back SA, Luo NL, Mallinson RA, et al. Selective vulnerability of preterm white matter to oxidative damage defined by F2-isoprostanes. Ann Neurol 2005; 58:108–120.
140. Inder T, Mocatta T, Darlow B, et al. Elevated free radical products in the cerebrospinal fluid of VLBW infants with cerebral white matter injury. Pediatr Res 2002; 52:213–218.

141. Haynes RL, Folkerth RD, Keefe RJ, et al. Nitrosative and oxidative injury to premyelinating oligodendrocytes in periventricular leucomalacia. J Neuropathol Exp Neurol 2003; 62:441–450.

142. Tin W, Gupta S. Optimum oxygen therapy in preterm babies. Arch Dis Child Fetal Neonatal Ed 2007; 92: F143–F147.

143. Saugstad OD. Optimal oxygenation at birth and in the neonatal period. Neonatology 2007; 91:319–322.

144. Turrens JF. Mitochondrial formation of reactive oxygen species. J Physiol 2003; 552:335–344.

145. Solberg R, Andresen JH, Escrig R, et al. Resuscitation of hypoxic newborn piglets with oxygen induces a dose-dependent increase in markers of oxidation. Pediatr Res 2007; 62:559–563.

146. Dohlen G, Carlsen H, Blomhoff R, et al. Reoxygenation of hypoxic mice with 100% oxygen induces brain nuclear factor-kappa B. Pediatr Res 2005; 58:941–945.

147. Munkeby BH, Borke WB, Bjornland K, et al. Resuscitation of hypoxic piglets with 100% oxygen increases pulmonary metalloproteinases and IL8. Pediatr Res 2005; 58:542–548.

148. Munkeby BH, Borke WB, Bjornland K, et al. Resuscitation with 100% O_2 increases cerebral injury in hypoxemic piglets. Pediatr Res 2004; 56:83–90.

149. Stevens JP, Churchill T, Fokkelman K, et al. Oxidative stress and matrix metalloproteinase-9 activity in the liver after hypoxia and reoxygenation with 21% or 100% oxygen in newborn piglets. Eur J Pharmacol 2008; 580:385–393.

150. Jantzie LL, Cheung PY, Obaid L, et al. Persistent neurochemical changes in neonatal piglets after hypoxia-ischemia and resuscitation with 100%, 21% or 18% oxygen. Resuscitation 2008; 77:111–120.

151. Cheung PY, Johnson ST, Obaid J, et al. The systemic pulmonary and regional hemodynamic recovery of asphyxiated newborn piglets resuscitated with 18%, 21% and 100% oxygen. Resuscitation 2008; 76:457–464.

152. Vento M, Sastre J, Asensi MA, et al. Room air resuscitation causes less damage to heart and kidney than 100% oxygen. Am J Respir Crit Care Med 2005; 172:1393–1398.

153. Saugstad OD, Ramji S, Soll R, et al. Resuscitation of newborn infants with 21% or 100% oxygen: an updated systematic review and meta-analysis. Neonatology 2008; 94:176–182.

154. Vento M, Roberts JL, Izquierdo I, et al. Monitorization of hypo-or-hyperoxia derived oxidative stress in extremely low birth weight (ELBW) infants using urinary F2-isoprostanes and isofurans. E-PAS 2008; 5851.9.

155. Tin W, Wiswell TE. Adjunctive therapies in chronic lung disease: examining the evidence. Semin Fetal Neonatal Med 2008; 13:44–52.

156. Ramanathan R. Optimal ventilatory strategies and surfactant to protect preterm lungs. Neonatology 2008; 93:302–308.

157. Ilizarov AM, Koo HC, Kazzaz JA, et al. Overexpression of manganese superoxide dismutase protects lung epithelial cells against oxidant injury. Am J Respir Cell Mol Biol 2001; 24:436–441.

158. Ahmed MN, Suliman HB, Folz RJ, et al. Extracellular superoxide dismutase protects lung development in hyperoxia-exposed newborn mice. Am J Respir Crit Care Med 2003; 167:400–405.

159. Chang LY, Subramaniam M, Yoder B, et al. A catalytic antioxidant attenuates alveolar structural remodelling in bronchopulmonary dysplasia. Am J Respir Crit Care Med 2003; 167:57–64.

160. Cotton RB, Sundell HW, Zeldin DC, et al. Inhaled nitric oxide attenuates hyperoxic lung injury in lambs. Pediatr Res 2006; 59:142–146.

161. Grover T. The diverse role of inhaled nitric oxide in experimental BPD: reduced fibrin deposition and improved lung growth. Am J Physiol Lung Cell Mol Physiol 2007; 293: L33–L34.

162. Kinsella JP, Cutter GR, Walsh WF, et al. Early inhaled nitric oxide therapy in premature newborns with respiratory failure. N Engl J Med 2006; 355:354–364.

163. Ballard RA, Truog WE, Cnaan A, et al. NO CLD Study Group. Inhaled nitric oxide in preterm infants undergoing mechanical ventilation. N Engl J Med 2006; 355:343–353.

164. Van Meurs KP, Hintz SR, Ehrenkranz RA, et al. Inhaled nitric oxide in infants > 1500 g and < 34 weeks gestation with severe respiratory failure. J Perinatol 2007; 27:347–352.

165. Truog WE. Inhaled nitric oxide for the prevention of bronchopulmonary dysplasia. Expert Opin Pharmacother 2007; 8:1505–1513.

166. Barrington KJ, Finer NN. Inhaled nitric oxide for respiratory failure in preterm infants. Cochrane Database Syst Rev 2007; (3):CD000509.

167. Asikainen TM, Schneider BK, Waleh NS, et al. Activation of hypoxia-inducible factors in hyperoxia through prolyl 4-hydroxylase blockade in cells and explants of primate lung. Proc Natl Acad Sci U S A 2005; 102:10212–10217.

168. Asikainen TM, Waleh NS, Schneider BK, et al. Enhancement of angiogenic effectors through hypoxia-inducible factor in preterm primate lung in vivo. Am J Physiol Lung Cell Mol Physiol 2006; 291:L588–L595.

169. Asikainen TM, White CW. HIF stabilizing agents: shotgun or scalpel? Am J Physiol Lung Cell Mol Physiol 2007; 293:L555–L556.

170. Ozer EA, Kumral A, Ozer E, et al. Effect of retinoic acid on oxygen-induced lung injury in the newborn rat. Pediatr Pulmonol 2005; 39:35–40.

171. Tyson JE, Wright LL, Oh W, et al. Vitamin A supplementation for extremely-low-birth-weight-infants. National Institute of Child Health and Human Development Neonatal Research Network. N Engl J Med 1999; 340:1962–1968.

172. Ambalavanan N, Wu TJ, Tyson JE, et al. A comparison of three vitamin A dosing regimens in extremely-low-birth-weight infants. J Pediatr 2003; 142:656–661.

173. Spears K, Cheney C, Zerzan J. Low plasma retinol concentrations increase the risk of developing bronchopulmonary dysplasia and long-term respiratory disability in very-low-birth-weight infants. Am J Clin Nutr 2004; 80:1589–1594.

174. Escobedo M. Moving from experience to evidence: changes in the US Neonatal Resuscitation Program based on International Liaison Committee on Resuscitation Review. J Perinatol 2008; 28(suppl 1):S35–S40.

175. Escrig R, Arruza L, Izquierdo I. Achievement of target saturation in extremely low gestational age neonates resuscitated with different oxygen concentrations: a prospective randomized clinical trial. Pediatrics 2008; 121:875–881.

176. Wang CL, Anderson C, Leone TA, et al. Resuscitation of preterm neonates using room air or 100% oxygen. Pediatrics 2008; 121:1083–1089.

17

Mechanical Ventilation: Early Strategies to Decrease BPD

TINA A. LEONE and NEIL N. FINER
University of California, San Diego, San Diego, California, U.S.A.

I. Introduction

Bronchopulmonary dysplasia (BPD) was first described by Northway et al. (1) in 1967 as a pathologic pulmonary consequence of treatment for respiratory distress syndrome. The initial description presented a timeline for the development of this chronic lung disease (CLD) on the basis of radiographic and pathologic findings in a cohort of 32 patients. The speculated pathogenesis of the findings included consequences of oxygen toxicity, the healing process of respiratory distress syndrome, and effects of ventilation and endotracheal intubation. Further evaluation of the pathogenesis of this disease has led to the understanding that this is a multifactorial process involving the degree of prematurity, individual host factors, prenatal environmental factors, and various treatment factors of which ventilatory support is among the most important. Over the 40 years since the recognition of this disease process, numerous changes have occurred in the care of preterm infants including the use of antenatal steroids and surfactant replacement, the availability of varieties of neonatal ventilators, and the addition of newer adjunctive medications and nutritional support. The modern era of neonatology is associated with increased survival of more immature infants with premature lung disease that is somewhat different from the initial BPD description. However, the continued significant occurrence of this neonatal CLD in surviving infants despite various changes in therapeutic approaches highlights the need for careful evaluation of all therapies and understanding of developmental physiology.

As artificial ventilation is a key component in the development of BPD, the overall goal in delivering ventilation should be to provide just enough assistance to maintain adequate physiologic status while minimizing lung injury. The quest to reduce the incidence of BPD has been the focus of much neonatal research over the 40 years since ventilator associated lung injury with subsequent BPD was recognized as a significant neonatal morbidity, but its incidence in the most premature infants remains essentially unchanged over the past 10 years (2). Approaches to dealing with this dilemma have involved limiting the use of invasive mechanical ventilation, altering the target of acceptable physiologic parameters, varying methods of delivering traditional ventilator breaths, and delivering ventilatory support through unique types of ventilators that alter the traditional concept of artificial ventilation. Unfortunately, there is currently a lack of evidence to demonstrate that one method of such support can successfully decrease the occurrence of BPD. It also seems unlikely that one approach would be suitable for all individuals. The ultimate goal may therefore be to identify the babies who truly need artificial ventilatory support and then provide support in the least injurious manner and for the shortest duration possible.

The evidence that mechanical ventilation may lead to lung injury resulting in bronchopulmonary dysplasia includes the recognition that all of the patients who initially developed the disease had been treated with mechanical ventilation. In Northway's original report every patient ventilated for more than six days developed the disease. In evaluations of populations of very low birth weight infants in North Carolina ventilation for >48 hours was identified as a risk factor for CLD with a relative risk of 8.5 (95% CI 5.5–13) (3). Currently, one of the strongest predictors for developing BPD is the duration of mechanical ventilation with each week increment in duration of ventilation associated with a 2.7 times increased odds (95% CI 1.76–4.18) (4).

II. The Need for Mechanical Ventilation

Perhaps the first issue to be addressed in discussing the role of mechanical ventilation in lung injury is the indication for intubation and mechanical ventilation. Some possible reasons preterm infants may require ventilation include apnea associated with perinatal asphyxia, hypoxia and/or hypercarbia secondary to lung immaturity, sepsis/pneumonia, or apnea of prematurity. During the transition from fetal to neonatal life, the infant must clear lung fluid and develop a functional residual capacity. With pulmonary immaturity and surfactant deficiency, the development of functional residual capacity is more difficult. The resultant clinical signs of respiratory distress caused by the various pathological processes may be indistinguishable. Treatment options for infants with signs of respiratory distress include mechanical ventilation and noninvasive modes of support such as nasal continuous positive airway pressure (CPAP).

In the early fetal transition process, some investigators have developed unique maneuvers for the immediate resuscitation process intended to help establish FRC. Lindner et al. described a method of delivering a prolonged (15 seconds) inflation by a single nasopharyngeal tube followed by CPAP (5). Compared with historical controls who were intubated early for signs of respiratory distress, the rate of intubation and mechanical ventilation was lower using this method. However, when compared in a randomized controlled fashion with nasopharyngeal positive pressure ventilation for signs of respiratory distress there was no difference in rate of intubation (6). When Harling et al. evaluated an initial inflation time of two seconds compared with five seconds no difference in inflammatory markers or ventilation parameters were noted (7). Recently, te Pas and Walther reported the results of a randomized trial comparing the delivery room respiratory management of 207 infants (8). The experimental group was treated with a sustained nasopharyngeal inflation (10 seconds) followed by CPAP, and the control group was treated with standard positive pressure ventilation performed with a self-inflating bag without PEEP or CPAP. The experimental group had fewer infants intubated by 72 hours of age and fewer cases of moderate to severe BPD ($p = 0.04$).

For at least 20 years, it has been recognized that the incidence of CLD varies substantially by center. In efforts to identify clinical factors associated with CLD, Avery et al. evaluated the incidence of oxygen use at 28 days among survivors at birth weights of 700 to 1500 g born at eight different centers (9). This report identified a large difference in the incidence of CLD among centers with one institution, Columbia, having much lower occurrence of the disease than any other center. The unique clinical care factors occurring at this institution included frequent use of nasal prong CPAP, no use of muscle relaxants, the acceptance of higher $PaCO_2$ values, and a single individual responsible for all ventilator management. More than 10 years later, in a further evaluation of the practice differences between Columbia and two Boston institutions, Columbia used significantly lower rates of mechanical ventilation and surfactant but used CPAP more frequently. Even the infants who were treated with mechanical ventilation at Columbia were ventilated for a median of 13 days compared with a median of 27 days in Boston. The rates of CLD in these populations of 500 to 1500 g birth weight infants were 4% at Columbia and 22% in Boston (10). A similar report compared infants less than 28 weeks' gestation treated at a neonatal intensive care unit in Boston with those treated at a unit in Stockholm. In Stockholm, 56% of the infants were initially treated with CPAP and 63% of those went on to be intubated within the first week of life. All infants treated in Boston were initially intubated, on average had higher mean airway pressures, and were less likely to be extubated within the first week of life. At 36 weeks more infants in the Boston unit were on mechanical ventilation and at 40 weeks more infants in this unit were treated with oxygen (11).

The respiratory management approach used at Columbia has been the subject of much speculation, emulation, and recently clinical research. One of the central ideas of the Columbia approach is that a premature baby does not need mechanical ventilation simply because of prematurity. Using this approach a premature infant is supported with CPAP (specifically "bubble CPAP") from the first minutes of life if the infant is making any spontaneous respiratory effort. In a recent observational report of their experiences with this approach, which described the treatment of all infants ≤1250 g, all but 12% were started on CPAP (12). Birth weight was one of the most significant factors in predicting success of CPAP. Among the smallest birth weight group identified, ≤750 g, 74% were started on CPAP and 50% of those were ultimately intubated and mechanically ventilated within the first 72 hours of life.

Other centers have adopted the Columbia approach to try to improve their own rates of CLD. These centers have described their experiences comparing new treatment techniques with historical controls and described reductions in CLD rates after making these practice changes (13–15). While retrospective reviews have suggested that such management changes are associated with reductions in BPD (16), other prospective quality improvement practice changes have not been successful in achieving a significant reduction in CLD rate, as evidence by the NICHD benchmarking trial. This trial, however, did not specify increased use of early CPAP as a practice change. And though centers were successful in achieving practice changes they were not successful in improving CLD rates (17).

The retrospective experience reported with early CPAP is difficult to reconcile with the evidence for benefit from exogenous surfactant administration. The early surfactant trials generally compared intubated and ventilated infants treated with surfactant to control infants mechanically ventilated and treated with placebo (18,19). Surfactant was not compared with any noninvasive therapy such as early CPAP. These trials consistently demonstrated that surfactant significantly decreased mortality and improved short-term respiratory parameters including decreases in mean airway pressure, oxygen administration, pneumothoraces, and pulmonary interstitial emphysema (20,21). Studies that have evaluated the use of prophylactic surfactant and early surfactant compared with the use of surfactant after establishment of respiratory distress syndrome (RDS) also reported improvements in short-term respiratory parameters, decreased rates of pneumothoraces, pulmonary interstitial emphysema, and mortality (22,23). Surfactant administered either in a prophylactic or in a treatment approach has improved rates of the combined outcome of BPD or death though not BPD alone with natural surfactant showing a greater benefit than synthetic products (24).

It is only within the last 10 years that early surfactant and early CPAP for preterm respiratory management have begun to be compared to each other. The first of the current trials to begin addressing this question (COIN trial) was a multicenter, international trial that randomized 610 infants of 25 to 28 weeks' gestation to treatment with either CPAP or intubation at five minutes of life if the infant was spontaneously breathing (25). Importantly, there were no protocol requirements for the administration of surfactant for infants in either arm, and no specific extubation criteria as both of these followed local practice. No differences were found in the rates of death or BPD at 36 weeks' gestational age, but there was a significantly higher number of pneumothoraces in the CPAP group, which may be related to the use of CPAP levels of 8 cm H_2O. In this trial, 77% of infants randomized to the intubation arm received surfactant. It seems likely that universal surfactant administration for all ventilated infants could have improved outcome in this group. It is encouraging that neither approach as practiced seems more detrimental during the hospitalization period, though longer-term outcomes are not yet available.

Two additional large ongoing trials are aimed at further evaluating the comparison of surfactant versus CPAP. The Vermont Oxford Network has stopped enrolling infants of 26 0/7th to 29 6/7th weeks' gestation in a three-arm trial in which infants are randomized to (*i*) intubation, early prophylactic surfactant with subsequent stabilization on ventilator support, (*ii*) intubation, early prophylactic surfactant with rapid extubation to CPAP, and (*iii*) early stabilization with nasal CPAP with selective intubation and surfactant administration for clinical indications (26). The SUPPORT trial which completed enrollment by March, 2009 enrolled infants of 24 0/7th weeks to 27 6/7th weeks, and these infants were randomized to either CPAP beginning in the delivery room with criteria for subsequent intubation or intubation with surfactant treatment within one hour of birth with continuing ventilation with criteria for extubation (27). While the specific criteria for intubating an infant assigned to CPAP in these trials were not identical, they are remarkably similar and include a $PaCO_2 > 60$ to 65 torr, or an FiO_2 requirement of greater than 0.4 to 0.6 or significant apnea. Thus, the answer to the question of whether early CPAP is superior or equivalent to early surfactant for the ELBW infant (infants of 1000 g or less) may be available within the next two to three years.

Some investigators have taken an alternate approach in an effort to provide the benefit of surfactant and still minimize the risk associated with mechanical ventilation with mixed results. The first suggestion of this strategy was described by Verder et al. in 1994 (28). Infants of 25 to 35 weeks' gestation were randomized to early intubation and treatment with surfactant with planned extubation within one hour of the dose or to later intubation once more significant signs of respiratory distress syndrome developed. Mechanical ventilation was used less frequently in the experimental group. Several small studies have been conducted to evaluate this approach and reviewed in a Cochrane

Collaboration meta-analysis (29). None of the currently available trials individually has been large enough to evaluate the effect on the outcome of BPD. However, the meta-analysis that combined six trials with slightly different approaches found decreased use of mechanical ventilation, decreased air leaks, and less BPD in the groups that received surfactant earlier and were extubated quickly. Two small studies evaluated early surfactant administration in both the control and experimental groups followed by either very rapid extubation or continued mechanical ventilation (30,31). Both studies found decreased overall use of mechanical ventilation in infants extubated early with no recognized adverse effects of early extubation.

A few small reports of alternate delivery techniques for surfactant administration without intubation have been published. These have included case series descriptions of intrapartum nasopharyngeal administration and laryngeal mask airway administration of surfactant (32,33). Another recent report describes a technique of administration of surfactant through a small caliber tube (feeding tube) inserted into the trachea under direct laryngoscopy (34,35). Using this method, infants are maintained on nasal CPAP before and after surfactant administration. These methods in theory limit the risks of the endotracheal tube and mechanical ventilation including direct trauma from the intubation procedure, ventilator associated lung injury, and nosocomial pneumonia associated with mechanical ventilation. There is also interest and one preliminary trial evaluating the use of aerosolized delivery of surfactant to infants receiving CPAP (36,37). Though these reports are intriguing, none are controlled trials and therefore require further investigation.

III. Limiting Ventilation

Whether attempting to limit the initiation of mechanical ventilation or the duration of mechanical ventilation, additional interventions may be able to help maintain adequate respiratory parameters. Noninvasive support can be delivered in the form of CPAP or nasal ventilation, which allows positive pressure breaths to be delivered through nasal prongs. One small study compared the early use of nasal CPAP with nasal intermittent mechanical ventilation (NIMV) in preterm infants with RDS and found that intubation was performed nearly half as often in the group initially treated with NIMV (25% vs. 49%, $p < 0.05$) and a decreased incidence of BPD (2% vs. 17%, $p < 0.05$) (38). Nasal CPAP after extubation has been shown to prevent extubation failure more than treatment with headbox oxygen (39) though synchronized nasal ventilation is more effective than CPAP (40).

There are many devices for the administration of CPAP, which include ventilators, flow drivers, and simple underwater "bubble-like" devices. To the present time it would appear that CPAP is best administered using short binasal prongs, and there is no proven advantage to any of the differing available systems for CPAP delivery (41). In addition, there are no studies that have evaluated the effects of differing levels of CPAP administered to determine if there is an optimal level related to important clinical outcomes, and by convention, most units defer to a level of 5 cm H_2O. Increasing levels of CPAP do increase lung volume (42), but higher levels may be a risk for air leaks and may adversely affect hemodynamics as has been reported in animal studies (43).

Methylxanthines have been shown to effectively treat apnea of prematurity, decrease the need for mechanical ventilation, and decrease extubation failure (44,45). A recent large trial evaluated the use of caffeine in infants of 500 to 1250 g birth weight with the primary purpose of evaluating long-term outcome (46). In this placebo-controlled trial, infants who received caffeine were treated with less open-label respiratory stimulant therapy, were successfully extubated one week earlier, received less duration of all positive pressure and oxygen, less postnatal corticosteroids, and fewer red blood cell transfusions. Additionally, the rate of BPD was significantly less in the caffeine group compared with the placebo group, 36% vs. 47%, $p < 0.001$. Finally, caffeine-treated infants were treated less often for patent ductus arteriosus and had more frequent survival without neurodevelopmental disabilities (47). The beneficial effect of caffeine in this group was quite significant although it should be noted that the incidence of BPD remained substantial.

IV. Mechanical Ventilation Strategies

The most important factor in preventing BPD may be avoiding the need for mechanical ventilation. However, since it would not be possible to completely eliminate the need for mechanical ventilation we must also evaluate different methods of providing ventilation to determine how to deliver breaths in the least injurious manner. As various clinical practices have been examined in relation to the incidence of BPD, different ventilator parameters and ventilation targets have been implicated in the development of this CLD. In the initial report by Avery et al. (9) describing the incidence of BPD in different neonatal units, it was noted that average arterial carbon dioxide levels ($PaCO_2$) above the physiologic range were associated with lower BPD rates. Wung et al. first described the technique of "gentle ventilation" in infants with persistent pulmonary hypertension of the newborn (PPHN), aiming for $PaCO_2$ levels up to 60 mmHg (48). Kraybill et al. published a multicenter historical cohort analysis of 235 infants with birth weights of 751 to 1000 g and reported that a $PaCO_2$ of less than 40 mmHg at 48 or 96 hours of life was the best predictor of BPD (49). They also noted that a mean $PaCO_2$ in those infants receiving mechanical ventilation at 48 and 96 hours strongly correlated with subsequent BPD rates. Garland et al. later noted a significant association between low $PaCO_2$ levels prior to the first dose of surfactant and the subsequent development of BPD; infants whose lowest $PaCO_2$ level was 29 mmHg or less were 5.6 times more likely to develop BPD than those whose lowest $PaCO_2$ level was 40 mmHg or more (50). Hypocapnia was also reported as a risk factor for increased neurodevelopmental impairment in preterm infants. Calvert et al. reported that infants with cystic periventricular leukomalacia (PVL) had longer durations with $PaCO_2$ levels <25 mmHg and lower mean $PaCO_2$ levels (51). Graziani et al. found that in ventilated infants, $PaCO_2$ levels of less than 17 mmHg during the first three days of life were associated with a significantly increased risk of moderate to severe periventricular echodensity, large periventricular cysts, grade 3 or 4 intracranial hemorrhage, and cerebral palsy (52). Fujimoto et al. reported a strong correlation between a $PaCO_2$ <20 mmHg and cystic PVL in infants without significant perinatal complications (53). The association between the use of the high-frequency jet ventilator and cystic PVL was reported by Wiswell et al. (54) and was also found to be related by logistic regression analysis to the duration of $PaCO_2$ <25 mmHg during day 1 of life (55).

Observations that the effects of moderate hypercapnia appear to be well tolerated in animal models led to the approach of allowing $PaCO_2$ values to be maintained higher than normal in the management of the ventilated adult patients with respiratory failure (56). Subsequently, two randomized trials of a strategy of permissive hypercapnia and a limitation of airway pressures and tidal volumes in adults were reported. Neither study found that such a strategy was associated with a higher rate of survival to hospital discharge (57,58). A subsequent large randomized, multicenter trial in adults with acute respiratory distress syndrome (ARDS), which targeted specific tidal volumes rather than $PaCO_2$ or pH ranges, reported that there were significant reductions in mortality and number of days without ventilator use in the group treated with lower tidal volumes (59). A recent meta-analysis of the use of low tidal volume ventilation for adults with ARDS, which compared a tidal volume ≤ 7 mL/kg with tidal volumes of 10 to 15 mL/kg, concluded that mortality was significantly reduced at day 28 and at the end of hospital stay. The authors noted that the effects on long-term mortality are unknown, although the possibility of a clinically relevant benefit could not be excluded (60).

In view of this information, it is not surprising that there has been a trend to accepting higher levels of $PaCO_2$ for the ventilated very preterm neonate. Two previous prospective randomized trials failed to demonstrate a benefit of this approach, although both were smaller trials (61–63). A more recent trial randomized preterm infants between 23 and 28 weeks requiring mechanical ventilation within six hours of birth to be managed with either a $PaCO_2$ target between 55 and 65 mmHg (minimal ventilation) or 35 and 45 mmHg for the first seven days of life. The trial was stopped early after enrolling 31% of the projected sample size. Enrolled infants had a median birth weight of 640 g. BPD or death occurred in 21/33 (64%) infants after minimal ventilation and 19/32 (59%) infants after routine ventilation. Minimal ventilation was associated with trends toward higher mortality and higher incidence of neurodevelopmental impairment, and a significantly increased combined outcome of mental impairment or death ($p < 0.05$) (64).

The larger question is whether preterm infants can safely tolerate such increases in $PaCO_2$ without significant neuromorbidity. The most recent experience in this area is that of Fabres et al. who reported that both high and low $PaCO_2$ values in VLBW infants are associated with severe IVH (65). Thus, in the absence of good evidence from randomized trials, it would appear prudent to avoid both very high and very low $PaCO_2$ values in the first few days of life in the very preterm infant.

Neonatal ventilation has generally been delivered in a pressure-controlled, time-cycled fashion where inspiratory and expiratory pressure levels, inspiratory time, and breath rates are set. Synchronized modes allow the ventilator to match the mechanical breath with the infant's own effort and have been associated with fewer air leaks and shorter duration of ventilation (66). Though some retrospective evaluations have suggested associations between higher mean airway pressure, peak inspiratory pressure, and ventilator rates with BPD, no particular ventilation method has been prospectively shown to be superior. More recently volume-controlled neonatal ventilators have become available, which allow the clinician to set the desired volume of each breath, and the ventilator adjusts the pressure to deliver that volume. A few small studies have evaluated volume versus pressure-controlled ventilation and have demonstrated a shorter duration of ventilation using volume-controlled ventilation and a nonsignificant trend toward lower BPD rates in the groups treated with volume ventilation (67). In a small trial, preterm infants ventilated at tidal volumes of 5 mL/kg versus 3 mL/kg had fewer days of ventilation and markers of inflammation (68). Volume guarantee ventilation is still a relatively new method of neonatal ventilation and different versions of this design appear to deliver differing inspiratory pressures and durations when set to the same tidal volume (69). The overview of volume targeted versus pressure targeted ventilation for newborn infants concluded that while there was no difference in death or BPD with either approach, the volume-targeted ventilation resulted in shorter duration of ventilation, fewer pneumothoraces, and less frequent severe (grade 3 or 4) intraventricular hemorrhage (67). Further studies with adequate power to address longer-term outcomes are required before any definite recommendations can be made.

With the recognition that mechanical ventilation was associated with ongoing pulmonary morbidity, alternate methods of providing ventilation were developed with the hope that they would decrease lung injury. High-frequency ventilators exist in two basic forms: high-frequency oscillators and high-frequency jet ventilators. High-frequency oscillatory ventilation (HFOV) as a primary ventilation method has been evaluated in several large trials. The first of these trials randomized 673 infants of 750 to 2000 g birth weight to HFOV or to conventional ventilation (70). The incidence of BPD was not different between the groups (40% vs. 41%, $p = 0.79$). This study also raised a concern because more infants in the high-frequency group developed grade 3 or 4 IVH. This study however took place in a time before the widespread use of antenatal steroids and surfactant and thus the relevance to current practice is questionable. Conflicting results were found in subsequent studies exemplified by two recent large trials conducted in multiple centers throughout the world. Johnson et al. evaluated 797 infants of 23 to 28 weeks gestation and found no difference in death or CLD (71). Courtney et al. enrolled 500 infants of 600 to 1200 g birth weight and found that infants treated with HFOV had a slightly decreased rate of death or BPD and shorter duration of ventilation, 13 vs. 21 days ($p < 0.001$) (72). A meta-analysis of 15 trials comparing HFOV with conventional ventilation found minimal differences between the two types of ventilation (73). These trials have been noted to be heterogeneous in respect to specific ventilators, general strategies of ventilation, and time of trial entry. When results were evaluated by these subgroups, rates of BPD were lower for HFOV particularly when piston oscillators and a higher mean airway pressure strategy of oscillation was used. Other findings among these trials include a higher incidence of air leak with HFOV and no difference in intracranial hemorrhage.

Similarly, high-frequency jet ventilation (HFJV) has been evaluated as a primary ventilation strategy for preterm infants. A meta-analysis of three trials examining this therapy compared with conventional ventilation found a small improvement in BPD rates with the use of HFJV (74). However, the largest trial (54) making this comparison found a significantly higher rate of PVL in the HFJV-treated infants. Therefore, the risk of this therapy used as the primary ventilation mode seems to outweigh any possible limited benefit.

V. Conclusion

Bronchopulmonary dysplasia or CLD of prematurity remains a significant morbidity for preterm infants and a dilemma for neonatologists. Some components of the pathogenesis of this disease process are not likely to be modifiable making persistence of the disease

Table 1 Summary of Evidence from Meta-analyses: Effects on Risk of BPD

Intervention	Source	Number of patients	BPD: O_2 at 28 days	Number of patients	BPD: O_2 at 36 wk
NCPAP after extubation	Davis and Henderson-Smart, 2003 (39)	433	RR: 1.00 (0.81, 1.24)	–	–
Nasal intermittent ventilation vs. NCPAP	Davis et al., 2001 (40)	–	–	118	RR: 0.73 (0.49, 1.07)
Prophylactic natural surfactant	Soll, 1997 (20)	932	RR: 0.93 (0.8, 1.07)	–	–
Prophylactic vs. treatment surfactant	Soll and Morley, 2001 (22)	2816	RR: 0.96 (0.82, 1.12)	–	–
Early vs. delayed selective surfactant	Yost and Soll, 1999 (23)	3039	RR: 0.97 (0.88, 1.06)	3007	RR: 0.70 (0.55, 0.88)
Volume-targeted vs. pressure-limited ventilation	McCallion, 2005 (67)	110	RR: 0.87 (0.39, 1.96)	103	RR: 0.34 (0.11, 1.05)
Elective HFOV	Henderson-Smart et al., 2007 (73)	1043	RR: 0.98 (0.88, 1.10)	2310	RR: 0.89 (0.81, 0.99)
Elective HFJV	Bhuta and Henderson-Smart, 1998 (74)	204	RR: 0.90 (0.74, 1.09)	170	RR: 0.59 (0.35, 0.99)

Abbreviations: BPD, bronchopulmonary dysplasia; HFJV, high-frequency jet ventilation; NCPAP, nasal continuous positive airway pressure.

probable. However, it is encouraging that low BPD rates have been able to be achieved in some situations. When interventions have been evaluated in a prospective manner, few effects on BPD rates have been identified. A summary of the available evidence that has been reviewed by Cochrane meta-analyses is available in the Table 1. Though adequate evidence is not available to guide all management decisions, a general approach can be developed based on our current knowledge. Care of preterm infants should include administration of antenatal steroids to the mother whenever possible (75). Such treatment reduces neonatal death, RDS and the need for respiratory support as well as intracranial hemorrhages, and necrotizing enterocolitis. The next consideration in the provision of respiratory support includes determining when the need for mechanical ventilation exists. Attempting to limit the use of mechanical ventilation whenever possible while not restricting its use in critical circumstances may help prevent ventilator associated injury. When the need for ventilation in the first days after birth does exist, surfactant should be used as early as possible for treatment of RDS as this is a proven method of improving mortality rates and air leak syndromes. Clinicians then should make every attempt to limit the duration of ventilation by extubating infants early and using adjunctive therapies to maintain extubation including caffeine and noninvasive mechanical ventilation modes. Alternate ventilation methods may be helpful in some circumstances but no ventilation method has at this point been demonstrated to be superior to others. There are many types of newer neonatal ventilators that incorporate a number of modalities including pressure support and volume versus pressure modes of support that are not intuitive. Each individual and unit should become familiar with a small number of devices and understand their limits and idiosyncrasies. The most difficult decision may be determining when a particular infant truly needs mechanical ventilation. Current indications for ventilation vary by center and probably need to be determined more clearly as do protocols and strategies for weaning and extubating infants who require mechanical ventilation. The risks and benefits of surfactant compared with those of primary support with CPAP need to be further evaluated in well-designed prospective trials with an emphasis on determining which populations of infants would benefit in the short and long term from either therapy. The smallest preterm infants ($\leq$750 g) are at highest risk of mortality and at highest risk for failing CPAP and therefore may benefit most from early surfactant. The overall incidence of BPD remains high and thus the possibility for improvement also remains high. Continued prospective evaluations of various techniques with the assessment of significant short and long term outcomes are essential to clarify future best practices.

References

1. Northway WH, Rosan RC, Porter DY. Pulmonary disease following respirator therapy of hyaline-membrane disease. N Engl J Med 1967; 276:357–368.
2. Kobaly K, Schluchter M, Minich N, et al. Outcomes of extremely low birth weight (<1 kg) and extremely low gestational age (<28 weeks) infants with bronchopulmonary dysplasia: Effects of practice changes in 2000 to 2003. Pediatrics 2008; 121(1):73–81.
3. Young TE, Kruyer LS, Marshall DD, et al. Population-based study of chronic lung disease in very low birth weight infants in North Carolina in 1994 with comparisons with 1984. Pediatrics 1999; 104:e17.
4. Serenius F, Ewald U, Farooqi A, et al. Short-term outcome after active perinatal management at 23–25 weeks of gestation. A study from two Swedish perinatal centres. Part 3: neonatal morbidity. Acta Paediatr 2004; 93:1090–1097.
5. Lindner W, Vossbeck S, Hummler H, et al. Delivery room management of extremely low birth weight infants: spontaneous breathing or intubation? Pediatrics 1999; 103:961–967.
6. Lindner W, Hogel J, Pohlandt F. Sustained pressure-controlled inflation or intermittent mandatory ventilation in preterm infants in the delivery room? A randomized, controlled trial on initial respiratory support via nasopharyngeal tube. Acta Paediatr 2005; 94:303–309.
7. Harling AE, Beresford MW, Vince GS, et al. Does sustained lung inflation at resuscitation reduce lung injury in the preterm infant? Arch Dis Child Fetal Neonatal Ed 2005; 90:406–410.
8. te Pas AB, Walther FJ. A randomized, controlled trial of delivery-room respiratory management in very preterm infants. Pediatrics 2007; 120:322–329.
9. Avery ME, Tooley WH, Keller JB, et al. Is chronic lung disease in low birth weight infants preventable? A survey of eight centers. Pediatrics 1987; 79:26–30.
10. Van Marter LJ, Allred EN, Pagano M, et al. Do clinical markers of barotraumas and oxygen toxicity explain interhospital variation in rates of chronic lung disease? Pediatrics 2000; 105:1194–1201.

11. Vanpee M, Walfridsson-Schultz U, Katz-Salamon M, et al. Resuscitation and ventilation strategies for extremely preterm infants: a comparison study between two neonatal centers in Boston and Stockholm. Acta Paediatr 2007; 96:10–16.

12. Ammari A, Suri M, Milisavljevic V, et al. Variables associated with the early failure of nasal CPAP in very low birth weight infants. J Pediatr 2005; 147:341–347.

13. Aly H, Milner JD, Patel K, et al. Does the experience with the use of nasal continuous positive airway pressure improve over time in extremely low birth weight infants? Pediatrics 2004; 114:697–702.

14. Narendran V, Donovan EF, Hoath SB, et al. Early bubble CPAP and outcomes in ELBW preterm infants. J Perinatol 2003; 23:195–199.

15. De Klerk AM, de Klerk RK. Nasal continuous positive airway pressure and outcomes of preterm infants. J Paediatr Child Health 2001; 37:161–167.

16. Geary C, Caskey M, Fonseca R, et al. Decreased incidence of bronchopulmonary dysplasia after early management changes, including surfactant and nasal continuous positive airway pressure treatment at delivery, lowered oxygen saturation goals, and early amino acid administration: a historical cohort study. Pediatrics 2008; 121:89–96.

17. Walsh M, Laptook A, Kazzi N, et al. A cluster randomized trial of benchmarking and multimodal quality improvement to improve rates of survival free of bronchopulmonary dysplasia for infants with birth weights less than 1250 grams. Pediatrics 2007; 119:876–890.

18. Horbar JD, Soil RF, Sutherland JM, et al. A multicentre, randomized, placebo controlled trial of surfactant therapy for respiratory distress syndrome. N Engl J Med 1989; 320:959–965.

19. Merritt TA, Hallman M, Bloom BT, et al. Prophylactic treatment of very premature infants with human surfactant. N Engl J Med 1986; 315:785–790.

20. Soil RF. Prophylactic natural surfactant extract for preventing morbidity and mortality in preterm infants. Cochrane Database Syst Rev 1997; (2):CD000511.

21. Soil RF. Prophylactic synthetic surfactant for preventing morbidity and mortality in preterm infants. Cochrane Database Syst Rev 2000; (2):CD001079.

22. Soil RF. Morley CJ. Prophylactic versus selective use of surfactant in preventing morbidity and mortality in preterm infants. Cochrane Database Syst Rev 2001; (2):CD000510.

23. Yost CC, Soil RF. Early versus delayed selective surfactant treatment for neonatal respiratory distress syndrome. Cochrane Database Syst Rev 1999; (4):CD001456.

24. Soil RF, Blanco F. Natural surfactant extract versus synthetic surfactant for neonatal respiratory distress syndrome. Cochrane Database Syst Rev 2001; (2):CD000144.

25. Morley CJ, Davis PG, Doyle LW, et al. Nasal CPAP or intubation at birth for very preterm infants. N Engl J Med 2008; 358:700–708.

26. DRM Trial. Comparing methods of post-delivery stabilization. Available at: http://www.vtoxford.org/home.aspx?p=research/drm/index.htm. Also available at: http://clinicaltrials.gov/ct2/show/NCT00244101?term=vermont+oxford+network&rank=1. Both accessed on July 7, 2009.

27. SUPPORT. Available at: http://www.clinicaltrials.gov/ct/show/NCT00233324?order=13. Accessed on July 7, 2009.

28. Verder H, Robertson B, Griesen G, et al. Surfactant therapy and nasal continuous positive airway pressure for newborns with respiratory distress syndrome. N Engl J Med 1994; 331:1051–1055.

29. Stevens TP, Blennow M, Myers EW, et al. Early surfactant administration with brief ventilation vs. selective surfactant and continued mechanical ventilation for preterm infants with or at risk for respiratory distress syndrome. Cochrane Database Syst Rev 2007; (4):CD003063.

30. Tooley J, Dyke M. Randomized study of nasal continuous positive airway pressure in the preterm infant with respiratory distress syndrome. Acta Paediatr 2003; 92:1170–1174.

31. Dani C, Bertini G, Pezzati M, et al. Early extubation and nasal continuous positive airway pressure after surfactant treatment for respiratory distress syndrome among preterm infants <30 weeks' gestation. Pediatrics 2004; 113:e560–e563.

32. Kattwinkel J, Robinson M, Bloom BT, et al. Technique for intrapartum administration of surfactant without requirement for an endotracheal tube. J Perinatol 2004; 24:360–365.

33. Trevisanuto D, Grazzina N, Ferrarese P, et al. Laryngeal mask airway used as a delivery conduit for the administration of surfactant to preterm infants with respiratory distress syndrome. Biol Neonate 2005; 87:217–220.

34. Kribs A, Pillekamp F, Hunsler C, et al. Early administration of surfactant in spontaneous breathing with nCPAP: feasibility and outcome in extremely premature infants (postmenstrual age ≤27 weeks). Pediatr Anesth 2007; 17:364–369.

35. Kribs A, Vierzig A, Hunsler C, et al. Early surfactant in spontaneously breathing with nCPAP in ELBW infants—a single centre four year experience. Acta Paediatr 2008; 97:293–298.

36. Finer NN, Merritt TA, Bernstein G, et al. A multicenter pilot study of Aerosurf™ delivered via nasal continuous positive airway pressure (nCPAP) to prevent respiratory distress syndrome in preterm neonates. Pediatr Res 2006; 59: PAS2006: 4840.138.

37. Mazela J, Merritt TA, Finer NN. Aerosolized surfactants. Curr Opin Pediatr 2007; 19: 155–162.

38. Kugelman A, Feferkorn I, Riskin A, et al. Nasal intermittent mandatory ventilation versus nasal continuous positive airway pressure for respiratory distress syndrome: a randomized, controlled, prospective study. J Pediatr 2007; 150(5):521–526, 526.e1.

39. Davis PG, Henderson-Smart DJ. Nasal continuous positive airway pressure immediately after extubation for preventing morbidity in preterm infants. Cochrane Database Syst Rev 2003; (2):CD000143.

40. Davis PG, Lemyre B, De Paoli AG. Nasal intermittent positive pressure ventilation (NIPPV) versus nasal continuous positive airway pressure (NCPAP) for preterm neonates after extubation. Cochrane Database Syst Rev 2001; (3):CD003212.

41. De Paoli AG, Davis PG, Faber B, et al. Devices and pressure sources for administration of nasal continuous positive airway pressure (NCPAP) in preterm neonates. Cochrane Database Syst Rev 2008; (1):CD002977.

42. Courtney SE, Pyon KH, Saslow JG, et al. Lung recruitment and breathing pattern during variable versus continuous flow nasal continuous positive airway pressure in premature infants: an evaluation of three devices. Pediatrics 2001; 107:304–308.

43. Polglase GR, Morley CJ, Crossley KJ, et al. Positive end-expiratory pressure differentially alters pulmonary hemodynamics and oxygenation in ventilated, very premature lambs. J Appl Physiol 2005; 99:1453–1461.

44. Henderson-Smart DJ, Steer P. Methylxanthine treatment for apnea in preterm infants. Cochrane Database Syst Rev 2001; (3):CD000140.

45. Henderson-Smart DJ, Davis PG. Prophylactic methylxanthines for extubation in preterm infants. Cochrane Database Syst Rev 2003; (1):CD000139.

46. Schmidt B, Roberts RS, Davis P, et al. Caffeine therapy for apnea of prematurity. N Engl J Med 2006; 354:2112–2121.

47. Schmidt B, Roberts RS, Davis P, et al. Long-term effects of caffeine therapy for apnea of prematurity. N Engl J Med 2007; 357:1893–1902.

48. Wung JT, James LS, Kilchevsky E, et al. Management of infants with severe respiratory failure and persistence of the fetal circulation without hyperventilation. Pediatrics 1985; 76:488–494.

49. Kraybill EN, Runyan DK, Bose CL, et al. Risk factors for chronic lung disease in infants with birth weights of 751 to 1000 grams. J Pediatr 1989; 115:115–120.

50. Garland JS, Buck RK, Allred EN, et al. Hypocarbia before surfactant therapy appears to increase bronchopulmonary dysplasia risk in infants with respiratory distress syndrome. Arch Pediatr Adolesc Med 1995; 149:617–622.

51. Calvert SA, Hoskins EM, Fong KW, et al. Etiologic factors associated with the development of periventricular leukomalacia. Acta Paediatr Scand 1987; 76:254–259.

52. Graziani LJ, Spitzer AR, Mitchell DG, et al. Mechanical ventilation in preterm infants: neurosonographic and developmental studies. Pediatrics 1992; 90:515–522.
53. Fujimoto S, Togari H, Yamagichi N, et al. Hypocarbia and cystic periventricular leukomalacia in premature infants. Arch Dis Child 1994; 71:F107–F110.
54. Wiswell TE, Graziani LJ, Kornhauser MS, et al. High frequency jet ventilation in the early management of respiratory distress syndrome is associated with a greater risk for adverse outcomes. Pediatrics 1996; 98:1035–1043.
55. Wiswell TE, Graziani LJ, Kornhauser MS, et al. Effects of hypocarbia on the development of cystic periventricular leukomalacia in premature infants treated with high-frequency jet ventilation. Pediatrics 1996; 98:918–924.
56. Dries DJ. Permissive hypercapnia. J Trauma 1995; 39:984–989.
57. Amato MB, Barbas CS, Medeiros DM, et al. Effect of a protective-ventilation strategy on mortality in the acute respiratory distress syndrome. New Eng J Med 1998; 338:347–354.
58. Stewart TE, Meade MO, Cook DJ, et al. Evaluation of a ventilation strategy to prevent barotrauma in patients at high risk for acute respiratory distress syndrome. N Engl J Med 1998; 338:355–361.
59. The Acute Respiratory Distress Syndrome Network. Ventilation with lower tidal volumes as compared with traditional tidal volumes for acute lung injury and the acute respiratory distress syndrome. N Engl J Med 2000; 342:1301–1308.
60. Petrucci N, Iacovelli W. Lung protective ventilation strategy for the acute respiratory distress syndrome. Cochrane Database Syst Rev 2007; (3):CD003844.
61. Carlo WA, Stark AR, Bauer C, et al. Effects of minimal ventilation in a multicenter randomized controlled trial of ventilator support and early corticosteroid therapy in extremely low birthweight infants. Pediatrics 1999; 104(3 suppl):738–739.
62. Mariani G, Cifuentes J, Carlo WA. Randomized trial of permissive hypercapnia in preterm infants. Pediatrics 1999; 104:1082–1088.
63. Woodgate PG, Davies MW. Permissive hypercapnia for the prevention of morbidity and mortality in mechanically ventilated newborn infants. Cochrane Database Syst Rev 2001; (2): CD002061.
64. Thome UH, Carroll W, Wu TJ, et al. Outcome of extremely preterm infants randomized at birth to different PaCO2 targets during the first seven days of life. Biol Neonate 2006; 90:218–225.
65. Fabres J, Carlo WA, Phillips V, et al. Both extremes of arterial carbon dioxide pressure and the magnitude of fluctuations in arterial carbon dioxide pressure are associated with severe intraventricular hemorrhage in preterm infants. Pediatrics 2007; 119:299–305.
66. Greenough A, Dimitiou G, Prendergast M, Milner AD. Synchronized mechanical ventilation for respiratory support in newborn infants. Cochrane Database Syst Rev 2008; (1): CD000456.
67. McCallion N, Davis PG, Morley CJ. Volume-targeted versus pressure-limited ventilation in the neonate. Cochrane Database Syst Rev 2005; (3):CD003666.
68. Lista G, Castoldi F, Fontana P, et al. Lung inflammation in preterm infants with respiratory distress syndrome: effects of ventilation with different tidal volumes. Pediatr Pulmonol 2006; 41:357–363.
69. Sharma A, Milner AD, Greenough A. Performance of neonatal ventilators in volume targeted ventilation mode. Acta Paediatrica 2007; 96:176–180.
70. HIFI Study Group. High-frequency oscillatory ventilation compared with conventional mechanical ventilation in the treatment of respiratory failure in preterm infants. N Engl J Med 1989; 320:88–93.
71. Johnson AH, Peacock JL, Greenough A, et al. High-frequency oscillatory ventilation for the prevention of chronic lung disease of prematurity. N Engl J Med 2002; 347:633–642.

72. Courtney SE, Durand DJ, Asselin JM, et al. High-frequency oscillatory ventilation versus conventional mechanical ventilation for very low birth weight infants. N Engl J Med 2002; 347:643–652.
73. Henderson-Smart DJ, Cools F, Bhuta T, et al. Elective high-frequency oscillatory ventilation versus conventional ventilation for acute pulmonary dysfunction in preterm infants. Cochrane Database Syst Rev 2007; (3):CD000104.
74. Bhuta T, Henderson-Smart DJ. Elective high frequency jet ventilation versus conventional ventilation for respiratory distress syndrome in preterm infants. Cochrane Database Syst Rev 1998; (2):CD000328.
75. Roberts D, Dalziel S. Antenatal corticosteroids for accelerating fetal lung maturation for women at risk of preterm birth. Cochrane Database Syst Rev 2006; (3):CD004454.

18
Lung Function, Structure and the Physiologic Basis for Mechanical Ventilation of Infants with Established BPD

ROBERT G. CASTILE and LEIF D. NELIN
The Ohio State University, Columbus, Ohio, U.S.A.

I. Lung Function in Established BPD

In 1967 Northway et al. (1) first described bronchopulmonary dysplasia (BPD), a chronic lung disease occurring in premature infants with respiratory distress syndrome treated with supplemental oxygen and mechanical ventilation. Widespread airway inflammation and injury were prominent findings in these infants. Respiratory epithelial cell metaplasia, peribronchial fibrosis, airway smooth muscle hypertrophy, and lung parenchymal fibrosis alternating with emphysema were common pathologic findings. At that time, the majority of infants developing BPD were over 30 weeks of gestational age and had birth weights greater than 1000 g. BPD as a long-term complication was uncommon in younger, less mature infants because they did not survive. Recent advances in neonatal care including the widespread use of maternal antenatal steroids, exogenous surfactant replacement therapy, and gentler modes of ventilatory support have resulted in striking changes in both the gestational ages of infants presenting with BPD and the pathologic findings seen in infants with this syndrome. While the incidence of BPD in infants greater than 1000 g has decreased, there have been dramatic increases in survival rates and the incidence of BPD in very premature infants. The incidence of BPD defined as a need for supplement oxygen at 36 weeks of postmenstrual age is about 30% for infants with birth weights less than 1000 g and around 50% for infants less than 750 g (2–4).

Pathologically, this new form of BPD (now termed "new BPD" to distinguish it from the classical or "old" form of BPD described by Northway) is characterized by a disruption and delay in acinar development with reduced alveolar and parenchymal complexity, abnormal parenchymal elastin deposition, and disturbed microvascular angiogenesis (5). In contradistinction to the classical BPD described by Northway et al. (1), minimal intrinsic changes are seen in the airways. This difference in pathologies between the old and the new BPDs most likely reflects the very different phases of lung development, which are occurring when these infants are born. Currently, the majority of infants who develop BPD are born at 24 to 28 weeks of gestational age, during the transition from the canalicular to the saccular stage of lung development. Most infants with old BPD were born at 28 or more weeks gestation, at a time when their lungs were more mature and in transition from the saccular to the alveolar stage of development.

New BPD is characterized by the need for supplemental oxygen at 28 days of life with level of severity defined by the degree of respiratory support required at 36 weeks of postmenstrual age. Having had respiratory distress syndrome as a consequence of early surfactant deficiency is no longer part of the definition, and some infants develop BPD without having required mechanical ventilatory support or supplemental oxygen immediately following birth. Despite enormous advancements in the care of prematurely born infants, rates of occurrence of BPD have not declined. With increases in the absolute numbers of very premature infants being born and surviving, the total numbers of infants with BPD have remained the same or may in fact be increasing (3,6,7). New BPD is now the most common cause of chronic respiratory disease in infants.

Very little has been written about ventilation strategies in infants with established BPD. This is an important issue as it is clear that the risk of mortality in these infants increases with the duration of mechanical ventilation. In one study, death occurred in 35% of infants requiring mechanical ventilation for two months and in 90% of those requiring support for greater than four months (8). Most authors agree that a strategy of larger tidal volumes delivered at slower rates with longer inspiratory and expiratory times is likely to improve distribution of ventilation in the nonhomogeneously obstructed lung and thus decrease physiologic dead space and gas trapping and improve gas exchange (9,10). This represents a distinct change in strategy from the higher rates and lower tidal volumes commonly utilized early in the course of respiratory distress in the premature infant. No objective studies have however been published to substantiate this approach. The purpose of this chapter is to summarize what is known about lung function and structure in infants with established BPD and based on that knowledge to describe a physiologically based ventilatory support strategy for these infants. The goal of this ventilatory strategy is to provide support while preventing complications and optimizing lung growth and recovery. The large majority of the investigations of lung function and structure in infants with established BPD have been carried out in infants with old BPD, and thus their relevance to the nature of the respiratory abnormalities in infants with new BPD needs to be interpreted with some caution. Recently published studies describing infants in the new BPD era have been noted in the text and given greatest weight in drawing conclusions.

II. Resistance and Compliance

Numerous methods have been used to assess lung mechanics in infants with established BPD during tidal breathing. These include dynamic resistance and compliance of the lung measured using an esophageal pressure catheter, the single-breath occlusion method for measuring resistance and compliance of the respiratory system, plethysmographic measurement of airway resistance, the interrupter and forced oscillation techniques for measuring respiratory system resistance, and the multiple occlusion and weighted spirometer methods for estimating respiratory system compliance. Changes in level of airway obstruction have also been inferred from respiratory inductive plethysmographic surface measurements of phase angle differences in chest wall and abdominal dimensions. The advantages and limitations of these methods have been recently reviewed in detail (11). A method for obtaining quasistatic expiratory pressure volume curves over the full vital capacity range in sedated infants that includes normal values for compliance has been published. No reports using this approach to assess compliance in infants with BPD have yet appeared (12).

Compliance is a direct function of lung size, and both resistance and compliance change rapidly in infants in relation to somatic growth. To compare groups or individuals of different sizes, specific compliance and conductance (the reciprocal of resistance) are calculated by dividing compliance and conductance by functional residual capacity (FRC). Body weight and length have also been used to adjust for the effects of growth. Normalized measures of lung compliance have generally been found to be reduced in established BPD, indicating the presence of increased lung elastic recoil (13–15). Resistance assessed using various methods has consistently been found to be increased and conductance decreased in infants with established BPD (14–17). Specific compliance and conductance have been found to improve in infants with BPD over the first two to three years of life (14,15,17). Gerhardt et al. (14) reported that in infants with old BPD lung compliance and conductance improved between 6 and 36 months of age but remained modestly below levels of function measured in normal infants at three years of age. Baraldi et al. (15) in 1997 found that in infants with new BPD, abnormalities in resistance and compliance measured using the single-breath occlusion method also improved over time reaching normal levels by two years of age. Recently, Hjalmarson and Sandberg (18), studying infants with new BPD at 39 to 40 of postconceptual age, measured no differences in specific compliance of the respiratory system between infants with mild, moderate and severe BPD, and healthy preterm control infants suggesting that parenchymal elastic dysfunction may be less prominent in new compared to old BPD. Respiratory system resistance also did not differ between groups. Specific conductance was found to be significantly higher in the infants with severe BPD than in the control infants, but this appeared to be a reflection of the much smaller functional residual capacities measured by nitrogen washout rather than a real increase in airway function. This result illustrates the limitations of these tidal range measurements. Measures of compliance and resistance are variable because they are measured over a limited volume range and depend on the lung volume at which they are measured. End expiratory lung volume levels are actively controlled in infants and change in response to changing levels of respiratory dysfunction. In patients with airway obstruction measurements made during tidal breathing are in addition affected by breathing rate (frequency dependence). Estimates of resistance and compliance measured by the single-breath method may not be entirely reliable because of the substantial curvilinearity of the passive expiratory flow volume relationship in infants with BPD. Jarriel et al. (19) have pointed out that respiratory system mechanics in these patients are much better characterized by a two compartment rather than a linear one-compartment resistance/compliance model. Measurements of resistance in infants are also thought to reflect predominantly upper and central airways making it difficult to infer the location of the obstruction. Although the methodologies are problematic and the number of recent publications limited, available data suggest that resistive and elastic abnormalities may be milder and improve more rapidly in new than in old BPD.

III. Lung Volumes

FRC has been measured in infants with BPD both plethysmographically and using nitrogen washout and gas dilution methods. Washout and gas dilution methods measure only gas that communicates with the airway opening during tidal breathing. These measurements thus often underestimate the actual lung volume at FRC because they do not measure volumes of gas behind closed airways and can underestimate volumes in severely obstructed poorly ventilated areas. Plethysmographic methods measure all gas within the lungs including gas that is trapped behind closed airways. Plethysmographic measurements in patients with airway obstruction are subject to artifactual increases that occur when there is flow between central and peripheral airways during airway occlusion (20). Flow-related pressure losses result in an underestimation of alveolar pressure by measurements made at the airway opening and overestimation of FRC. An extensive review of these methods and results of measurements made on infants with BPD has recently been published (21). Guidelines for both methods have been published (22,23).

Measurements of FRC made before one year of age using gas dilution and washout methods have been consistently reported to be reduced in infants with both old and new BPD (14,15,21,24,25). Mahut et al. in 2007 (26) reported that mean FRC measured by helium dilution was normal in patients with new BPD between 10 and 20 months of age. In most studies, FRC measured by washout and dilution methods has been shown to improve rapidly, reaching normal levels by early in the second year of life (14,15,24). Plethysmographic measurements have demonstrated normal or elevated measures of FRC (27,28). This difference in FRC measurements by the two methods was examined by Wauer et al. (29) who measured FRC both plethysmographically and by nitrogen washout in infants with BPD at 36 weeks' postconceptual age (average age 60 days) and again near the time of hospital discharge (average age 149 days). At 36 weeks, mean FRC measured plethysmographically was found to be increased (138% of predicted), while mean FRC measured by nitrogen washout was found to be decreased (61% predicted). When compared to similar paired measurements made in normal newborn control infants, this difference in FRC between the two methods was five times greater in the infants with BPD. By the time of discharge this difference had declined to 2.5 times that of the control infants. Reductions in gas dilution and nitrogen washout in FRC measurements reported in infants with established BPD in the first year of life thus probably reflect the amount of noncommunicating trapped gas not measured in infants with obstructive disease rather than being indicative of a restrictive defect. Reduction in the difference between the two methods is probably indicative of improvements in airway function, less air trapping, and better gas exchange. The overall implication of these data is that the basic functional abnormalities in infants with established BPD are obstructive rather than restrictive. Introduction of the raised volume rapid thoracic compression (RVRTC) method for performing spirometry in sedated infants has also made possible the measurement of complete fractional lung volumes including total lung capacity (TLC) and residual volume (RV) (30). In this method, expiratory reserve volume (ERV) is measured following the RVRTC-forced vital capacity (FVC) maneuver and FRC is measured plethysmographically. Subtracting ERV from the RVRTC FVC provides RV and adding RV to the FVC yields TLC. Robin et al.

(28) have reported the results of fractional lung volume measurements in 28 patients with new BPD. Mean RV and RV/TLC ratio were found to be significantly elevated in infants with BPD compared with normal control infants while mean TLC was in the normal range. Plethysmographically measured FRC was found to be only marginally elevated compared with the normal control infants. A recent report from these authors reveals that although TLC continues to increase normally over the second year of life in infants with new BPD, levels of air trapping as reflected by the RV/TLC ratio remain unchanged (31). Infants with new BPD have obstructive airway disease with air trapping that persists over time. Again the available data suggest levels of dysfunction as reflected by measurements of FRC may be milder in patients with new versus old BPD.

IV. Forced Flows

Measurements of forced flows have been made in infants with BPD using the rapid thoracic compression (RTC) method to produce partial flow volume curves and the forced deflation and RVRTC techniques to produce forced expiratory flows over the full vital capacity range. The use of these tests in infants with BPD has recently been reviewed, and guidelines for the two RTC methods have been published (32–34). Measurements of forced flows in infants with established BPD were first reported by Tepper et al. in 1986 (24). Using the RTC or so-called "squeeze" technique to produce partial expiratory flow volume curves, they found that average maximal flows measured at FRC (V'_{maxFRC}) were reduced by approximately 50% in infants with BPD compared with those measured in normal infants. These authors also noted that the configuration of the partial flow volume curves obtained in infants with BPD was consistently concave in the direction of the flow and volume axes suggesting nonhomogeneous airway obstruction. A reduction in V'_{maxFRC} in infants with BPD has been a consistent finding in all subsequent studies including the publication by Hofhuis et al. (27) involving infants with new BPD. Measured longitudinally over the first two years of life, the infants with BPD reported by Tepper et al. (24) demonstrated very modest increases in absolute flows in individual infants with BPD. On average, however, the rate of increase for infants with BPD was substantially below that measured in normal infants over the same interval. Thus at follow-up, measurements of V'_{maxFRC} in the infants with BPD had fallen even farther below those measured in normal infants. Iles and Edmunds (35), who measured V'_{maxFRC} in infants with BPD every three months over the first year of life, reported a similar lack of recovery of airway function. Studying infants with new BPD, Hofhuis et al. (27) found that V'_{maxFRC} z-scores fell from −1.7 to −2.2 between 6 and 12 months of age. This decline was significantly greater in infants who had been treated using conventional mechanical ventilation compared with those treated using high-frequency ventilation.

In 1987 Motoyama et al. (36) measured forced flows in intubated infants with BPD over the full vital capacity range using the forced deflation method. They found that forced flows were markedly reduced and that the configuration of the full flow volume curves they produced scooped inwardly toward the flow and volume axes indicating nonhomogeneous airway obstruction. Using the same method Mallory et al. (37) measured forced expiratory flows in patients with severe BPD longitudinally over the first three years of life and, as in studies assessing airway function using V'_{maxFRC}, demonstrated persistent obstruction. Only infants weaned from ventilatory support prior to 10 months of age demonstrated limited recovery of airway function. FVC, however, reached normal levels in all infants by three years of age. Recently, Robin et al. (28) used the RVRTC method to assess lung function in 28 infants with moderate to severe new BPD (mean age 68 weeks, mean gestational age at birth 26 weeks, and mean days of ventilatory support 51). Although RVRTC spirometry revealed a wide variation in degrees of obstruction, the mean level of dysfunction was in the mild range. As noted above, measurements of fractional lung volumes revealed mild to moderate air trapping suggesting small airways as a primary contributor to the overall degree of obstruction. Additional studies from these authors (31) demonstrate no improvement in the degree of the deficit in forced flows between 14 and 22 months of age. This persistence of reduced forced flows in toddlers is not surprising, as almost all longer-term follow-up studies have detected a reduction in forced flows in children, adolescents, and young adults with BPD during voluntarily performed spirometry (38). Interestingly, Friedrich et al. (39), also using the RVRTC method, have shown that forced flows measured in the first year of life are substantially reduced in prematurely born infants without a history of neonatal respiratory disease. As in infants with BPD, they found that there was little recovery of airway function when studies were repeated early in the second year of life (40). Reductions in forced flows were found to be significantly associated with gestational age at birth, with each additional week of prematurity accounting for a 5% reduction in mid-volume forced flows (FEF25-75) (39). This result extrapolated to the mean 26 weeks of gestational age infants with BPD studied by Robin et al. (28) suggests that premature birth alone may account for a large fraction of the airway dysfunction measured in these infants with new BPD. This extrapolation is probably not entirely valid, but it does suggest that disruption of lung maturation plays a central role in the development of the persistent airway abnormalities observed in infants with new BPD. Although the presence of persistent air flow obstruction appears to be functionally similar in both new and old BPD, it is not as yet clear whether the structural determinants of that obstruction are similar. Studies of infants and toddlers with established BPD reveal persistence of airway obstruction with only modest, if any, recovery of function. Abnormal lung growth, development, remodeling and repair secondary to premature birth itself rather than oxygen toxicity and mechanical ventilation may now be the central cause of impaired lung function in infants with BPD.

V. Lung Imaging

The chest radiographic characteristics of infants with BPD have changed substantially since the original description by Northway et al. (1) in 1967 of the four-stage progression from RDS to BPD occurring over the first 30 days of life. These authors described chest X ray changes that progressed from the dense and then mottled granular ground glass appearances of acute and unresolving RDS through the classical pattern of diffuse reticular linear densities alternating with cystic lucencies diagnostic for BPD. Current definitions of BPD no longer include radiographic characteristics, as some infants meeting current criteria for this diagnosis have only fine interstitial changes by

36 weeks' postconceptual age. Although the chest X ray of BPD as classically described is still seen in many infants, this pattern may now appear later than 30 days or never appear at all. Radiographic changes in smaller, less mature infants with new BPD are much more variable and may be initially masked by other conditions (cardiac disease, pulmonary infection, interstitial emphysema, pneumothorax) that also alter the chest X ray and prolong the need for ventilatory support and oxygen supplementation. The chest X ray in these complicated patients may never demonstrate the bubbly cystic appearance of classical BPD but rather be characterized by irregularly distributed areas of streaky density and hyperlucency.

Chest radiographs have been shown to correlate poorly with and underestimate the extent of the pathologic changes in infants with established BPD (41,42). High-resolution computed tomography (HRCT) appears to be a more sensitive technique for detecting the structural abnormalities in the lungs of patients with established BPD than plain chest radiography (26,43–47). Only two reports describing the structural abnormalities seen in infants with established BPD have been published. In 1998 Kubota et al. (43) reported the HRCT findings from 22 infants not treated with surfactant whose mean age at the time of study was 11.6 months. Mean gestational age at birth was 29 weeks and birth weight averaged 1245 g. The duration of mechanical ventilation was 62 days and of supplemental oxygen was 120 days. Areas of hyperlucency were identified in 82%, linear opacities in 77%, triangular subplural opacities in 27%, and bronchovascular bundle distortion in 50% of these infants with old BPD. Similar structural abnormalities have been reported from long-term follow-up chest HRCT evaluations of children, adolescents, and adults with old BPD (44–47). The degree of hyperlucency on HRCT was found to correlate with clinical severity score. Mahut et al. (26) in 2007 reported HRCT findings on 41 infants with a mean age at time of study of 16 months, 62% of whom were treated with surfactant. Their mean gestational age at birth was 27 weeks and mean birth weight 914 g. The average time on ventilator support was relatively brief, 16 days, and over half were on room air by 36 weeks' postconceptual age suggesting that this was on average a group with mild BPD. On HRCT hyperlucent areas were seen in 88%, linear opacities in 95%, and triangular subplural opacities in 63% of patients. Measurements of FRC by helium dilution, as noted earlier, were on average in the normal range but correlated inversely with both number of linear opacities and number of triangular subplural opacities. The number of triangular subplural opacities also correlated with the duration of ventilation. Measurements of V'_{maxFRC} were substantially reduced but did not correlate with any HRCT characteristics. Although the numbers of studies available for comparison are limited, there appear to be no obvious differences in the type or frequency of abnormalities identified on HRCT in patients with old versus new BPD. Correlations between abnormalities seen on HRCT and measures of lung function and clinical severity suggest, however, that HRCT may be useful in clinical management and as an outcome measure in this population.

Long and Castile (48) have recently reported a method for obtaining high-quality motion-free images of the lungs at specific lung volumes in infants with minimal sedation and without intubation. In this method, the lungs of sedated infants are inflated two to five times in synchrony with spontaneous inspiratory efforts to pressures of 25 cm H_2O to produce a respiratory pause. The lungs are then inflated again to 25 cm H_2O and held at that pressure during imaging, thus simulating the deep breath and hold

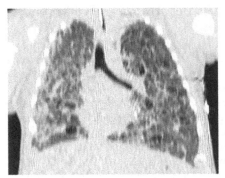 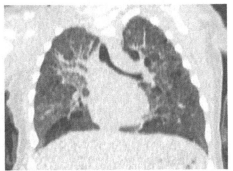

36 weeks Post-conceptual Age   75 weeks Post-conceptual Age

Figure 1 HRCT images (coronal views) obtained at 36 and 75 weeks of postconceptual age from a 25-week gestational age female premature infant. The child was one of twins and her course was complicated by early sepsis (total days of ventilatory support 299 days, total length of hospital stay 379 days). Full volumetric HRCT imaging was performed using a relatively low-dose protocol (100 kVp, 20 mAs, estimated exposure 0.5 mSv, equivalent to approximately 5–10 chest X rays).

maneuver performed voluntarily by older children and adults undergoing CT imaging of the chest. Imaging can also be done during the induced respiratory pause without inflation (i.e., at 0 cm H_2O) to assess homogeneity of lung emptying (air trapping). This technique can be performed using a face mask or via an endotracheal or tracheostomy tube. In patients on ventilators, small and even moderate air leaks do not compromise the method as long as a constant inflation pressure can be maintained throughout the simulated breath hold. Airways as small as 0.5 mm in diameter can be resolved using this technique. In addition to improving resolution, imaging at specific inflation pressures (i.e., lung volumes) permits comparison of measurements over time and comparisons with measurements made in normal infants. Limited quantitative data on airway dimensions and lung parenchymal densities in normal infants have been reported (49,50). An HRCT scoring system for infants with BPD has also recently been published (51). Figure 1 shows coronal HRCT images obtained at 25 cm H_2O on a premature infant with BPD (born at 25 weeks of gestation with birth weight 949 g) obtained at 36 and again at 75 weeks of age. Changes in parenchymal structure suggest that serial HRCT imaging may be useful for assessing changes in lung growth and development over time. Increasing levels of complexity suggest that lung development has progressed from the saccular to the early alveolar phase. CT imaging is useful for identifying unsuspected abnormalities in the lungs of individual patients with BPD but its ultimate utility as a tool for clinical management and as an outcome measure for research investigations is not yet clear. Radiation exposure from CT imaging is substantially greater than that received from standard chest X rays (52). Thus, until imaging protocols that reduce exposure become more widely available, HRCT imaging in infants should be utilized judiciously. Approaches to HRCT chest imaging in infants that reduce exposure to near levels received during standard chest radiography have been proposed (53).

VI. Summary of Structure Function Measurements in BPD

The predominant functional abnormality in infants with established BPD is heterogeneous airway obstruction with air trapping. Early in life specific compliance is reduced but improves rapidly and in most studies normalizes by around one year of age. Although nonhomogeneously distributed interstitial linear densities and architectural distortion are commonly seen on HRCT images of the lungs of infants with BPD, lung volumes do not appear to be significantly restricted due to global reductions in compliance. In both old and new BPD, however, nonhomogeneities in lung elasticity probably play a role in determining maldistribution of ventilation and nonuniformity of airway emptying. Lung volumes improve rapidly and in studies of old BPD reach normal levels by the second year of life. Recent studies suggest that mild air trapping persists in infants with new BPD. TLC has been reported to be normal in infants with new BPD by early in the first year of life. Although premature birth disrupts alveolar development, it does not result in an overall reduction in lung volume. Airway function in both old and new BPD is reduced and improves less rapidly. Resistance, which probably measures predominantly central and upper airway function, improves and in some studies reaches normal levels by two to three years of age. In both old and new BPD, low- and mid-lung volume forced expiratory flows, which probably reflect both smaller and larger airway function, increase slowly in absolute terms but remain below normal levels. In follow-up studies of patients with old BPD, this reduction in forced flows persists into childhood and early adult life. Similar longer-term follow-up studies on patients with new BPD are not yet available. Injury to larger airways typified the pathology of old BPD. The pathology of new BPD is characterized by heterogeneous injury and repair occurring at the acinar/parencymal level. On the basis of the differences in lung pathology between old and new BPD, it seems likely that the sites of obstruction in new BPD are more peripheral than they were in old BPD. Currently, there are no functional or imaging data to support this speculation. The unmistakable differences in pathology between old and new BPD are not as clearly apparent when viewed functionally or radiographically.

VII. Mechanical Ventilation

The physiologic basis and suggested ventilator strategies discussed in this chapter are only meant for those patients with the most severe form of established BPD, that is, the patients who continue to require intermittent positive pressure ventilation (IPPV) many weeks into their initial hospitalization. This chapter does not deal with strategies to prevent BPD. Although the exact incidence of severe ventilator-dependent BPD is unclear, it represents only a small subset of those patients meeting the criteria for severe BPD by the NICHD/NHLBI/ORD consensus definition of BPD. In 2000, the NICHD/NHLBI/ORD developed their consensus definition of BPD on the basis of the severity of disease (5). The criteria outlined range from a diagnosis of no BPD, when there is no supplemental oxygen requirement at 28 days of age, to severe BPD when there is a $\geq 30\%$ supplemental oxygen requirement or a need for continuous positive airway pressure or a need for IPPV at 36 weeks' corrected postmenstrual age. Utilizing the consensus definition of BPD, Ehrenkranz et al. (4) in 2005 reported that in a cohort of

4866 patients with birth weight less than 1000 g and gestational age at birth less than 32 weeks approximately 76% of patients had some form of BPD and that approximately 16% of these patients had severe BPD. Carlo et al. (54) in a study of 220 patients with a birth weight between 501 and 1000 g found that only 17 (~8%) required mechanical ventilation at 36 weeks' postmenstrual age. Ballard et al. in 2006 (55) reported that of 582 patients with a birth weight of 500 to 1250 g and who were born at less than 32 weeks' postmenstrual age only 48 (~8%) continued to require mechanical ventilation at 40 weeks' postmenstrual age. Another important issue that remains unresolved is when patients should be considered to have established severe BPD and be ventilated using the principles described in this chapter. By the NICHD/NHLBI/ORD consensus definition, for a patient born at less than 32 weeks severe BPD is diagnosed at 36 weeks' postmenstrual age, and for a patient born at more than 32 weeks' severe BPD is diagnosed at 56 days of age (5). It has also been suggested that patients who require IPPV through four weeks of age have established BPD (2,56). Thus, while we await randomized controlled trials to determine when a patient can be considered to have established severe BPD, somewhere between 4 to 8 weeks of age or after 36 weeks' corrected postmenstrual age may represent the appropriate time to consider the ventilation principles discussed in this chapter.

The main purpose of mechanical ventilation is to improve ventilation-perfusion (V/Q) matching. In severe established BPD improving V/Q matching will decrease the requirement for supplemental oxygen and the frequency of hypoxemic episodes. Established ventilator-dependent BPD is a lung disease characterized by areas of overinflation. When this overinflation becomes large, the patient is then breathing on a relatively flat portion of their lung compliance curve such that generating large pressures results in only small tidal volumes. Furthermore, lung overinflation will increase pulmonary vascular resistance due to compression of the alveolar vessels. Thus, overinflation of the lung will lead to a worsening in V/Q matching and result in hypoxemia by impacting both ventilation and perfusion of the lungs. Consequently, care must be taken when utilizing a positive pressure ventilator in these patients to avoid lung overinflation. To effectively utilize mechanical ventilation in established severe BPD we must focus on exhalation. By providing adequate time for exhalation, the lungs will be able to empty, preventing or reducing areas of overinflation and in this manner improving both ventilation and perfusion within the lungs resulting in improved V/Q matching.

Alterations in airway and lung structure caused by both ventilator-induced airway injury and the alterations in lung development that underlie the pathogenesis of BPD lead to increased respiratory system resistance in patients with severe BPD. In patients on IPPV, inhalation is an active process driven by the ventilator, while exhalation is passive in terms of the ventilator. That is to say, that the ventilator will provide the inhaled tidal volume but the patient must exhale without any help from the ventilator. A typical volume-time curve is shown in Figure 2A for a patient on positive pressure ventilation. It can be seen that both inhalation and exhalation volumes depend on ventilator pressures and the time that those pressures are applied to the endotracheal tube. Exhalation in Figure 2A can be described by the following equation:

$$V(t) = V_0 e^{(-t/RC)} \tag{1}$$

where $V(t)$ is the volume in the lung at any time after exhalation begins, V_0 is the inspired tidal volume, t is the time in seconds, R is the resistance of the respiratory

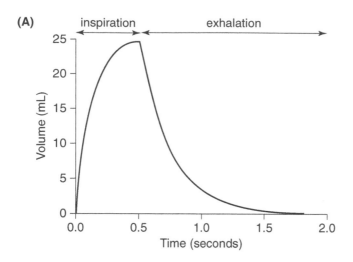

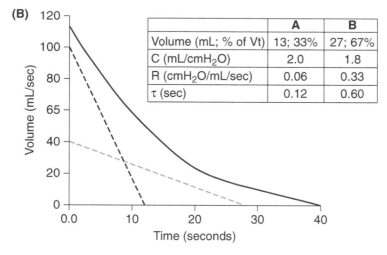

Figure 2 Examples of volume-time (**A**) and flow-volume curves (**B**), with most modern neonatal ventilators these curves are often readily available when a flow probe is placed in between the ventilator tubing and the endotracheal tube. The volume-time curve (**A**) is from a patient ventilated with an inspiratory time of 0.5 seconds. The passive flow-volume curve (**B**) is obtained following an inspiratory occlusion maneuver, and the parameter obtained using a 2-space model are shown in the table.

system, and C is the compliance of the respiratory system. Since exhalation is an exponential function the time necessary for exhalation can be derived from the time constant (τ) where

$$\tau = RC \qquad (2)$$

As with any exponential function, the time necessary to empty the inspired tidal volume will be a function of τ, where one time constant results in emptying of 63% of the inspired tidal volume, two time constants result in emptying of 86% of the inspired tidal volume, and five time constants result in emptying of 99% of the inspired tidal volume. Thus, five time constants are necessary to completely empty the inspired tidal volume. Providing less than five time constants for exhalation will result in inhalation beginning prior to complete emptying of the inspired tidal volume from the previous breath, this will result in gas trapping and eventually will lead to lung overdistension. Furthermore, from equation (2) it should be noted that lung diseases that increase R will result in longer time constants, particularly since the changes in C tend to be of much smaller magnitude than changes in R.

It is helpful to consider flow-volume curves when assessing lung function in these patients. Many ventilators used in the intensive care setting now have available flow probes that can be placed in-line between the endotracheal tube and the ventilator circuit allowing for convenient measurement and display of flow-volume loops in many of these patients. Figure 2B shows only the exhalation portion from peak flow to the end of exhalation of a passive flow-volume loop after an inspiratory occlusion maneuver in a patient with severe established BPD. In these types of passive exhalation flow-volume curves from normal subjects, the resultant curve is a straight line, and exhalation in normal subjects can be modeled using a single compartment, that is, a straight line fit to the data where the slope (m) of the straight line is the negative inverse of the time constant for exhalation (i.e., $m = -1/\tau$). However, in patients with abnormal exhalation, that is, patients with airway abnormalities such as seen in severe BPD, the exhalation flow-volume curve is often not a straight line but rather exhibits concavity in the direction of the flow and volume axes (19) as described above under section IV "Forced Flows". There are different approaches to modeling this concavity, including adding a second compartment to the model analysis shown in equation (1). For the purposes of this discussion these nonlinear exhalation flow-volume curves will be modeled using a two-compartment approach as shown below

$$V(t) = V_{A0}Ae^{-t/R_A C_A} + V_{B0}Be^{-t/R_B C_B} \tag{3}$$

where the subscript A refers to compartment A and subscript B refers to compartment B. As can be seen in Figure 2B, the fits for compartment A and compartment B have been resolved into two straight lines, such that adding these two lines together will fit the original curvilinear flow-volume loop. It can be seen that compartment A empties fairly quickly, and will be referred to as the "fast" compartment and compartment B empties relatively slowly and will be referred to as the "slow" compartment. It is important to point out that the slow compartment accounts for the majority of the exhaled tidal volume. In reality there are many slow compartments, however for the purposes of modeling, the use of one compartment as a global mean of all the slow compartments fits the data as well as using many slow compartments. Although modeling of the lung separates two very distinct compartments, anatomically in the lung of the vast majority of severe BPD patients there are many of these compartments intermingled throughout the parenchyma. Therefore, any ventilation strategy employed in severe BPD must take into account both compartments and pay particular attention to exhalation from the slow compartment.

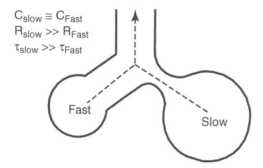

$C_{slow} \cong C_{Fast}$
$R_{slow} \gg R_{Fast}$
$\tau_{slow} \gg \tau_{Fast}$

Fast

Slow

Figure 3 A two-compartment model of the lung. Both compartments have comparable compliances (C). However, the slow compartment has a much higher resistance (R) than does the fast compartment resulting in a substantially longer time constants (τ) in the slow compartment compared with the fast compartment.

The patient with severe BPD has a maldistribution of ventilation, and for the purposes of this discussion that maldistribution can be represented as occurring between the fast and the slow compartments. This maldistribution of ventilation can be depicted as shown in Figure 3. The lung compliance between the two compartments is not very different, while the resistance is much higher in the slow space than in the fast space. Thus, by simple inspection of Figure 3, it is clear that the time constant for exhalation is much longer in the slow compartment than it is in the fast compartment. What then are the options for ventilating this type of lung disease? One could follow a ventilation strategy aimed at ventilating the fast compartment, which may be at the expense of the slow compartment. For example, if we use an inspiratory time of 0.5 seconds, which is reasonable considering that inspiratory time constants are faster than expiratory time constants given that R on inspiration is lower than R on expiration. If we consider a fast compartment with a time constant of 0.12 seconds (Fig. 2B) then to allow for five time constants for exhalation would require a minimum of 0.60 seconds in exhalation. The maximum rate that would allow for five time constants would be 60 (sec/min) divided by 0.5 + 0.60 seconds or a rate of 54 breaths per minute. Note that in this ventilation scheme, the slow compartment, which has an exhalation time constant of 0.60 seconds, would empty only about 63% of the inspired tidal volume before the next mechanical ventilator breath begins. Alternatively, one could follow a ventilation strategy aimed at ventilating the slow compartment, which may underventilate the fast compartment. Remembering that the majority of the exhaled tidal volume comes from the slow compartment, this may be a reasonable method to optimize V/Q matching and avoid overdistension of the lung. For this example, the inspiratory time will again be set at 0.5 seconds. The maximum set rate on the ventilator that will allow for five time constants is 60 (sec/min) divided by (5 × 0.60 seconds) + 0.5 seconds, which equals a maximum rate of 17 breaths per minute. Thus, in those few patients in the NICU who have severe ventilator-dependent established BPD, to optimize V/Q matching and minimize lung overinflation, these patients should be ventilated with a slow rate and a longer inspiratory time.

Patients with established BPD who require IPPV can be ventilated most effectively by using a slow rate and a longer inspiratory time. When the set rate on the ventilator is increased, the patient is unable to completely exhale the inspired tidal volume. In these patients if the set rate on the ventilator is increased beyond the maximum that will allow for five exhalation time constants, then the patient will develop air trapping and overdistension of the slow compartments in the lung (remember that the slow compartment accounts for the majority of the tidal volume in these patients). This will manifest clinically as an increased oxygen requirement, due to worsening V/Q mismatch, and in increasing PCO_2 levels due to decreased tidal volumes and increased physiologic dead space in the lung. Indeed, paradoxical to what is seen in most lung diseases, patients with established BPD usually have improvements in oxygenation and PCO_2 levels when the rates on the ventilator are decreased. To optimize V/Q matching and tidal volumes in the patients with severe established BPD adequate time must be given for exhalation, and this can only be accomplished in this long time constant disease by using relatively slow set rates on the ventilator.

Slow rate and long inspiratory time ventilation results in the ability to slowly wean the inspiratory pressures needed to inflate the lungs. The inspiratory pressures can be slowly weaned, since as the lung deflates areas of overinflation will decrease, which will bring the lung at end-expiration to a steeper portion of the compliance curve. Thereby, adequate tidal volumes can be generated at lower inspiratory pressures. Furthermore, in patients ventilated for relatively long periods of time with slow rates and long inspiratory times, lung development continues as evidenced by improvements both on lung CT scan and in pulmonary function testing. Thus, these patients that require mechanical ventilation need a strategy that optimizes V/Q matching while minimizing lung overdistension. Keep in mind that at this point there are no objective studies addressing optimal strategies for providing ventilatory support to patients with severe ventilator-dependent BPD. Until such a time as other modes and/or modalities for ventilating patients with established BPD can be developed and studied, ventilation with a slow rate and long inspiratory time is the strategy that best provides for V/Q matching and lung emptying. Furthermore, this ventilation strategy allows for interval lung growth as demonstrated in the serial CT scans shown in Figure 1 from a patient with severe established BPD ventilated using a slow rate and long inspiratory time.

VIII. Future Directions

The current state of the art for the evaluation of lung function and structure in infants has evolved such that the tests that can now be preformed parallel those available in older children and adults, differing only by the requirement for sedation. RVRTC spirometry, plethysmographic fractional lung volumes, and controlled ventilation HRCT imaging of the lungs are now being used at many large medical centers on a clinical and research basis. To date these tests have been utilized only on a limited basis for the investigation of the pathogenesis of BPD. We currently use these tests routinely for evaluating infants with BPD who are not progressing as anticipated. Figure 4 shows an infant with BPD with a tracheostomy tube undergoing plethysmographic measurement of FRC. Although standard testing is performed using a facemask sealed with therapeutic putty to prevent air leaks, accurate results can also be obtained in patients with tracheostomy tubes.

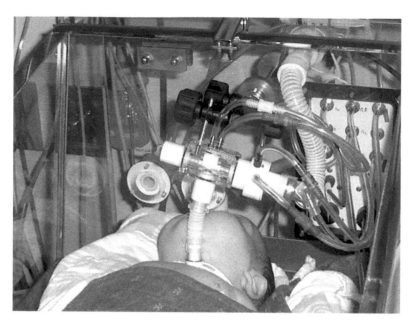

Figure 4 Sedated seven-month-old former premature infant with established BPD and cuffed trachostomy tube undergoing infant lung function testing. The infant is shown within the plethysmograph for measurement of FRC.

A cuffed tracheostomy tube is placed prior to testing to prevent air leaks and adjustments for differences in equipment and airway dead space are made in calculating results. If indicated, both controlled ventilation HRCT imaging and infant pulmonary function testing can be performed during a single period of sedation. Full evaluations take two to three hours depending on the extent of testing. Performing these tests in patients on chronic ventilatory support requires substantial experience in the management of critically ill infants. Figure 5 shows spirometry and fractional lung volume results, HRCT images at 25 and 0 cm H_2O, and flow-volume and pressure-volume curves obtained on an infant with established BPD. Tabulated pulmonary function and respiratory system compliance (Crs) results are shown both in absolute terms and as percents of predicted normal values for each test (13,23,57). Pre- and postbronchodilator studies can also be performed and evaluated in relation to published responses in normal infants (58). On a clinical basis, we have found these familiar tests to be useful in defining levels of dysfunction and assessing the effects of therapeutic interventions. These measures have played a central role in the investigation of lung disorders in children and adults and are likely to contribute similarly to our understanding of the nature of lung injury in very premature infants. These and other new tests of lung function and structure in infants including interrupter and oscillatory resistance, exhaled nitric oxide levels, carbon monoxide diffusion capacity, multiple breath washout measures of ventilatory heterogeneity, and hyperpolarized helium-3 MRI estimates of alveolar size and complexity are likely to contribute substantially to our understanding of the pathophysiology of new

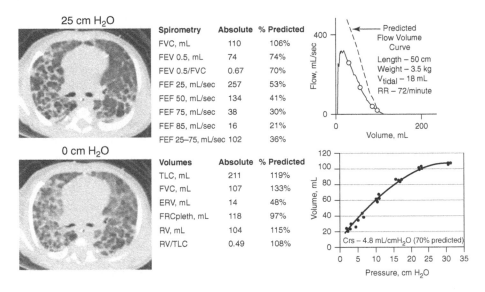

Figure 5 Lung function results and HRCT lung images obtained at 19 weeks of age from a former premature infant born at 25 weeks of gestation with birth weight 830 g. The child's early course was complicated by prolonged ruptured membranes and sepsis. Axial HRCT images at the level of the carina obtained near full lung inflation (*above*) and near FRC (*below*) are shown. The child had a tracheostomy and was on chronic ventilator support at the time the studies were performed.

BPD. Furthermore, these techniques will allow the clinician/researcher to determine the impact of postnatal interventions on subsequent lung development, which is an absolute requirement for "curing" patients with established severe BPD.

References

1. Northway W Jr., Rosan R, Porter D. Pulmonary disease following respirator therapy of hyaline-membrane disease: bronchopulmonary dysplasia. N Engl J Med 1967; 276:357–368.
2. Walsh MC, Wilson-Costello D, Zadell A, et al. Safety, reliability, and validity of a physiologic definition of bronchopulmonary dysplasia. J Perinatol 2003; 23:451–456.
3. Lemons JA, Bauer CR, Oh W, et al. Very low birth weight outcomes of the National Institute of Child health and human development neonatal research network, January 1995 through December 1996. NICHD Neonatal Research Network. Pediatrics 2001; 107:E1.
4. Ehrenkranz RA, Walsh MC, Vohr BR, et al. Validation of the National Institutes of Health consensus definition of bronchopulmonary dysplasia. Pediatrics 2005; 116:1353–1360.
5. Jobe AH, Bancalari E. NICHD/ NHLBI/ORF workshop summary: bronchopulmonary dysplasia. Am J Respir Crit Car Med 2001; 163:1723–1729.
6. Van Marter LJ, Allred EN, Leviton A, et al. Antenatal glucocorticoid treatment does not reduce chronic lung disease among surviving preterm infants. J Pediatr 2001; 138:198–204.
7. Langhoff-Roos J, Kesmodel U, Jacobsson B, et al. Spontaneous preterm delivery in primiparous women at low risk in Denmark: population based study. BMJ 2006; 332:937–939.

8. Overstreet DW, Jackson JC, van Belle G, et al. Estimation of mortality risk in chronically ventilated infants with bronchopulmonary dysplasia. Pediatrics 1991; 88:1153.

9. Abman SH, Groothius JR. Pathophysiology and treatment of bronchopulmonary dysplasia. Pediatr Clin North Am 1994; 41:277–315.

10. Abman SH, Davis JM. Bronchopulmonary dysplasia. In: Chernick V, Boat T, Wilmott RW, et al., eds. Kendig's Disorders of the Respiratory Tract in Children. 7th ed. Philadelphia: Saunders Elsevier, 2006:353.

11. Gappa M, Pillow J, Allen J, et al. Lung function tests in neonates and infants with chronic lung disease: lung and chest-wall mechanics. Pediatr Pulmonol 2006; 41:291–317.

12. Tepper RS, Williams T, Kisling J, et al. Static compliance of the respiratory system in healthy infants. Am J Respir Crit Care Med 2001; 163:91–94.

13. Tepper RS, Pagtakhan RD, Taussig LM. Noninvasive determination of total respiratory system compliance in infants by the weighted-spirometer method. Am Rev Respir Dis 1984; 130:461–466.

14. Gerhardt T, Hehre D, Feller R, et al. Serial determination of pulmonary function in infants with chronic lung disease. J Pediatr 1987; 110:448–456.

15. Baraldi E, Filippone M, Trevisanuto D, et al. Pulmonary function until two years of life in infants with bronchopulmonary dysplasia. Am J Respir Crit Care Med 1997; 155:149–155.

16. Moriette G, Gaudebout C, Clement A, et al. Pulmonary function at 1 year of age in survivors of neonatal respiratory distress: a multivariate analysis of factors associated with sequelae. Pediatr Pulmonol 1987; 3:242–250.

17. Farstad T, Brockmeier F, Bratlid D. Cardiopulmonary function in premature infants with bronchopulmonary dysplasia—a 2 year follow up. Eur J Pediatr 1995; 154:853–858.

18. Hjalmarson O, Sandberg K. Lung function at term reflects severity of bronchopulmonary dysplasia. J Pediatr 2005; 146:86–90.

19. Jarriel WS, Richardson P, Knapp RD, et al. A nonlinear regression analysis of nonlinear, passive-deflation flow-volume plots. Pediatr Pulmonol 1993; 15:175–182.

20. Mead J. Contribution of compliance of airways to frequency-dependent behavior of lungs. J Appl Physiol 1969; 26:670–673.

21. Hulskamp G, Pillow JJ, Dinger J, et al. Lung function in infants and young children with chronic lung disease of infancy: functional residual capacity. Pediatr Pulmonol 2006; 41: 1–22.

22. Stocks J, Godfrey S, Beardsmore C, et al. Standards for infant pulmonary function testing: plethysmographic measurements of lung volume and airway resistance. Eur Respir J 2001; 17:302–312.

23. Morris MG, Gustafsson P, Tepper R, et al. ERS/ATS Task Force on Standards for Infant Respiratory Function Testing. The bias flow nitrogen washout technique for measuring the functional residual capacity in infants. Eur Respir J 2001; 17:529–536.

24. Tepper RS, Morgan WJ, Cota K, et al. Expiratory flow limitation in infants with broncho-pulmonary dysplasia. J Pediatr 1986; 109:1040–1046.

25. Greenough A, Dimitriou G, Bhat RY, et al. Lung volumes in infants who had mild to moderate bronchopulmonary dysplasia. Eur J Pediatr 2005; 164:583.

26. Mahut B, De Blic J, Emond S, et al. Chest computed tomography findings in broncho-pulmonary dysplasia and correlation with lung function. Arch Dis Child 2007; 92: F459–F464.

27. Hofhuis W, Huysman MW, van der Wiel EC, et al. Worsening of V'_{maxFRC} in infants with chronic lung disease in the first year of life: a more favorable outcome after high-frequency oscillation ventilation. Am J Respir Crit Care Med 2002; 166:1539–1544.

28. Robin B, Kim YJ, Huth J, et al. Pulmonary function in bronchopulmonary dysplasia. Pediatr Pulmonol 2004; 37:236.

29. Wauer RR, Maurer T, Nowotny T, et al. Assessment of functional residual capacity using nitrogen washout and plethysmographic techniques in infants with and without bronchopulmonary dysplasia. Intensive Care Med 1998; 24:469–475.
30. Castile R, Filbrun D, Flucke R, et al. Adult-type pulmonary function tests in infants without respiratory disease. Pediatr Pulmonol 2000; 30:215–227.
31. Filbrun AG, Linn MJ, McIntosh NA, et al. Longitudinal measures of lung function in infants with bronchopulmonary dysplasia. Am J Respir Crit Care Med 2007; 175:A92.
32. Lum S, Hulskamp G, Merkus P, et al. Lung function tests in neonates and infants with chronic lung disease: forced expiratory maneuvers. Pediatr Pulmonol 2006; 41:199–214.
33. Sly PD, Tepper R, Henschen M, et al. Tidal forced expirations. ERS/ATS Task Force on Standards for Infant Respiratory Function Testing. European Respiratory Society/American Thoracic Society. Eur Respir J 2000; 16:741–748.
34. Lum S, Stocks J, Castile RG, et al. ATS/ERS Statement: raised volume forced expirations in infants: guidelines for current practice. Am J Respir Crit Care Med 2005; 172:1463–1471.
35. Iles R, Edmunds T. Assessment of pulmonary function in resolving chronic lung disease of prematurity. Arch Dis Child 1997; 76:F113–F117.
36. Motoyama EK, Fort MD, Klesh KW, et al. Early onset of airway reactivity in premature infants with bronchopulmonary dysplasia. Am Rev Respir Dis 1987; 136:50–57.
37. Mallory GB Jr., Chaney H, Mutich RL, et al. Longitudinal changes in lung function during the first three years of premature infants with moderate to severe bronchopulmonary dysplasia. Pediatr Pulmonol 1991; 11:8–14.
38. Baraldi E, Filippone M. Chronic lung disease after premature birth. N Engl J Med 2007; 357:1946–1955.
39. Friedrich L, Stein RT, Pitrez PMC, et al. Reduced lung function in healthy preterm infants in the first months of life. Am J Respir Crit Care Med 2006; 173:442–447.
40. Friedrich L, Pitrez PMC, Stein RT, et al. Growth rate of lung function in healthy preterm infants. Am J Respir Crit Care Med 2007; 176:1269–1273.
41. Opperman HC, Wille L, Bleyl U, et al. Bronchopulmonary dysplasia in premature infants. A radiological and pathological correlation. Pediatr Radiol 1977; 5:137–141.
42. Edwards DK, Colby TV, Northway WH. Radiographic-pathologic correlation in bronchopulmonary dysplasia. J Pediatr 1979; 95:834–836.
43. Kubota J, Ohki Y, Inoue T, et al. Ultrafast CT scoring system for assessing bronchopulmonary dysplasia: reproducibility and clinical correlation. Radiat Med 1998; 16:167–174.
44. Oppenheim C, Mamou-Mani T, Sayegh N, et al. Bronchopulmonary dysplasia: value of CT in identifying pulmonary sequelae. Am J Roentgenol 1994; 163:169–172.
45. Aquino SL, Schechter MS, Chiles C, et al. High-resolution inspiratory and expiratory CT in older children and adult with bronchopulmonary dysplasia. Am J Roentgenol 1999; 173: 963–967.
46. Howling SJ, Northway WH Jr., Hansel DM, et al. Pulmonary sequelae of bronchopulmonary dysplasia survivors: high-resolution CT findings. Am J Roentgenol 2000; 174:1323–1326.
47. Aukland SM, Halvorsen T, Fosse KR, et al. High-resolution CT of the chest in children and young adults who were born prematurely: findings in a population based study, Am J Roentgenol 2006; 187: 1012–1018.
48. Long F, Castile R. Technique and clinical applications of full inflation and end-exhalation controlled-ventilation chest CT in infants and young children. Pediatr Radiology 2001; 31: 413–422.
49. Long FR, Williams RS, Castile RG. Factors influencing CT lung density in infants and young children. Pediatr Radiol 2005; 35:1075–1080.
50. Long FR, Williams R, Castile RG. Structural airway abnormalities in infants and young children with cystic fibrosis. J Pediatr 2004; 144:154–161.

51. Ochiai M, Hikino S, Yabuuchi H, et al. A new scoring system for computed tomography of the chest for assessing the clinical status of bronchopulmonary dysplasia. J Pediatr 2008; 152:90–95.
52. de González AB, Kim KP, Samet JM. Radiation-induced cancer risk from annual computed tomography for patients with cystic fibrosis. Am J Respir Crit Care Med 2007; 176:970–973.
53. Long FR. High-resolution computed tomography of the lung in children with cystic fibrosis: technical factors. Proc Am Thorac Soc 2007; 4:306–309.
54. Carlo WA, Stark AR, Wright LL, et al. Barbara Stoll B for the National Institute of Child Health and Human Development Neonatal Research Network. J Pediatr 2002; 141:370–374.
55. Ballard RA, Truog WE, Cnaan A, et al. Inhaled nitric oxide in preterm infants undergoing mechanical ventilation. N Engl J Med 2006; 355:343–353.
56. Ambalavanan N, Carlo WA. Ventilatory strategies in the prevention and management of bronchopulmonary dysplasia. Semin Perinatol 2006; 30:192–199.
57. Jones M, Castile R, Davis S, et al. Forced expiratory flows and volumes in infants: normative data and lung growth. Am J Respir Crit Care Med 2000; 161:353–359.
58. Goldstein AB, Castile RG, Filbrun DA, et al. Bronchodilator responsiveness in normal infants and young children. Am J Respir Crit Care Med 2001; 164:447–454.

19
Pulmonary Vascular Disease in Bronchopulmonary Dysplasia: Physiology, Diagnosis, and Treatment

PETER M. MOURANI and STEVEN H. ABMAN
Pediatric Heart Lung Center, Sections of Critical Care and Pulmonary Medicine, Department of Pediatrics, University of Colorado Denver, School of Medicine and The Children's Hospital, Aurora, Colorado, U.S.A.

I. Introduction

Improvements in neonatal care have changed the nature and epidemiology of bronchopulmonary dysplasia (BPD) over the last four decades, but pulmonary hypertension (PH) continues to contribute significantly to high morbidity and mortality of premature infants. Past clinical studies demonstrated that early elevations of pulmonary artery pressure are associated with an increased risk for the development of BPD (1,2), and that sustained PH beyond three months of age is related to high mortality (40%) (3). Despite striking therapeutic advances throughout the "post–surfactant era," late PH continues to be strongly linked with poor survival, with a recent report suggesting mortality rates of nearly 70% for infants with severe PH (4).

In addition to the adverse effects of PH on the clinical course of infants with BPD, the lung circulation is further characterized by persistence of abnormal or "dysmorphic" growth of the pulmonary circulation, including a relative paucity of small pulmonary arteries with an altered pattern of distribution within the interstitium of the distal lung (5–7). In infants with severe BPD, decreased vascular growth occurs in conjunction with marked reductions in alveoli, suggesting that the "new BPD" is primarily characterized by growth arrest of the developing lung (8). This reduction of alveolar-capillary surface area impairs gas exchange, thereby increasing the need for prolonged supplemental oxygen and ventilator therapy, causing marked hypoxemia with acute respiratory infections and late exercise intolerance, and further increases the risk for developing severe PH. Experimental studies have further shown that the early injury to the developing lung can impair angiogenesis, which further contributes to decreased alveolarization and simplification of distal lung airspace (the "vascular hypothesis") (9). Thus, abnormalities of the lung circulation in BPD are not only related to the presence or absence of PH, but more broadly, *pulmonary vascular disease* after premature birth as manifested by decreased vascular growth and structure also contributes to the pathogenesis and abnormal cardiopulmonary physiology of BPD.

Overall, PH remains a major clinical concern in infants with BPD, and strategies that preserve and enhance lung vascular growth and function after premature birth may provide novel therapeutic approaches for the prevention of BPD. In addition, strategies to lower pulmonary artery pressure, including targeting higher oxygen saturations in infants with established BPD, aggressive management of the underlying lung disease, and pharmacological therapy with agents such as inhaled nitric oxide (iNO), sildenafil, and endothelin receptor antagonists may improve clinical outcomes.

This chapter briefly reviews the contribution of pulmonary vascular disease to the pathophysiology of BPD, with emphasis on our current approaches toward the diagnostic evaluation and therapy of PH in infants with BPD.

II. Abnormalities of the Pulmonary Circulation in BPD

From the earliest descriptions of BPD, PH and cor pulmonale were recognized as being associated with high mortality in BPD (3,10,11). Early injury to the lung circulation leads to the rapid development of PH after premature birth (12). Abnormalities of the pulmonary circulation in BPD include alterations of vascular function (tone and vasoreactivity), structure (hypertensive remodeling), and growth (dysmorphic structure with reduced angiogenesis) (Fig. 1). Structural changes in the lung vasculature contribute to high pulmonary vascular resistance (PVR) due to narrowing of the vessel diameter and decreased vascular compliance. The media of small pulmonary arteries undergo striking changes including smooth muscle cell proliferation, maturation of mesenchymal cells into mature smooth muscle cells, and incorporation of fibroblasts or myofibroblasts into the vessel wall (13). In addition to these structural changes, the pulmonary circulation is further characterized by abnormal vasoreactivity that, in addition to high tone, also contributes to clinical signs of PH in BPD (14–16). Physiological abnormalities of the pulmonary circulation in BPD include elevated PVR and abnormal vasoreactivity, as evidenced by the

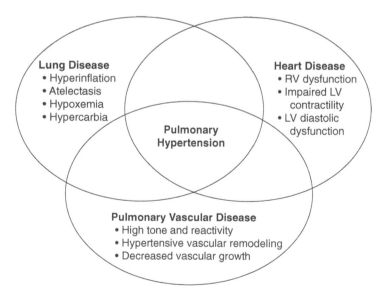

Figure 1 Schematic illustrating the components contributing to pulmonary hypertension in bronchopulmonary dysplasia.

marked vasoconstrictor response to acute hypoxia (14,15,17). Cardiac catheterization studies have shown that even mild hypoxia causes marked elevations in pulmonary artery pressure, including those infants with modest basal levels of PH. Elevation of vascular tone can contribute to high PVR even in older children with BPD without hypoxia, suggesting that abnormal vascular function persists late in the course (17).

More recently, the importance of decreased angiogenesis has been increasingly recognized as playing a key role in the pathogenesis and development of PH in BPD. Reduced vascular growth limits vascular surface area, causing further elevations of PVR, especially in response to high cardiac output with exercise or stress. The ability of the lung to achieve normal gas exchange requires ongoing growth and maintenance of an intricate system of airways and vessels, including the establishment of a thin yet vast blood-gas interface. In animal models, disruption of angiogenesis during lung development not only increases the risk for PH but also impairs alveolarization (18). Disruption of lung angiogenesis plays a critical role in the pathogenesis of BPD; however, little is known about basic mechanisms of pulmonary vascular injury in the immature lung and the impact of this injury on subsequent lung vascular growth and function.

Of diverse growth factors and signaling pathways that contribute to normal lung development, vascular endothelial growth factor (VEGF) plays an especially prominent role in growth and development of the pulmonary circulation. As suggested from experimental models (18–21), impaired VEGF signaling was subsequently associated with the pathogenesis of BPD in the clinical setting. Bhatt et al. first demonstrated decreased lung expression VEGF and VEGFR-1 in the lungs of premature infants who died with BPD (22). Tracheal fluid VEGF levels were lower in samples from premature neonates who subsequently develop BPD than those who do not develop chronic lung disease (23). Experimentally, lung VEGF expression is decreased in rodent, primate, and ovine models of BPD induced by neonatal hyperoxia or mechanical ventilation after premature birth (20,21,24). Pharmacological inhibition of VEGF signaling in newborn rats impairs lung vascular growth and inhibits alveolarization (18,19,25), further supporting the hypothesis that impaired VEGF signaling contributes to the pathogenesis of BPD. Thus, inhibition of lung vascular growth during a critical period of postnatal lung growth impairs alveolarization, suggesting that endothelial-epithelial cross-talk, especially via VEGF signaling, is critical for normal lung growth following birth.

Clinically, this decrement in lung vascular surface area also suggests that even relatively minor increases in left-to-right shunting of blood flow through a patent foramen ovale, atrial septal defect, or patent ductus arteriosus may induce a far greater hemodynamic injury in infants with BPD than in infants with normal lung vascular growth. This would suggest the need for earlier closure of such shunt lesions, prior to the development of progressive PH.

Prominent bronchial or other systemic-to-pulmonary collateral vessels were noted in early morphometric studies of infants with BPD, and can be readily identified in many infants during cardiac catheterization (12). Although these collateral vessels are generally small, large collaterals may contribute to significant shunting of blood flow to the lung, causing edema and need for higher FiO_2. Collateral vessels have been associated with high mortality in some patients with severe BPD who also had severe PH (16). Some infants have improved after embolization of large collateral vessels, as reflected by a reduced need for supplemental oxygen, ventilator support, or diuretics.

III. Approach to the Diagnosis and Treatment of PH in BPD

Although the exact incidence of PH in BPD is uncertain, moderate PH beyond the first few months of life has been associated with 47% mortality within two years after diagnosis (4). PH is not only a marker of more advanced BPD, but high PVR also causes poor right ventricular function, impaired cardiac output, limited oxygen delivery, increased pulmonary edema, and possibly a higher risk for sudden death. The diagnosis of PH and other cardiovascular complications in infants with BPD can be difficult because clinical signs and symptoms of PH can be subtle or overlap with respiratory signs, even in patients with moderate or severe PH. For example, infants with BPD on low-flow nasal cannula oxygen therapy can have marked PH, even in the absence of cyanotic spells, severe distress, and related signs.

On the basis of the strong correlations between PH and survival in BPD (3,4), early detection of PH may provide helpful prognostic information and lead to earlier application of more aggressive respiratory support, cardiac medications, vasodilators, and surgical or interventional cardiac catheterization procedures to improve late outcomes. Unfortunately, prospective data regarding the precise incidence and natural history of PH in BPD are lacking, and most information on diagnostic and therapeutic strategies are based on clinical observations, rather than rigorous, randomized clinical trials. While recognizing these limitations, we present a general approach to screening, diagnosis, and management of PH in infants with BPD, while highlighting gaps in our knowledge and the need for further research in this field.

A. Diagnosis of PH in BPD

Who, when, and how to screen patients for PH is controversial, and broadly accepted screening guidelines do not exist for PH in premature infants or in the setting of established BPD. Confusing this issue even further is the lack of a data-derived definition of PH in BPD, and the level of pulmonary artery pressure or PVR above which predictable adverse consequences occur remains uncertain. Thus, defining the levels of pulmonary artery pressure to identify the presence and severity of PH and to guide therapy remains uncertain. With this in mind, we present recommendations for an approach to the evaluation and treatment of PH in infants with BPD, which is primarily based on clinical experience (Fig. 2; Table 1).

In general, we recommend early echocardiograms for the diagnosis of PH in preterm infants with severe RDS who require high levels of ventilator support and supplemental oxygen (26), especially in the setting of oligohydramnios and intrauterine growth restriction. Similarly, infants with particularly slow rates of clinical improvement, as manifested by persistent or progressively increased need for high levels of respiratory support, should be assessed for PH (27). In the setting of established BPD, preterm infants who at 36 weeks' postconceptual age still require positive pressure ventilation support are not weaning consistently from oxygen, have oxygen needs at levels disproportionate to their degree of lung disease, or have recurrent cyanotic episodes warrant screening for PH or related cardiovascular sequelae. Other clinical markers often associated with more severe disease include feeding dysfunction and poor growth, recurrent hospitalizations, and elevated $PaCO_2$. High $PaCO_2$ is a marker of disease severity and reflects significant airways obstruction, abnormal lung compliance

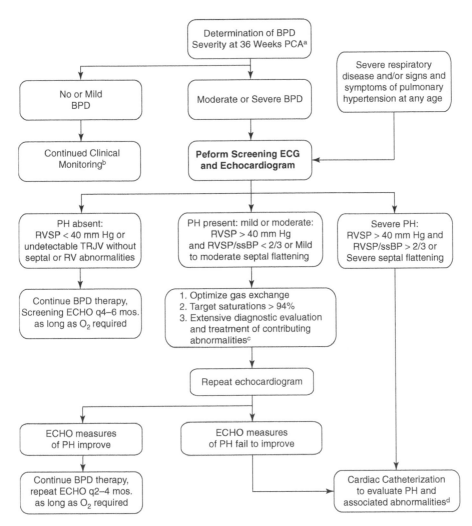

Figure 2 Proposed clinical approach to screening and evaluation of pulmonary hypertension in bronchopulmonary dysplasia. (a) As defined by NICHD/NHLBI/ORD Workshop (8). (b) See text. (c) See Table 4. (d) See Tables 2 and 3. *Abbreviations*: BPD, bronchopulmonary dysplasia; PH, pulmonary hypertension; RVSP, right ventricular systolic pressure; TRJV, tricuspid regurgitant jet velocity; ssBP, systemic systolic blood pressure; RV, right ventricle; ECHO, echocardiogram.

with heterogeneous parenchymal disease, or reduced surface area, and is an indication for PH screening (28). Persistent pulmonary edema requiring frequent diuretic use can be a sign of pulmonary venous obstruction or left-sided cardiac diastolic dysfunction (29). A more liberal strategy would be to screen every patient at 36 weeks of age diagnosed with moderate or severe BPD, according to NIH consensus criteria (8).

Table 1 Indications for Echocardiogram Evaluation in BPD

Screening at 36 wk PCA for moderate and severe BPD
At any time the following indications exist:

  Severe respiratory disease, failing to improve
  Respiratory disease out of proportion to situation
  Failure to wean oxygen support
  Recurrent cyanotic episodes or respiratory deteriorations
  Persistent hypercarbia
  Lack of overall improvement
  Poor growth despite stable respiratory status
  Other clinical reasons to suspect pulmonary hypertension or cardiac disease

The relative utility of electrocardiograms (ECG) or echocardiogram for screening for PH in infants with BPD also remains controversial. Serial ECGs may have inadequate sensitivity and positive predictive value for identification of right ventricular hypertrophy (RVH) as a marker of PH. A recent study found no relationship between ECG changes and echocardiogram estimates of pulmonary artery pressure (30), and some patients can have significant RVH and PH despite minimal or normal ECG findings. Therefore, we recommend serial echocardiograms as the predominant approach for screening PH in patients with BPD (Table 1).

Estimated systolic pulmonary artery pressure (sPAP) derived from the tricuspid regurgitant jet (TRJV) measured by echocardiogram has become one of the most utilized findings for evaluating PH (31–34). Past studies have shown excellent correlation coefficients (r values between 0.93 and 0.97) when compared with cardiac catheterization measurements in children less than two years old with congenital heart disease (33,35). However, these studies evaluated echocardiogram and cardiac catheterization performed simultaneously under the same hemodynamic conditions, and the utility of echocardiograms in predicting disease severity as applied in the clinical setting is less clear.

A recent study examined the utility of echocardiogram assessments of PH in infants with BPD with subsequent cardiac catheterization measurements of pulmonary artery pressure (36). Systolic PAP could be estimated in only 61% of studies, but there was poor correlation between echocardiogram and cardiac catheterization measures of sPAP in these infants (Fig. 3). Echocardiogram estimates of sPAP correctly identified the presence or absence of PH in 79% of these studies, but the severity of PH was correctly assessed in only 47% of those studies. Seven of 12 children (58%) without PH by echocardiogram had PH during subsequent cardiac catheterization. In the absence of a measurable TRJV, qualitative echocardiogram findings of PH, including right atrial enlargement, right ventricular hypertrophy, right ventricular dilation, pulmonary artery dilation, and septal flattening, either alone or in combination have relatively poor predictive value. However, the best of these appears to septal flattening. It has been postulated that factors associated with chronic lung disease, specifically marked pulmonary hyperinflation, expansion of the thoracic cage, and alteration of the position of the heart, adversely affect the ability to detect and measure TRJV (37). Thus, as used in clinical practice, echocardiography often identifies PH in infants with BPD, but

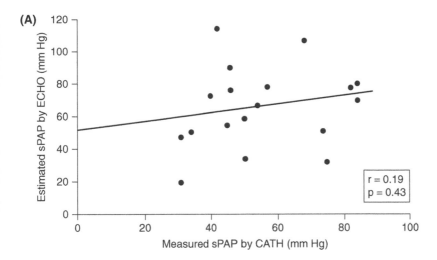

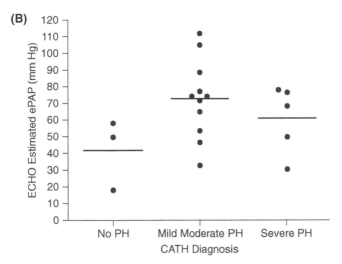

Figure 3 Clinical utility of echocardiogram for evaluation of pulmonary hypertension in infants and toddlers with lung disease (36). (**A**) Relationship between sPAP estimated by ECHO and directly measured by cardiac catheterization (CATH). (**B**) ECHO estimates of sPAP displayed by severity of PH as diagnosed by CATH. PH was defined as mPAP > 25 mm Hg; mild to moderate PH was PH with an mPAP/MAP < 0.67; severe PH was defined as mPAP/MAP ≥ 0.67. There were no significant differences between the mean sPAP of the three groups by ANOVA. *Abbreviations*: sPAP, systolic pulmonary artery pressure; ECHO, echocardiogram; CATH, catheterization; PH, pulmonary hypertension.

estimates of sPAP were not obtained consistently and were often not reliable for determining disease severity.

Other measures of right ventricular strain and PH, including AT/ET ration and the Tei index could be helpful in the absence of a measurable TRJV, but have not been fully evaluated in infants with BPD. Echocardiographic assessment of anatomic cardiac disease, especially shunt lesions, is an important aspect of cardiovascular evaluation of BPD infants. Infants with moderate to severe BPD may not tolerate even relatively small atrial or ventricular level shunting, and may be at higher risk for the development of pulmonary vascular disease and PH. Echocardiograms can also be useful for identifying pulmonary venous lesions and large aortopulmonary collateral vessels, but are not as sensitive as cardiac catheterization. Additionally, decreased shortening fraction, left ventricular ejection fraction, or signs of left ventricular hypertrophy may be signs of left ventricular dysfunction, which may require catheterization for diagnosis (29,38).

In summary, despite its limitations, echocardiography remains the best available screening tool for PH in BPD patients. We recommend a baseline screening echocardiogram at 36 weeks for any patient still requiring oxygen therapy. If the echocardiogram is normal or shows subtle signs of PH, we recommend serial echocardiograms be performed on a bimonthly basis as long as patients require oxygen therapy, and then once again one to two months after weaning off oxygen therapy (Fig. 1).

B. Role of Cardiac Catheterization in BPD

Whether echocardiogram correctly identifies infants with BPD who should undergo cardiac catheterization for further evaluation of PH, provides sufficient information regarding disease severity that required intervention, and provides sufficient information to effectively monitor patients with established PH without cardiac catheterization remains highly controversial. In general, we recommend cardiac catheterization for patients with BPD who (*i*) have persistent signs of severe cardiorespiratory disease or clinical deterioration not directly related to airways disease; (*ii*) are suspected of having significant PH despite optimal management of their lung disease and associated morbidities; (*iii*) are candidates for PH drug therapy; (*iv*) have unexplained, recurrent pulmonary edema; (*v*) and others. The goals of cardiac catheterization are to assess the severity of PH; exclude or document the severity of associated anatomic cardiac lesions; define the presence of systemic-pulmonary collateral vessels, pulmonary venous obstruction, or left heart dysfunction; and to assess pulmonary vascular reactivity in patients who fail to respond to oxygen therapy alone (Table 2).

Acute vasoreactivity testing (AVT) is important to determine the relative safety and potential efficacy of vasodilating agents that may be initiated in patients with

Table 2 Role of Cardiac Catheterization in BPD

Assess severity of pulmonary hypertension
Evaluate for anatomic heart disease/shunt lesions
Evaluate for structural vascular abnormalities, e.g., arterial stenosis, pulmonary venous stenosis,
    obstruction, others
Assess cardiac function (left ventricular dysfunction)
Acute vasoreactivity/hypoxia testing for selection of chronic therapy
Cather-based interventions, e.g., collaterals, stenosis, shunt

significant PH despite adequate oxygen and ventilation therapy. AVT is generally performed with iNO, usually at doses of 20 to 40 ppm, and often in combination with 100% oxygen to assess maximal vasodilator potential. Prolonged iNO therapy for PH may be considered for hospitalized patients who are ventilated or by nasal cannula delivery. In such patients, dose-response studies may help to optimize the level of iNO therapy during the catheterization study. Assessing AVT during acute hypoxia may also have therapeutic implications. Exaggerated pulmonary vascular constriction in response to hypoxia, even in the absence of baseline PH, is often seen in infants with BPD and can persist in older children (15,17). In some patients, marked increases in PVR occur even with relatively mild levels of hypoxia, suggesting the need for targeting higher oxygen saturations during chronic therapy to avoid hypoxemia.

Other critical information can be acquired during cardiac catheterization that may significantly aid in the management of infants with BPD (Table 3). In particular, assessment of shunt lesions; the presence, size, and significance of bronchial or systemic collateral arteries; determining the presence of pulmonary artery stenosis; and structural assessments of the pulmonary arterial and venous circulation by angiography are among several key factors that may affect cardiopulmonary function. A recent report highlighted the importance of pulmonary vein stenosis or veno-occlusive disease in premature infants (39). Most importantly, elevated pulmonary capillary wedge (PCWP) or left atrial pressure (LAP) may signify left-sided systolic or diastolic dysfunction. LV diastolic dysfunction can contribute to PH, recurrent pulmonary edema, or poor iNO responsiveness in infants with BPD, and measuring changes in PCWP and LAP during AVT may help with this assessment (29).

C. Treatment of PH in BPD

The initial clinical strategy for the management of PH in infants with BPD begins with treating the underling lung disease. This includes an extensive evaluation for chronic reflux and aspiration, structural airway abnormalities (such as tonsillar and adenoidal hypertrophy, vocal cord paralysis, subglottic stenosis, tracheomalacia, and other lesions), assessments of bronchoreactivity, improving lung edema and airway function, and others (Table 4). Periods of acute hypoxia whether intermittent or prolonged are the most likely causes of persistent PH in BPD (27). Brief assessments of oxygenation ("spot checks") are not sufficient for decisions on the level of supplemental oxygen needed. Targeting oxygen saturations to 92% to 94% should be sufficient to prevent the adverse effects of hypoxia in most infants, without increasing the risk of additional lung inflammation and injury.

Growth failure during home oxygen therapy may be the result of poor parental compliance or premature discontinuation of supplemental oxygen, as previously reported (40). A sleep study may be necessary to determine the presence of noteworthy episodes of hypoxia and whether hypoxemia has predominantly obstructive, central, or mixed causes. Additional studies that may be required include flexible bronchoscopy for the diagnosis of anatomical and dynamic airway lesions (such as tracheomalacia) that may contribute to hypoxemia and poor clinical responses to oxygen therapy. Upper gastrointestinal series, pH or impedance probe, and swallow studies may be indicated to evaluate for gastroesophageal reflux and aspiration that can contribute to ongoing lung injury. If findings are positive or even if clinical suspicion remains high in the face of

Table 3 Cardiac Catheterization Protocol for BPD Infants

Initial hemodynamics performed under baseline conditions[a]
  Hemodynamic measurements
    Right atrial pressures
    Right ventricular pressures
    Pulmonary artery pressures (main, left, and right pulmonary arteries)
    Systemic arterial pressures
    Left atrial or pulmonary capillary wedge pressure[b]
    Cardiac Index (by thermodilution for patients without shunt lesions)
    Oximetry (SVC, PA, pulmonary veins, and systemic artery)
    Systemic arterial blood gas

  Hemodynamic calculations
    Pulmonary vascular resistance (PVR)
    Systemic vascular resistance (SVR)
    PVR/SVR
    Qp and Qs (by method of Fick for patients with shunt lesions)
    Qp:Qs

Assess hemodynamic in response to[c]
  1. Hypoxia (systemic saturations of 80–85%)
  2. 100% oxygen (systemic saturation target > 95%)
  3. 100% oxygen + inhaled nitric oxide (20 ppm)
  4. Potential therapeutic medication(s)[d]

Pulmonary angiograms to assess pulmonary artery stenosis
Pulmonary venograms to assess for stenosis/obstruction
Aortogram to assess for aortopulmonary collateral vessels

[a]Consideration should be given to whether procedure is performed under conscious sedation or general anesthesia based on patient safety. However, effort should be directed to using the minimum sedation possible to maintain hemodynamic and gas exchange targets that mimic the patient's baseline state.
[b]Consideration should be given to the amount of diuretic the patient receives when interpreting these values. High normal pressures in the faces of high-dose diuretics may be suggestive of LV dysfunction.
[c]All hemodynamic measurements and calculations should be repeated for every condition.
[d]If calcium channel blocker therapy is considered, the hemodynamic response should be assessed during catheterization secondary to risks of systemic hypotension and hemodynamic compromise. Enteric administration of sildenafil and bosentan may require extended period of time for onset of action, and is not recommended.
Abbreviations: Qp, pulmonary blood flow; Qs, systemic blood flow.

Table 4 Evaluation for Factors Contributing to BPD Lung Disease

Diagnosis	Evaluation
Intermittent hypoxia/insufficient oxygen supplementation	Sleep Study
Gastro-Esophageal Reflux	Upper gastrointestinal series
	pH probe
	Esophageal Impedance study
Aspiration	Swallow study
Upper airway abnormalities/obstruction	Sleep study
	Bronchoscopy
Tracheobronchomalacia	Bronchoscopy
	Fluoroscopic PEEP study

negative findings and in the setting of lung disease that fails to improve, consideration should be given to Nissen fundoplication and gastrostomy tube placement. For patients with BPD and severe PH who fail to maintain near-normal ventilation or require high levels of FiO$_2$ despite conservative treatment, consideration should be given to chronic mechanical ventilatory support.

Despite the growing use of pulmonary vasodilator therapy for the treatment of PH in BPD, data demonstrating efficacy are extremely limited, and the use of these agents should only follow thorough diagnostic evaluations and aggressive management of the underlying lung disease. Current therapies used for PH therapy in infants with BPD generally include inhaled NO, sildenafil, endothelin-receptor antagonists, and calcium channel blockers (CCBs).

iNO causes selective pulmonary vasodilation (17) and improves oxygenation in infants with established BPD (41), and may decrease the incidence of chronic lung disease in some premature infants with respiratory distress syndrome (42–44). Although acute improvement in pulmonary hemodynamics during cardiac catheterization has been reported in infants with BPD (17), the role of long-term, low-dose iNO treatment has not been adequately studied.

The acute hemodynamic response to iNO in patients with BPD and PH has been shown to be greater than to CCBs (17) with doses as low as 2 ppm demonstrating near normalization of pulmonary pressures. Thus, it has been suggested that iNO may be useful for long-term therapy of PH (45–47). Indeed, long-term iNO therapy has been used in limited numbers of BPD infants, especially for those who require continued mechanical ventilatory support (36,48) or remain in the intensive care unit setting. Initiating iNO for PH therapy at doses of 10 to 20 ppm is recommended, utilizing frequent echocardiograms to assess response to therapy. Many patients subsequently tolerate weaning of the iNO dose to a range of 2 to 10 ppm. Methemoglobinemia, a possible side effect, is rare in the recommend dose range of 1 to 20 ppm. As these patients approach extubation or transfer out of the intensive care setting, consider transition to alternate vasodilator medications if PH therapy is still required.

Mechanisms underlying a poor acute response to iNO include poor lung inflation and inadequate delivery of iNO to the alveolar space, anatomic cardiac disease with high-flow shunt lesions, left ventricular dysfunction leading to persistent pulmonary edema, structural vascular disease with severe arterial remodeling or pulmonary venous obstruction, and biochemical alterations within the lung such as increased phosphodiesterase-5 (PDE-5) activity and increased superoxide production. Some of these factors like poor lung inflation can be corrected with changes in vent strategy; others may require interventional procedures, such as cardiac catheterization or the use of other medications.

Sildenafil, a highly selective PDE-5 inhibitor, augments cyclic GMP content in vascular smooth muscle, and has been shown to benefit adults with PH as monotherapy (49) and in combination with standard treatment regimens (50,51). Studies of sildenafil therapy in children with PH have been limited, but include a demonstration of its efficacy in the treatment of persistent PH of the newborn (52), and its safety and efficacy during long-term therapy in older children with PH (53). By prolonging cGMP levels during iNO induced vasodilation, PDE-5 inhibitors may be useful to augment the response to iNO therapy or to prevent rebound PH after abrupt withdrawal of iNO (54). In a study of 25 infants with chronic lung disease and PH (18 with BPD), prolonged

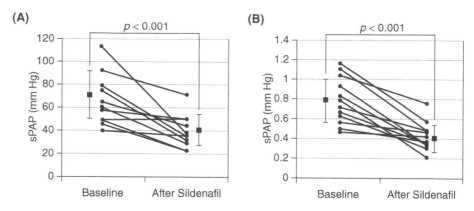

Figure 4 Changes in systolic pulmonary artery pressures (**A**) and pulmonary/systemic systolic artery pressure (**B**) as determined by echocardiogram in response to prolonged sildenafil therapy. Median duration of treatment between studies was 58 days (range: 25–334). Individual data plotted together with mean ± SD; *n* = 13 patients (48).

sildenafil therapy as part of an aggressive program to treat PH was associated with improvement in PH by echocardiogram in most (88%) patients without significant rates of adverse events (48) (Fig. 4). Although the time to improvement was variable, many patients were able to wean off mechanical ventilator support and other PH therapies, especially iNO, during the course of sildenafil treatment without worsening of PH. The recommended starting dose for sildenafil is 0.5 mg/kg/dose every eight hours. If there is no evidence of systemic hypotension, this dose can be gradually increased over two weeks to achieve desired pulmonary hemodynamic effect or a maximum of 2 mg/kg/dose every six hours.

Endothelin-1 is potent vasoconstrictor and smooth muscle mitogen that has been implicated in the pathogenesis of PH in neonates with severe pulmonary hypertension of the newborn (55), and may play a role in the pathogenesis of BPD (56,57). The effects of ET-1 are mediated through two receptors, ET_A and ET_B. ET_A is present on vascular smooth muscle cells and, when activated, promotes vasoconstriction and proliferation. ET_B receptors are located on endothelial cells and mediate vasodilation through nitric oxide and prostacyclin release. Bosentan, an oral agent that inhibits both ET receptors, is commonly used in older patients with PH. A retrospective study suggested that bosentan may be safe and effective for the treatment of PH in children as young as nine months (58), but data are limited to case reports regarding its use in BPD infants. Systemic hypotension, peripheral edema, systemic arterial desaturation, fatigue, and increases in liver transaminases have been reported with its use in children (58). Monthly liver enzyme tests are required with bosentan use. Sitaxsentan, a selective ET_A receptor blocker, has potential benefit for patients with PH by blocking the vasoconstrictor effects of endothelin-A while maintaining the vasodilator functions of ET_B receptors, but has even less experience in children compared with bosentan (59).

CCBs benefit some patients with PH, and short-term effects of CCB in infants with BPD have been reported (60,61). Nifedipine can acutely lower pulmonary artery pressure and PVR in children with BPD; however, some patients were hypoxemic during their evaluation, and the effects of nifedipine on pulmonary artery pressure were not different from the effects of supplemental oxygen alone (60). In comparison with an acute study of iNO reactivity in infants with BPD, the acute response to CCB was poor, and some infants developed systemic hypotension (17). In general, we generally use sildenafil or bosentan for chronic therapy of PH in infants with BPD.

Intravenous prostacyclin (PGI$_2$; epoprostenol) therapy has been used extensively in older patients with severe PH, and has been shown to improve survival of patients with advanced disease (62,63). PgI$_2$ has been used in some infants with BPD and late PH (64,65), but concerns regarding its potential to worsen gas exchange due to increased ventilation-perfusion mismatching in the setting of chronic lung disease and systemic hypotension have limited its use in this setting. In addition, the half-life of PgI$_2$ is extremely short, necessitating the use of a pump and central line for continuous, chronic infusion. As a result, line infections, cracking of the central venous catheter and related tubing, malfunction of the delivery system, and high risk of rebound PH with sudden withdrawal have limited enthusiasm for its long-term use in children. Treprostinil, a more stable PgI$_2$ analogue, has been delivered by intravenous and subcutaneous infusion, but has limited use in younger children. Although another stable PgI$_2$ analogue, iloprost, is available for inhalational use, the need for frequent treatments (6–8 times daily) and occasional bronchospasm may be significant factors restricting its use in the setting of BPD (66).

In addition to close monitoring of pulmonary status, infants with BPD and PH should be followed by serial echocardiograms, which should be obtained at least every two to four weeks with the initiation of therapy and at four- to six-month intervals with stable disease. Abrupt worsening of PH may reflect several factors including the lack of compliance with oxygen therapy or medication use, but can be related to the progressive development of pulmonary vein stenosis or veno-occlussive disease (39). Repeat cardiac catheterization may be indicated for patients being treated for PH with vasodilator therapy who experience clinical deterioration, worsening PH by echocardiogram, or when echocardiogram measurements fail to provide adequate hemodynamic assessment of sicker patients. We recommend that weaning of medications may be considered when normal or near-normal echocardiogram findings have been demonstrated on successive evaluations. Whether the addition of such biomarkers as brain natriuretic peptide levels are useful to follow in the setting of BPD is unknown.

IV. Conclusions

In summary, pulmonary vascular disease plays a key role in the pathogenesis and pathophysiology of BPD, and PH remains a major cause of morbidity and mortality in infants with BPD. Novel strategies that enhance lung vascular growth and function after premature birth may attenuate the severity of BPD. Although new therapies are now available for the treatment of PH, their role in the clinical care of severe BPD and improving long-term outcomes requires more thorough investigation.

References

1. Evans NJ, Archer LNJ. Doppler assessment of pulmonary artery pressure during recovery from hyaline membrane disease. Arch Dis Child 1991; 66:802–824.
2. Subhedar NV, Shaw NJ. Changes in pulmonary arterial pressure in preterm infants with chronic lung disease. Arch Dis Child 2000; 82:F243–F247.
3. Fouron JC, Le Guennec JC, Villemant D, et al. Value of echocardiography in assessing the outcome of bronchopulmonary dysplasia of the newborn. Pediatrics 1980; 65(3):529–535.
4. Khemani E, McElhinney DB, Rhein L, et al. Pulmonary artery hypertension in formerly premature infants with bronchopulmonary dysplasia: clinical features and outcomes in the surfactant era. Pediatrics 2007; 120(6):1260–1269.
5. Coalson JJ. Pathology of chronic lung disease of early infancy. In: Bland RD, Coalson JJ, eds. Chronic Lung Disease of Early Infancy. New York: Marcel Dekker, 2000:85–124.
6. De Paepe ME, Mao Q, Powell J, et al. Growth of pulmonary microvasculature in ventilated preterm infants. Am J Respir Crit Care Med 2006; 173(2):204–211.
7. Hussain AN, Siddiqui NH, Stocker JT. Pathology of arrested acinar development in post-surfactant BPD. Hum Pathol 1998; 29:710–717.
8. Jobe AH, Bancalari E. Bronchopulmonary dysplasia. Am J Respir Crit Care Med 2001; 163 (7):1723–1729.
9. Abman SH. BPD: a vascular hypothesis. Am J Respir Crit Care Med 2001; 164:1755–1756.
10. Hislop AA, Haworth SG. Pulmonary vascular damage and the development of cor pulmonale following hyaline membrane disease. Pediatr Pulmonol 1990; 9(3):152–161.
11. Tomashefski JF, Opperman HC, Vawter GF. BPD: a morphometric study with emphasis on the pulmonary vasculature. Pediatr Pathol 1984; 2:469–487.
12. Abman SH. Pulmonary hypertension in chronic lung disease of infancy. Pathogenesis, pathophysiology and treatment. In: Bland RD, Coalson JJ, eds. Chronic Lung Disease of Infancy. New York: Marcel Dekker, 2000:619–668.
13. Jones R, Zapol WM, Reid LM. Pulmonary artery remodeling and pulmonary hypertension after exposure to hyperoxia for 7 days. Am J Pathol 1984; 117:273–285.
14. Halliday HL, Dumpit FM, Brady JP. Effects of inspired oxygen on echocardiographic assessment of pulmonary vascular resistance and myocardial contractility in BPD. Pediatrics 1980; 65:536–540.
15. Abman SH, Wolfe RR, Accurso FJ, et al. Pulmonary vascular response to oxygen in infants with severe BPD. Pediatrics 1985; 75:80–84.
16. Goodman G, Perkin R, Anas N. Pulmonary hypertension in infants with BPD. J Pediatr 1988; 112:67–72.
17. Mourani PM, Ivy DD, Gao D, et al. Pulmonary vascular effects of inhaled NO and oxygen tension in BPD. Am J Respir Crit Care Med 2004; 170(9):1006–1013.
18. Jakkula M, Le Cras TD, Gebb S, et al. Inhibition of angiogenesis decreases alveolarization in the developing rat lung. Am J Physiol Lung Cell Mol Physiol 2000; 279:L600–L607.
19. Le Cras TD, Markham NE, Tuder RM, et al. Treatment of newborn rats with a VEGF receptor inhibitor causes pulmonary hypertension and abnormal lung structure. Am J Physiol Lung Cell Mol Physiol 2002; 283:L555–L562.
20. Klekamp JG, Jarzecka K, Perkett EA. Exposure to hyperoxia decreases the expression of vascular endothelial growth factor and its receptors in adult rat lungs. Am J Pathol 1999; 154:823–831.
21. Maniscalco WM, Watkins RH, D'Angio CT, et al. Hyperoxic injury decreases alveolar epithelial cell expression of vascular endothelial growth factor (VEGF) in neonatal rabbit lung. Am J Respir Cell Mol Biol 1997; 16:557–567.

22. Bhatt AJ, Pryhuber GS, Huyck H, et al. Disrupted pulmonary vasculature and decreased VEGF, flt-1, and Tie 2 in human infants dying with BPD. Am J Respir Crit Care Med 2000; 164:1971–1980.
23. Lassus P, Turanlahti M, Heikkila P, et al. Pulmonary vascular endothelial growth factor and Flt-1 in fetuses, in acute and chronic lung disease, and in persistent pulmonary hypertension of the newborn. Am J Respir Crit Care Med 2001; 164:1981–1987.
24. Bland RD, Mokres LM, Ertsey R, et al. Mechanical ventilation with 40% oxygen reduces pulmonary expression of genes that regulate lung development and impairs alveolar septation in newborn mice. Am J Physiol 2007; 293:L1099–L1110.
25. Thebaud B, Ladha F, Michelakis ED, et al. VEGF gene therapy increases survival, promotes lung angiogenesis, and prevents alveolar damage in hyperoxia-induced lung injury: evidence that angiogenesis participates in alveolarization. Circulation 2005; 112(16):2477–286.
26. Walther FJ, Benders MJ, Leighton JO. Persistent pulmonary hypertension in premature neonates with severe respiratory distress syndrome. Pediatrics 1992; 90(6):899–904.
27. Abman SH. Monitoring cardiovascular function in infants with chronic lung disease of prematurity. Arch Dis Child Fetal Neonatal Ed 2002; 87(1):F15–F18.
28. Kovesi T, Abdurahman A, Blayney M. Elevated carbon dioxide tension as a predictor of subsequent adverse events in infants with bronchopulmonary dysplasia. Lung 2006; 184 (1):7–13.
29. Mourani PM, Ivy DD, Rosenberg AA, et al. Left ventricular diastolic dysfunction in bronchopulmonary dysplasia. J Pediatr 2008; 152(2):291–293.
30. Puchalski MD, Lozier JS, Bradley DJ, et al. Electrocardiography in the diagnosis of right ventricular hypertrophy in children. Pediatrics 2006; 118(3):1052–1055.
31. Yock PG, Popp RL. Noninvasive estimation of right ventricular systolic pressure by Doppler ultrasound in patients with tricuspid regurgitation. Circulation 1984; 70(4):657–662.
32. Berger M, Haimowitz A, Van Tosh A, et al. Quantitative assessment of pulmonary hypertension in patients with tricuspid regurgitation using continuous wave Doppler ultrasound. J Am Coll Cardiol 1985; 6(2):359–365.
33. Currie PJ, Seward JB, Chan KL, et al. Continuous wave Doppler determination of right ventricular pressure: a simultaneous Doppler-catheterization study in 127 patients. J Am Coll Cardiol 1985; 6(4):750–756.
34. Skjaerpe T, Hatle L. Noninvasive estimation of systolic pressure in the right ventricle in patients with tricuspid regurgitation. Eur Heart J 1986; 7(8):704–710.
35. Skinner JR, Stuart AG, O'Sullivan J, et al. Right heart pressure determination by Doppler in infants with tricuspid regurgitation. Arch Dis Child 1993; 69(2):216–220.
36. Mourani PM, Sontag MK, Younoszai A, et al. Clinical utility of echocardiography for the diagnosis and management of pulmonary vascular disease in young children with chronic lung disease. Pediatrics 2008; 121(2):317–325.
37. Arcasoy SM, Christie JD, Ferrari VA, et al. Echocardiographic assessment of pulmonary hypertension in patients with advanced lung disease. Am J Respir Crit Care Med 2003; 167 (5):735–740.
38. Yates AR, Welty SE, Gest AL, et al. Myocardial tissue Doppler changes in patients with BPD. J Pediatr 2008; 152:766–770.
39. Drossner DM, Kim DW, Maher KO, et al. Pulmonary vein stenosis: prematurity and associated conditions. Pediatrics 2008; 122:e656–e661.
40. Groothuis JR, Rosenberg AA. Home oxygen promotes weight gain in infants with bronchopulmonary dysplasia. Am J Dis Child 1987; 141(9):992–995.
41. Banks BA, Seri I, Ischiropoulos H, et al. Changes in oxygenation with inhaled nitric oxide in severe bronchopulmonary dysplasia. Pediatrics 1999; 103(3):610–618.
42. Schreiber MD, Gin-Mestan K, Marks JD, et al. Inhaled nitric oxide in premature infants with the respiratory distress syndrome. N Engl J Med 2003; 349(22):2099–2107.

43. Kinsella JP, Cutter GR, Walsh WF, et al. Early inhaled nitric oxide therapy in premature newborns with respiratory failure. N Engl J Med 2006; 355(4):354–364.
44. Ballard RA, Truog WE, Canaan A, et al. Inhaled nitric oxide in preterm infants undergoing mechanical ventilation. N Engl J Med 2006; 355(4):343–353.
45. Channick RN, Newhart JW, Johnson FW, et al. Pulsed delivery of inhaled nitric oxide to patients with primary pulmonary hypertension: an ambulatory delivery system and initial clinical tests. Chest 1996; 109(6):1545–1549.
46. Kitamukai O, Sakuma M, Takahashi T, et al. Hemodynamic effects of inhaled nitric oxide using pulse delivery and continuous delivery systems in pulmonary hypertension. Intern Med 2002; 41(6):429–434.
47. Ivy DD, Parker D, Doran A, et al. Acute hemodynamic effects and home therapy using a novel pulsed nasal nitric oxide delivery system in children and young adults with pulmonary hypertension. Am J Cardiol 2003; 92(7):886–890.
48. Mourani PM, Sontag MK, Lui G, et al. Effects of long-term sildenafil treatment for pulmonary hypertension in infants with chronic lung disease. J Pediatr 2009; 154(3):379–384.
49. Galie N, Ghofrani HA, Torbicki A, et al. Sildenafil citrate therapy for pulmonary arterial hypertension. N Engl J Med 2005; 353(20):2148–2157.
50. Ghofrani HA, Rose F, Schermuly RT, et al. Oral sildenafil as long-term adjunct therapy to inhaled iloprost in severe pulmonary arterial hypertension. J Am Coll Cardiol 2003; 42 (1):158–164.
51. Bhatia S, Frantz RP, Severson CJ, et al. Immediate and long-term hemodynamic and clinical effects of sildenafil in patients with pulmonary arterial hypertension receiving vasodilator therapy. Mayo Clin Proc 2003; 78(10):1207–1213.
52. Baquero H, Soliz A, Neira F, et al. Oral sildenafil in infants with persistent pulmonary hypertension of the newborn: a pilot randomized blinded study. Pediatrics 2006; 117 (4):1077–1083.
53. Humpl T, Reyes JT, Holtby H, et al. Beneficial effect of oral sildenafil therapy on childhood pulmonary arterial hypertension: twelve-month clinical trial of a single-drug, open-label, pilot study. Circulation 2005; 111(24):3274–3280.
54. Namachivayam P, Theilen U, Butt WW, et al. Sildenafil prevents rebound pulmonary hypertension after withdrawal of nitric oxide in children. Am J Respir Crit Care Med 2006; 174(9):1042–1047.
55. Rosenberg AA, Kennaugh J, Koppenhafer SL, et al. Elevated immunoreactive endothelin-1 levels in newborn infants with persistent pulmonary hypertension. J Pediatr 1993; 123 (1):109–114.
56. Kojima T, Hattori K, Hirata Y, et al. Endothelin-1 has a priming effect on production of superoxide anion by alveolar macrophages: its possible correlation with bronchopulmonary dysplasia. Pediatr Res 1996; 39(1):112–116.
57. Allen SW, Chatfield BA, Koppenhafer SL, et al. Circulating immunoreactive endothelin-1 in children with pulmonary hypertension associated with acute hypoxic pulmonary vasoreactivity. Am Rev Respir Dis 1993; 148:519–522.
58. Rosenzweig EB, Ivy DD, Widlitz A, et al. Effects of long-term bosentan in children with pulmonary arterial hypertension. J Am Coll Cardiol 2005; 46(4):697–704.
59. Benza RL, Mehta S, Keogh A, et al. Sitaxsentan treatment for patients with pulmonary arterial hypertension discontinuing bosentan. J Heart Lung Transplant 2007; 26(1):63–69.
60. Brownlee JR, Beekman RH, Rosenthal A. Acute hemodynamic effects of nifedipine in infants with bronchopulmonary dysplasia and pulmonary hypertension. Pediatr Res 1988; 24 (2):186–190.
61. Johnson CE, Beekman RH, Kostyshak DA, et al. Pharmacokinetics and pharmacodynamics of nifedipine in children with bronchopulmonary dysplasia and pulmonary hypertension. Pediatr Res 1991; 29(5):500–503.

62. Barst RJ, Rubin LJ, Long WA, et al. A comparison of continuous epoprotenol (prostacyclin) with conventional therapy for primary pulmonary hypertension. N Engl J Med 1996; 334:296–302.
63. Barst RJ, Maislin G, Fishman AP. Vasodilator therapy for primary pulmonary hypertension in children. Circulation 1999; 99(9):1197–1208.
64. Zaidi AN, Dettorre MD, Ceneviva GD, et al. Epoprostenol and home mechanical ventilation for pulmonary hypertension associated with chronic lung disease. Pediatr Pulmonol 2005; 40 (3):265–269.
65. Rugolotto S, Errico G, Beghini R, et al. Weaning of epoprostenol in a small infant receiving concomitant bosentan for severe pulmonary arterial hypertension secondary to broncho-pulmonary dysplasia. Minerva Pediatr 2006; 58(5):491–494.
66. Ivy DD, Doran AK, Smith KJ, et al. Short- and long-term effects of inhaled iloprost therapy in children with pulmonary arterial hypertension. J Am Coll Cardiol 2008; 51(2):161–169.

20
Drug Therapies in the Management of BPD

HENRY L. HALLIDAY

Queen's University Belfast and Royal Maternity Hospital, Belfast, Northern Ireland, U.K.

I. Introduction

Bronchopulmonary dysplasia (BPD) is a chronic lung disease primarily affecting preterm infants needing respiratory support after birth. In the post–surfactant era, BPD is even more important because of increased survival of very preterm infants. Furthermore, the spectrum of BPD has changed since Northway et al. (1) published their classic description in 1967. BPD follows abnormal repair processes after inflammatory lung injury, leading to remodeling of the lung (2). Inflammation may be initiated by many stimuli including mechanical ventilation, oxidative stress, and infection. Neutrophil chemotaxis and degranulation release enzymes that may cause proteolysis of lung extracellular matrix. Abnormal healing with remodeling leads to poorly compliant lungs with reduced capacity for gas exchange.

Recently described "new" BPD, a less severe form, occurs in very preterm infants who survive following gentler types of assisted ventilation, including CPAP. Usually they have not been exposed to high ventilation pressures or volumes and high oxygen concentrations, the major factors in pathogenesis of "classic" BPD (1). Infection and inflammation are critically important in the pathogenesis of new BPD (3).

A. Prenatal Infection and Lung Inflammation

There is a well-established association between chorioamnionitis and preterm labor (4). Subclinical infection often is responsible for preterm birth but chorioamnionitis may also cause serious neonatal multiorgan morbidity following a systemic fetal inflammatory response (5). Inflammation, however, may be confined to the fetal lung and predispose to development of BPD (6). How chorioamnionitis-induced lung inflammation affects alveolarization and pulmonary angiogenesis in preterm babies is unknown, but it has been hypothesized that destruction of lung extracellular matrix by inflammatory collagenases may be important (7).

The pathophysiology of BPD may be thought of as separate processes of inflammation, architectural disruption, fibrosis, and disordered or delayed development. Classic BPD is represented by inflammation and fibrosis whereas new BPD is primarily an arrest of lung development (8,9). A spectrum exists with classic BPD representing lung injury and new BPD representing disordered and delayed pulmonary development.

Once developed, BPD is difficult to treat, and emphasis should therefore be on prevention. Drugs that may influence lung modeling and remodeling can be broadly divided into three groups:

1. Those administered prenatally to induce lung maturation thereby reducing need for mechanical ventilation and oxygen exposure
2. Those administered postnatally to prevent or minimize the initiation and effects of inflammatory stimuli
3. Those that may influence the inflammatory response to limit airways remodeling

II. Prevention of BPD

Prevention has been attempted with interventions ranging from the ideal of prevention of preterm birth to the more realistic minimization of lung injury.

A. Prenatal Interventions

Prevention of Preterm Birth

This aspiration will be difficult to fulfill as there are so many causes of preterm birth. Most studies have targeted at-risk women such as those with a previous preterm birth. Intervention programs to prevent preterm labor based on identification of women at risk have no effect on frequency of preterm birth (10,11).

Progesterone has also been used to prevent preterm birth in at-risk women. A systematic review and meta-analysis of progesterone supplementation for preventing preterm birth identified seven randomized controlled trials (RCTs) (12) (Table 1).

Table 1 Drug Therapies for Prevention of BPD: Prenatal Interventions

Intervention (Ref.)	Outcome	No. of studies	No. of subjects	RR (95% CI)	NNT (95% CI)
Progesterone (12)	Preterm birth	7	1020	0.58 (0.48–0.70)	8 (5–14)
Antibiotic treatment of asymptomatic bacteriuria (14)	Low birth weight	14	1923	0.66 (0.49–0.89)	20 (13–50)
Treatment of bacterial vaginosis before 20 wk (15)	Preterm birth	5	2387	0.63 (0.48–0.84)	37 (29–50)
Antibiotics for preterm, prelabor rupture of membranes (16)	Preterm birth	3	4931	1.00 (0.97–1.03)	–
	BPD 28 day	4	5597	0.75 (0.53–1.06)	–
	BPD 36 wk	1	4809	0.91 (0.70–1.17)	–
Prenatal glucocorticoids (21)	RDS	21	4038	0.66 (0.59–0.73)	11 (9–15)
	BPD	6	818	0.86 (0.61–1.22)	–
Prenatal thyrotropin-releasing hormone (33)	BPD 28 day	5	2511	1.01 (0.85–1.19)	–
	Death/BPD 28 day	6	3694	1.08 (0.94–1.25)	–

Abbreviations: RR, relative risk; CI, confidence interval; NNT, number needed to treat; BPD, bronchopulmonary dysplasia; RDS, respiratory distress syndrome.

Women who receive progesterone are significantly less likely to give birth at <37 weeks (7 studies, 1020 women, RR 0.58; 95% CI, 0.48–0.70), to have an infant with birth weight ≤2.5 kg (6 studies, 872 infants, RR 0.62; 95% CI, 0.49–0.78), or to have an infant with intraventricular hemorrhage (IVH) (1 study, 458 infants, RR 0.25; 95% CI, 0.08–0.82). Progesterone treatment leads to a 50% decreased risk of preterm birth, but has minimal effect on neonatal outcomes. Also, there is currently insufficient information to allow recommendations regarding its optimal dose, route, and timing of administration (13).

Antibiotic treatment of asymptomatic bacteriuria reduces the incidence of low birth weight babies (RR 0.66; 95% CI, 0.49–0.89) but not preterm birth (14). However, in women with a previous preterm birth treatment for bacterial vaginosis does not affect risk of subsequent preterm birth (RR 0.89; 95% CI, 0.71–1.11) or risk of preterm prelabor rupture of membranes (15). Treatment <20 weeks' gestation, however, may reduce preterm birth (RR 0.63; 95% CI, 0.48–0.84). There is little evidence that screening and treating all pregnant women with asymptomatic bacterial vaginosis will prevent preterm birth and its consequences (15). Another approach based on antibiotic treatment after onset of labor or after membrane rupture does not reduce preterm birth (RR 1.00; 95% CI, 0.97–1.03), although it decreases risk of chorioamnionitis (RR 0.57; 95% CI, 0.37–0.86), neonatal sepsis (RR 0.68; 95% CI, 0.53–0.87), and cerebral abnormalities (RR 0.82; 95% CI, 0.68–0.98) after preterm rupture of membranes (16). Antibiotic treatment does not affect need for oxygen at 28 days (RR 0.75; 95% CI, 0.53–1.06) or at 36 weeks' corrected age (RR 0.91; 95% CI, 0.70–1.17), nor does it decrease need for assisted ventilation (RR 0.90; 95% CI, 0.8–1.02) despite reducing surfactant use (RR 0.83; 95% CI, 0.72–0.96) (16).

Prevention of RDS—Prenatal Glucocorticoids

These promote maturation of the surfactant system (17), increase antioxidant capacity (18) and activity of lung endothelial nitric oxide synthase (19), and histologic lung maturation with increased size of air spaces and thinner more mature epithelium (20). The net result is a decreased risk of respiratory distress syndrome (RDS) (RR 0.66; 95% CI, 0.59–0.73) (21). Ideally glucocorticoids should be given between one and seven days before birth. However, although the effect on RDS is well established there is no clear evidence that glucocorticoids reduce the risk of BPD (RR 0.86; 95% CI, 0.61–1.22) (21), and indeed in an earlier meta-analysis there was a trend toward an increased risk (RR 1.38; 95% CI, 0.90–2.11) (22). Furthermore, another earlier meta-analysis showed that multiple courses of glucocorticoids increased the incidence of BPD (RR 3.01; 95% CI, 1.54–5.88) (23). Animal studies suggest that while glucocorticoids are necessary for normal lung development, excess inhibits normal lung maturation (20). Although there is improved lung compliance, changes in lung elastin and collagen content during this abnormal modeling increase the risk of mechanical ventilation–induced alveolar disruption (24).

The most recent meta-analysis shows that repeat courses of prenatal glucocorticoids for women at risk of preterm birth compared to a single course do not increase BPD (RR 0.95; 95% CI, 0.75–1.21; 4 trials, 2155 infants) (25). Currently available evidence suggests that repeat courses of prenatal glucocorticoids reduce severity of acute neonatal lung disease. However, there is insufficient evidence on longer-term benefits and risks (25). The National Institutes of Health recommend that no more than one course of glucocorticoids be used routinely outside clinical trials (26).

Glucocorticoids and inflammation appear to work synergistically to induce lung maturation. The combination may lead to more functionally mature lungs enabling preterm infants to survive, but this is offset, in part, by an increased susceptibility to ventilation-induced lung injury (2). This may explain why improved early pulmonary outcome is not associated with a reduction in BPD (21).

Prevention of RDS—Prenatal Thyrotrophin-Releasing Hormone

Thyroid hormones are involved in fetal lung growth and maturation acting synergistically with glucocorticoids to improve surfactant synthesis in sheep (27). Early small clinical trials of thyrotrophin-releasing hormone (TRH) were promising but had conflicting results (28,29). In the large Australian ACTOBAT study (30) and a subsequent North American clinical trial involving 996 women, prenatal TRH given with glucocorticoids was no more effective in preventing RDS or death than glucocorticoids alone (31). Furthermore, in the ACTOBAT study infants of mothers treated with TRH had an increased risk of motor and sensory impairment at 12-month follow-up (32). In a meta-analysis of 13 trials with over 4600 women, prenatal TRH increased the need for neonatal ventilation (RR 1.16; 95% CI, 1.03–1.29; 3 trials, 1969 infants) (33). TRH administration to women expected to deliver prematurely cannot be recommended.

B. Postnatal Interventions

Surfactant Therapy

Since its introduction in the early 1990s surfactant therapy has improved survival particularly for the smallest preterm infants who are at greatest risk of developing BPD. Surfactant also allows more gentle forms of ventilation with fewer pneumothoraces and as a result more neonates are surviving with mainly new BPD (8,9). This has skewed the population of infants with BPD to the more preterm end of the scale. Early trials of surfactant show increase in survival without BPD. The prevalence of BPD at 28 days of age is about 40% in infants with birth weights between 500 to 1000 g who require ventilation (34). Several RCTs have confirmed the safety and efficacy of surfactant therapy. Several meta-analyses (35–41) of various approaches to surfactant replacement have been performed (Table 2). Surfactant treatment significantly reduces mortality, but without a statistically significant effect on rates of BPD. As with prenatal glucocorticoids, the effects of surfactant replacement may have been concealed because of increased survival of extremely immature infants.

Inositol

Inositol, a six-carbon sugar alcohol found widely throughout mammalian tissues, is an essential nutrient required by human cells in culture for growth and survival. It promotes maturation of several components of surfactant and may play a critical role in fetal and early neonatal life. Three RCTs of inositol supplementation after birth, one using oral inositol for 10 days (42), a second intravenous inositol in the first 5 days of life (43), and a third a formula high in inositol (44), have been reported. A recent meta-analysis of

Table 2 Prevention of BPD: Postnatal Interventions—Surfactant Therapy

Intervention (Ref.)	Outcome	No. of patients	No. of studies	RR (95% CI)	NNT (95% CI)
Early surfactant and	BPD 28 day	68	1	0.94 (0.20–4.35)	–
short ventilation vs.	Death before	68	1	0.38 (0.08–1.81)	–
ongoing ventilation (35)	28 day				
Early vs. delayed	BPD 28 day	3039	3	0.97 (0.88–1.06)	–
selective	BPD 36 wk	3007	2	0.70 (0.55–0.88)	33 (20–100)
surfactant (40)	Mortality	3039	3	0.90 (0.79–1.01)	–
Multiple vs. single	BPD 28 day	343	1	1.10 (0.63–1.93)	–
dose of surfactant (37)	Mortality	394	2	0.63 (0.39–1.02)	–
Natural vs. synthetic	BPD 28 day	3515	8	1.02 (0.93–1.11)	–
surfactant (36)	BPD 36 wk	3179	5	1.01 (0.90–1.12)	–
	Mortality	4588	10	0.86 (0.76–0.98)	50 (20–100)
Prophylactic natural	BPD 28 day	932	7	0.93 (0.80–1.07)	–
surfactant (38)	Mortality	932	7	0.60 (0.44–0.83)	14 (8–33)
Prophylactic synthetic	BPD 28 day	1086	4	1.06 (0.83–1.36)	–
surfactant (39)	Mortality	1500	7	0.70 (0.58–0.85)	–
Prophylactic surfactant	BPD 28 days	2816	8	0.96 (0.82–1.12)	–
vs. selective	Mortality	2613	7	0.61 (0.48–0.77)	14 (9–33)
surfactant (40)					
Synthetic surfactant for	BPD 28 day	2248	5	0.75 (0.61–0.92)	25 (16–100)
RDS (41)	Mortality	2352	6	0.73 (0.61–0.88)	20 (14–50)

Abbreviations: RR, relative risk; CI, confidence interval; NNT, number needed to treat; BPD, bronchopulmonary dysplasia; RDS, respiratory distress syndrome.

these trials showed a strong trend favoring a reduction in BPD at 28 days (RR 0.68; 95% CI, 0.45–1.02; NNT 12; 95% CI, 6–1000) (45). Other effects of inositol supplementation include reductions in rates of death, death or BPD, IVH of grades III or IV, and retinopathy of prematurity of stage 4 or needing treatment. However, these findings are based on a limited number of patients. They require confirmation in large multicenter trials before inositol supplementation can be recommended as a routine part of nutritional management of preterm infants with RDS (45) (Table 3).

Early Systemic Postnatal Glucocorticoids

The history of postnatal glucocorticoids has evolved from one of potential short-term benefit to one of long-term harm, and it is a warning against adoption of new neonatal treatments without long-term follow-up studies to establish risk-benefit ratio. In the early 1980s, high-dose dexamethasone was used to successfully wean babies with BPD from ventilation (46,47). In 1989, Cummings et al. treated 36 infants, at high risk of BPD on ventilation at 14 days, with either an 18-day or a prolonged 42-day tapering course of dexamethasone and both regimens resulted in faster weaning from ventilation and reductions in supplemental oxygen (48). The prolonged course was associated with fewer long-term neurodevelopmental sequelae and thus high-dose dexamethasone became almost standard practice during the 1990s. There were acute adverse effects such as hypertension, hyperglycemia, gastrointestinal bleeding, infection, cardiac hypertrophy, and poor growth, but these were felt to be manageable and reversible once

Table 3 Prevention of BPD: Postnatal Interventions Other Than Surfactant

Intervention (Ref.)	Outcome	No. of studies	No. of patients	RR (95% CI)	NNT (95% CI)
Inositol (45)	BPD 28 day	3	336	0.68 (0.45–1.02)	–
	Death/BPD 28 day	2	295	0.56 (0.42–0.77)	5 (3–9)
Early steroids (54)	BPD 28 day	16	2621	0.85 (0.79–0.92)	14 (9–25)
	BPD 36 wk	15	2415	0.69 (0.60–0.80)	11 (8–20)
Inhaled steroids (66)	BPD 28 day	5	429	1.05 (0.84–1.32)	–
	BPD 36 wk	5	429	0.97 (0.62–1.52)	–
Bronchodilators (70)	BPD 28 day	1	173	1.03 (0.78–1.37)	–
Ibuprofen (73)	BPD 28 day	1	41	0.88 (0.32–2.42)	–
	BPD 36 wk	3	626	1.10 (0.91–1.33)	–
Prophylactic	BPD 28 day	9	1022	1.08 (0.92–1.22)	–
indomethacin (71)	BPD 36 wk	1	999	1.06 (0.92–1.22)	–
Caffeine (75)	BPD	1	2006	0.22 (0.13–0.30)	10 (7–18)
Vitamin A (84)	BPD 36 wk	2	793	0.87 (0.77–0.99)	14 (7–100)
Superoxide	BPD 28 day	1	33	3.65 (0.10–9.86)	–
dismutase (93)	BPD 36 wk	1	33	1.00 (0.21–65.05)	–
α1-Antitrypsin (100)	BPD 28 day	2	151	0.81 (0.64–1.01)	–
	BPD 36 wk	2	151	1.56 (0.58–4.17)	–
Nitric oxide (120)	BPD 36 wk	7	748	0.89 (0.78–1.02)	–
	Death/BPD 36 wk	5	460	0.96 (0.77–1.18)	–

Abbreviations: RR, relative risk; CI, confidence interval; NNT, number needed to treat; BPD, bronchopulmonary dysplasia.

treatment was discontinued. Many neonatologists believed that the benefit of improved lung function, earlier extubation, and less BPD outweighed these adverse effects.

All this changed after 1998 with the publication of three follow-up studies reporting increases in adverse neurodevelopmental sequelae, including cerebral palsy, in infants who had been treated with dexamethasone (49–51). In 2001 and 2002, the European Association of Perinatal Medicine (52) and the American Academy of Pediatrics with the Canadian Paediatric Society (53) recommended that glucocorticoids should not be used for treatment of preterm infants unless as a last resort or as part of a well-designed RCT with long-term follow-up.

Glucocorticoids were used early in RDS to prevent BPD (54) or later when BPD was developing (55) or had developed (56). Later use of glucocorticoids is discussed under section III "Treatment of BPD." The rationale for use of early postnatal glucocorticoids was the belief that the course of RDS could be altered despite a study in 1972 showing no apparent benefits from early hydrocortisone in babies with RDS (57). Moreover, there were long-term adverse neurologic effects including severe IVH (58) and abnormal EEG (59) in two follow-up studies. More recently infants with RDS have been found to have higher endogenous glucocorticoid levels, probably due to a stress response, but levels in those who later develop BPD are reduced (60). This provides a second rationale for early glucocorticoid treatment.

A third rationale for early treatment was the knowledge that inflammation begins early in RDS and treatment soon after birth may help prevent progression to BPD. Early glucocorticoid treatment reduces levels of proinflammatory cytokines in tracheal aspirates from ventilated preterm infants (61). In the 1980s and 1990s there were about 20 RCTs of early glucocorticoids to prevent BPD in preterm babies with RDS, and these have been summarized in a meta-analysis (54). Dexamethasone, starting at 0.5 mg/kg/ day halving every 3 days for a total of 12 days, was the most usual drug regimen, but hydrocortisone was also used as were other dosing regimens. Acute adverse effects of raised blood pressure and blood glucose were confirmed, but in addition there was an increased risk of cerebral palsy (RR 1.69; 95% CI, 1.20–2.38) (54). Early glucocorticoid treatment led to earlier extubation (risk of extubation failure before day 28) (RR 0.84; 95% CI, 0.72–0.98) and reduced risk of BPD at 28 days (RR 0.85; 95% CI, 0.79–0.92) and 36 weeks' corrected age (RR 0.69; 95% CI, 0.60–0.80), but had no effect on neonatal mortality (RR 1.05; 95% CI, 0.90–1.22).

Early Inhaled Postnatal Glucocorticoids

These offer an attractive option of obtaining the beneficial pulmonary effects of glucocorticoids while avoiding adverse systemic side effects. Several studies of inhaled glucocorticoids in neonates at risk of developing BPD compared beclomethasone (62), budesonide (63), flunisolide (64), and fluticasone (65) with placebo. Some studies showed a trend toward reduced time on ventilation and need for oxygen at 36 weeks, but they were insufficiently powered to detect significant differences. A systematic review of inhaled glucocorticoids given in the first two weeks of life showed a trend toward reduced mortality, earlier extubation, and reduced BPD without significant side effects, but the results were not statistically significant (66).

More research is needed to determine if there is a role for inhaled glucocorticoids, and studies assessing effects of lower systemic doses of other glucocorticoids in physiologic rather than pharmacologic doses are also warranted (66,67).

Other Anti-inflammatory Agents

Sodium cromoglycate with a nebulized dose of 20 mg, 6 hourly, lowered levels of proinflammatory cytokines in bronchoalveolar lavage fluid but did not reduce incidence of BPD at 28 days in 26 infants at high risk of developing it (68).

Bronchodilators

One RCT of inhaled salbutamol 200 µg given every four hours or a placebo for 28 days from the 10th day to 173 preterm infants at risk of developing BPD showed no statistically significant difference in duration of ventilatory support or age of weaning from respiratory support (69,70).

Prostaglandin Synthetase Inhibitors

The effectiveness of indomethacin-induced closure of a persistent ductus arteriosus (PDA) in preventing BPD has been confirmed in a systematic review (71). Earlier therapy, when symptoms of PDA first appear, may be more effective in preventing pulmonary morbidity than therapy after signs of congestive heart failure are present (71). However, prophylactic therapy with indomethacin did not decrease incidence of oxygen need at 36 weeks' corrected age in 1202 infants of 500 to 999 g birth weight despite reducing the incidence of symptomatic PDA (72). With easy availability and high efficacy of indomethacin for PDA closure, prompt medical or surgical closure of symptomatic PDA is a reasonable method of BPD prevention.

Two recent systematic reviews of ibuprofen for prevention (73) and treatment (74) of PDA in preterm infants showed that it did not prevent BPD at 28 days (RR 0.88; 95% CI, 0.32–2.42) or at 36 weeks (RR 1.10; 95% CI, 0.91–1.33) (73). However, there was a statistically significant increased incidence of BPD at 28 days with ibuprofen compared to indomethacin (RR 1.37; 95% CI, 1.01–1.86). The incidence of BPD at 36 weeks was not significantly different (RR 1.28; 95% CI, 0.77–2.10) (74).

Caffeine

Caffeine and similar drugs known as methylxanthines have been used for over 35 years to treat apnea of prematurity. The Caffeine for Apnea of Prematurity (CAP) study enrolled 2006 preterm infants between 1999 and 2004. This RCT compared 1000 control infants receiving placebo with 1006 infants treated with an initial dose of 20 mg/kg of caffeine citrate. At 36 weeks' corrected age there was a significant reduction in BPD in the caffeine treated group (RR 0.22; 95% CI, 0.13–0.30; NNT 10; 95% CI, 7–18) (75), possibly due to the placebo group having longer exposure to positive pressure ventilation. However, caffeine also reduces pulmonary resistance and increases lung compliance in infants with BPD (76). Reducing ventilator-induced lung damage may be important in preventing BPD, but caffeine also acts as a diuretic and reduced lung fluid would improve lung mechanics and gas exchange. Caffeine also has anti-inflammatory effects and others have hypothesized that methylxanthines act as antioxidants (77). Schmidt et al. recently concluded that compared to vitamin A and glucocorticoids, caffeine was the drug of choice for prevention of BPD (78).

Antibiotic Treatment of Chorioamnionitis

Chorioamnionitis appears to decrease the risk of RDS but increase the risk of BPD in intubated preterm infants (60). Infection with *Ureaplasma urealyticum* is specifically related to subsequent increased risk of BPD (79), and this is especially so in infants weighing less than 1000 g (80). Colonization with ureaplasma is associated with an increased risk of developing BPD (RR 1.72; 95% CI, 1.50–1.96) compared with uncolonized neonates. However, RCTs of erythromycin treatment do not show any reduction in BPD (81). This may be because erythromycin fails to eliminate airway colonization with *U. urealyticum* in very low birth weight infants (82).

Antioxidant Therapy

Since immature infants are deficient in endogenous pulmonary antioxidants and are exposed to multiple sources of oxidative stress (83), a number of antioxidant therapies have been used to prevent BPD. Antioxidants, such as vitamins A (84) and E (85) and superoxide dismutase (86) as well as the free radical scavenger *N*-acetylcysteine (87) and allopurinol (88), an inhibitor of xanthine oxidase (an enzyme capable of generating superoxide radicals following hypoxia ischemia), have been given to preterm babies at risk of BPD to try to reduce oxygen free radical–induced lung damage. To date only vitamin A treatment has shown encouraging results, with a statistically significant if modest reduction in BPD (RR 0.89; 95% CI, 0.80–0.99) in babies treated with intramuscular vitamin A (84,89). Vitamin A is a retinoid and its benefits may not be due entirely to antioxidant effects. Retinoic acid promotes alveolar septation (90), and rats treated with trans-retinoic acid in the postnatal period of alveolarization show a 50% increase in lung septation (91). The beneficial effect of vitamin A may be due to a reduction in prenatal glucocorticoid-induced alveolar hypoplasia.

Recombinant human superoxide dismutase (rh SOD) given intratracheally to piglets reduces lung damage caused by hyperoxia and hyperventilation (92). However, studies in preterm babies have produced disappointing results. In a multicenter, placebo-controlled RCT intratracheal human copper zinc SOD (CuZnSOD) administered every 48 hours for up to 1 month in mechanically ventilated extremely preterm infants did not reduce mortality or oxygen-dependence at 36 weeks (93). At one year treated infants had lower rates of hospitalization, emergency room visits, and treatment with asthma medications, suggesting a potential pulmonary benefit that was not evident on earlier assessment (94). Clearly further trials will be needed before this drug can be recommended for prevention of BPD.

Although the antioxidant and free radical scavenger N-acetylcysteine reduces markers of injury in a rat model of endotoxin-mediated acute lung injury (87), a Nordic RCT of six days of intravenous treatment with N-acetylcysteine in mechanically ventilated infants of 500 to 999 g birth weight showed no significant improvement in lung function (95) or reduction in mortality or supplemental oxygen at 28 days or 36 weeks' corrected age (96).

In 400 infants between 24 and 32 weeks' gestation randomly allocated to receive either enteral allopurinol (20 mg/mL) or placebo for 7 daily doses, the rate of BPD was not reduced despite plasma hypoxanthine concentrations at birth being significantly higher in infants who subsequently developed BPD (88).

More effective antioxidant therapies now being tested in animals might offer greater short-term benefits. In the moderately preterm baboon model of BPD, an intravenous infusion of a catalytic antioxidant metalloporphyrin, AEOL 10113, partially reversed the morphologic changes induced by 100% oxygen exposure and inhibited hyperoxia-induced increases in pulmonary neuroendocrine cells and urine bombesin-like peptide (97). This compound has yet to be evaluated in clinical trials. Oxygen free radicals play a role in cell signaling during tissue growth and differentiation, and for this reason others have cautioned against using antioxidant therapy in newborn (98).

Proteinase Inhibitors

Lung injury by proteolytic enzymes accompanies unopposed antioxidant stress and pulmonary inflammation, and disruption of the pulmonary proteinase-antiproteinase balance is associated with development of BPD (99). Neutrophil elastase is released in the lungs as part of the inflammatory process and α1-proteinase inhibitor forms a complex with it preventing destruction of the extracellular matrix. In a RCT, intravenous α1-proteinase inhibitor (60 mg/kg) or placebo was infused on four occasions during the first two weeks of life (100). The reduction in BPD at 36 weeks (RR 0.48; 95% CI, 0.23–1.00) in the treated group just failed to reach statistical significance, but there was a significant reduction in pulmonary hemorrhage (RR 0.22; 95% CI, 0.05–0.98). Neutrophil elastase excess and proteinase-antiproteinase imbalance might be of less importance in the pathogenesis of new BPD (101). However, benefits of antiproteinase therapy are biologically plausible, the number of infants studied to date is small, and no adverse effects of treatment have been observed, making this a preventive therapy for BPD worthy of larger-scale clinical trials.

Inhaled Nitric Oxide

Inhaled NO (iNO) is a selective pulmonary vasodilator reversing pulmonary hypertension and improving oxygenation without affecting the systemic circulation. iNO is of proven benefit in term and near-term infants with persistent pulmonary hypertension, reducing need for ECMO (102). In preterm babies with early lung disease, iNO may reduce pulmonary vascular resistance and selectively increase blood flow to areas of lung that are adequately ventilated, thereby improving oxygenation and reducing ventilatory requirements and risk of oxygen toxicity. Moreover, in animal studies, iNO reduces pulmonary inflammation directly (103) and decreases pulmonary artery remodeling in rat pups (104). The capacity of iNO to improve ventilation-perfusion matching as well as its anti-inflammatory (105) and antioxidant (106) effects offer potential benefit to preterm infants at risk of BPD.

Three early studies of iNO showed no benefit for prevention of BPD either independently (107–109) or in a meta-analysis (RR 0.93, 95% CI, 0.79–1.09) (102). However, in a recent RCT, low-dose (10 ppm) iNO in preterm infants with mild or moderate RDS reduced risk of death or BPD from 64% to 49% (110). The effect was greater among infants whose respiratory illness was less severe (oxygenation index <6.94). Any benefits must be weighed against potential adverse effects of iNO including prolonged bleeding time (111), surfactant dysfunction (112), and increased pulmonary inflammation (113), all more likely at higher doses. However, no adverse effects of iNO were detected with respect to rates of severe IVH or periventricular leukomalacia (PVL), although the study protocol did not provide standardized assessment of these outcomes (110). At 24-month follow-up of 138 of 168 (82%) survivors, improved outcomes were found among the iNO treated group (24% abnormal neurodevelopment vs. 46% in the placebo group) (114).

A multicenter RCT of iNO treatment of extremely preterm infants at 15 NICHD Neonatal Network centers enrolled 420 newborns with gestations <34 weeks and birth weights of 401 to 1500 g who had signs of ongoing respiratory failure more than 4 hours after receiving surfactant (115). There was no difference in the primary outcome, death or BPD at 36 weeks' corrected age, between study groups (80% in iNO group and 82% in placebo group; RR 0.97; 95% CI, 0.86–1.08). There were no apparent effects of iNO treatment on rates of IVH or PVL. Post hoc analyses suggested that iNO effects differed by birth weight. For infants >1000 g iNO was associated with improved primary outcome (death or BPD); however, infants at or <1000 g birth weight who were treated with iNO had higher rates of mortality and IVH than controls and the study was eventually terminated due to this increase (115).

In a U.K. trial of very preterm infants with severe lung disease after surfactant replacement, iNO did not improve either short- or long-term outcomes and because death occurred later in the treated group iNO had significant cost implications (116).

A recent meta-analysis (117) of five RCTs involving a total of 808 infants <34 weeks' gestation showed a reduction in BPD with iNO (RR 0.83; 95 % CI, 0.72–0.95).

Results of two further quite large RCTs have recently been published (118,119). The first involving 793 infants, 398 treated with iNO (5 ppm) and 395 with placebo, found no overall difference in death or BPD between groups (118). However, iNO therapy reduced the incidence of BPD in infants with birth weight $\geq$1000 g by 50% ($p = 0.001$) in a post hoc analysis, a result that should be treated with caution. The second RCT enrolled 582 infants $\leq$1250 g birth weight requiring ventilatory support at 7 to 21 days of age (119). Treated infants received decreasing concentrations of iNO, beginning at 20 ppm, for a minimum of 24 days. Severity of lung disease, based on hospitalization and need for ventilatory support, was less at 36 ($p = 0.012$), 40 ($p = 0.014$), and 44 ($p = 0.033$) weeks' corrected age. There were no differences between groups with regard to comorbidities occurring after entry apart from an increased survival without BPD at 36 weeks' postmenstrual age in the iNO group (43.9% vs. 36.8%; $p = 0.042$). In post hoc analyses, iNO improved survival without BPD for infants enrolled at 7 to 14 days (49.1% vs. 27.8%, $p = 0.001$) but not for infants enrolled at 15 to 21 days (40.7% vs. 42.8%), and benefit was restricted to infants with less severe lung disease at entry (119).

Recently RCTs of iNO in preterm infants have been assessed in three groups: early prophylaxis, early rescue, and late treatment (120). Only infants treated with early prophylaxis derived any benefit with reduction in severe IVH/PVL (RR 0.70; 95% CI, 0.53–0.91), death (RR 0.77; 95% CI, 0.61–0.98), and death or BPD (RR 0.92; 0.85–0.99). However, BPD at 36 weeks was not significantly reduced (RR 0.92; 95% CI, 0.83–1.02) in this most recent meta-analysis.

iNO may not be the magic bullet that was hoped for, and its role, if any, is likely to be early, in low dose, for babies with mild or moderate lung disease. Its use in babies <1000 g birth weight remains uncertain. Further studies with long-term neuro-developmental and respiratory follow-up are ongoing and results should be awaited before iNO can be recommended as routine therapy to prevent BPD in very preterm infants.

Cytokines and Anticytokines

Future preventive interventions for BPD are likely to include targeted cytokine or anticytokine therapies aimed at upregulating beneficial and blocking harmful humoral factors. Lung maturation is induced by administration of low dose proinflammatory cytokines. Endotoxin is a potent inducer of synthesis of proinflammatory cytokines. Prenatal endotoxin causes lung maturational effects in preterm sheep similar to those following prenatal glucocorticoids (121). This effect is not mediated by upregulation of endogenous cortisol (122), acts synergistically with the glucocorticoid effect (121), and requires direct contact of lung epithelium with endotoxin (123). However, inflammation also leads to remodeling and alveolar hypoplasia, so concerns about longer-term adverse effects may limit usefulness of endotoxin as a therapeutic agent.

Another potential therapy is antimacrophage chemokine (anti-MCP-1). In a newborn model of lung injury at one week, anti-MCP-1 treated rats had reduced pulmonary macrophages and neutrophils in BAL fluid, suggesting suppression of harmful inflammatory factors (124). Other candidates for future therapies include anti-inflammatory agents (such as interleukin-10), surfactant proteins (125), Clara cell secretory protein (126), and bombesin-blocking molecules (97).

III. Treatment of BPD

A. Introduction

The major postnatal risk factors for BPD include overventilation, nosocomial infection, oxidative stress, and PDA. Avoiding fluid overload and maintaining good nutrition are of importance in reducing lung damage and aiding repair. Mechanical ventilation is associated with an increased risk of BPD probably because of overdistension of the lung. Babies with the lowest arterial carbon dioxide levels at 48 hours appear to be at greatest risk of BPD, implying that overventilation may be a key causative factor (127).

Preterm babies are at risk of oxidative stress and they are often exposed to high concentrations of inspired oxygen for resuscitation and to maintain normal arterial oxygen tensions after birth. High oxygen exposure leads to generation of oxygen free radicals that can cause oxidative damage to tissues and trigger an inflammatory response. The presence of lipid peroxidation products in BAL fluid has been linked to development of BPD (128,129). Preterm babies have low levels of antioxidant protection and an inability to increase antioxidant production in response to oxidative stress. The aim of management of preterm infants has traditionally been to maintain arterial oxygen saturations in the range that is normal for a term baby (94–97%), believing that this is optimal for growth and brain development and for promoting closure of the ductus arteriosus. These saturations are much higher than those needed for maintenance of well-being in utero. Acceptance of lower oxygen saturations might reduce risk of BPD. The STOP-ROP trial was designed to see if maintaining preterm babies with prethreshold retinopathy of prematurity at higher oxygen saturations (96–99% vs. 89–94%) would reduce progression of retinopathy of prematurity (130). There were no differences in ophthalmologic outcomes but the group maintained at lower oxygen saturations had less respiratory morbidity suggesting that further studies are warranted to define safe oxygen saturation targets for the very preterm baby (131).

As previously discussed prenatal infections increase risk of BPD, as do postnatal infections (132). There is an association between respiratory colonization of premature infants with organisms such as *U. urealyticum* and later development of BPD (80,81,133).

Interstitial edema is a pathological feature of infants with BPD, and PDA and excessive fluid administration may contribute to its development and worsening of respiratory status (134). Symptomatic PDA has also been associated with development of BPD (34). Both PDA and systemic infection increase proinflammatory cytokines and this may be the mechanism of action (135).

Preterm infants are born before they can maximally accumulate nutrients. Their limited stores, inadequate postnatal nutrient intake, simultaneous use of other medications such as glucocorticoids and diuretics, oxidative stress, and infections may result in a prolonged hypercatabolic state, which may further impair the process of healing (135). Thus, the interactions of several factors, such as proinflammatory cytokines, mechanical ventilation, oxygen, relative lack of antioxidant defenses, and release of cytotoxic enzymes such as elastases and proteinases, interfere with normal developmental signals and may lead to BPD. In this section drug management of established BPD will be discussed.

Late Systemic Postnatal Glucocorticoids

Two systematic reviews of the numerous RCTs examining benefits and risks of systemic glucocorticoids for babies with or developing BPD are based on timing of treatment after

Table 4 Drug Treatment of BPD

Intervention (Ref.)	Outcome	No. of studies	No. of patients	RR (95% CI)	NNT (95% CI)
Moderately early	BPD 28 day	6	623	0.87 (0.81–0.94)	9 (6–20)
glucocorticoids (55)	BPD 36 wk	5	247	0.62 (0.47–0.82)	5 (3–11)
Late glucocorticoids (56)	BPD 36 wk	1	118	0.76 (0.58–1.00)	6 (3–100)
	Death or BPD 36 wk	1	118	0.73 (0.58–0.93)	5 (3–14)

Abbreviations: RR, relative risk; CI, confidence interval; NNT, number needed to treat; BPD, bronchopulmonary dysplasia.

birth: moderately early treatment (7–14 days) (55) and late treatment (>3 weeks) (56) (Table 4). With moderately early glucocorticoids there is a reduction in neonatal mortality before 28 days and a clear trend toward reduction in mortality before discharge in treated babies. Treatment started between 7 to 14 days also facilitates earlier extubation and significantly reduces the risk of BPD at 36 weeks. However, side effects include hypertension and cardiac hypertrophy. Late systemic glucocorticoids also lead to more rapid weaning from mechanical ventilation but mortality is not affected and there is also an increased risk of side effects. Overall glucocorticoid treatment exerts short-term beneficial effects on the neonatal lung, with improved lung mechanics and gas exchange facilitating earlier extubation, perhaps through a reduction of pulmonary inflammation. The additional benefit of a reduction in supplemental oxygen only occurs when treatment is given within the first 14 days of life. Side effects occur regardless of timing of treatment. However, as with prenatal glucocorticoids there is evidence from rat studies that postnatal treatment also inhibits alveolarization and reduces lung growth (136). There is conflicting evidence regarding duration of this effect with one study showing persistence into adulthood (136), but another with doses more similar to those used in neonates showing resolution (137).

Late Inhaled Glucocorticoids

Inhaled glucocorticoids are an alternative method for delivering anti-inflammatory activity locally without risks associated with systemic administration. When given to intubated infants with BPD for periods of one to four weeks, inhaled glucocorticoids significantly improve rate of successful extubation during treatment (RR 0.12; 95% CI, 0.03–0.43) (138). They seem to be as good as systemic steroids for weaning babies from the ventilator (139,140). Although studies that assessed adverse effects such as adrenal dysfunction, infection, retinopathy of prematurity, and IVH generally did not find an increase in glucocorticoid-treated infants, they were small and lacked power to detect clinically significant differences. A recent study of adrenal function in preterm infants treated with inhaled glucocorticoids showed decreases in basal cortisol levels, but normal responses to stimulation (141). Further RCTs are needed to address risk-benefit ratios of different delivery techniques, dosing schedules, and long-term effects of inhaled steroids, with particular attention to neurodevelopmental outcome.

Diuretics

These could potentially improve pulmonary compliance and airway resistance by reducing lung edema. Two Cochrane reviews assessed effects of enteral loop diuretics (such as furosemide) (142) and those acting on the distal renal tubule (such as thiazides and spironolactone) (143) in either preventing or treating BPD in preterm infants. Chronic administration of furosemide improves oxygenation and lung compliance in infants with BPD (144). A small study of 17 infants with BPD suggested that furosemide (1 mg/kg 12 hourly intravenously or 2 mg/kg 12 hourly orally) also hastens ventilator weaning when compared with placebo (144). However, because of the scarcity of RCTs, a recent systematic review concluded that routine use of furosemide could not be recommended in BPD (142). Although a single dose of aerosolized furosemide improves lung mechanics, lack of data on important clinical outcomes means that routine or sustained use of this therapy cannot be recommended (145).

Treatment of BPD with distal tubular diuretics (thiazides and spironolactone) has also been assessed in a systematic review (143). A one-week course improved pulmonary function in some studies, but not in others (146,147). A four-week course improved pulmonary function and decreased need for concomitant furosemide in a study of 43 infants with BPD (148). These diuretics and theophylline have additive effects on pulmonary function in infants with BPD (149). Although distal tubular diuretics may cause significant electrolyte abnormalities, incidence of nephrocalcinosis and hearing loss do not appear to be increased by these drugs (150,151).

Beneficial effects of diuretics on lung function in BPD cannot be solely explained by increased diuresis. Diuretics may directly affect lung fluid balance by altering ion water transport or pulmonary vascular tone (152). While both types of diuretic result in short-term improvements of lung compliance, there is little evidence of reductions in ventilatory support, length of hospital stay, or other important long-term outcomes. Their use in BPD remains empirical, although they may improve lung compliance and airway resistance as a short-term measure during acute exacerbations.

Bronchodilators

Infants with severe BPD frequently have airway smooth muscle hypertrophy and hyperreactivity, and both systemic and inhaled bronchodilators have been used to treat them. However, most of the literature deals with short-term effects on pulmonary function, and little new research has been done (153,154). Up-to-date evidence for a long-term benefit of bronchodilators both in prevention and treatment of BPD does not exist (155). Inhaled bronchodilators used in BPD include β-agonists and anticholinergic agents alone or in combination. There is some acute improvement of lung function in ventilated preterm infants early in life and in non-ventilator-dependent infants with overt BPD, but response rates are variable (155). The inhaled β-agonists, salbutamol, isoprenaline, orciprenaline, and albuterol, all lead to acute improvement in airflow (156). The inhaled anticholinergic agents, atropine and ipratropium bromide, also cause bronchodilation and improve pulmonary function in BPD in the short term (154), but long-term efficacy has not been studied for any of these drugs (155).

Other Anti-inflammatory Drugs

Methylxanthines (aminophylline and caffeine) reduce airway resistance in infants with BPD and have other potential beneficial effects, such as respiratory stimulation and a mild diuretic effect. Aminophylline may also improve respiratory muscle contractility.

Like other drugs that inhibit phosphodiesterases, they may also have anti-inflammatory effects. Improvement in pulmonary function in infants with BPD is additive to the effects of diuretics (149). Although methylxanthines lead to improved weaning of infants from mechanical ventilation, long-term studies of effectiveness in BPD have not been performed (157). Methylxanthines also have significant side effects, such as gastroesophageal reflux, clearly undesirable in preterm infants with BPD. However, the recently reported short- (75) and long-term (158) results of the CAP study demonstrating significant reductions in BPD, PDA, and cerebral palsy may lead to even greater use of caffeine to treat very preterm infants soon after birth.

Mucolytics

Recombinant human deoxyribonuclease (rhDNase, dornase alfa), administered by inhalation, is used as a mucolytic agent in cystic fibrosis. There have been several case reports of use of dornase alfa, administered intratracheally or by nebulization, to relieve mucus plugging in BPD. It appears to improve radiographic evidence of plugging and decrease oxygen requirements (159), but no RCTs have been performed (156).

Antibiotics for Postnatal Infection

Prevention of nosocomial infection is important but there is no evidence that antibiotics affect the incidence of BPD. In a study of 28 infants of <30 weeks' gestation colonized with *U. urealyticum*, although erythromycin treatment was effective in reducing colonization, there was no evidence that treatment altered the severity of lung disease (133). However, some antibiotics such as erythromycin fail to eliminate airway colonization with this organism in very low birth weight infants (82).

Immunization and Monoclonal Antibodies

Infants with BPD are at increased risk of recurrent respiratory tract infections especially those due to respiratory syncitial virus (RSV). In a meta-analysis of RCTs of RSV immunoglobulin or RSV monoclonal antibody, these were effective in preventing readmission to hospital and to pediatric intensive care units (160). A large multicenter study of palivizumab, a humanized monoclonal antibody against RSV, found that monthly injections of 15 mg/kg for five months reduced hospitalization rate for RSV infection by 4.9% (12.8–7.9%) in infants with BPD (160). Thus 20 infants with BPD need to receive a course of palivizumab to prevent one admission to hospital with RSV. Many centers now routinely administer palivizumab either to all preterm infants or all those with BPD who are likely to be discharged home prior to or during their first annual encounter with the peak RSV season. American Academy of Pediatrics recommendations are that palivizumab or RSV-IGIV prophylaxis should be considered for infants and children <2 years of age with BPD who required medical therapy for their lung disease within 6 months before the anticipated RSV season. Infants with more severe BPD may benefit from prophylaxis for two RSV seasons (161).

New Treatments

Sildenafil, a cGMP-specific phosphodiesterase inhibitor, improves alveolar growth and reduces pulmonary hypertension in hyperoxia-induced lung injury in rats (162). Rat pups were randomly exposed from birth to normoxia, hyperoxia (95% FiO_2; BPD model), and hyperoxia plus sildenafil (100 mg/kg/day subcutaneously). Those exposed to hyperoxia showed fewer and enlarged air spaces as well as decreased capillary density, mimicking pathologic features in human BPD. Sildenafil preserved alveolar growth and lung angiogenesis and decreased pulmonary vascular resistance, right ventricular hypertrophy, and medial wall thickness (162).

Pentoxifylline is a methylxanthine with anti-inflammatory and anticytokine effects. Its anti-inflammatory effects include inhibition of neutrophils, macrophages, and monocytes. In a small, uncontrolled trial of five infants with BPD, seven days of therapy with nebulized pentoxifylline was associated with a trend to reduction in oxygen requirement and improved pulmonary mechanics, but there have been no RCTs (163). An interim analysis of a prophylactic trial (164) suggested pentoxifylline may reduce treatment requirements after the neonatal period and that, in established BPD, pentoxifylline and dexamethasone may be of similar efficacy.

IV. Conclusions

It is over 40 years since Northway et al. (1) published the classic description of BPD in 1967. BPD continues to be a major complication of preterm birth as well as a major therapeutic challenge. Future developments will depend on a combination of understanding the interplay between lung injury and lung development, and the development of novel treatments to interrupt the pathogenesis of BPD and deal with its sequelae. It is unlikely that one single intervention will be found to prevent BPD (165), but more likely that treatments will involve a cocktail of anti-inflammatory, antioxidant, and anti-apoptotic agents. Since genetic and prenatal factors are important in pathogenesis, postnatal interventions may be too late (165), although a recent historical cohort study suggests that a combination of early surfactant, nasal CPAP at delivery, lowered oxygen saturation goals, and early amino acid administration may decrease rate of BPD (166). Further, basic science research combined with appropriate clinical trials will hopefully lead to prevention or amelioration of the effects of BPD in the future. It is important that all interventions are tested in adequately sized trials with long-term pulmonary and neurodevelopmental follow-up.

References

1. Northway WH, Rosan RC, Porter DY. Pulmonary disease following respirator therapy of hyaline-membrane disease. Bronchopulmonary dysplasia. N Engl J Med 1967; 276:357–368.
2. Sweet DG, Halliday HL. Modeling and remodeling of the lung in neonatal chronic lung disease: implications for therapy. Treat Respir Med 2005; 4:347–359.
3. Halliday HL, O'Neill CP. What is the evidence for drug therapy in the prevention and management of bronchopulmonary dysplasia? In: Bancalari E, ed. The Newborn Lung: Neonatology Questions and Controversies. Philadelphia: Saunders Elsevier, 2008.
4. Goldenberg RL, Hauth JC, Andrews WW, et al. Intrauterine infection and preterm delivery. N Engl J Med 2000; 342:1500–1507.
5. Yoon BH, Jun JK, Romero R, et al. Amniotic fluid inflammatory cytokines (interleukin-6, interleukin-1beta, and tumor necrosis factor-alpha), neonatal brain white matter lesions, and cerebral palsy. Am J Obstet Gynecol 1997; 177:19–26.

6. Schmidt B, Cao L, Mackensen-Haen S, et al. Chorioamnionitis and inflammation of the fetal lung. Am J Obstet Gynecol 2001; 185:173–177.

7. Curley AE, Sweet DG, Thornton CM, et al. Chorioamnionitis and increased neonatal lung lavage fluid matrix metalloproteinase-9 levels: implications for antenatal origins of chronic lung disease. Am J Obstet Gynecol 2003; 188:871–875.

8. Jobe AH. The new BPD: an arrest of lung development. Pediatr Res 1999; 46:641–643.

9. Coalson JJ. Pathology of new bronchopulmonary dysplasia. Semin Neonatol 2003; 8:73–81.

10. Alexander GR, Weiss J, Hulsey TC, et al. Preterm birth prevention: an evaluation of programs in the United States. Birth 1991; 18:160–169.

11. Goldenberg RL, Rouse DJ. Prevention of premature birth. N Engl J Med 1998; 339:313–320.

12. Dodd JM, Crowther CA, Cincotta R, et al. Progesterone supplementation for preventing preterm birth: a systematic review and meta-analysis. Acta Obstet Gynecol Scand 2005; 84:526–533.

13. Dodd JM, Flenady V, Cincotta R, et al. Prenatal administration of progesterone for preventing preterm birth. Cochrane Database Syst Rev 2006; (1):CD004947.

14. Smaill F, Vazquez JC. Antibiotics for asymptomatic bacteriuria in pregnancy. Cochrane Database Syst Rev 2007; (2):CD000490.

15. McDonald H, Brocklehurst P, Gordon A. Antibiotics for treating bacterial vaginosis in pregnancy. Cochrane Database Syst Rev 2007; (1):CD000262.

16. Kenyon S, Boulvain M, Neilson J. Antibiotics for preterm rupture of membranes. Cochrane Database Syst Rev 2003; (4):CD001058.

17. Ballard PL, Ning Y, Polk D, et al. Glucocorticoid regulation of surfactant components in immature lambs. Am J Physiol 1997; 273:1048–1057.

18. Keeney SE, Mathews MJ, Rassin DK, et al. Antioxidant enzyme responses to hyperoxia in preterm and term rats after prenatal dexamethasone administration. Pediatr Res 1993; 33:177–180.

19. Asoh K, Kumai T, Murano K, et al. Effect of antenatal dexamethasone treatment on Ca^{2+}-dependent nitric oxide synthase activity in rat lung. Pediatr Res 2000; 48:91–95.

20. Willet KE, Jobe AH, Ikegami M, et al. Lung morphometry after repetitive antenatal glucocorticoid treatment in preterm sheep. Am J Respir Crit Care Med 2001; 163:1437–1443.

21. Roberts D, Dalziel S. Antenatal corticosteroids for accelerating fetal lung maturation for women at risk of preterm birth. Cochrane Database Syst Rev 2006; (3):CD000065.

22. Crowley P. Prophylactic corticosteroids for preterm birth. Cochrane Database Syst Rev 2000; (2):CD000065.

23. Banks BA, Macones G, Cnaan A, et al. Multiple courses of antenatal corticosteroids are associated with early severe lung disease in preterm neonates. J Perinatol 2002; 22:101–107.

24. Willet KE, Jobe AH, Ikegami M, et al. Pulmonary interstitial emphysema 24 hours after antenatal betamethasone treatment in preterm sheep. Am J Respir Crit Care Med 2000; 162:1087–1094.

25. Crowther CA, Harding J. Repeat doses of prenatal corticosteroids for women at risk of preterm birth for preventing neonatal respiratory disease. Cochrane Database Syst Rev 2007; (3):CD003935.

26. National Institutes of Health Consensus Development Panel. Antenatal corticosteroids revisited: repeat courses—National Institutes of Health Consensus Development Conference Statement. Obstet Gynecol 2001; 98:144–150.

27. Ballard PL. Hormones and lung maturation. Monogr Endocrinol 1986; 28:1–354.

28. Ballard PL, Ballard RA, Ning Y, et al. Plasma thyroid hormones in premature infants: effect of gestational age and antenatal thyrotropin-releasing hormone treatment. TRH Collaborative Trial Participants. Pediatr Res 1998; 44:642–649.

29. Knight DB, Liggins GC, Wealthall SR, et al. A randomized, controlled trial of antepartum thyrotropin-releasing hormone and betamethasone in the prevention of respiratory disease in preterm infants. Am J Obstet Gynecol 1994; 171:11–16.

30. Anonymous. Australian collaborative trial of antenatal thyrotropin-releasing hormone (ACTOBAT) for prevention of neonatal respiratory disease. Lancet 1995; 345:877–882.

31. Ballard RA, Ballard PL, Cnaan A, et al. Antenatal thyrotropin-releasing hormone to prevent lung disease in preterm infants. North American Thyrotropin-Releasing Hormone Study Group. N Engl J Med 1998; 338:493–498.

32. Crowther CA, Hiller JE, Haslam RR, et al. Australian Collaborative Trial of Antenatal Thyrotropin-Releasing Hormone: adverse effects at 12-month follow-up. ACTOBAT Study Group. Pediatrics 1997; 99:311–317.

33. Crowther CA, Alfirevic Z, Haslam RR. Thyrotropin-releasing hormone added to corticosteroids for women at risk of preterm birth for preventing neonatal respiratory disease. Cochrane Database Syst Rev 2004; (2):CD000019.

34. Rojas MA, Gonzalez A, Bancalari E, et al. Changing trends in the epidemiology and pathogenesis of neonatal chronic lung disease. J Pediatr 1995; 126:605–610.

35. Stevens TP, Blennow M, Soll RF. Early surfactant administration with brief ventilation vs selective surfactant and continued mechanical ventilation for preterm infants with or at risk for respiratory distress syndrome. Cochrane Database Syst Rev 2004; (3):CD003063.

36. Soll RF, Blanco F. Natural surfactant extract versus synthetic surfactant for neonatal respiratory distress syndrome. Cochrane Database Syst Rev 2001; (2):CD000144.

37. Soll RF. Multiple versus single dose natural surfactant extract for severe neonatal respiratory distress syndrome. Cochrane Database Syst Rev 2000; (2):CD000141.

38. Soll RF. Prophylactic natural surfactant extract for preventing morbidity and mortality in preterm infants. Cochrane Database Syst Rev 2000; (2):CD000511.

39. Soll RF. Prophylactic synthetic surfactant for preventing morbidity and mortality in preterm infants. Cochrane Database Syst Rev 2000; (2):CD001079.

40. Soll RF, Morley CJ. Prophylactic versus selective use of surfactant in preventing morbidity and mortality in preterm infants. Cochrane Database Syst Rev 2001; (2):CD000510.

41. Soll RF. Synthetic surfactant for respiratory distress syndrome in preterm infants. Cochrane Database Syst Rev 2000; (2):CD001149.

42. Hallman M, Jarvenpaa AL, Pohjavuori M, et al. Respiratory distress syndrome and inositol supplementation in preterm infants. Arch Dis Child 1986; 61:1076–1083.

43. Hallman M, Bry K, Hoppu K, et al. Inositol supplementation in premature infants with respiratory distress syndrome. N Engl J Med 1992; 326:1233–1239.

44. Friedman CA, McVey J, Borne MJ, et al. Relationship between serum inositol concentration and development of retinopathy of prematurity: a prospective study. J Pediatr Ophthalmol Strabismus 2000; 37:79–86.

45. Howlett A, Ohlsson A. Inositol for respiratory distress syndrome in preterm infants. Cochrane Database Syst Rev 2003; (4):CD000366.

46. Mammel MC, Green TP, Johnson DE, et al. Controlled trial of dexamethasone therapy in infants with bronchopulmonary dysplasia. Lancet 1983; 1:1356–1358.

47. Avery GB, Fletcher AB, Kaplan M, et al. Controlled trial of dexamethasone in respirator-dependent infants with bronchopulmonary dysplasia. Pediatrics 1985; 75:106–111.

48. Cummings JJ, D'Eugenio DB, Gross SJ, et al. A controlled trial of dexamethasone in preterm infants at high risk for bronchopulmonary dysplasia. N Engl J Med 1989; 320:1505–1510.

49. Yeh TF, Lin YJ, Huang CC, et al. Early dexamethasone therapy in preterm infants: a follow-up study. Pediatrics 1998; 101:E7.

50. O'Shea TM, Kothadia JM, Klinepeter KL, et al. Randomized placebo-controlled trial of a 42-day tapering course of dexamethasone to reduce the duration of ventilator dependency in very low birth weight infants: outcome of study participants at 1-year adjusted age. Pediatrics 1999; 104:15–21.

51. Shinwell ES, Karplus M, Reich D, et al. Early postnatal dexamethasone treatment and increased incidence of cerebral palsy. Arch Dis Child Fetal Neonatal Ed 2000; 83:F177–F181.

52. Halliday HL. Guidelines on neonatal steroids. Prenat Neonatal Med 2001; 6:371–373.
53. American Academy of Pediatrics, Committee on Fetus and Newborn, and Canadian Paediatric Society, Fetus and Newborn Committee. Postnatal corticosteroids to treat or prevent chronic lung disease in preterm infants. Pediatrics 2002; 109:330–338.
54. Halliday HL, Ehrenkranz RA, Doyle LW. Early postnatal (<96 hours) corticosteroids for preventing chronic lung disease in preterm infants. Cochrane Database Syst Rev 2003; (1): CD001146.
55. Halliday HL, Ehrenkranz RA, Doyle LW. Moderately early (7–14 days) postnatal corticosteroids for preventing chronic lung disease in preterm infants. Cochrane Database Syst Rev 2003; (1):CD001144.
56. Halliday HL, Ehrenkranz RA, Doyle LW. Delayed (>3 weeks) postnatal corticosteroids for chronic lung disease in preterm infants. Cochrane Database Syst Rev 2003; (1):CD001145.
57. Baden M, Bauer CR, Colle E, et al. A controlled trial of hydrocortisone therapy in infants with respiratory distress syndrome. Pediatrics 1972; 50:526–534.
58. Taeusch HW Jr., Wang NS, Baden M, et al. A controlled trial of hydrocortisone therapy in infants with respiratory distress syndrome: II. Pathology. Pediatrics 1973; 52:850–854.
59. Fitzhardinge PM, Eisen A, Lejtenyi C, et al. Sequelae of early steroid administration to the newborn infant. Pediatrics 1974; 53:877–883.
60. Watterberg K. Anti-inflammatory therapy in the neonatal intensive care unit: present and future. Semin Fetal Neonatal Med 2006; 11:378–384.
61. Groneck P, Reuss D, Gotze-Speer B, et al. Effects of dexamethasone on chemotactic activity and inflammatory mediators in tracheobronchial aspirates of preterm infants at risk for chronic lung disease. J Pediatr 1993; 122:938–944.
62. Zimmerman JJ, Gabbert D, Shivpuri C, et al. Meter-dosed, inhaled beclomethasone attenuates bronchoalveolar oxyradical inflammation in premature infants at risk for bronchopulmonary dysplasia. Am J Perinatol 1998; 15:567–576.
63. Merz U, Kusenbach G, Hausler M, et al. Inhaled budesonide in ventilator-dependent preterm infants: a randomized, double-blind pilot study. Biol Neonate 1999; 75:46–53.
64. Konig P, Shatley M, Levine C, et al. Clinical observations of nebulized flunisolide in infants and young children with asthma and bronchopulmonary dysplasia. Pediatr Pulmonol 1992; 13:209–214.
65. Dugas MA, Nguyen D, Frenette L, et al. Fluticasone inhalation in moderate cases of bronchopulmonary dysplasia. Pediatrics 2005; 115:e566–e572.
66. Shah V, Ohlsson A, Halliday HL, et al. Early administration of inhaled corticosteroids for preventing chronic lung disease in ventilated very low birth weight preterm neonates (review). Cochrane Database Syst Rev 2007; (4):CD001969.
67. Grier DG, Halliday HL. Management of bronchopulmonary dysplasia in infants: guidelines for corticosteroid use. Drugs 2005; 65:15–29.
68. Viscardi RM, Hasday JD, Gumpper KF, et al. Cromolyn sodium prophylaxis inhibits pulmonary proinflammatory cytokines in infants at high risk for bronchopulmonary dysplasia. Am J Respir Crit Care Med 1997; 156:1523–1529.
69. Denjean A, Paris-Llado J, Zupan V, et al. Inhaled salbutamol and beclomethasone for preventing broncho-pulmonary dysplasia: a randomised double-blind study. Eur J Pediatr 1998; 157:926–931.
70. Ng GY, da Silva O, Ohlsson A. Bronchodilators for the prevention and treatment of chronic lung disease in preterm infants. Cochrane Database Syst Rev 2001:CD003214.
71. Cooke L, Steer P, Woodgate P. Indomethacin for asymptomatic patent ductus arteriosus in preterm infants. Cochrane Database Syst Rev 2003; (2):CD003745.
72. Clyman RI. Recommendations for the postnatal use of indomethacin: an analysis of four separate treatment strategies. J Pediatr 1996; 128:601–607.

73. Shah SS, Ohlsson A. Ibuprofen for the prevention of patent ductus arteriosus in preterm and/or low birth weight infants. Cochrane Database Syst Rev 2006; (1):CD004213.
74. Ohlsson A, Walia R, Shah S. Ibuprofen for the treatment of patent ductus arteriosus in preterm and/or low birth weight infants. Cochrane Database Syst Rev 2005; (4):CD003481.
75. Schmidt B, Roberts RS, Davis P, et al. Caffeine therapy for apnea of prematurity. N Engl J Med 2006; 354:2112–2121.
76. Davis JM, Bhutani VK, Stefano JL, et al. Changes in pulmonary mechanics following caffeine administration in infants with bronchopulmonary dysplasia. Pediatr Pulmonol 1989; 6:49–52.
77. Lapenna D, De Gioia S, Mezzetti A, et al. Aminophylline: could it act as an antioxidant in vivo? Eur J Clin Invest 1995; 25:464–470.
78. Schmidt B, Roberts R, Millar D, et al. Evidence-based neonatal drug therapy for prevention of bronchopulmonary dysplasia in very-low-birth-weight infants. Neonatology 2008; 93:284–287.
79. Lyon A. Chronic lung disease of prematurity. The role of intra-uterine infection. Eur J Pediatr 2000; 159:798–802.
80. Wang EE, Ohlsson A, Kellner JD, et al. Association of Ureaplasma urealyticum colonization with chronic lung disease of prematurity: results of a meta-analysis. J Pediatr 1995; 127:640–644.
81. Iles R, Lyon A, Ross P, et al. Infection with Ureaplasma urealyticum and Mycoplasma hominis and the development of chronic lung disease in preterm infants. Acta Paediatr 1996; 85:482–484.
82. Baier RJ, Loggins J, Kruger TE, et al. Failure of erythromycin to eliminate airway colonization with Ureaplasma urealyticum in very low birth weight infants. BMC Pediatrics 2003; 3:10.
83. Collard KJ, Godeck S, Holley JE, et al. Pulmonary antioxidant concentrations and oxidative damage in ventilated premature babies. Arch Dis Child Fetal Neonatal Ed 2004; 89:F412–F416.
84. Darlow BA, Graham PJ. Vitamin A supplementation for preventing morbidity and mortality in very low birthweight infants. Cochrane Database Syst Rev 2007(4):CD000501.
85. Watts JL, Milner R, Zipursky A, et al. Failure of supplementation with vitamin E to prevent bronchopulmonary dysplasia in infants less than 1,500 g birth weight. Eur Respir J 1991; 4:188–190.
86. Davis JM. Superoxide dismutase: a role in the prevention of chronic lung disease. Biol Neonate 1998; 74:29–34.
87. Kao SJ, Wang D, Lin HI, et al. N-acetylcysteine abrogates acute lung injury induced by endotoxin. Clin Exp Pharmacol Physiol 2006; 33:33–40.
88. Russell GA, Cooke RW. Randomised controlled trial of allopurinol prophylaxis in very preterm infants. Arch Dis Child Fetal Neonatal Ed 1995; 73:F27–F31.
89. Tyson JE, Wright LL, Oh W, et al. Vitamin A supplementation for extremely-low-birth-weight infants. National Institute of Child Health and Human Development Neonatal Research Network. N Engl J Med 1999; 340:1962–1968.
90. Ross SA, McCaffery PJ, Drager UC, et al. Retinoids in embryonal development. Physiol Rev 2000; 80:1021–1054.
91. Massaro GD, Massaro D. Postnatal treatment with retinoic acid increases the number of pulmonary alveoli in rats. Am J Physiol 1996; 270:305–310.
92. Nakamura T, Ogawa Y. Prophylactic effects of recombinant human superoxide dismutase in neonatal lung injury induced by the intratracheal instillation of endotoxin in piglets. Biol Neonate 2001; 80:163–168.
93. Davis JM, Rosenfeld W, Richter SE, et al. Safety and pharmacokinetics of multiple doses of recombinant human CuZn superoxide dismutase administered intratracheally to premature neonates with respiratory distress syndrome. Pediatrics 1997; 100:24–30.

94. Davis JM, Parad RB, Michele T, et al. Pulmonary outcome at 1 year corrected age in premature infants treated at birth with recombinant human CuZn superoxide dismutase. Pediatrics 2003; 111:469–476.

95. Sandberg K, Fellman V, Stigson L, et al. N-acetylcysteine administration during the first week of life does not improve lung function in extremely low birth weight infants. Biol Neonate 2004; 86:275–279.

96. Ahola T, Lapatto R, Raivio KO, et al. N-acetylcysteine does not prevent bronchopulmonary dysplasia in immature infants: a randomized controlled trial. J Pediatr 2003; 143:713–719.

97. Chang LY, Subramaniam M, Yoder BA, et al. A catalytic antioxidant attenuates alveolar structural remodeling in bronchopulmonary dysplasia. Am J Respir Crit Care Med 2003; 167:57–64.

98. Jankov RP, Negus A, Tanswell AK. Antioxidants as therapy in the newborn: some words of caution. Pediatr Res 2001; 50:681–687.

99. Merritt TA, Cochrane CG, Holcomb K, et al. Elastase and alpha 1-proteinase inhibitor activity in tracheal aspirates during respiratory distress syndrome. Role of inflammation in the pathogenesis of bronchopulmonary dysplasia. J Clin Invest 1983; 72:656–666.

100. Stiskal JA, Dunn MS, Shennan AT, et al. Alpha1-proteinase inhibitor therapy for the prevention of chronic lung disease of prematurity: a randomized, controlled trial. Pediatrics 1998; 101:89–94.

101. Sveger T, Ohlsson K, Polberger S, et al. Tracheobronchial aspirate fluid neutrophil lipocalin, elastase- and neutrophil protease-4-alpha1-antitrypsin complexes, protease inhibitors and free proteolytic activity in respiratory distress syndrome. Acta Paediatr 2002; 91:934–937.

102. Barrington KJ, Finer NN. Inhaled nitric oxide for respiratory failure in preterm infants. Cochrane Database Syst Rev 2006; (1):CD000509.

103. Kinsella JP, Parker TA, Galan H, et al. Effects of inhaled nitric oxide on pulmonary edema and lung neutrophil accumulation in severe experimental hyaline membrane disease. Pediatr Res 1997; 41:457–463.

104. Roberts JD Jr., Chiche JD, Weimann J, et al. Nitric oxide inhalation decreases pulmonary artery remodeling in the injured lungs of rat pups. Circ Res 2000; 87:140–145.

105. Wang T, El Kebir D, Blaise G, et al. Inhaled nitric oxide in 2003: a review of its mechanisms of action. Can J Anaesth 2003; 50:839–846.

106. Hamon I, Fresson J, Nicolas MB, et al. Early inhaled nitric oxide improves oxidative balance in very preterm infants. Pediatr Res 2005; 57:637–643.

107. Kinsella JP, Walsh WF, Bose CL, et al. Inhaled nitric oxide in premature neonates with severe hypoxaemic respiratory failure: a randomised controlled trial. Lancet 1999; 354:1061–1065.

108. Anonymous. Early compared with delayed inhaled nitric oxide in moderately hypoxaemic neonates with respiratory failure: a randomised controlled trial. The Franco-Belgium Collaborative NO Trial Group. Lancet 1999; 354:1066–1071.

109. Subhedar NV, Ryan SW, Shaw NJ, et al. Open randomised controlled trial of inhaled nitric oxide and early dexamethasone in high risk preterm infants. Arch Dis Child Fetal Neonatal Ed 1997; 77:F185–F190.

110. Schreiber MD, Gin-Mestan K, Marks JD, et al. Inhaled nitric oxide in premature infants with the respiratory distress syndrome. N Engl J Med 2003; 349:2099–2107.

111. Hogman M, Frostell C, Arnberg H, et al. Bleeding time prolongation and NO inhalation. Lancet 1993; 341:1664–1665.

112. Hallman M, Waffarn F, Bry K, et al. Surfactant dysfunction after inhalation of nitric oxide. J Appl Physiol 1996; 80:2026–2034.

113. Robbins CG, Davis JM, Merritt TA, et al. Combined effects of nitric oxide and hyperoxia on surfactant function and pulmonary inflammation. Am J Physiol 1995; 269:545–550.

114. Mestan KK, Marks JD, Hecox K, et al. Neurodevelopmental outcomes of premature infants treated with inhaled nitric oxide. N Engl J Med 2005; 353:23–32.

115. Van Meurs KP, Wright LL, Ehrenkranz RA, et al. Inhaled nitric oxide for premature infants with severe respiratory failure. N Engl J Med 2005; 353:13–22.

116. Field D, Elbourne D, Truesdale A, et al. Neonatal ventilation with inhaled nitric oxide versus ventilatory support without inhaled nitric oxide for preterm infants with severe respiratory failure: the INNOVO multicentre randomised controlled trial (ISRCTN 17821339). Pediatrics 2005; 115:926–936.

117. Hoehn T, Krause MF, Buhrer C, et al. Meta-analysis of inhaled nitric oxide in premature infants: an update. Klin Padiatr 2006; 218:57–61.

118. Kinsella JP, Cutter GR, Walsh WF, et al. Early inhaled nitric oxide therapy in premature newborns with respiratory failure. N Engl J Med 2006; 355:354–364.

119. Ballard RA, Truog WE, Cnaan A, et al. Inhaled nitric oxide in preterm infants undergoing mechanical ventilation. N Engl J Med 2006; 355:343–353.

120. Subhedar N, Dewhurst C. Is nitric oxide effective in preterm infants? Arch Dis Child Fetal Neonatal Ed 2007; 92:F337–F341.

121. Jobe AH, Newnham JP, Willet KE, et al. Effects of antenatal endotoxin and glucocorticoids on the lungs of preterm lambs. Am J Obstet Gynecol 2000; 182:401–408.

122. Jobe AH, Newnham JP, Willet KE, et al. Endotoxin-induced lung maturation in preterm lambs is not mediated by cortisol. Am J Respir Crit Care Med 2000; 162:1656–1661.

123. Moss TJ, Nitsos I, Kramer BW, et al. Intra-amniotic endotoxin induces lung maturation by direct effects on the developing respiratory tract in preterm sheep. Am J Obstet Gynecol 2002; 187:1059–1065.

124. Vozzelll MA, Mason SN, Whorton MH, et al. Antimacrophage chemokine treatment prevents neutrophil and macrophage influx in hyperoxia-exposed newborn rat lung. Am J Physiol Lung Cell Mol Physiol 2004; 286:488–493.

125. Chiba H, Piboonpocanun S, Mitsuzawa H, et al. Pulmonary surfactant proteins and lipids as modulators of inflammation and innate immunity. Respirology 2006; 11:S2–S6.

126. Levine CR, Gewolb IH, Allen K, et al. The safety, pharmacokinetics, and anti-inflammatory effects of intratracheal recombinant human Clara cell protein in premature infants with respiratory distress syndrome. Pediatr Res 2005; 58:15–21.

127. Kraybill EN, Runyan DK, Bose CL, et al. Risk factors for chronic lung disease in infants with birth weights of 751 to 1000 grams. J Pediatr 1989; 115:115–120.

128. Buss IH, Darlow BA, Winterbourn CC, et al. Elevated protein carbonyls and lipid peroxidation products correlating with myeloperoxidase in tracheal aspirates from premature infants. Pediatr Res 2000; 47:640–645.

129. Schock BC, Sweet DG, Halliday HL, et al. Oxidative stress in lavage fluid of preterm infants at risk of chronic lung disease. Am J Physiol Lung Cell Mol Physiol 2001; 281: L1386–L1391.

130. Anonymous. Supplemental therapeutic oxygen for prethreshold retinopathy of prematurity (STOP-ROP), a randomized, controlled trial. I: primary outcomes. Pediatrics 2000; 105:295–310.

131. Cole CH, Wright KW, Tarnow-Mordi W, et al. Resolving our uncertainty about oxygen therapy. Pediatrics 2003; 112:1415–1419.

132. Gonzalez A, Sosenko IR, Chandar J, et al. Influence of infection on patent ductus arteriosus and chronic lung disease in premature infants weighing 1000 grams or less. J Pediatr 1996; 128:470–478.

133. Jonsson B, Rylander M, Faxelius G, et al. Ureaplasma urealyticum, erythromycin and respiratory morbidity in high-risk preterm neonates. Acta Paediatr 1998; 87:1079–1084.

134. Van Marter LJ, Leviton A, Allred EN, et al. Hydration during the first days of life and the risk of bronchopulmonary dysplasia in low birth weight infants. J Pediatr 1990; 116:942–949.

135.   Frank L. Antioxidants, nutrition, and bronchopulmonary dysplasia. Clin Perinatol 1992; 19:541–562.
136.   Blanco LN, Frank L. The formation of alveoli in rat lung during the third and fourth postnatal weeks: effect of hyperoxia, dexamethasone, and deferoxamine. Pediatr Res 1993; 34:334–340.
137.   Schwyter M, Burri PH, Tschanz SA, et al. Geometric properties of the lung parenchyma after postnatal glucocorticoid treatment in rats. Biol Neonate 2003; 83:57–64. Erratum in: Biol Neonate 2003; 84:141.
138.   Lister P, Iles R, Shaw B. Inhaled steroids for neonatal chronic lung disease. Cochrane Database Syst Rev 2000(3):CD002311.
139.   Shah SS, Ohlsson A, Halliday H, et al. Inhaled versus systemic corticosteroids for the treatment of chronic lung disease in ventilated very low birth weight preterm infants. Cochrane Database Syst Rev 2003; (2):CD002057.
140.   Shah SS, Ohlsson A, Halliday H, et al. Inhaled versus systemic corticosteroids for preventing chronic lung disease in ventilated very low birth weight preterm neonates. Cochrane Database Syst Rev 2003; (1):CD002058.
141.   Cole CH. Inhaled glucocorticoid therapy in infants at risk for neonatal chronic lung disease. J Asthma 2000; 37:533–543.
142.   Brion LP, Primhak RA. Intravenous or enteral loop diuretics for preterm infants with (or developing) chronic lung disease. Cochrane Database Syst Rev 2002; (1):CD001453.
143.   Brion LP, Primhak RA, Ambrosio-Perez I. Diuretics acting on the distal renal tubule for preterm infants with (or developing) chronic lung disease. Cochrane Database Syst Rev 2002; (1):CD001817.
144.   McCann EM, Lewis K, Deming DD, et al. Controlled trial of furosemide therapy in infants with chronic lung disease. J Pediatr 1985; 106:957–962.
145.   Brion LP, Primhak RA, Yong W. Aerosolized diuretics for preterm infants with (or developing) chronic lung disease. Cochrane Database Syst Rev 2001; (2):CD001694.
146.   Engelhardt B, Blalock WA, Donlevy S, et al. Effect of spironolactone-hydrochlorothiazide on lung function in infants with chronic bronchopulmonary dysplasia. J Pediatr 1989; 114:619–624.
147.   Kao LC, Warburton D, Cheng MH, et al. Effect of oral diuretics on pulmonary mechanics in infants with chronic bronchopulmonary dysplasia: results of a double-blind crossover sequential trial. Pediatrics 1984; 74:37–44.
148.   Kao LC, Durand DJ, McCrea RC, et al. Randomized trial of long-term diuretic therapy for infants with oxygen-dependent bronchopulmonary dysplasia. J Pediatr 1994; 124:772–781.
149.   Kao LC, Durand DJ, Phillips BL, et al. Oral theophylline and diuretics improve pulmonary mechanics in infants with bronchopulmonary dysplasia. J Pediatr 1987; 111:439–444.
150.   Davis JM, Sinkin RA, Aranda JV, et al. Drug therapy for bronchopulmonary dysplasia. Pediatr Pulmonol 1990; 8:117–125.
151.   Farrell PA, Fiascone JM. Bronchopulmonary dysplasia in the 1990s: a review for the pediatrician. Curr Probl Pediatr 1997; 27:129–163.
152.   Thomas W, Speer CP. Management of infants with bronchopulmonary dysplasia in Germany. Early Hum Dev 2005; 81:155–163.
153.   Sosulski R, Abbasi S, Bhutani VK, et al. Physiologic effects of terbutaline on pulmonary function of infants with bronchopulmonary dysplasia. Pediatr Pulmonol 1986; 2:269–273.
154.   Wilkie RA, Bryan MH. Effect of bronchodilators on airway resistance in ventilator-dependent neonates with chronic lung disease. J Pediatr 1987; 111:278–282.
155.   D'Angio CT, Maniscalco WM. Bronchopulmonary dysplasia in preterm infants: pathophysiology and management strategies. Pediatr Drugs 2004; 6:303–330.
156.   Allen J, Zwerdling R, Ehrenkranz R, et al. Statement on the care of the child with chronic lung disease of infancy and childhood. Am J Respir Crit Care Med 2003; 168:356–396.

157. Henderson-Smart DJ, Davis PG. Prophylactic methylxanthines for extubation in preterm infants. Cochrane Database Syst Rev 2003; (1):CD000139.
158. Schmidt B, Roberts RS, Davis P, et al. Long-term effects of caffeine therapy for apnea of prematurity. N Engl J Med 2007; 357:1893–1902.
159. Reiter PD, Townsend SF, Velasquez R, et al. Dornase alfa in premature infants with severe respiratory distress and early bronchopulmonary dysplasia. J Perinatol 2000; 20:530–534.
160. Wang EE, Tang NK. Immunoglobulin for preventing respiratory syncytial virus infection. Cochrane Database Syst Rev 2000; (2):CD001725.
161. American Academy of Pediatrics Committee on Infectious Diseases and Committee on Fetus and Newborn. Revised indications for the use of palivizumab and respiratory syncytial virus immune globulin intravenous for the prevention of respiratory syncytial virus infections. Pediatrics 2003; 112:1442–1446.
162. Ladha F, Bonnet S, Eaton F, et al. Sildenafil improves alveolar growth and pulmonary hypertension in hyperoxia-induced lung injury. Am J Respir Crit Care Med 2005; 172:750–756.
163. Lauterbach R, Szymura-Oleksiak J. Nebulized pentoxifylline in successful treatment of five premature neonates with bronchopulmonary dysplasia. Eur J Pediatr 1999; 158:607.
164. Lauterbach R, Pawlik D, Zembala M, et al. Pentoxyfylline in and prevention and treatment of chronic lung disease. Acta Paediatr Suppl 2004; 93:20–22.
165. Thomas W, Speer CP. Nonventilatory strategies for prevention and treatment of bronchopulmonary dysplasia—what is the evidence? Neonatology 2008; 94:150–159.
166. Geary C, Caskey M, Fonesca R, et al. Decreased incidence of bronchopulmonary dysplasia after early management changes, including surfactant and nasal continuous positive airway pressure treatment at delivery, lowered oxygen saturation goals, and early amino acid administration: a historical cohort study. Pediatrics 2008; 121:89–96.

21
Lung Function Abnormalities in Infants and Children with Bronchopulmonary Dysplasia

MARCO FILIPPONE and EUGENIO BARALDI
University of Padua, School of Medicine, Padua, Italy

I. Introduction

A considerable scientific effort has been produced in the last few decades to expand our knowledge in the field of lung function in newborns and infants delivered prematurely, with and without bronchopulmonary dysplasia (BPD). Despite a strong research commitment and the production of large amounts of data, considerable uncertainty still surrounds a number of aspects of lung development after premature birth, and ongoing research continues to seek answers to several unsolved questions (1).

Interest in pulmonary health after premature birth has recently been fueled by emerging evidence that unfavorable effects on pulmonary development and lung injuries sustained in infancy and early childhood may affect respiratory health for life (2). Even small reductions in lung function early on may have significant long-term consequences, so survivors of prematurity should be considered at risk of long-term respiratory problems later in their lives (3). A new chronic obstructive pulmonary disease (COPD)-like phenotype is probably destined to emerge over the next few years, having its origins in neonatal intensive care units or even before birth (3,4). Adult physicians will presumably have to contend more and more often with this problem, since premature infants who would once have died are now increasingly surviving into adulthood.

When BPD was first described, the technical equipment needed to assess pulmonary function in uncooperative children was not yet readily available, and that is why BPD was initially described simply as a clinical and pathological entity (5), without any functional correlates. It soon became apparent, however, that objective lung function measurements were needed in BPD infants to assess the extent and severity of their pulmonary disease, to follow up its natural course, and to evaluate the effects of any preventive or therapeutic measures, as is routinely done in older children with asthma or other chronic pulmonary diseases. Innovative approaches to assessing pulmonary function in newborns, infants, and young children have progressively been developed and applied to both term and premature infants, in healthy or diseased. With time, these pulmonary function–testing methods have helped to significantly improve our understanding of the respiratory consequences of prematurity (1).

However, interpreting data on pulmonary function in premature infants is not always easy. The continuous epidemiological evolution of prematurity and the evolving principles of neonatal care have considerably changed the characteristics, and even the very nature, of pulmonary disease following premature delivery. Problems concerning the definition of BPD and the lack of homogeneity of the populations considered make it tough to compare the findings of different studies. In addition, inconsistencies in theoretical approach and technical weaknesses inherent in the various study methods adopted cast doubts on the reliability of the data and influence their interpretation (6).

This chapter briefly reviews the main techniques currently available for assessing lung function and summarizes the most important information available to date on pulmonary function in preterm infants and children with and without BPD.

II. Static Lung Volumes—Functional Residual Capacity

The only static lung volume readily measurable in infants and young children is functional residual capacity (FRC), that is, the resting lung volume at the end of expiration. FRC is highly relevant in physiological terms because it is crucial to gas exchange. It is an important indicator of lung development and growth and enables a normalized interpretation of volume-dependent lung function parameters (i.e., compliance, resistance, forced expiratory flows, and gas-mixing efficiency indices) (7).

A. Technical Aspects

FRC is currently measured by two different methods, that is, whole-body plethysmography (FRC_{pleth}) and gas dilution/washout techniques (FRC_{gas}) (7).

Whole-body plethysmography involves placing infants in an airtight, inextensible container and occluding their airway opening (connected to a flowmeter) with a shutter to keep the lung at a constant volume, despite the infant's respiratory efforts. According to Boyle's law, FRC_{pleth} is calculated by correlating the changes in the alveolar pressure during the occlusion with the changes in alveolar volume (extrapolated from the changes in plethysmographic pressure). This is based on the assumption that a rapid pressure balancing occurs during airway occlusion, so alveolar pressure is accurately reflected by the airway opening pressure. This is not always the case, however, especially in infants with significant airway obstruction. Whole-body plethysmography is quick to perform, reproducible, and relatively noninvasive (though the infant usually has to be sedated), but the method is unsuitable for bedside use in tiny, sick infants. FRC_{pleth} [formerly referred to as thoracic gas volume (TGV)] measures the whole gas volume remaining in the lungs at the end of expiration, including the gas potentially trapped behind obstructed airways, thus enabling the detection of hyperinflation and air trapping.

Conversely, gas dilution/washout techniques only measure the end-expiratory gas volume in direct communication with the central airways during tidal breathing. FRC_{gas} values are consequently usually lower than FRC_{pleth} values, and it has been suggested that measuring both values in the same individual is a useful way to evaluate gas trapping (8–10). FRC_{gas} is measured from the concentration of an inert gas used as a tracer. In the *helium (He) dilution technique*, infants are connected, at the end of expiration, to a closed circuit containing a gas mixture with a known He concentration. Helium is then inhaled and a balance is gradually established between the circuit and the infant lung; FRC_{He} is calculated from the initial and final He concentrations in the system, providing the initial volume of the circuit is known and the total amount of He remains constant. In the *open-circuit washout method*, a tracer gas (e.g., nitrogen N_2, sulfur hexafluoride SF_6, or He) is inhaled until a preset concentration is reached in the lungs, then it is washed out by making the infant breathe a gas mixture that does not contain the tracer. Continuous measurements of tracer gas concentrations and airflow at the airway opening are needed to calculate the volume of tracer gas being washed out, and thus determine FRC_{gas}.

Gas dilution/washout methods are more time consuming than plethysmography but can usually be performed on unsedated infants. FRC_{gas} can even be measured in ventilated infants, though leaks around the uncuffed tracheal tubes used in newborns may interfere with gas balancing and therefore significantly affect the measurements. There is also the problem of an uneven gas distribution and subsequently difficult equilibration in subjects with significant bronchial obstruction.

B. FRC Studies in Premature Infants

A crucial pathophysiological component of respiratory distress syndrome (RDS) is lung volume loss. Infants with RDS are usually unable to expand their lungs normally at birth and maintain an adequate FRC later on. Surfactant deficiency is important in this context, but several adjunctive factors may contribute to further reducing lung volume, including excessive chest wall compliance and relative muscular weakness. Such factors may interfere with the maintenance of an effective FRC in preterm neonates without RDS too, who indeed often require some kind of respiratory support (e.g., CPAP), during the initial pulmonary adaptation at least. FRC is probably also "naturally" lower in very preterm neonates than in more mature infants, because of the primitive, simplified shape of their distal airspaces. FRC is therefore expected to change with gestational age (i.e., with progressive pulmonary maturation), but there are currently no studies establishing adequate reference data for different stages of maturity.

Most of the information available on FRC in neonatal age comes from studies in infants ventilated for RDS. As expected, these patients' FRC is lower than in reference cohorts of healthy, spontaneously breathing infants (11–14), but the data are difficult to interpret because different measuring conditions considerably influence results. Further evidence of infants with RDS having a reduced FRC comes from studies assessing the effects of surfactant treatment, which induces a rapid clinical response associated with a significant increase in FRC (15–19) before any improvement in respiratory system compliance. Surfactant treatment is thought to reduce the typical alveolar instability of RDS, facilitating the subsequent recruitment of newly aerated alveoli.

Ventilator settings can obviously affect FRC, as shown by studies assessing the impact of different positive end-expiratory pressure (PEEP) levels in infants with RDS or evolving toward BPD (20–23). Substantial technical improvements will be needed, however, before we can obtain clinically relevant lung volume measurements in newborns requiring respiratory support (including CPAP). FRC monitoring in such patients would represent a considerable advance, since an optimal level of lung inflation is considered fundamental to ensuring an adequate gas exchange with the least injury to the lung, whatever the ventilation method used.

In several studies, infants with established BPD still had lower FRC_{He} or FRC_{N2} values at near-term postmenstrual age by comparison with reference data (24) or healthy controls (25,26). When followed up for two to three years, low FRC values persisted during the first few months of life, but a progressive increase and final normalization were seen thereafter. This was interpreted as evidence of pulmonary recovery over time in subjects with BPD, with lung growth catching up during the first year of life, followed by a rise in FRC until it parallels that of normal controls by the age of three years (26). On the other hand, some studies found significant lung hyperinflation on measuring FRC_{pleth} in survivors of BPD. At a mean age of 15 months, FRC_{pleth} was reportedly significantly higher in survivors of BPD than in controls born at term (27). This finding was associated with airflow obstruction and was interpreted as an indicator of air trapping. Wauer et al. (8) recorded lung hyperinflation in infants with BPD as soon as near term; however, the infants with BPD revealing a higher FRC_{pleth} and lower FRC_{N2} than controls born at term. Such findings might indicate a relative excess volume of gas not communicating directly with the central airways, which again means air trapping.

It is not clear whether premature infants without BPD have abnormal lung volumes too. Some studies report no difference in lung volume between such infants and controls born at term (28). Preterm infants who never had respiratory symptoms, or who recovered from RDS, have likewise been shown to have higher FRC_{He} values than infants with BPD, at term equivalent (29). Conversely, Hjalmarson and Sandberg (30) found that "healthy" premature infants studied near term had a significantly lower FRC_{N2} than full-term controls; they also found pulmonary mechanics and gas mixing efficiency indices abnormal in preterm infants, suggesting that premature birth may in itself impair the development of the terminal respiratory units, even in infants experiencing no notable respiratory distress or given any form of respiratory support early in life. More recently, the same authors showed that lung function anomalies are qualitatively similar in preterm infants with no history of respiratory problems and in those with BPD (31), though infants with severe BPD had the lowest FRC and more severely disrupted gas mixing and pulmonary mechanics than those with mild or no BPD. Taken together, these data suggest that prematurity per se may induce significant developmental anomalies in the respiratory system, and that BPD simply represents the worst end of a wide spectrum of clinical and functional anomalies due to preterm birth (and intrauterine exposures relating or leading to premature delivery).

III. Respiratory System Mechanics

Respiratory mechanics are concerned with the interaction of resistive, elastic, and inertial forces during breathing, assessing the properties of all the components of the respiratory system (airways, lung tissues, and chest wall) in terms of changes in pressure, flow, and volume during the respiratory cycle. The most important indexes of respiratory mechanics are compliance (Δvolume/Δpressure) and resistance (Δpressure/Δflow), usually measured using dynamic and passive techniques, respectively during the breathing cycle or in the absence of any respiratory effort (32).

A. Technical Aspects

In earlier studies, dynamic lung mechanics were generally assessed by *esophageal manometry*. A catheter is used to measure esophageal pressure, which is assumed to reflect pleural pressure and used to calculate transpulmonary pressure from the difference between the esophageal and the airway opening pressures. Flow and volume are measured at the airway opening with a flowmeter. Significant inaccuracies may derive from incorrect esophageal catheter placement, since the manometer may sample only regional changes in pleural pressure, especially in premature or sick infants. More recently, this method has been largely replaced by less-invasive (passive) occlusion techniques. The single-breath occlusion technique (SOT) is based on measuring alveolar pressure as reflected by the airway opening pressure recorded during a brief airway occlusion at the end of inspiration. The flow-volume curve obtained during the exhalation following the occlusion is used to calculate compliance (C_{rs}), resistance (R_{rs}), and the time constant (T_{rs}) of the respiratory system. The plateau phase during the occlusion and the subsequent expiratory phase are assumed to be passive as a result of eliciting the Hering–Breuer inflation reflex, which makes respiratory muscles relax when the airways are occluded at volumes above FRC. Much the same theoretical principles apply to the multiple occlusion technique (MOT) in which the airway is occluded repeatedly at different volumes, enabling C_{rs} measurement.

SOT describes the respiratory system as a single-compartment model, which is inappropriate in most cases. This is particularly important in sick infants, whose increased respiratory drive and strong respiratory reflexes may interfere with proper pressure balancing or respiratory muscle relaxation, thus yielding inaccurate measurements. MOT probably has fewer theoretical drawbacks, but it does not enable R_{rs} or T_{rs} to be measured and it is used much less than SOT.

The occlusion techniques are unable to distinguish between the relative contributions of the airway and lung parenchyma to the respiratory system mechanics as a whole. Methods aiming to assess partitioned airway and tissue mechanics have recently been developed, for example, the interrupter technique and the low-frequency forced-oscillation technique. Though they have contributed little to our current knowledge, these are promised methods for future research (32). The low-frequency forced-oscillation technique, in particular, has potential for future applications in lung function monitoring already in the neonatal intensive care units, enabling an assessment of the effects of maturation or of different diseases and treatments in the developing lung.

B. Respiratory Mechanics Studies in Premature Infants

Data from prospective follow-up studies of respiratory mechanics show that infants with BPD have reduced compliance and increased resistance values early in their lives; significant recovery occurs over time with ongoing lung growth and development, leading to near-normal values of pulmonary mechanics at two to three years of age (24,26). The early respiratory mechanics derangement has been interpreted as the result of the morphological changes occurring in the classic form of BPD and related to interstitial edema, atelectasis, parenchymal scarring, airway fibrosis, epithelial metaplasia, and smooth muscle hypertrophy (33). However, altered compliance and resistance might in part derive from a disturbed pattern of lung development, acquired in the perinatal period due to prematurity and/or its causes. As discussed earlier, indeed, data collected in cohorts of premature infants without clinically significant respiratory disease suggest that reduced C_{rs} and increased R_{rs} may be associated with premature delivery irrespective of any neonatal respiratory symptoms or treatment received (30).

Accordingly, dynamic compliance and resistance showed comparable changes in very immature neonates (24–25 weeks of gestation) with and without RDS, studied longitudinally up to 35 postmenstrual weeks, suggesting that lung immaturity outweighs RDS in disrupting pulmonary function in these subjects (34).

The early changes in lung mechanics have been tested as potential predictors of long-term prognosis after premature birth (development of BPD, later oxygen dependence) by several authors (35–38). Results have been conflicting, however, and none of the parameters studied seems accurately predictive of subsequent respiratory health in these patients.

IV. Forced Expiratory Maneuvers

Several studies have suggested that survivors of BPD have significant airflow anomalies persisting through their early years of life, despite a progressive improvement in respiratory system mechanics. The documented gradual decrease in R_{rs} probably reflects the progressive structural and functional development of the large extrathoracic airways in these infants, but R_{rs} is a rather insensitive index of the smaller intrathoracic airways' functioning (39). Judging from pathological data obtained from infants who died of BPD, these more distal airways are among the most severely injured lung structures (40), so it is hardly surprising that they should also be a crucial point of airflow limitation in survivors of BPD.

A. Technical Aspects

Functional intrathoracic airway limitations in survivors of BPD have come to light since the introduction of methods for studying forced expiratory flow in uncooperative children. Although infants cannot be trained to perform forced expiratory maneuvers, from total lung capacity to residual volume, as in school-age children, their forced expiratory flow-volume loops can be obtained by substituting voluntary effort with a pressure applied externally to the airways or chest and abdomen to force exhalation (41). In the forced deflation technique (FD), the infant's lung is first inflated to total lung capacity, then rapidly deflated by applying a negative pressure of -40 cm H_2O to the airway opening to produce a maximal forced expiratory flow-volume loop. FD is accurate and reproducible, but its invasiveness makes it suitable only for intubated and deeply sedated subjects, and prevented its wide diffusion. The most commonly used method for measuring forced expiratory flow in premature infants is the rapid thoracoabdominal compression technique (RTC), whereby forced expiratory flow-volume curves are obtained by rapidly inflating a pneumatic jacket wrapped around the infant's chest and abdomen at the end of a tidal inspiration. Inflating the jacket brings an external positive pressure to bear on the chest and abdomen, forcing expiration through a face mask and a pneumotachograph. The thoracoabdominal pressure is stepped up until the maximal expiratory flow is generated (i.e., until flow limitation is achieved). The forced expiratory volume usually exceeds the tidal end-expiratory level, thus enabling flow detection at FRC level. The maximal expiratory flow at FRC (V_{maxFRC}) is the most commonly reported parameter using this technique and reflects the airways' functional status at low lung volumes. RTC produces only a "partial" flow-volume curve because expiration begins from the tidal end-inspiratory level, so the raised volume RTC technique (RVRTC) was developed to extend the volume range that can be studied: in RVRTC, the thoracoabdominal compression is preceded by a positive-pressure lung inflation maneuver (usually at 30 cm H_2O) to force expiration from a level closer to total lung capacity. Indices commonly measured by RVRTC are forced vital capacity (FVC), forced expiratory volume in 0.5 seconds ($FEV_{0.5}$), and the forced expiratory flows at different FVC levels, which are conceptually similar to the typical expiratory flow-volume curves obtained by spirometry in collaborating subjects.

B.   Forced Expiratory Flow Studies in Premature Infants

Data collected cross sectionally or longitudinally invariably show a lower V_{maxFRC} in subjects with BPD by comparison with normative values or control groups of healthy premature or term infants (24,25,42–48). Most such data relate to infants with BPD in their first year of life (25,42–45,47). The first study was published in 1986 by Tepper et al. (25), who studied a group of 20 infants with BPD, some of them followed up to a postnatal age of about 12 months: these infants had a significantly lower V_{maxFRC} than a control group of healthy premature and term-born infants during their first year of life, and the difference in V_{maxFRC} values between the BPD cases and the healthy infants increased toward the end of the study, indicating that BPD was associated with poor airway growth. This failure to catch up in terms of airway growth during the first year of life has been documented again more recently, in a group of tinier and more immature survivors of BPD (45). Other studies have shown a high prevalence of significant airflow limitation in survivors of BPD up to two years of age (24,44), and similar results were reported in infants with BPD up to three years of age using RVRTC (27) and FD (49). Finally, a low V_{maxFRC}—indicating persistent airway obstruction—was recorded in a series of technology-dependent children with BPD up to four years of age (46).

   Although these studies were conducted over two decades, and the BPD subjects considered differed in gestational age and birth weight and received different neonatal care (e.g., surfactant, antenatal steroids), their V_{maxFRC} results look remarkably homogeneous. There are several possible explanations for this situation. One important point to make is that the above-mentioned studies often report on selected cohorts of neonates with severe respiratory disease (24,46): having excluded cases with a better neonatal course or milder BPD may have made it impossible to note any beneficial effects of improved neonatal care on subsequent airway function in the population of survivors of BPD as a whole. The mean duration of the BPD infants' oxygen dependence was very high in several studies and prolonged positive-pressure ventilation was invariably required in all cohorts, so it is reasonable to assume that current data overestimate the incidence of significant airflow limitation in infants and young children with BPD. The need for prolonged mechanical ventilation also suggests that direct iatrogenic insult may have significantly contributed to these infants' airway injury, and most of these cases should probably be classified as having "old BPD." Several studies found that mechanical ventilation had an important influence on V_{maxFRC}. As an example, Hofhuis et al. (47) showed a different severity of airflow limitation in infants given conventional or high-frequency ventilation, indicating that iatrogenic insult clearly affected the magnitude of later airway functional derangements in their cohort. Baraldi et al. (24) found a significant correlation between V_{maxFRC} at two years of age and C_{rs} measured during mechanical ventilation in the first 10 to 20 days of life, and this was interpreted as meaning that chronic airway injury was more severe in infants who, whatever the reason, were not ventilated in the linear portion of the pressure-volume loop. Hence, factors such as distorted or thickened airway walls, increased smooth muscle layers, or a disturbed development of airway caliber (as seen in old BPD) probably had a role in determining the airflow limitations documented in the above-mentioned cohorts (41). Some of these pathological aspects are lacking or less pronounced in subjects who develop new BPD, so caution is warranted when applying currently available data to the more recent populations of newborn intensive care unit (NICU) graduates. We need V_{maxFRC} data specifically concerning cohorts of very tiny, immature infants with new BPD. While the use of less invasive approaches to neonatal respiratory failure (e.g., the early use of surfactant, early extubation attempts, extensive use of nCPAP) may improve functional airway outcome in these infants, there is currently nothing to corroborate this hypothesis. Indeed, there is concern that the increasingly lengthy survival of ever more immature babies will be associated with significant long-term airway dysfunction. It is becoming increasingly apparent that prematurity per se may considerably impact on airway function and development, regardless of any iatrogenic complications or clinical signs in neonatal age (3). This first emerged in a study longitudinally measuring V_{maxFRC} in a group of healthy infants who were born slightly premature (mean gestational age around 33 weeks), but had never required respiratory support (50). V_{maxFRC} (expressed as a z-score) was within the normal range shortly after birth, but decreased significantly over the first year of life, suggesting that preterm birth is detrimental to subsequent lung development. In a group of 62 infants born at 33 weeks of gestation and studied by RVRCT at 2 months old, Friedrich et al. recently found that flow rates and expiratory volumes were about 30% lower than in normal term-born controls (51); here again, a neonatal history of mechanical ventilation and oxygen supplementation >48 hours were among the exclusion criteria, which rules out any direct iatrogenic impact on subsequent airway function. Twenty-six of these infants were reassessed at a mean 15 months old (52) and showed no signs of catching up in terms of their forced expiratory flows.

The pathogenic mechanisms behind airflow limitation in such "healthy" preterm infants have yet to be clarified. It has been speculated that premature delivery induces disorganized patterns of airway growth and maturation, leading to narrow and/or excessively compliant airways (53). A limited secondary septation would also result in fewer alveolar attachments to the terminal airways, meaning a weaker mechanical support and greater collapsibility (54). Such a "developmental" mechanism of airflow limitation would naturally be even more important in neonates born at extremely low gestational ages. A possible implication of these findings is that although reducing iatrogenic lung injury remains a fundamental aim of advances in neonatal critical care, it may not be enough to guarantee a "normal" airway development in premature infants (3), while the longer survival of more and more immature newborns may further expand the population heading for significant, inevitable airway disease.

Whether airflow limitation early in life precedes long-term airway obstruction remains to be seen due to the shortage of pulmonary function data collected longitudinally right from the first months of age in premature infants with and without BPD. In the only study available, however, which monitored lung function prospectively from birth in a small group of children with moderate BPD, a close correlation emerged between V_{maxFRC} at 24 months of life and FEV_1 and FEF_{25-75} at a mean age of around

9 years (55). These findings suggest that airway function tracks over time in infants born prematurely, with no detectable functional recovery up to school age. Similarly, V_{maxFRC} measured shortly after birth was able to predict impaired pulmonary function in young adulthood in a large unselected cohort of individuals born healthy and followed up to 22 years of age (56). On the basis of these data, poor airway function in the early years of life should be seen as an important risk factor for airflow obstruction up to young adulthood, which is in turn considered one of the strongest predictors of the onset of COPD later in life (56).

V. Long-Term Lung Function in Survivors of BPD and Prematurity

In the last two decades, several studies based on spirometry or static lung volume measurements have assessed long-term respiratory outcome after premature birth, particularly in survivors of BPD.

Spirometry is considered the "gold standard" for understanding respiratory physiology, detecting airway obstructions, and providing prognostic information (57–59). Expiratory airflow is a function of muscle effort, elastic recoil of the lungs and chest, small and large airway function, and the interdependence between the small airways and the surrounding alveolar attachments. With adequate coaching, children as young as four years can be taught to perform the maneuver of forced expiration needed for spirometry. FEV_1 and the FEV_1/FVC ratio are the most reproducible parameters for detecting airflow limitation. Ideally, spirometry should be done serially to identify children at risk of impaired lung function development.

Figure 1 summarizes the FEV_1 values reported in 18 studies published since 1990 in which cohorts of 6- to 19-year-old survivors of BPD were compared with control groups of healthy individuals born at term (60–77). The results of these studies clearly show that survivors of BPD have significant airflow obstruction at any age: their mean FEV_1 values (% pred.) are generally around or below 80% predicted, and severely compromised lung function was reported in individuals in virtually every cohort. Only four studies reported on cases nearing young adulthood (74–77), and no information currently exists on lung function beyond the second decade of life in subjects with BPD. Other important lung function anomalies reported in survivors of BPD up to late adolescence are (*i*) a higher residual volume and residual volume to total lung capacity ratio, suggesting air trapping; (*ii*) a limited ventilatory reserve during exercise; and (*iii*) a significant airway hyperreactivity to histamine, methacholine, or exercise (78).

The studies in Figure 1 give us the best available estimate of the impact of BPD on pulmonary function in the long term, but several methodological issues should be taken into account when interpreting their results and applying currently available data to the more recent populations of NICU graduates. For instance, study populations are often rather heterogeneous and difficult to compare, due to the use of different definitions of BPD or arbitrary selection criteria. Difficulties in selecting appropriate control groups may likewise influence data interpretation, and differences in neonatal care at different centers and over time may further interfere with any comparisons between the studies.

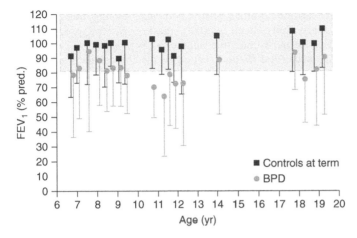

Figure 1 FEV$_1$ values (% pred.) in children, adolescents, and young adults surviving BPD, compared with controls born at term. Data (presented as mean −2SD) from 18 studies, published since 1990, comparing BPD survivors from 6 to 19 years of age with a reference population born at term (60–77). In all but two studies mean FEV$_1$ was significantly lower in BPD patients than in healthy controls. Eighty percent of the predicted FEV$_1$ is the accepted lower limit of normal. *Source*: From Ref. 2.

An important point to make is that most of the available data refer mainly to cases of old BPD. Survivors of BPD studied in the medium and longer term were almost invariably delivered before exogenous surfactants were introduced and antenatal steroid administration became widespread, and they will have had prolonged mechanical ventilation. Acute lung injury was therefore likely to have a major role in their chronic lung disease, so their functional outcome is not comparable with the situation in more recent cases of BPD, which often concerns preterm newborns who may have needed little or no ventilatory support in the early days after birth (79). New BPD is primarily a developmental disease of the terminal airspaces and its symptoms are usually milder, during the neonatal age, than in old BPD (80). Since patients with mild BPD reportedly usually have better long-term spirometric results than those with a severe neonatal course (74), new BPD patients will presumably have a better ultimate respiratory outcome. Whether this is actually the case remains to be seen, however, as no data referring specifically to cohorts of subjects with new BPD are available as yet (80). Clinical observations on more recent populations of NICU graduates (born after the introduction of antenatal corticosteroids and surfactants) have shown that the prevalence of respiratory symptoms and the need for inhaled drugs remain high in early childhood (81) and up to six years of age in extremely premature individuals (82). Moreover, there is no evidence of children with BPD born since the introduction of surfactant replacement therapy having better spirometric results at school age than those born earlier (63,64,66,67,83). Two recent studies (64,84) on successive cohorts of infants born under 1000 g or up to 28 weeks of gestation also found that the advent of surfactant therapy and generally improved neonatal care did not reduce airflow limitation at school age, though the benefits associated with better care may have been partially masked by the progressive improvement in the survival of the most immature infants (64,84).

An additional aspect that makes it difficult to anticipate the clinical and functional evolution of BPD with age is that we do not really know the exact nature of airway obstruction in those patients. No information is available on lung pathology in survivors of BPD (and prematurity) beyond infancy, so we lack the anatomical correlates of their functional anomalies (2,53). Survivors of BPD usually have considerable respiratory disturbances (cough, recurrent wheezing, respiratory tract infections) in the first two to three years of life; though such problems tend to subside progressively over time (2), respiratory symptoms as well as spirometric evidence of airway obstruction are common in individuals with BPD until young adulthood (74–76) and are often referred to as "asthma." The assumption that the well-known pathological features of asthma underlie the clinical manifestations of BPD, however, is arbitrary, to say the least. Available evidence suggests that BPD is a separate condition resulting from specific pathogenic mechanisms. To give an example, eosinophil-driven inflammation is central in childhood asthma, but exhaled nitric oxide (high levels of which are a biomarker of eosinophilic inflammation and responsiveness to corticosteroids) is reportedly normal in children with BPD (66). What's more, preterm babies do not have a higher prevalence of atopy (75,85), which is a major risk factor for childhood asthma. Another difference is that airflow limitation is only partially reversed by β_2-agonists in children with BPD, suggesting a stabilized remodeling process (66,67,74). High-resolution computed tomographic studies have also documented specific morphological differences between the lungs of children with asthma and those with BPD (86). On the basis of these observations, the common practice of giving anti-asthma medication (e.g., inhaled glucocorticosteroids) to survivors of BPD should be considered neither effective nor safe. Establishing the pathological features of long-standing BPD has become a research priority to gain insight to guide patient management and anticipate the respiratory outcome with aging (2,53). It is likely, however, that multiple patterns of airway and parenchymal involvement will characterize the various forms of BPD, depending on the mutual influence of prematurity and early acute lung injury in defining the phenotype.

Until further information becomes available, studies on patients in early adulthood give us the best idea of the ultimate respiratory outcome of BPD (74–77): these studies show that survivors of BPD have substantially lower airflows than subjects born at term, and they usually have a worse spirometric performance than controls of similar birth weights or gestational ages. A better understanding of the mechanisms controlling normal intrauterine and postnatal lung growth would help us to develop strategies to prevent COPD in adult life (56). As discussed earlier in this chapter, it has been claimed that preterm birth may be a factor independently associated with abnormal lung function, irrespective of any BPD and iatrogenic influences. Prematurity is certainly an important risk factor for respiratory morbidity during the first years of life, and altered lung volumes, airway hyperresponsiveness, and airflow limitations have been reported even in infants born only slightly preterm and with no significant neonatal lung disease or iatrogenic influences. Whether such anomalies are relevant to these subjects' respiratory future is debatable. Children born premature without BPD may still have airway obstruction at school age (66–69), although to a lesser extent than survivors of BPD. Data available on adolescents or young adults tend to confirm significant differences in airflow parameters between survivors of prematurity without BPD and controls born at term (76,77,87). Again, these data emphasize that premature delivery may be associated per se with long-term respiratory disorders, these problems simply being more evident and severe in subjects who develop BPD as a result of additional early lung injuries.

More reassuring data have recently been reported in a group of individuals born preterm (mean gestational age 31.5 weeks) studied at about 22 years of age, (88% of them without BPD) (88): these subjects showed no evidence of airflow obstruction or airway hyperresponsiveness, and their lung function had improved vis-à-vis a previous assessment in mid-childhood. But despite this favorable functional picture, their prevalence of respiratory symptoms was significantly higher than that in a group of healthy controls born at term. Persistent respiratory symptoms or long-term lung function anomalies raise concern about the prospects of respiratory outcome with aging.

Burrows et al. (89) first observed, 30 years ago, that adults with a history of respiratory disease during childhood had lower lung function levels and higher risk of developing obstructive lung disease, introducing the hypothesis that obstructive pulmonary disease has its origins in fetal life (56). In fact, there is some concern that survivors of preterm birth and BPD will be susceptible to COPD in later life (74–76,79,90). The pulmonary derangement characterizing many BPD survivors may remain latent in most of them as they grow up, but a reduced respiratory reserve could increase their risk of a COPD-like phenotype later on. There may be an overlap in the clinical and physiological features of BPD and COPD, but a longer follow-up and data on lung pathology in long-term survivors of BPD will be needed before any conclusions can be reached. Lung function, as reflected by FEV_1, normally increases to a maximal level in early adulthood, then remains stable for some years before it begins to decline (by about 30 mL a year) into senescence, generally never reaching disabling values (Fig. 2) (91). This is true of people with a normal lung development, but may not apply to some survivors of prematurity, and especially those with a history of BPD, whose maximal FEV_1 is suboptimal due to damage sustained in the perinatal period (55,76).

In some young adult survivors of BPD, maximal FEV_1 is well below 80% of the predicted value (Fig. 2), and the natural decline in FEV_1 may make these subjects reach a critical threshold for the onset of respiratory symptoms already in mid-adulthood. It is also not clear whether the rate of this decline in respiratory function will be normal or early, or accelerated, in survivors of prematurity and/or BPD. A significantly worsening FEV_1/FVC ratio from the age of 8 to 18 was recently reported in a group of survivors of BPD (76). Respiratory diseases in childhood may be associated with chronic airflow obstruction later in life (92), and a faster rate of decline in lung function has been reported in people who had wheezy bronchitis as children, even though their lung function became normal in early adulthood (93). A recent study on young adults demonstrated that the main predictors of COPD are early respiratory signs and a lung function below the normal range (57). Smoking is another well-known risk factor for a more rapid age-related decline in lung function (91) and the onset of COPD in later life. Almost 30% of people born prematurely smoke as young adults (73,74,88), and the reduction in their respiratory function is several times greater than it is for smokers who were born at term (94), so every effort should be made to prevent smoking among people born prematurely.

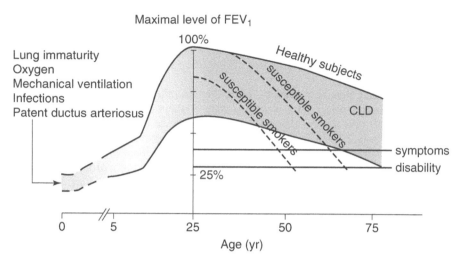

Figure 2 Model of the natural history and time-related changes in FEV_1 by age. Theoretical FEV_1 curves in healthy normal subjects and BPD survivors (*gray area*). BPD survivors may have variable airflow limitation from the first years of life with little evidence of "catch-up" growth in lung function. Most of these patients fail to attain a maximal level of FEV_1 in early adulthood and will start the declining phase from substantially reduced FEV_1 values. The dashed lines represent the potential impact of smoking in susceptible subjects on the rate of decline of FEV_1. Forced expiratory flows in the first three years of life are extrapolated from measurements of maximal flow at functional residual capacity. *Source*: From Ref. 2.

References

1. Stocks J, Coates A, Bush A. Lung function in infants and young children with chronic lung disease of infancy: the next steps? Pediatr Pulmonol 2007; 42(1):3–9.
2. Baraldi E, Filippone M. Chronic lung disease after premature birth. N Engl J Med 2007; 357(19):1946–1955.
3. Bush A. Update in pediatric lung disease 2007. Am J Respir Crit Care Med 2008; 177(7):686–695.
4. Bentham JR, Shaw NJ. Some chronic obstructive pulmonary disease will originate in neo-natal intensive care units. Paediatr Respir Rev 2005; 6:29–32.
5. Northway WH Jr., Rosan RC, Porter DY. Pulmonary disease following respirator therapy of hyaline-membrane disease: bronchopulmonary dysplasia. N Engl J Med 1967; 276:357–368.
6. Hülskamp G, Pillow JJ, Stocks J. Lung function testing in acute neonatal respiratory disorders and chronic lung disease of infancy: a review series. Pediatr Pulmonol 2005; 40:467–470.
7. Hülskamp G, Pillow JJ, Dinger J, et al. Lung function tests in neonates and infants with chronic lung disease of infancy: functional residual capacity. Pediatr Pulmonol 2006; 41(1): 1–22.
8. Wauer RR, Maurer T, Nowotny T, et al. Assessment of functional residual capacity using nitrogen washout and plethysmographic techniques in infants with and without broncho-pulmonary dysplasia. Intensive Care Med 1998; 24:469–475.

9. Castile RG, Iram D, McCoy KS. Gas trapping in normal infants and in infants with cystic fibrosis. Pediatr Pulmonol 2004; 37:461–469.
10. Gustafsson PM, Kallman S, Ljungberg H, et al. Method for assessment of volume of trapped gas in infants during multiple-breath inert gas washout. Pediatr Pulmonol 2003; 35:42–49.
11. Kavvadia V, Greenough A, Dimitriou G, et al. Lung volume measurements in infants with and without chronic lung disease. Eur J Pediatr 1998; 157:336–339.
12. Richardson P, Bose CL, Carlstrom JR. The functional residual capacity of infants with respiratory distress syndrome. Acta Paediatr Scand 1986; 75:267–271.
13. Edberg KE, Sandberg K, Silberberg A, et al. Lung volume, gas mixing, and mechanics of breathing in mechanically ventilated very low birth weight infants with idiopathic respiratory distress syndrome. Pediatr Res 1991; 30:496–500.
14. Dimitriou G, Greenough A. Measurement of lung volume and optimal oxygenation during high frequency oscillation. Arch Dis Child 1995; 72:180–183.
15. Edberg KE, Ekstrom-Jodal B, Hallman M, et al. Immediate effects on lung function of instilled human surfactant in mechanically ventilated newborn infants with IRDS. Acta Paediatr Scand 1990; 79:1750–1755.
16. Goldsmith LS, Greenspan JS, Rubenstein SD, et al. Immediate improvement in lung volume after exogenous surfactant: alveolar recruitment versus increased distension. J Pediatr 1991; 119:424–428.
17. Cotton RB, Olsson T, Law AB, et al. The physiologic effects of surfactant treatment on gas exchange in newborn premature infants with hyaline membrane disease. Pediatr Res 1993; 34:495–501.
18. Farstad T, Bratlid D. Pulmonary effects after surfactant treatment in premature infants with severe respiratory distress syndrome. Biol Neonate 1995; 68:246–253.
19. Dinger J, Topfer A, Schaller P, et al. Functional residual capacity and compliance of the respiratory system after surfactant treatment in premature infants with severe respiratory distress syndrome. Eur J Pediatr 2002; 161:485–490.
20. da Silva WJ, Abbasi S, Pereira G, et al. Role of positive end-expiratory pressure changes on functional residual capacity in surfactant treated preterm infants. Pediatr Pulmonol 1994; 18:89–92.
21. Bjorklund LJ, Vilstrup CT, Larsson A, et al. Changes in lung volume and static expiratory pressure-volume diagram after surfactant rescue treatment of neonates with established respiratory distress syndrome. Am J Respir Crit Care Med 1996; 154:918–923.
22. Thome U, Topfer A, Schaller P, et al. Comparison of lung volume measurements by antero-posterior chest X-ray and the SF6 washout technique in mechanically ventilated infants. Pediatr Pulmonol 1998; 26:265–272.
23. Dinger J, Topfer A, Schaller P, et al. Effect of positive end expiratory pressure on functional residual capacity and compliance in surfactant-treated preterm infants. J Perinat Med 2001; 29:137–143.
24. Baraldi E, Filippone M, Trevisanuto D, et al. Pulmonary function until two years of life in infants with bronchopulmonary dysplasia. Am J Respir Crit Care Med 1997; 155: 149–155.
25. Tepper RS, Morgan WJ, Cota K, et al. Expiratory flow limitation in infants with broncho-pulmonary dysplasia. J Pediatr 1986; 109(6):1040–1046.
26. Gerhardt T, Hehre D, Feller R, et al. Serial determination of pulmonary function in infants with chronic lung disease. J Pediatr 1987; 110:448–456.
27. Robin B, Kim YJ, Huth J, et al. Pulmonary function in bronchopulmonary dysplasia. Pediatr Pulmonol 2004; 37:236–242.
28. Merth IT, de Winter JP, Borsboom GJJM, et al. Pulmonary function during the first year of life in healthy infants born prematurely. Eur Respir J 1995; 8:1141–1147.

29. de Winter JP, Merth IT, Brand R, et al. Functional residual capacity and static compliance during the first year in preterm infants treated with surfactant. Am J Perinatol 2000; 17: 377–384.

30. Hjalmarson O, Sandberg K. Abnormal lung function in healthy preterm infants. Am J Respir Crit Care Med 2002; 165:83–87.

31. Hjalmarson O, Sandberg KL. Lung function at term reflects severity of bronchopulmonary dysplasia. J Pediatr 2005; 146:86–90.

32. Gappa M, Pillow JJ, Allen J, et al. Lung function tests in neonates and infants with chronic lung disease: lung and chest-wall mechanics. Pediatr Pulmonol 2006; 41(4):291–317.

33. Eichenwald EC, Stark AR. Pulmonary function in BPD and its aftermath. In: Bland RD, Coalson JJ, eds. Chronic Lung Disease in Early Infancy. USA: Informa Healthcare, 1999.

34. Fitzgerald DA, Mesiano G, Brosseau L, et al. Pulmonary outcome in extremely low birth weight infants. Pediatrics 2000; 105:1209–1215.

35. Lui K, Lloyd J, Ang E, et al. Early changes in respiratory compliance and resistance during the development of bronchopulmonary dysplasia in the era of surfactant therapy. Pediatr Pulmonol 2000; 30:282–290.

36. Kavvadia V, Greenough A, Dimitriou G. Early prediction of chronic oxygen dependency by lung function test results. Pediatr Pulmonol 2000; 29:19–26.

37. Snepvangers Y, deWinter JP, Burger H, et al. Respiratory outcome in preterm ventilated infants: importance of early respiratory system resistance. Eur J Pediatr 2004; 163:378–384.

38. Bhutani VK, Bowen FW, Sivieri EM. Postnatal changes in pulmonary mechanics and energetics of infants with respiratory distress syndrome following surfactant treatment. Biol Neonate 2005; 87:323–331.

39. Bancalari E, Gonzalez A. Clinical course and lung function abnormalities during development of neonatal chronic lung disease. In: Bland RD, Coalson JJ, eds. Chronic Lung Disease in Early Infancy. Informa Healthcare, 1999.

40. Coalson JJ. Pathology of bronchopulmonary dysplasia. Semin Perinatol 2006; 30:179–184.

41. Lum S, Hülskamp G, Merkus P, et al. Lung function tests in neonates and infants with chronic lung disease: forced expiratory maneuvers. Pediatr Pulmonol 2006; 41:199–214.

42. Nickerson BG, Durand DJ, Kao LC. Short-term variability of pulmonary function tests in infants with bronchopulmonary dysplasia. Pediatr Pulmonol 1989; 6:36–41.

43. Kao LC, Durand DJ, Nickerson BG. Effects of inhaled metaproterenol and atropine on the pulmonary mechanics of infants with bronchopulmonary dysplasia. Pediatr Pulmonol 1989; 6:74–80.

44. Farstad T, Brockmeier F, Bratlid D. Cardiopulmonary function in premature infants with bronchopulmonary dysplasia—a 2-year follow up. Eur J Pediatr 1995; 154:853–858.

45. Iles R, Edmunds AT. Assessment of pulmonary function in resolving chronic lung disease of prematurity. Arch Dis Child Fetal Neonatal Ed 1997; 76:113–117.

46. Talmaciu I, Ren CL, Kolb SM, et al. Pulmonary function in technology-dependent children 2 years and older with bronchopulmonary dysplasia. Pediatr Pulmonol 2002; 33:181–188.

47. Hofhuis W, Huysman MW, van der Wiel EC, et al. Worsening of VmaxFRC in infants with chronic lung disease in the first year of life: a more favorable outcome after high-frequency oscillation ventilation. Am J Respir Crit Care Med 2002; 166:1539–1543.

48. Mahut B, De Blic J, Emond S, et al. Chest computed tomography findings in bronchopulmonary dysplasia and correlation with lung function. Arch Dis Child Fetal Neonatal Ed 2007; 92(6):459–464.

49. Mallory GB Jr., Chaney H, Mutich RL, et al. Longitudinal changes in lung function during the first three years of premature infants with moderate to severe bronchopulmonary dysplasia. Pediatr Pulmonol 1991; 11(1):8–14.

50. Hoo AF, Dezateux C, Henschen M, et al. Development of airway function in infancy after preterm delivery. J Pediatr 2002; 141:652–658.

51. Friedrich L, Stein RT, Pitrez PMC, et al. Reduced lung function in healthy preterm infants in the first months of life. Am J Respir Crit Care Med 2006; 173:442–447.
52. Friedrich L, Pitrez PMC, Stein RT, et al. Growth rate of lung function in healthy preterm infants. Am J Respir Crit Care Med 2007; 176:1269–1273.
53. Jobe AH. An unknown: lung growth and development after very preterm birth. Am J Respir Crit Care Med 2002; 166:1529–1530.
54. Gappa M, Stocks J, Merkus P. Lung growth and development after preterm birth: further evidence. Am J Respir Crit Care Med 2003; 168:399–400.
55. Filippone M, Sartor M, Zacchello F, et al. Flow limitation in infants with bronchopulmonary dysplasia and respiratory function at school age. Lancet 2003; 361:753–754.
56. Stern DA, Morgan WJ, Wright AL, et al. Poor airway function in early infancy and lung function by age 22 years: a non-selective longitudinal cohort study. Lancet 2007; 370(9589):758–764.
57. Albers M, Schermer T, Heijdra Y, et al. Predictive value of lung function below the normal range and respiratory symptoms for progression of chronic obstructive pulmonary disease. Thorax 2008; 63(3):201–207.
58. Beydon N, Davis SD, Lombardi E, et al. An official American Thoracic Society/European Respiratory Society statement: pulmonary function testing in preschool children. Am J Respir Crit Care Med 2007; 175(12):1304–1345.
59. Young RP, Hopkins R, Eaton TE. Forced expiratory volume in one second: not just a lung function test but a marker of premature death from all causes. Eur Respir J 2007; 30:616–622.
60. Mitchell SH, Teague WG. Reduced gas transfer at rest and during exercise in school-age survivors of bronchopulmonary dysplasia. Am J Respir Crit Care Med 1998; 157:1406–1412.
61. Gross SJ, Iannuzzi DM, Kveselis DA, et al. Effect of preterm birth on pulmonary function at school age: a prospective controlled study. J Pediatr 1998; 133:188–192.
62. Hakulinen AL, Heinonen K, Länsimies E, et al. Pulmonary function and respiratory morbidity in school-age children born prematurely and ventilated for neonatal respiratory insufficiency. Pediatr Pulmonol 1990; 8:226–232.
63. Korhonen P, Laitinen J, Hyödynmaa E, et al. Respiratory outcome in school-aged, very-low-birth-weight children in the surfactant era. Acta Paediatr 2004; 93:316–321.
64. Doyle LW. Respiratory function at age 8-9 years in extremely low birthweight/very preterm children born in Victoria in 1991-1992. Pediatr Pulmonol 2006; 41:570–576.
65. Santuz P, Baraldi E, Zaramella P, et al. Factors limiting exercise performance in long-term survivors of bronchopulmonary dysplasia. Am J Respir Crit Care Med 1995; 152:1284–1289.
66. Baraldi E, Bonetto G, Zacchello F, et al. Low exhaled nitric oxide in school-age children with bronchopulmonary dysplasia and airflow limitation. Am J Respir Crit Care Med 2005; 171:68–72.
67. Pelkonen AS, Hakulinen AL, Turpeinen M. Bronchial lability and responsiveness in school children born very preterm. Am J Respir Crit Care Med 1997; 156:1178–1184.
68. Jacob SV, Lands LC, Coates AL, et al. Exercise ability in survivors of severe bronchopulmonary dysplasia. Am J Respir Crit Care Med 1997; 155:1925–1929.
69. Kennedy JD, Edward LJ, Bates DJ, et al. Effects of birthweight and oxygen supplementation on lung function in late childhood in children of very low birth weight. Pediatr Pulmonol 2000; 30:32–40.
70. Kilbride HW, Gelatt MC, Sabath RJ. Pulmonary function and exercise capacity for ELBW survivors in preadolescence: effect of neonatal chronic lung disease. J Pediatr 2003; 143:488–493.
71. Giacoia GP, Venkataraman PS, West-Wilson KI, et al. Follow-up of school-age children with bronchopulmonary dysplasia. J Pediatr 1997; 130:400–408.
72. Pianosi PT, Fisk M. Cardiopulmonary exercise performance in prematurely born children. Pediatr Res 2000; 47:653–658.

73. Doyle LW, Cheung MMH, Ford GW, et al. Birth weight <1501 g and respiratory health at age 14. Arch Dis Child 2001; 84:40–44.
74. Halvorsen T, Skadberg BT, Eide GE, et al. Pulmonary outcome in adolescents of extreme preterm birth: a regional cohort study. Acta Paediatr 2004; 93:1294–1300.
75. Northway WH Jr., Moss RB, Carlisle KB, et al. Late pulmonary sequelae of broncho-pulmonary dysplasia. N Engl J Med 1990; 323:1793–1799.
76. Doyle LW, Faber B, Callanan C, et al. Bronchopulmonary dysplasia in very low birth weight subjects and lung function in late adolescence. Pediatrics 2006; 118:108–113.
77. Vrijlandt EJ, Gerritsen J, Boezen HM, et al. Lung function and exercise capacity in young adults born prematurely. Am J Respir Crit Care Med 2006; 173:890–896.
78. Allen J, Zwerdling R, Ehrenkranz R, et al. Statement on the care of the child with chronic lung disease of infancy and childhood. Am J Respir Crit Care Med 2003; 168:356–396.
79. Kinsella JP, Greenough A, Abman SH. Bronchopulmonary dysplasia. Lancet 2006; 367: 1421–1431.
80. Abman SH, Davis JM. Bronchopulmonary dysplasia. In: Chernick V, Boat TF, Wilmott RW, et al., eds. Disorders of the Respiratory Tract in Children. 7th ed. Philadelphia: Saunders/ Elsevier, 2006:342–358.
81. Vrijlandt EJ, Boezen HM, Gerritsen J, et al. Respiratory health in prematurely born preschool children with and without bronchopulmonary dysplasia. J Pediatr 2007; 150:256–261.
82. Hennessy EM, Bracewell M, Wood N, et al. Respiratory health in pre-school and school age children following extremely preterm birth. Arch Dis Child 2008; 93(12):1037–1043.
83. Gappa M, Berner MM, Hohenschild S, et al. Pulmonary function at school-age in surfactant-treated preterm infants. Pediatr Pulmonol 1999; 27(3):191–198.
84. Halvorsen T, Skadberg BT, Eide GE, et al. Better care of immature infants: has it influenced longterm pulmonary outcome? Acta Paediatr 2006; 95:547–554.
85. Vrijlandt EJ, Gerritsen J, Boezen HM, et al. Gender differences in respiratory symptoms in 19-year-old adults born preterm. Respir Res 2005; 6:117.
86. Aukland SM, Halvorsen T, Fosse KR, et al. High-resolution CT of the chest in children and young adults who were born prematurely: findings in a population-based study. AJR Am J Roentgenol 2006; 187:1012–1018.
87. Anand D, Stevenson CJ, West CR, et al. Lung function and respiratory health in adolescents of very low birth weight. Arch Dis Child 2003; 88:135–138.
88. Narang I, Rosenthal M, Cremonesini D, et al. Longitudinal evaluation of airway function 21 years after preterm birth. Am J Respir Crit Care Med 2008; 178(1):74–80.
89. Burrows B, Knudson RJ, Lebowitz MD. The relationship of childhood respiratory illness to adult obstructive airway disease. Am Rev Respir Dis 1977; 115:751–760.
90. Eber E, Zach MS. Long term sequelae of bronchopulmonary dysplasia (chronic lung disease of infancy). Thorax 2001; 56:317–323.
91. Fletcher C, Peto R. The natural history of chronic airflow obstruction. Br Med J 1977; 1:1645–1648.
92. Samet JM, Tager IB, Speizer FE. The relationship between respiratory illness in childhood and chronic air-flow obstruction in adulthood. Am Rev Respir Dis 1983; 127:508–523.
93. Edwards CA, Osman LM, Godden DJ, et al. Wheezy bronchitis in childhood: a distinct clinical entity with lifelong significance? Chest 2003; 124:18–24.
94. Doyle LW, Olinsky A, Faber B, et al. Adverse effects of smoking on respiratory function in young adults born weighing less than 1000 grams. Pediatrics 2003; 112:565–569.

22
Long-Term Outcomes of Infants with BPD

ANNE GREENOUGH
Division of Asthma, Allergy & Lung Biology, MRC-Asthma U.K. Centre in Allergic Mechanisms of
Asthma, King's College London, London, U.K.

I. Introduction

In this chapter, the long-term outcomes of infants who developed BPD are described. It is important to emphasize that the reports of older children and adults include patients with "classical" BPD. Such patients often had severe respiratory failure in the neonatal period, but also had more nonpulmonary acute complications such as intracerebral hemorrhage, which would have adversely affected their long-term outcome. Nowadays, infants can become chronically oxygen dependent despite minimal or even no respiratory distress immediately after birth and are described as suffering from "new" BPD (1). Such infants suffer less pulmonary inflammation and fibrosis but have reduced alveolarization (2). Whether affected children experience catch-up growth is not known, if they do not then their long-term pulmonary outcome could potentially be worse than that of those who had classical BPD.

II. Rehospitalization

In the first two years after birth, rehospitalization is common in BPD infants with rates varying from 40% to 60% (3). In the first year, the rehospitalization rate is at least twice that of prematurely born infants without BPD (4). Rehospitalization is usually for respiratory problems (Table 1). In one study (5), reactive airways disease, pneumonia, and respiratory syncytial virus (RSV) infection were responsible for 65% of the admissions in the first year and 81% in the second year. The length of the total hospital stay over the two-year period was associated with the severity of BPD and the total duration of oxygen dependency (5). Multiple admissions are common; in one series, 73% of BPD infants required at least one readmission and 27% had three or more readmissions in the first two years (6). The hospitalization rate declines after the second year with very few readmissions in the preschool years (7) and hospitalization is infrequent in prematurely born teenagers, regardless of BPD status (8).

Table 1 Health Care Utilization and Cost of Care in BPD Infants in the First Two Years After Birth Related to Type of Rehospitalization

	RSV proven ($n = 45$)	Probable bronchiolitis ($n = 24$)	Other respiratory ($n = 60$)	Non-respiratory ($n = 106$)
Hospital admission rate per infant	4 (1–20)	2 (1–11)	3 (1–14)	0 (0–5)
Days in hospital	21 (4–282)	6.5 (1–70)	8 (1–114)	0 (0–25)
Total cost of care (£) (mean, 95% CI)	12,638 (8041, 17,235)	6059 (3427, 8690)	5683 (3427, 6775)	2461 (2074, 2849)

Data are presented as median (range).
Abbreviation: RSV, respiratory syncytial virus.
Source: From Ref. 6.

III. Pulmonary Outcome

A. Chronic Oxygen Dependence

Prematurely born BPD infants can require supplementary oxygen for many months or even years (9), although few remain oxygen dependent beyond two years of age (10). Those who have prolonged oxygen dependence are frequently sent home on supplementary oxygen. The American Academy of Pediatrics' Guidelines for Pediatric Home Health Care suggested use of supplementary oxygen in infants with BPD with oxygen saturation levels less than 95% and that therapy should be targeted to maintain saturation levels between 95% and 98% (11). Similarly, the American Thoracic Society in a statement on the Care of the Child with Chronic Lung Disease of Infancy and Childhood recommended oxygen saturation levels should be kept greater than 94% once the risk of retinopathy of prematurity (ROP) was past (12). There is, however, variation in the oxygen saturation threshold used as criteria to institute home oxygen (13). A survey of the Vermont Oxford Network highlighted that although 43% of respondents used a pulse oximetry saturation threshold of less than 90% for the initiation of home oxygen therapy, thresholds varied from less than 84% to less than 98% (13). Once on home oxygen, the target oxygen to achieve saturation also varied from greater than 84% to greater than 98%. Infants are usually discharged home on supplementary oxygen when they have no other medical problem, but some units allow infants home on supplementary oxygen who also require nasogastric tube feeding if there is appropriate support in the community. The latter policy allows earlier discharge from the neonatal unit with cost savings as, in a four-center study, no increase in subsequent hospital readmission was demonstrated (14). Provision of supplementary oxygen may also result in improved growth, particularly if higher oxygen saturations are used (15). It can, however, adversely impact on the family's quality of life (16). Analysis of parental completed quality of life questionnaires highlighted that after controlling for gestational age, postnatal age, birth weight, and type of residence, parents of infants on home oxygen compared with those whose infants no longer required home oxygen or had never required it, had less desire to go out, saw their friends and family less often, and were more likely to complain of fatigue (16). Infants requiring supplementary oxygen at home have twice the requirement for hospital readmission in the first two years after birth than infants with BPD not depending on home oxygen (9), likely reflecting they had more severe pulmonary disease. In addition, even when no longer home oxygen dependent, in one series (10), BPD infants who had required home oxygen had significantly more outpatient attendances (Table 2) and were more likely to wheeze and require an inhaler when aged between two and five years than BPD children who had never required home oxygen.

B. Respiratory Symptoms

Recurrent respiratory symptoms requiring treatment are common in prematurely born infants, children, and young adults who had BPD. BPD was a significant risk factor for wheeze in the first two years [odds ratio (OR) 6.0, 95% confidence intervals (CI) 2.6, 13.6] among infants born after 26 weeks of gestation; 20% of those who had RDS had wheeze. Similarly, examination of 492 infants born prior to 29 weeks of gestational age from the United Kingdom Oscillation Study revealed that 27% were coughing and 20% wheezing at both 6 and 12 months, 6% were coughing and 3% wheezing more than once a week, and 14% had taken bronchodilators and 8% inhaled steroids (17). BPD was demonstrated to be a significant risk factor for both wheeze (OR 2.7) and medication requirement (OR 2.4) (17). Wheezing in the first two years after birth in prematurely born infants is associated with lung function abnormalities including a high airways resistance and gas trapping (18). In very prematurely born infants, including those who had BPD, the number of days of wheeze significantly correlated with the degree of gas trapping, as evidenced by a reduced functional (measured by gas dilution) to thoracic (measured by plethysmography) lung volume (19). Lung function abnormalities in BPD infants and children are described in detail in another chapter.

At preschool age, respiratory symptoms remain common. In one BPD cohort, 28% coughed and 7% wheezed more than once a week; this was associated on average with 10 (maximum 68) attendances to the general practitioners' surgeries during the three-year period (10). In another study (20), approximately one-third of prematurely born preschool children, regardless of BPD status, coughed in the last 12 months and more than 10% wheezed. At school age, prematurely born children, particularly if they had BPD, are more likely to be symptomatic than their classroom colleagues born at term. In a cohort of seven- to eight-year-olds, 30% of BPD children and 24% of prematurely born children without BPD were wheezing, but only 7% of term controls were so affected (21). In one series (22), 23% of young adults who had had BPD had current respiratory symptoms, wheeze, and

Table 2 Health Care Utilization and Cost of Care in Years Two to Four Inclusive Related to Home Oxygen Status

	Home oxygen	No home oxygen	p
n	70	120	
Outpatient attendances (n)	8 (0–39)	5 (0–39)	0.0021
Specialist attendances (n)	3 (0–104)	1 (0–62)	0.0023
Respiratory prescriptions (n)	5.5 (0–46)	4 (0–29)	<0.0001
Total cost of care (£)	10,683 (1367–84,350)	4044 (277–87,285)	<0.0001

Data are presented as median (range).
Source: From Ref. 10.

need for long-term medication. Significantly more of the "BPD" adults had respiratory symptoms and need for medication than both the adults born prematurely but without BPD ($p = 0.047$) and the term controls ($p = 0.0001$). Similarly, in a nationwide follow-up study in the Netherlands, the prevalence of doctor-diagnosed asthma was significantly higher in 19-year-olds born prior to 32 weeks of gestational age with or without BPD than age-matched controls (23). There was, however, an effect of gender. Whereas the women who had had BPD were more likely to have asthma (24% vs. 5%, $p = 0.001$) and shortness of breath during exercise (43% vs. 16%, $p = 0.008$) than the controls, the prevalence of reported symptoms by the men who had had BPD was similar to the controls (23). Different patterns of thoracic growth in term children results at the end of puberty in approximately 25% higher lung function in males than females. The authors (23), therefore, speculated that a similar process may take place in the prematurely born population and explain the differences they found in symptoms according to gender.

C. Upper Airway Problems

Infants with BPD frequently require prolonged intubation and are at risk of laryngo-tracheal stenosis, laryngomalacia, tracheomalacia, unilateral vocal cord paralysis and granulation tissue, and subglottic cyst formation (24). The prevalence of trachea/bron-chomalacia in prematurely born infants with BPD had been reported to vary from 16% to 45%. The incidence of laryngotracheal stenosis has declined in the last 10 years (25) but is a significant risk factor for tracheostomy requirement (26). Other risk factors for tracheostomy in prematurely born infants include the severity of pulmonary disease (27), the duration of intubation, and the number of reintubations (26). The tracheostomy-related complication rate is between 26% and 63% and prematurely born infants have lower decannulation rates and spend twice the average time with a tracheostomy than the overall population of children (28). Disorders of speech, language, and swallowing are common in prematurely born children with tracheostomies (26).

D. Abnormalities on Chest Imaging

The severe chest radiograph abnormalities described by Northway in infants with classical BPD are now uncommon. Review of chest radiographs obtained at 28 days and 36 weeks' postmenstrual age (PMA) from 60 infants born before 29 weeks of gestation, however, demonstrated that there was no abnormality on only three of the chest radiographs (29). Hyperinflation and interstitial but not cystic shadows were common (29) (Fig. 1) and the presence of interstitial abnormalities at 28 days' and 36 weeks' PMA were particularly predictive of frequent wheeze in the first six months (30). At follow-up, computed tomograph (CT) scan examinations of the chest are particularly useful, demonstrating that the majority of children and young adults who had BPD and ongoing respiratory insufficiency have marked abnormalities. In one series (31), all 23 children with a mean age of 4 (range 2–13) months had abnormal CT scan appearances with multifocal areas of hyperexpansion, linear opacities, and triangular subpleural opacities. Similarly, review of the CT scan findings of 41 infants with BPD aged between 10 and 20 months demonstrated none had normal findings; 88% had hyper-lucent areas, 95% linear opacities, and 63% triangular subpleural opacities (32). Cor-relations were found between the CT findings and the duration on mechanical ventilation and neonatal oxygen exposure (32). Twenty-four of 26 young adults (mean

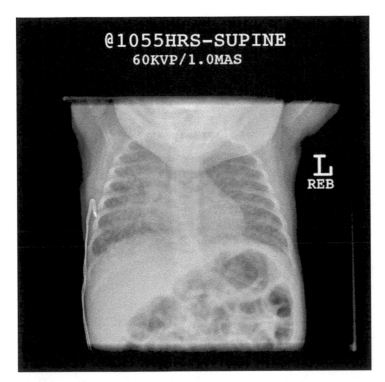

Figure 1 Chest radiograph of a 26-week-gestation infant who at two months of age was CPAP dependent and required 30% oxygen, although had required minimal support in the perinatal period. The chest radiograph demonstrates bilateral interstitial shadows greater on the right side. *Abbreviation*: CPAP, continuous positive airway pressure.

age of 19 years) had abnormal CT scans with reticular opacities, architectural distortion, and/or gas trapping; the CT abnormalities significantly correlated with pulmonary function test results (33). In addition, in a study of 25-year-old adults who had BPD, multifocal areas of reduced lung attenuation and perfusion and bronchial wall thickening were highlighted (34).

IV. Cardiovascular Problems

Systemic hypertension is commoner in infants with BPD (affecting between 13% and 43%) than in prematurely born infants with RDS but no BPD (1–9%) and in infants born at term (0.7–3%) (35), and it is more common in those with severe BPD (36). Causes include renal damage due to nephrocalcinosis or prolonged umbilical catheterization and use of medications such as systemic corticosteroids. Systemic hypertension may contribute to the development of left ventricular hypertrophy, which may be important in the pathogenesis of pulmonary edema in BPD (37). Pulmonary hypertension is discussed in another chapter.

V. Renal Problems

Infants with BPD are at increased risk of nephrocalcinosis. The etiology of nephrocalcinosis is multifactorial and includes immaturity, low glomerular filtration rate resulting in low urinary output, high intakes of calcium and phosphate (to prevent rickets with high excretion of calcium), low citrate excretion, and use of medications, particularly diuretics commonly used in the treatment of BPD infants. Frusemide has a hypercalcuric effect, but corticosteroids, xanthines, and gentamicin also contribute to the development of nephrocalcinosis. In infants with nephrocalcinosis, proximal tubular function is unaffected, but there is impaired glomerular and distal tubular function (38,39). Urinary tract infection is more common in infants with nephrocalcinosis, and in one series (39), the systolic blood pressure was above the 95th percentile in 39% of affected infants at one year and in 30% at two years (39). In rare cases, nephrocalcinosis leads to renal calculi or renal insufficiency. It usually resolves within months but is still present in 15% of affected infants at the age of 30 months.

VI. Growth Failure

Growth failure in the initial postdischarge period may affect between 30% and 67% of BPD infants (40). They have altered body composition with deficit in free fat mass and total body fat, which may persist throughout infancy (41). Growth failure and malnutrition in BPD infants is due to decreased nutrient intake, hypoxia, and increased energy requirements (12). There is often delay in both starting enteral feeds and advancing to full enteral nutrition, as well as enteral feeds are often interrupted because of concerns about feeding intolerance and intercurrent illnesses (42). Infants with BPD can have oral aversion secondary to intubation-related injuries, prolonged orotracheal intubation, palatal groove formation, and tube feeding (43). Fractures together with generalized bone demineralization are frequently observed in patients with BPD (Fig. 2) and are usually secondary to dietary or parenteral deficiency of calcium or vitamin D and excessive calciuria resulting from chronic diuretic therapy. It is controversial whether school children who had BPD remain smaller than controls (44,45).

VII. Gastroesophageal Reflux

Gastroesophageal reflux is common in BPD infants; rates of between 18% and 63% have been reported, although diagnostic criteria have not been consistent (46). Risk factors include prolonged gastric tube use (46). Chronic respiratory disorders such as BPD predispose patients to gastroesophageal reflux because of the increased negative intrathoracic pressure needed to overcome increased airways resistance, the decreased lower oesophageal sphincter pressure resulting from flattened diaphragms, and the increased forced exhalation as occurs in coughing (24). Gastroesophageal reflux is associated with xanthine-resistant apneic spells, bradycardic spells, frequent emesis, nasal-oral regurgitation, and exacerbation of BPD. In addition, infants with gastroesophageal reflux may develop esophagitis leading to aversion to feeding or inability to take adequate volumes

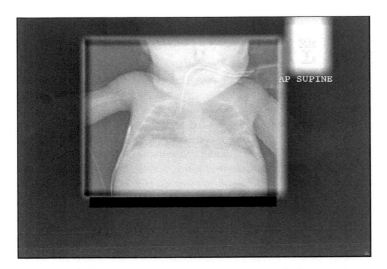

Figure 2 A chest radiograph of a 24-week-gestation infant who at four months of age remained ventilator dependent. The chest radiograph demonstrates small-volume lungs and bilateral shadows. Note fracture of the upper end of the humerus and osteopenia.

orally (47). Not surprisingly then, in comparison to controls matched for gestational age, birth weight, gender and severity of BPD, infants with gastroesophageal reflux were demonstrated to take significantly longer to achieve full feeds and had a longer hospital stay (47). Aspiration can play an important role in the ongoing respiratory difficulties of patients with BPD, as demonstrated by positive lipid-laden macrophages being found in the bronchoalveolar lavage fluid of BPD children aged three months to five years (24). The prevalence of gastroesophageal reflux is so high in prematurely born children with BPD that those who have persistent respiratory difficulties not responding to therapy and with persistent vomiting or failure to thrive should undergo evaluation for gastroesophageal reflux and aspiration.

VIII. Neurodevelopmental Problems

Neurodevelopmental outcome is poorer in infants with BPD. Cerebral palsy rates are higher in BPD infants (48). The association remains significant even among the most high-risk infants; the odds ratio for BPD infants developing cerebral palsy among 827 infants born prior to 25 weeks of gestation in the NICHD Network was 1.66 (49). In the Trial of Indomethacin Prophylaxis in Preterm Infants (TIPP) in which infants of birth weight of 500 to 999 g were recruited, BPD was independently correlated with poor outcome (death or cerebral palsy, cognitive delay, hearing loss requiring amplification and/or bilateral blindness) at 18 months (OR 2.4) (50). Unfortunately, comparison of two time periods (1996 to 1999 vs. 2000 to 2003) revealed that although, among extremely low birth weight (ELBW) and extremely low gestational age infants, neurosensory abnormalities were less common (29% vs. 16% and 31% vs. 16%, respectively), there were no significant changes overall in the proportions with developmental impairment

(51% vs. 49% and 50% vs. 51%, respectively) or in an MDI score less than 70 (42% vs. 42% and 37% vs. 45%, respectively) (51). For the ELBW group, predictors were multiple birth, ventilator dependence, and severe cranial ultrasound abnormalities and for the extremely low gestational age group, predictors of overall impairment were severe cranial ultrasound abnormalities, ventilator dependence, postnatal steroid therapy, and patent ductus arteriosus ligation (51). Other studies have demonstrated that postnatal dexamethasone worsens neurodevelopmental outcome in infants less than 28 weeks of gestation, particularly if the course is prolonged (52). At school age, BPD children still perform less well. At 8 to 10 years of age, BPD was associated with significantly worse cognitive performance (53). Others (54) have demonstrated impaired psychoeducational performance, especially with regard to language abilities and reading skills, in BPD children compared with controls; 41% of BPD children versus 21% of the controls had a verbal IQ score below one standard deviation from the norm. Comparison at approximately 10 years of age highlighted that 27 subjects with BPD compared to preterm controls matched for gestational age were more likely (71% vs. 19%) to have neurological abnormalities including neurological signs, cerebral palsy microcephaly, and behavioral difficulties (54). Over half the BPD cohort had difficulties in gross and/or fine motor kills (54). Durations of hospitalization and home oxygen, as markers of severity of illness, have been shown to correlate with motor outcomes (55). Others (56) have demonstrated that more than 50% of VLBW infants with BPD received occupational or physical therapy at eight years of age. The IQ of BPD children generally falls in the low average range (80–90) and the difference between their IQ and that of controls is between one quarter to two-thirds of a standard deviation (48). BPD children are also at greater risk of attentional impairments; in one series, the proportion with scores greater than one standard deviation below the mean was 59% versus 32% in the controls (49). Attention deficit hyperactive disorder is also increased, affecting 15% of eight-year-old, VLBW, BPD children, that is double that of controls (56). In addition, 15% of BPD children were reported to have significant receptive language impairment and 9% were reported to have significant expressive language impairment, which is more than double the occurrence found in non-BPD, VLBW born children (57). Spatial memory impairments are also more common (58); 65% of BPD children had memory impairment equivalent to one standard deviation below the expected compared with 29% of non-BPD controls (59). BPD children may also suffer from executive dysfunction; measures of planning ability, mental flexibility, and working memory have been shown to negatively correlate with weeks of oxygen requirement (60). They also perform poorer at school reading and mathematics (53), and this may affect as many as 47% of BPD children (59).

IX. Hearing Problems

Approximately 4% of BPD babies have sensorineural hearing loss (61). In the first year after birth, BPD infants also have an increased risk of conductive hearing loss; 22% of one series compared with 8% of controls of similar gestational age required myringotomy and grommet insertion (62). Auditory brainstem responses at neonatal unit discharge, however, did not accurately predict later conductive hearing loss (62) and thus it is recommended that infants with BPD should have audiological assessment at least at one year of age.

X. Visual Problems

BPD infants have an increased risk for compromised long-term development of functional vision, particularly amblyopic like effects on spatial vision, but only a minority are profoundly affected (63). BPD, however, is a major risk factor for strabismus at school age (64) and visual spatial perceptual deficits are reported even when such children are 16 years of age (60).

Summary

Infants with bronchopulmonary dysplasia (BPD) can remain oxygen dependent for many months and frequently require hospital readmissions in the first two years after birth. Troublesome, recurrent respiratory symptoms requiring treatment are common even in young adulthood in the most severely affected. Upper airway problems include laryngotracheal stenosis, laryngomalacia, tracheomalacia, unilateral vocal cord paralysis, granulation tissue, and subglottic cyst formation. Nonpulmonary abnormalities are also common and include systemic hypertension resulting from renal damage due to nephrocalcinosis or prolonged umbilical catheterization and use of medications such as systemic corticosteroids. Growth failure and malnutrition in BPD infants are due to decreased nutrient intake, hypoxia, and increased energy requirements. Neurodevelopmental outcome is poorer in infants with BPD, including increased cerebral palsy rates, worse cognitive and psychoeducational performance (especially language abilities and reading skills), difficulties in gross and/or fine motor skills, and lower intelligence quotient and executive dysfunction.

References

1. Jobe AH. The new bronchopulmonary dysplasia: an arrest of lung development. Pediatr Res 1999; 46(6):641–643.
2. Husain AN, Siddiqui NH, Stocker JT. Pathology of arrested acinar development in post-surfactant bronchopulmonary dysplasia. Hum Pathol 1998; 29(7):710–717.
3. Doyle LW, Ford G, Davis N. Health and hospitalisations after discharge in extremely low birth weight infants. Semin Neonatol 2003; 8(2):137–145.
4. Smith VC, Zupancic JAF, McCormick MC, et al. Reshospitalization in the first year of life among infants with bronchopulmonary dysplasia. J Pediatr 2004; 144(6):799–803.
5. Furman L, Baley J, Borawski-Clark E, et al. Hospitalisation as a measure of morbidity among very low birth weight infants with chronic lung disease. J Pediatr 1996; 128(4):447–452.
6. Greenough A, Alexander J, Burgess S, et al. Health care utilisation of chronic lung disease infants related to hospitalisation for respiratory syncytial virus infection. Arch Dis Child 2001; 85(6):463–468.
7. Greenough A, Alexander J, Burgess S, et al. Health care utilisation of prematurely born, preschool children related to hospitalisation for RSV infection. Arch Dis Child 2004; 89(7):673–678.
8. Doyle LW, Cheun MMH, Ford GW, et al. Birth weight < 1501 g and respiratory health at age 14. Arch Dis Child 2001; 84(1):40–44.
9. Greenough A, Alexander J, Burgess S, et al. Home oxygen status and rehospitalisation and primary care requirements of chronic lung disease infants. Arch Dis Child 2002; 86(1):40–43.

10. Greenough A, Alexander J, Burgess S, et al. Preschool health care utilisation related to home oxygen status. Arch Dis Child Fetal Neonatal Ed 2006; 91(5):F337–F341.

11. Panitch H. Bronchopulmonary dysplasia. In: McConnell Ms, Imaizumi SO, eds. Guidelines for Pediatric Home Health Care. Elk Grove Village, Illinois: American Academy of Pediatrics, 2002:323–342.

12. Allen J, Zwerlding R, Ehrenkrantz R, et al. Statement on the care of the child with chronic lung disease of infancy and childhood. Am J Respir Crit Care Med 2003; 168(3):356–396.

13. Ellsbury DL, Acarregui MJ, McGuinness GA, et al. Controversy surrounding the use of home oxygen for premature infants with bronchopulmonary dysplasia. J Perinatol 2004; 24(1): 36–40.

14. Greenough A, Alexander J, Burgess S, et al. High versus restricted use of home oxygen therapy, health care utilization and the cost of care in CLD infants. Eur J Pediatr 2004; 163 (6):292–296.

15. Hudak BB, Allen MC, Hudak ML, et al. Home oxygen therapy for chronic lung disease in extremely low birthweight infants. Am J Dis Child 1989; 143(3):357–360.

16. McLean A, Townsend A, Clark J, et al. Quality of life of mothers and families caring for preterm infants requiring home oxygen therapy: a brief report. J Paediatr Child Health 2000; 36(5):440–444.

17. Greenough A, Limb E, Marston L, et al. Risk factors for respiratory morbidity in infancy following very premature birth. Arch Dis Child 2005; 90(4):F320–F323.

18. Yuksel B, Greenough A. Relationship of symptoms to lung function abnormalities in preterm infants at follow-up. Pediatr Pulmonol 1991; 11(3):202–206.

19. Broughton S, Thomas MR, Marston L, et al. Very prematurely born infants wheezing at follow up—lung function and risk factors. Arch Dis Child 2007; 92(9):776–780.

20. Vrijlandt EJ, Boezen KM, Gerritsen J, et al. Respiratory health in prematurely born school children with and without bronchopulmonary dysplasia. J Pediatr 2007; 150(3):256–261.

21. Gross SJ, Iannuzzi DM, Kveselis DA, et al. Effect of preterm birth on pulmonary function at school age: a prospective controlled study. J Pediatr 1998; 133(2):188–192.

22. Northway WH Jr., Moss RB, Carlisle KB, et al. Late pulmonary sequelae of bronchopulmonary dysplasia. N Engl J Med 1990; 323(26):1793–1799.

23. Vrijlandt EJ, Gerritsen J, Boezen HM, et al., and the Dutch POPS-19 Collaborative Study Group. Gender differences in respiratory symptoms in 19-year-old adults born preterm. Respir Res 2005; 6:117.

24. Radford PJ, Stillwell PC, Blue B, et al. Aspiration complicating bronchopulmonary dysplasia. Chest 1995; 107(1):185–188.

25. Walner DL, Loewen MS, Kimura RE. Neonatal subglottic stenosis: incidence and trends. Laryngoscope 2001; 111(1):48–51.

26. Sisk EA, Kim TB, Schumacher R, et al. Tracheotomy in very low birth weight neonates: indications and outcomes. Laryngoscope 2006; 116(6):928–933.

27. Pereira KC, MacGregor AR, McDuffie CM, et al. Tracheostomy in preterm infants. Arch Otolaryngol Head Neck Surg 2003; 129(12):1268–1271.

28. Tantinikorn W, Alper CM, Bluestone CD, et al. Outcome in pediatric tracheotomy. Am J Otolaryngol 2003; 24(3):131–137.

29. Greenough A, Dimitirou G, Johnson AH, et al. The chest radiograph appearances of very premature infants at 36 weeks post conceptional age. Br J Radiol 2000; 73(868):366–369.

30. Thomas MR, Greenough A, Johnson A, et al. Frequent wheeze at follow up of very preterm infants—which factors are predictive? Arch Dis Child Fetal Neonatal Ed 2003; 88(4): F329–F332.

31. Oppenheim C, Mamou-Mani T, Sayegh N, et al. Bronchopulmonary dysplasia: value of CT in identifying pulmonary sequelae. AJR Am J Roentgenol 1994; 163(1):169–172.

32. Mahut B, De Blic J, Emond S, et al. Chest computed tomography findings in broncho-pulmonary dysplasia and correlation with lung function. Arch Dis Child Fetal Neonatal Ed 2007; 92(6):F459–F464.
33. Aquino SL, Schechter MS, Chiles C, et al. High resolution inspiratory and expiratory CT in older children and adults with bronchopulmonary dysplasia. Am J Roentgenol 1999; 173 (4):963–972.
34. Howling SJ, Northway WH Jr., Hansell DM, et al. Pulmonary sequelae of bronchopulmonary dysplasia survivors: high resolution CT findings. AJR Am J Roentgenol 2000, 174(5), 1323–1326.
35. Abman SH, Warady BA, Lum GM, et al. Systemic hypertension in infants with broncho-pulmonary dysplasia. J Pediatr 1984, 104(6), 928–931.
36. Alagappan A, Malloy MH. Systemic hypertension in very low birthweight infants with bronchopulmonary dysplasia. AJR Am J Perinatol 1998; 15(1):3–8.
37. Melnick G, Pickoff AS, Ferrer PL, et al. Normal pulmonary vascular resistance and left ventricular hypertrophy in young infants with bronchopulmonary dysplasia: an echocardio-graphic and pathologic study. Pediatrics 1980; 66(4):589–596.
38. Kist van Holthe JE, van Zwieten PH, Schell-Feith EA, et al. Is nephrocalcinosis in preterm neonates harmful for long term blood pressure and renal function? Pediatrics 2007; 119(3): 468–475.
39. Schell-Feith EA, Kist van Holthe JE, van Zwieten PH, et al. Preterm neonates with neph-rocalcinosis: natural course and renal function. Pediatr Nephrol 2003; 18(11):1102–1108.
40. Johnson DB, Cheney C, Monsen ER. Nutrition and feeding in infants with bronchopulmonary dysplasia after initial hospital discharge: risk factors for growth failure. J Am Diet Assoc 1998; 98(6):649–656.
41. Huysman WA, de Ridder M, de Bruin NC, et al. Growth and body composition in preterm infants with bronchopulmonary dysplasia. Arch Dis Child Fetal Neonatal Ed 2003; 88(1): F46–F51.
42. Biniwale MA, Ehrenkranz RA. The role of nutrition in the prevention and management of bronchopulmonary dysplasia. Semin Neonatol 2006; 30(4):200–208.
43. Bier JA, Ferguson A, Cho C, et al. The oral motor development of low birthweight infants who underwent orotracheal intubation during the neonatal period. Am J Dis Child 1993; 147 (8):858–862.
44. Bott L, Beghin L, Devos P, et al. Nutritional status at 2 years in former infants with bron-chopulmonary dysplasia influences nutrition and pulmonary outcomes during childhood. Pediatr Res 2006; 60(3):340–344.
45. Korhonen P, Hyodynmaa E, Lenko HL, et al. Growth and adrenal androgen status at 7 years in very low birthweight survivors with and without bronchopulmonary dysplasia. Arch Dis Child 2004; 89(4):320–324.
46. Mendes TB, Mezzacappa MA, Toro AA, et al. Risk factors for gastroesophageal reflux disease in very low birthweight infants with bronchopulmonary dysplasia. J Pediatr (Rio J) 2008; 84(2):154–159.
47. Frakaloss G, Burke G, Sanders MR. Impact of gastroesophageal reflux on growth and hos-pital stay in premature infants. J Pediatr Gastroenterol Nutr 1998; 26(2):146–150.
48. Anderson PJ, Doyle LW. Neurodevelopmental outcome of bronchopulmonary dysplasia. Semin Neonatol 2006; 30(4):227–232.
49. Hintz SR, Kendrick DE, Stoll BJ, et al. Neurodevelopmental and growth outcomes of extremely low birth weight infants after necrotising enterocolitis. Pediatrics 2005; 115(3):696–703.
50. Schmidt B, Asztalow EV, Roberts RS, et al. Impact of bronchopulmonary dysplasia, brain injury, and severe retinopathy on the outcome of extremely low birthweight infants at 18 months. JAMA 2003; 289(9):1124–1129.

51. Kobaly K, Schluchter M, Minich N, et al. Outcomes of extremely low birthweight (<1 kg) and extremely low gestational age (<28 weeks) infants with bronchopulmonary dysplasia: effects of practice changes in 2000 to 2003. Pediatrics 2008; 121(1):73–81.

52. Needelman H, Evans M, Roberts H, et al. Effects of postnatal dexamethasone exposure on the developmental outcome of premature infants. J Child Neurol 2008; 23(4):421–424.

53. Hughes C, O'Gorman L, Shyr Y, et al. Cognitive performance at school age of very low birthweight infants with bronchopulmonary dysplasia. J Dev Behav Pediatr 1999; 20(1):1–8.

54. Gray PH, O'Callaghan MJ, Rogers YM. Psychoeducational outcome at school age of preterm infants with bronchopulmonary dysplasia. J Paediatr Child Health 2004; 40(3):114–120.

55. Majnemer A, Riley P, Shevell M, et al. Severe bronchopulmonary dysplasia increases risk for later neurological and motor sequelae in preterm survivors. Dev Med Child Neurol 2000; 42(1):53–60.

56. Short EJ, Klein NK, Lewis BA, et al. Cognitive and academic consequences of bronchopulmonary dysplasia and very low birthweight: 8 year old outcomes. Pediatrics 2003; 112(5):e359.

57. Lewis BA, Singer LT, Fulton S, et al. Speech and language outcomes of children with bronchopulmonary dysplasia. J Commun Disord 2002; 35(5):393–406.

58. Vicari S, Caravale B, Carelesimo G, et al. Spatial working memory deficits in children at ages 3-4 who were low birth weight, preterm infants. Neuropsychol 2004; 18(4):673–678.

59. Farel AM, Hooper SR, Teplin SW, et al. Very low birthweight infants at seven years: an assessment of the health and nuerodevelopmental risk conveyed by chronic lung disease. J Learn Disabil 1998; 31(2):118–126.

60. Taylor HG, Minich N, Bangert B, et al. Long term neuropsychological outcomes of very low birth weight: associations with early risks for periventricular brain insults. J Int Neuropsychol Soc 2004; 10(7):987–1004.

61. Leslie G, Kalaw MB, Bowen JR, et al. Risk factors for sensorineural hearing loss in extremely premature infants. J Paediatr Child Health 1995; 31(4):312–316.

62. Gray PH, Sarkar S, Young J, et al. Conductive hearing loss in preterm infants with bronchopulmonary dysplasia. J Paediatr Child Health 2001; 37(3):278–282.

63. Adams RJ, Hall HL, Courage ML. Long term visual pathology in children with significant perinatal complications. Dev Med Child Neurol 2005; 47(9):598–602.

64. McGinnity FG, Halliday HL. Perinatal predictors of ocular morbidity in school children who were very low birthweight. Paediatr Perinat Epidemiol 1993; 7(4):417–425.

23

Neurodevelopmental Outcomes of Children with Bronchopulmonary Dysplasia

JOY V. BROWNE
University of Colorado Denver School of Medicine and The Children's Hospital, Aurora, Colorado, U.S.A.

I. Introduction

Since the early studies that documented development in infants diagnosed with bronchopulmonary dysplasia (BPD), a number of significant changes have ensued to alter our perspectives on their neurodevelopmental outcomes. Survival rates of earlier born and medically more complex infants, enhanced technological and pharmacological treatment modalities, utilization of early and comprehensive developmental assessment, and even the working definition of BPD have changed. In 1992, Bregman and Farrell (1) reviewed neurodevelopmental outcomes in children with BPD and stated:

> It appears that the survivor of BPD is at risk for neurodevelopmental compromise, but not necessarily to any greater extent than are prematurely born infants in general. (p. 691)

However, in a more recent review of current research on neurodevelopmental outcomes, Anderson and Doyle (2) stated:

> Children born preterm are vulnerable for long-term cognitive, educational and behavioral impairments but research clearly demonstrates that BPD is an additional risk factor which exacerbates these problems. (p. 227)

Early measurement of neurodevelopmental outcomes focused primarily on neurosensory, cognitive, and motor outcomes; however, a wider perspective on how to evaluate neurodevelopmental outcomes has evolved to include not only those more commonly studied domains but also communication, psychological, socioemotional, learning, executive, and adaptive functioning; in essence, areas that contribute to children's daily activities, learning, and quality of life. The impact of the family's socioeconomic resources and the parent's education contribute to outcomes of these already medically and developmentally compromised infants, further complicating our understanding of how many of these infants fare neurodevelopmentally as they grow into early childhood, school age, and adolescence (3).

Neurosensory outcomes include outcomes such as cerebral palsy, visual impairments, hearing impairments, and intracranial hemorrhage. Cerebral palsy, from mild to severe, is found in a small but consistent proportion of infants born prematurely. BPD is now thought to be a significant risk factor for moderate or severe cerebral palsy. Infants weighing less than 1500 g and who were on oxygen for <28 days have a rate of 3% to 4% of moderate to severe cerebral palsy compared with 15% in infants with BPD who were on oxygen for >28 days (4–6).

Visual impairments include not only poor vision but also strabismus and retinopathy of prematurity. The rates of visual impairments are declining, but still there is an increased incidence for very low birth weight (VLBW) infants. BPD adds an additional risk factor for ophthalmologic problems (7). Similarly, children with a history of BPD have more conductive hearing problems and diminished auditory brain stem responses. The brain stem auditory–evoked responses differ in children with BPD when matched with VLBW infants (8,9).

Neurodevelopmental outcomes that have been typically described for the population of children with BPD include cognitive and psychomotor scores on standardized developmental assessment. Cognitive function is known to decline in the preterm population with decreasing birth weight. As the numbers of infants who develop BPD are now typically the youngest and sickest of the babies admitted to newborn intensive care units, it is consistent for them to have lower cognitive scores than the older population studied in previous years. Cognitive deficits are more common when babies have neonatal complications such as BPD as demonstrated by early developmental testing. In fact, cognitive and motor delays are reported to be more than double that of similar VLBW infants (10) without a diagnosis of BPD.

Many professionals have promoted the belief that developmental delay in the early months and years after initial hospitalization will be overcome as the child grows and catches up with other peers. However, for many of the children with a diagnosis of BPD, problems do not dissipate, and may only be identified and perhaps exacerbated as the child enters the school setting. As the child meets school demands, many cognitive deficits are uncovered that previously had been undocumented or downplayed. In general, children once tested as they enter the school setting, have lower IQs than VLBW children who did not develop BPD. The average IQ for school-age children with BPD in general falls into the low average range (80–90), with approximately one-fourth to two-thirds of a standard deviation or more below average, that is, an IQ below 85. A significant proportion of infants with a diagnosis of BPD have IQ scores indicative of significant cognitive impairment with scores less than 70 (2).

Learning is challenging for most children with a history of BPD. Attention problems that affect a child's ability to attend to, take in, and process information are significantly higher in children with BPD than in children born VLBW. Some studies indicate that in eight-year-old children with BPD, a diagnosis of attention deficit hyperactivity disorder is double that of their VLBW born peers. Children with BPD also made more errors, which suggests that their attention is impaired (11). Associated with learning is the ability to remember. Although few studies are available, indications are that children with BPD have twice as many errors in memory than do children born VLBW. The problems seem most significant for auditory—listening and remembering— and for working memory—holding information in their mind while working on a problem (12). Taylor (13) questions if the number of weeks on oxygen therapy can be correlated with poor memory and learning. Clearly, more research is needed in this area.

Academic performance is similarly affected in children with BPD, with almost half being challenged in particular by reading and math problems. They perform significantly less well than their VLBW peers in reading, arithmetic, and spelling (14), needing additional educational assistance. Up to 50% of children with BPD receive special education in the school setting (11).

Speech, language, and communication deficits are more common in preterm than in term born children. However, having a diagnosis of BPD is associated with more significant speech and language deficits. Singer et al. (15) identified almost half of preschool children with BPD who were significantly delayed in receptive and expressive language. Similar findings for school-age childrens' receptive language were described. Others, finding similar speech and language outcomes, identified significant delays which were double those of children without BPD (7,11). Additionally, 50% of school-age children with BPD had speech therapy when compared with only 20% of their VLBW peers (11,16).

Adverse motor outcomes are more likely in infants and young children with BPD. Early reports of a movement disorder described motor involvement of infants with BPD during initial hospitalization (17,18). Children with BPD develop poorer fine and gross motor skills when compared with their VLBW peers (3,11), and more than 50% of children with BPD are reported to receive motor therapies at eight years of age (19). Some research suggest poorer articulation skills due to oral motor involvement (16).

Visual-spatial skills affect children's abilities to attend to and coordinate motor movements with looking, a particularly necessary skill as the child enters the school system. Up to 30% of children with a diagnosis of BPD perform poorly on visual-spatial testing (20), and difficulties with perceptual motor tasks are associated with BPD (21). Taylor and colleagues documented an association between the number of weeks on oxygen and measures that are associated with optimal visual-spatial perception skills in children with BPD.

Psychological and socioemotional development has only recently been included in neurodevelopmental outcome studies. Issues of attention, hyperactivity, disorganized behavior, social interactions, and psychological adaptation can significantly impact other areas of development. Social and relational challenges can significantly interfere with relationships with caregivers, teachers, or peers, consequently affecting cognition and learning. Internalizing or externalizing behaviors such as anxiety, depression, hyperactivity, or poor attention can similarly interfere with learning, motor development, self-regulation, and self-esteem.

Infants with BPD have been noted to have significant irritability, sleep disturbances, flat affect, poor eye contact for social interaction, erratic or subdued body movement during interactions, and poor relationship development. These behaviors during infancy make the infant difficult to manage medically and pharmacologically, difficult to console, and challenging to interact with, greater than the typical VLBW growing infant (22). The "acquired behavior pattern of BPD" that includes physiological, motor, state, and self-regulatory disorganization (23) is reemerging in this population of infants with BPD to make medical management and caregiving interactions challenging, and significantly impacts neurodevelopmental outcomes as the child grows.

Mental health diagnoses are now being identified more frequently in the population of VLBW children, and in particular in children with BPD. Recent evidence indicates that the incidence of psychological problems in the VLBW infant population is high as they grow into preschool and childhood, and even higher in infants with BPD. More behavior problems have been consistently identified in infants with medical complications such as BPD when compared with their peers (13,24). Up to 75% show hyperactivity (12), and more children with BPD have internalizing symptoms (25). Of great concern are higher rates of diagnosed attention deficit hyperactivity disorder, autism, and schizophrenia in children also diagnosed with BPD (26,27).

Adaptive functioning in children refers to the ability to perform everyday expected activities in the home and community. For infants, these adaptive functions are in the context of typical daily activities such as eating, sleeping, and self-regulation. Early eating behavior and state regulation are typically challenging for infants, particularly if they have had medical/physiological compromise and early hospital experiences that did not lay the foundation for predictable, consistent daily routines.

Early eating behavior is one of the most complex neurobehavioral activities that a young infant is asked to manage in a coordinated way (28,29). Infants with BPD are known to have significantly delayed oral feeding that may reflect poor neurodevelopmental status and predict adverse outcomes. Typical respiratory complications of VLBW infants include delayed coordination of sucking, swallowing, and breathing (30,31), as well as clinically unidentified hypoxia (32). In infants who have compromised respiratory status, coordination of sucking, swallowing, and breathing is exceptionally challenging (32–34). Infants often compensate by using weak sucking pressures to maintain adequate ventilation during feeding (35). Apneic swallows and the swallow-breathe phase relationships involving apnea are significantly increased in infants with BPD over 35 weeks resulting in less rhythmic and predictable coordination of swallowing and breathing during feeding (36,37).

Extremely low birth weight (ELBW) infants who develop chronic lung disease have significantly longer times both to start feedings and to accomplish full feedings (38), reflecting less neurodevelopmental organization during early infancy. Nutrition and eating in infants with BPD continue to be challenging after discharge, and are known risk factors for growth failure (33,39,40), which further impacts neurodevelopmental outcomes.

Sleep cycles and identifiable sleep stability emerge late in gestation and are impacted by both the environment in which the infant is sleeping and the interactions with caregivers and NICU caregiving practices (41). Clinically, infants with BPD are known to have poor sleep cycle development, frequent behavioral arousals, and significant irritability (22,23). Their sleep architecture is different from typical preterm infants with increases in indeterminate sleep, numbers of arousals, and body movements (42,43), and their hypoxic arousal response in quiet sleep is impacted (44,45). Decreased rapid eye movement (REM) sleep has been described in infants with chronic lung disease (43,46), particularly those with severe BPD. Significant time in REM sleep is necessary for neurological organization during this phase of brain development (44, 47–49). Implications for supporting functional sleep organization and increased duration of REM sleep including both environmental modifications to avoid sleep disturbances and insuring adequate oxygen saturations are warranted.

Possible explanations for poor neurodevelopmental organization and outcomes vary with the perspective of the professional who evaluates this diverse group of infants. During early infancy and childhood, neurodevelopment is likely impacted by a variety of factors including medically related procedures and course during early hospitalization, postnatal growth deficiencies, and altered socioemotional and environmental stimulation (50,51). Some attribute neurodevelopmental deficits to disrupted brain growth and development, which would have been significantly different should the infant have had more time in the expected environment of the uterus. Once born, the experience expected by the early born infant is vastly different from a variety of supports for brain growth that would have been available in the womb. Some of these expected experiences include an organized and appropriately timed sensory environment, physiological regulation, motor supports and liquid suspension, and entrained cyclicity of the mother's activity. A vast literature supports the importance of organized and appropriately provided experiences for optimal brain development.

Brain injury has also been proposed as contributing to poor neurobehavioral outcomes associated with BPD. Aside from potential insults such as intraventricular hemorrhage, repeated hypoxic and bradycardic episodes that are characteristic of the experience of infants with BPD may have a cumulative effect on the organization of the brain and ultimately on developmental outcomes (8). However, currently, there are few data to explain complex effects of repeated episodes of hypoxemia on outcomes of early born infants. Scher et al. (52) hypothesized that infants with BPD who have altered sleep architecture, possibly due to frequent arousals during hypoxemic sleep episodes, have abnormal or delayed neurological development. Recently, Wilkinson et al. (8) found impaired myelinization and decreased efficacy of synaptic transmission with measurement of brain stem auditory–evoked responses in infants with BPD. They hypothesized that these neurological deficits are likely attributable to frequent and chronic hypoxic events during early infancy.

Environmental stress may also contribute to hypoxic events. Repeated stressful and painful events for a young infant may bring on an escalation of reactivity and irritability, cumulating in physiological changes that result in further brain insults. Many infants with BPD are described as reactive to sound, bright light, handling, and caregiving procedures, more than would be expected by growing VLBW infants (22,23).

Constitutional factors may also play a role in severity of outcomes for infants with BPD. Although there are not currently adequate explanations of heritability in the development of BPD, temperament and reactivity may be related to a familial trait. What is known about families who experience significant social and economic stress is that as the number of stressful conditions increase, adverse developmental outcomes for infants and children increase as well (53,54). One of the most powerful predictors of developmental outcome is the environment in which the child develops, impacted significantly by the mother's level of education, where the fewer number of years of school are related to poorer child outcome. Consideration for family supports both during hospitalization and after discharge has the potential for influencing neurodevelopmental outcomes in children compromised by both low birth weight and medical compromise such as BPD.

II. Medical Management Changes and Neurodevelopmental Outcomes

In the last 20 years, significant improvement in medical management of ELBW infants has been made with the hope of decreasing the incidence of poor outcomes for infants with BPD. Differences between ELBW infants (<1 kg) and extremely low gestational age infants (<28 weeks) were studied by Kobaly et al. (55); infants were from the period of 1996 to 1999 and 2000 to 2003, respectively. Although there was a significant decrease in cranial ultrasound abnormalities from the first to the second time period, the rate of BPD in the population of ELBW infant's rate stayed relatively the same. Significant neurosensory abnormalities including deafness decreased, but when neurodevelopmental outcomes were studied, no cognitive or overall developmental impairment changes were identified.

Severity classifications of BPD were validated in 2005 by the National Institutes of Health consensus definition of BPD (56). One of the hopes of this classification system was that it would determine the predictive validity of severity of BPD during infancy and neurodevelopmental outcomes. BPD severity successfully predicted poor one-year clinical and developmental outcomes in VLBW infants (57). Additionally, children classified as having severe BPD in the perinatal period had significant cognitive, perceptual, language and visual-spatial deficits and required more school-based special education interventions at eight years of age than did children with BPD who were described as mild or moderately affected (19). Thus, the early classification system may have the potential of leading to enhanced prediction of which infants will need more resources and supports during early development.

Further studies that identify and study medical, technological, and pharmacological interventions to decrease the incidence and severity of BPD are necessary with the hope that better medical outcomes will obtain with better neurodevelopmental outcomes. Other strategies to manage behavioral and physiologic organization early in the infant's life may also contribute to more optimal development. One particular early intervention strategy that has been shown to decrease the incidence and severity of BPD is the Newborn Individualized Developmental Care and Assessment Program (NIDCAP) (58,59). Randomized controlled studies of this comprehensive program of environmental modification, support for physiological, motor, and state organization, as well as enhancing parental confidence and resources have documented significantly fewer days on the ventilator or continuous positive airway pressure, fewer days on supplemental oxygen, fewer apneic episodes, and less chronic lung disease (60–62). Further, brain organization and behavior of infants studied at term, and neurodevelopmental outcomes to five years were significantly more positive in the infants receiving this type of intervention (63–67). This low tech, behavioral organizing and parent supportive intervention may address many of the neurobehavioral challenges that professionals face in caring for the VLBW infant at risk for the development of BPD and subsequent adverse neurodevelopmental outcomes.

III. Conclusion

Over the last two decades, medical, therapeutic, and pharmacological advances have provided significant changes in intervention strategies for infants at risk for developing BPD. With more comprehensive and carefully implemented interventions, it appeared that the incidence and severity of BPD had diminished. However, with these improvements came the survival of more complex and fragile ELBW infants and a subsequent increase of infants with a diagnosis of BPD.

Evaluation of neurodevelopmental outcomes of children has also become more sophisticated and comprehensive, and has expanded to encompass the assessment of complex learning, adaptive and communication needs that face children as they grow into their preschool and school age years. Comparative studies of infants diagnosed with BPD in the 1980s and early 1990s with those born in the later 1990s and 2000s reveal that when compared with their VLBW and ELBW peers, children with BPD fare significantly worse, used more services in the school years, and had more complex needs in almost every neurodevelopmental area studied. Professionals who treat these vulnerable infants and families in the hospital are furthering their understanding of the causes of the development of BPD and developing strategies for medical and pharmacological intervention. In addition, proven NICU early intervention programs that have shown promise in prevention of adverse neurodevelopmental outcomes should be coupled with appropriate medical interventions to maximize the cognitive, perceptual, motor, communication, and visual-spatial outcomes of this vulnerable population. Family programs that support parents to consistently be with their infants, develop strong social networks, ease economic hardships, and facilitate their confidence will contribute to an enriched environment in which infants will grow. Provision of seamless in-home support programs that provide continuity for the recovering infant can improve neurodevelopmental outcomes by enhancing the family's confidence, advocacy, and responsiveness for their infant.

References

1. Bregman J, Farrell EE. Neurodevelopmental outcome in infants with bronchopulmonary dysplasia. Clin Perinatol 1992; 19:673–694.
2. Anderson PJ, Doyle LW. Neurodevelopmental outcome of bronchopulmonary dysplasia. Semin Perinatol 2006; 30:227–232.
3. Vohr BR, Coll CG, Lobato D, et al. Neurodevelopmental and medical status of low-birth-weight survivors of bronchopulmonary dysplasia at 10 to 12 years of age. Dev Med Child Neurol 1991; 33:690–697.
4. Skidmore MD, Rivers A, Hack M. Increased risk of cerebral palsy among very low-birth-weight infants with chronic lung disease. Dev Med Child Neurol 1990; 32:325–332.
5. Vohr BR, Wright LL, Poole WK, et al. Neurodevelopmental outcomes of extremely low birth weight infants <32 weeks' gestation between 1993 and 1998. Pediatrics 2005; 116:635–643.
6. Hintz SR, Kendrick DE, Stoll BJ, et al. Neurodevelopmental and growth outcomes of extremely low birth weight infants after necrotizing enterocolitis. Pediatrics 2005; 115:696–703.
7. McGinnity FG, Halliday HL. Perinatal predictors of ocular morbidity in school children who were very low birthweight. Paediatr Perinat Epidemiol 1993; 7:417–425.
8. Wilkinson AR, Brosi DM, Jiang ZD. Functional impairment of the brainstem in infants with bronchopulmonary dysplasia. Pediatrics 2007; 120:362–371.
9. Gray PH, Sarkar S, Young J, et al. Conductive hearing loss in preterm infants with bronchopulmonary dysplasia. J Paediatr Child Health 2001; 37:278–282.
10. Singer L, Yamashita T, Lilien L, et al. A longitudinal study of developmental outcome of infants with bronchopulmonary dysplasia and very low birth weight. Pediatrics 1997; 100:987–993.
11. Short EJ, Klein NK, Lewis BA, et al. Cognitive and academic consequences of bronchopulmonary dysplasia and very low birth weight: 8-year-old outcomes. Pediatrics 2003; 112:e359.
12. Farel AM, Hooper SR, Teplin SW, et al. Very-low-birthweight infants at seven years: an assessment of the health and neurodevelopmental risk conveyed by chronic lung disease. J Learn Disabil 1998; 31:118–126.
13. Taylor HG, Klein N, Schatschneider C, et al. Predictors of early school age outcomes in very low birth weight children [comment]. J Dev Behav Pediatr 1998; 19:235–243.
14. Hughes CA, O'Gorman LA, Shyr Y, et al. Cognitive performance at school age of very low birth weight infants with bronchopulmonary dysplasia. J Dev Behav Pediatr 1999; 20:1–8.

15. Singer LT, Siegel AC, Lewis B, et al. Preschool language outcomes of children with history of bronchopulmonary dysplasia and very low birth weight. J Dev Behav Pediatr 2001; 22:19–26.
16. Lewis BA, Singer LT, Fulton S, et al. Speech and language outcomes of children with bronchopulmonary dysplasia. J Commun Disord 2002; 35:393–406.
17. Perlman JM, Volpe JJ. Movement disorder of premature infants with severe broncho-pulmonary dysplasia: a new syndrome. Pediatrics 1989; 84:215–218.
18. Hadders-Algra M, Bos AF, Martijn A, et al. Infantile chorea in an infant with severe bronchopulmonary dysplasia: an EMG study. Dev Med Child Neurol 1994; 36:177–182.
19. Short EJ, Kirchner HL, Asaad GR, et al. Developmental sequelae in preterm infants having a diagnosis of bronchopulmonary dysplasia: analysis using a severity-based classification system. Arch Pediatr Adolesc Med 2007; 161:1082–1087.
20. Gray PH, O'Callaghan MJ, Rogers YM. Psychoeducational outcome at school age of preterm infants with bronchopulmonary dysplasia. J Paediatr Child Health 2004; 40:114–120.
21. Taylor HG, Minich N, Bangert B, et al. Long-term neuropsychological outcomes of very low birth weight: associations with early risks for periventricular brain insults. J Int Neuropsychol Soc 2004; 10:987–1004.
22. Vandenberg K, Franck LS. Behavioral issues for infants with BPD. In: Lund CH, ed. Bronchopulmonary Dysplasia: Strategies for Total Patient Care. Petaluma: Neonatal Network, 1990:113–152.
23. Browne JV. Developmental interventions in the neonatal ICU for neonates with broncho-pulmonary dysplasia: acquired patterns of behavior in the infant with BPD. In: Blair M, ed. Developmental Interventions in Neonatal Care. Anaheim, CA: Contemporary Forums, 1996.
24. Robertson CM, Etches PC, Goldson E, et al. Eight-year school performance, neuro-developmental, and growth outcome of neonates with bronchopulmonary dysplasia: a comparative study. Pediatrics 1992; 89:365–372.
25. Gray PH, O'Callaghan MJ, Poulsen L. Behaviour and quality of life at school age of children who had bronchopulmonary dysplasia. Early Hum Dev 2008; 84:1–8.
26. Wilkerson DS, Volpe AG, Dean RS, et al. Perinatal complications as predictors of infantile autism. Int J Neurosci 2002; 112:1085–1098.
27. Botting N, Powls A, Cooke RW, et al. Attention deficit hyperactivity disorders and other psychiatric outcomes in very low birthweight children at 12 years. J Child Psychol Psychiatry 1997; 38:931–941.
28. Hanlon MB, Tripp JH, Ellis RE, et al. Deglutition apnoea as indicator of maturation of suckle feeding in bottle-fed preterm infants. Dev Med Child Neurol 1997; 39:534–542.
29. Medoff-Cooper B, Ratcliffe SJ. Development of preterm infants: feeding behaviors and brazelton neonatal behavioral assessment scale at 40 and 44 weeks' postconceptional age. ANS Adv Nurs Sci 2005; 28:356–363.
30. Gewolb IH, Vice FL, Schwietzer-Kenney EL, et al. Developmental patterns of rhythmic suck and swallow in preterm infants. Dev Med Child Neurol 2001; 43:22–27.
31. Mizuno K, Ueda A. The maturation and coordination of sucking, swallowing, and respiration in preterm infants. J Pediatr 2003; 142:36–40.
32. Garg M, Kurzner SI, Bautista DB, et al. Clinically unsuspected hypoxia during sleep and feeding in infants with bronchopulmonary dysplasia. Pediatrics 1988; 81:635–642.
33. Singer L, Martin RJ, Hawkins SW, et al. Oxygen desaturation complicates feeding in infants with bronchopulmonary dysplasia after discharge. Pediatrics 1992; 90:380–384.
34. Craig CM, Lee DN, Freer YN, et al. Modulations in breathing patterns during intermittent feeding in term infants and preterm infants with bronchopulmonary dysplasia. Dev Med Child Neurol 1999; 41:616–624.
35. Mizuno K, Nishida Y, Taki M, et al. Infants with bronchopulmonary dysplasia suckle with weak pressures to maintain breathing during feeding. Pediatrics 2007; 120:e1035–e1042.

36. Gewolb IH, Bosma JF, Taciak VL, et al. Abnormal developmental patterns of suck and swallow rhythms during feeding in preterm infants with bronchopulmonary dysplasia. Dev Med Child Neurol 2001; 43:454–459.
37. Gewolb IH, Bosma JF, Reynolds EW, et al. Integration of suck and swallow rhythms during feeding in preterm infants with and without bronchopulmonary dysplasia. Dev Med Child Neurol 2003; 45:344–348.
38. Itani O, Kornhauser M, Kirkby S, et al. Enteral nutritional failure is a critical developmental factor in "New" BPD. Pediatric Res 2004; 55:438A.
39. Johnson DB, Cheney C, Monsen ER. Nutrition and feeding in infants with bronchopulmonary dysplasia after initial hospital discharge: risk factors for growth failure. J Am Diet Assoc 1998; 98:649–656.
40. Kurzner SI, Garg M, Bautista DB, et al. Growth failure in infants with bronchopulmonary dysplasia: nutrition and elevated resting metabolic expenditure. Pediatrics 1988; 81:379–384.
41. Graven SN, Browne JV. Sleep and brain development: The critical role of sleep in fetal and early neonatal brain development. Newborn Infant Nurs Rev 2008; 8(4):173–179.
42. Harris MA, Sullivan CE. Sleep pattern and supplementary oxygen requirements in infants with chronic neonatal lung disease. Lancet 1995; 345:831–832.
43. Scher MS, Richardson GA, Salerno DG, et al. Sleep architecture and continuity measures of neonates with chronic lung disease. Sleep 1992; 15:195–201.
44. Garg M, Kurzner SI, Bautista D, et al. Hypoxic arousal responses in infants with bronchopulmonary dysplasia. Pediatrics 1988; 82:59–63.
45. Bhat RY, Hannam S, Pressler R, et al. Effect of prone and supine position on sleep, apneas, and arousal in preterm infants. Pediatrics 2006; 118:101–107.
46. Fitzgerald D, Van Asperen P, Leslie G, et al. Higher SaO$_2$ in chronic neonatal lung disease: does it improve sleep? Pediatr Pulmonol 1998; 26:235–240.
47. Zinman R, Blanchard PW, Vachon F. Oxygen saturation during sleep in patients with bronchopulmonary dysplasia. Biol Neonate 1992; 61:69–75.
48. Sekar KC, Duke JC. Sleep apnea and hypoxemia in recently weaned premature infants with and without bronchopulmonary dysplasia. Pediatr Pulmonol 1991; 10:112–116.
49. Rome ES, Miller MJ, Goldthwait DA, et al. Effect of sleep state on chest wall movements and gas exchange in infants with resolving bronchopulmonary dysplasia. Pediatr Pulmonol 1987; 3:259–263.
50. Kurzner SI, Garg M, Bautista DB, et al. Growth failure in bronchopulmonary dysplasia: elevated metabolic rates and pulmonary mechanics. J Pediatr 1988; 112:73–80.
51. Meisels SJ, Plunkett JW, Pasick PL, et al. Effects of severity and chronicity of respiratory illness on the cognitive development of preterm infants. J Pediatr Psychol 1987; 12:117–132.
52. Scher MS, Steppe DA, Dahl RE, et al. Comparison of EEG sleep measures in healthy full-term and preterm infants at matched conceptional ages. Sleep 1992; 15:442–448.
53. Sameroff A, Seifer R, Zax M, et al. Early indicators of developmental risk: Rochester Longitudinal Study. Schizophr Bull 1987; 13:383–394.
54. Sameroff A, Fiese B. Transactional regulation: the developmental ecology of early intervention. In: Shonkoff JP, Meisels SJ, eds. Handbook of Early Childhood Intervention. 2nd ed. New York: Cambridge University Press, 2000:135–139.
55. Kobaly K, Schluchter M, Minich N, et al. Outcomes of extremely low birth weight (<1 kg) and extremely low gestational age (<28 weeks) infants with bronchopulmonary dysplasia: effects of practice changes in 2000 to 2003. Pediatrics 2008; 121:73–81.
56. Ehrenkranz RA, Walsh MC, Vohr BR, et al. Validation of the National Institutes of Health consensus definition of bronchopulmonary dysplasia. Pediatrics 2005; 116:1353–1360.
57. Jeng SF, Hsu CH, Tsao PN, et al. Bronchopulmonary dysplasia predicts adverse developmental and clinical outcomes in very-low-birthweight infants. Dev Med Child Neurol 2008; 50:51–57.

58. Als H, Duffy FH, McAnulty GB. Effectiveness of individualized neurodevelopmental care in the newborn intensive care unit (NICU). Acta Paediatr Suppl 1996; 416:21–30.
59. Als H. Earliest intervention for preterm infants in the newborn intensive care unit. In: Guralnick M, ed. The Effectiveness of Early Intervention. Baltimore: Brookes Publishing Co, 1996:47–76.
60. Als H, Lawhon G, Duffy FH, et al. Individualized developmental care for the very low-birth-weight preterm infant. Medical and neurofunctional effects. JAMA 1994; 272:853–858.
61. Westrup B, Kleberg A, von Eichwald K, et al. A randomized, controlled trial to evaluate the effects of the newborn individualized developmental care and assessment program in a Swedish setting. Pediatrics 2000; 105:66–72.
62. Fleisher BE, VandenBerg K, Constantinou J, et al. Individualized developmental care for very-low-birth-weight premature infants. Clin Pediatr 1995; 34:523–529. Erratum in: Clin Pediatr (Phila) 1996; 35(3):172.
63. Als H, Lawhon G, Brown E, et al. Individualized behavioral and environmental care for the very low birth weight preterm infant at high risk for bronchopulmonary dysplasia: neonatal intensive care unit and developmental outcome. Pediatrics 1986; 78:1123–1132.
64. Als H, Duffy FH, McAnulty GB, et al. Early experience alters brain function and structure. Pediatrics 2004; 113:846–857.
65. Kleberg A, Westrup B, Stjernqvist K. Developmental outcome, child behaviour and mother-child interaction at 3 years of age following Newborn Individualized Developmental Care and Intervention Program (NIDCAP) intervention. Early Hum Dev 2000; 60:123–135.
66. Kleberg A, Westrup B, Stjernqvist K, et al. Indications of improved cognitive development at one year of age among infants born very prematurely who received care based on the Newborn Individualized Developmental Care and Assessment Program (NIDCAP). Early Hum Dev 2002; 68:83–91.
67. Westrup B, Böhm B, Lagercrantz H, et al. Preschool outcome in children born very prematurely and cared for according to the Newborn Individualized Developmental Care and Assessment Program (NIDCAP). Acta Paediatr Scand Suppl 2004; 93:498–507.

24

Inhaled Nitric Oxide in Premature Infants for the Prevention and Treatment of BPD

JOHN P. KINSELLA
The Children's Hospital and University of Colorado School of Medicine, Aurora, Colorado, U.S.A.

PHILIP L. BALLARD and ROBERTA A. BALLARD
University of California at San Francisco, San Francisco, California, U.S.A.

MICHAEL D. SCHREIBER
University of Chicago, Chicago, Illinois, U.S.A.

I. Introduction

Early reports of inhaled nitric oxide (iNO) therapy in near-term and term newborns with hypoxemic respiratory failure and persistent pulmonary hypertension described marked improvements in gas exchange (1,2), and subsequent randomized trials demonstrated that iNO decreased the need for extracorporeal life support in this population (3,4). iNO is uniquely suited to the treatment of persistent pulmonary hypertension of the newborn due to its selectivity for the pulmonary circulation and the absence of apparent short-term toxicities when used at low doses.

Laboratory and clinical studies have also shown that in addition to its effects on reducing pulmonary artery pressure, other beneficial effects of iNO may include improvements in ventilation/perfusion matching, decreasing lung inflammation and oxidant stress, and favorably modulating angiogenesis and growth in the immature lung. Thus, there is also considerable interest in the potential role of iNO in premature newborns with respiratory failure. However, persistent concerns about potential toxicity have limited the use of iNO in premature newborns to controlled, clinical trials. The results of recent clinical trials have helped to more clearly define the potential role of iNO in the premature newborn with respiratory failure, particularly as it relates to the prevention of bronchopulmonary dysplasia (BPD) (5) and its effects on brain injury. This chapter reviews the rationale for the use of iNO in premature infants, summarizes the results of recent clinical trials and follow-up studies, and describes the proper role of iNO in premature newborns as informed by current evidence.

II. Rationale for iNO Therapy in the Premature Newborn

The rationale for the use of iNO in premature newborns is based on laboratory and clinical studies that suggest important roles for both (*i*) endogenous NO production in fetal lung development and (*ii*) exogenous (inhaled) NO in pulmonary vasoregulation, lung-specific immunomodulation, protection against oxidant injury, and alveolarization. Studies in animal models have determined the developmental patterns for synthesis of endogenous NO in the lung, which provide evidence for a developmental deficiency of NO production in lungs of prematurely born infants. Endogenous NO is produced by three isoforms of nitric oxide synthase (NOS), designated neuronal (nNOS), inducible (iNOS), and endothelial (eNOS); all three isoforms are expressed in respiratory epithelium and likely interact to regulate alveolar development, airway tone, and epithelial immunological activity and response to inflammation and injury (6). In the lung of rats and baboons, expression of nNOS and eNOS, as well as total NOS activity, increase in the second half of gestation and postnatally after term birth (7–9). By contrast, activity of arginases, which compete with NOSs for L-arginine as substrate, is highest in fetal lung and likely contributes to low production of NO (10). Infant baboons delivered prematurely (at the end of the second trimester) are therefore deficient in endogenous NOS production and activity compared with term animals. Moreover, lung NOS activity decreased markedly during the first two weeks after birth as the animals developed chronic lung disease (CLD). The deficiency in NOS primarily reflected the activity of nNOS, which is expressed throughout the lung epithelium from upper airways to the alveolus (11). In a pneumonectomy model, eNOS-deficient mice were markedly impaired in compensatory alveolar and total lung growth, indicating that eNOS is required for normal lung growth under these injury conditions (12). Mice deficient in eNOS also demonstrated abnormal lung structure after exposure to hyperoxia compared with eNOS$^{+/+}$ animals (13). These observations suggest that the use of iNO to prevent BPD represents replacement therapy for a developmental deficiency, similar to replacement surfactant treatment to prevent respiratory distress syndrome (RDS).

After laboratory studies in term-gestation animal models confirmed that the low-dose iNO caused selective and sustained pulmonary vasodilation in the transitional and neonatal pulmonary circulation (14,15); parallel studies showed that endogenous NO modulates pulmonary vascular tone and contributes to pulmonary vasodilation at birth in extremely preterm sheep, and that low-dose iNO (5 ppm) causes sustained improvements in gas exchange and reduces pulmonary vascular resistance during mechanical ventilation of premature lambs with RDS (16,17).

In addition to its effects on pulmonary hemodynamics and gas exchange during inhalation, endogenous NO may regulate vascular permeability and neutrophil adhesion in the microcirculation (18). In premature lambs, low-dose iNO increases pulmonary blood flow and improves gas exchange without increasing pulmonary edema, and decreases lung neutrophil accumulation (19). The effects of low-dose iNO on reducing early neutrophil accumulation in the lung may have important clinical implications because the neutrophil plays an important role in the inflammatory cascade that contributes to acute lung injury and the development of BPD (20–23). Therapies that reduce neutrophil accumulation in the lung in RDS could potentially modify the early inflammatory process that amplifies acute lung injury and contributes to the development of BPD.

iNO may also play a role in reducing oxidant stress in the premature newborn exposed to high inspired oxygen concentrations. In lambs delivered at 130 days' gestation and mechanically ventilated for 5 hours with iNO showed no evidence of lung oxidative stress injury (lung malondialdehyde, reduced glutathione, and glutathione reductase) compared to controls (24), consistent with other studies on the role of iNO in reducing oxidant stress (25–27).

In addition to the acute effects of iNO on pulmonary vasodilation, lung inflammation, and oxidant stress, there is increasing evidence that impaired endogenous NO production contributes to the pathogenesis of BPD. For example, lung eNOS expression is decreased in ovine and primate models of BPD (28,29), and mice genetically deficient for eNOS have abnormal distal lung architecture (30,31). The potential for iNO to modulate the evolution of lung injury in animal models of BPD has been the focus of recent studies, providing further experimental rationale for the role of iNO in premature subjects (32). Lin et al. found that hyperoxia exposure of neonatal rats inhibited lung vascular growth and impaired alveolarization, and that treatment with iNO after neonatal hyperoxia enhanced late lung growth and improved alveolarization in this model of BPD (33). McCurnin et al. studied the effects of iNO in a baboon model of BPD over the first 14 days of life (34). They found that iNO improved early pulmonary function, and favorably altered lung growth and extracellular matrix deposition in mechanically ventilated premature baboons with evolving BPD. In chronically ventilated premature lambs, Bland et al. found that iNO administration preserved structure and function of airway smooth muscle and enhanced alveolar development (35). Thus, compelling evidence suggests that endogenous NO plays a vital role in pulmonary vascular and alveolar development in the immature lung, and that low-dose iNO may have beneficial effects on both the acute and chronic perturbations that are associated with the pathogenesis of BPD in the premature newborn (Fig. 1).

III. iNO Therapy in Premature Newborns with Respiratory Failure

The effects of iNO on the pulmonary circulation in infants with severe pulmonary hypertension were evident in early clinical studies where iNO caused marked improvement in oxygenation by decreasing extrapulmonary right-to-left shunting in term newborns (37,38). Early reports of iNO therapy in a premature newborn with pulmonary hypertension demonstrated marked improvement in oxygenation caused by effective treatment of severe pulmonary hypertension and resolution of extrapulmonary right-to-left shunting (39), as well as other preterm infants with severe respiratory failure (40,41). Subsequently, several randomized, controlled trials (RCTs) have confirmed the acute improvement in oxygenation caused by iNO treatment in the term infant. However, in contrast to the direct pulmonary vasodilator effects of iNO, the focus of the most recently published studies has been on the potential beneficial effects of prolonged iNO administration on lung parenchymal and vascular development (42).

Early case reports also raised speculation about potential adverse effects including intracranial hemorrhage (ICH) (40,41). Such speculation was based, in part, on laboratory and clinical studies suggesting that high doses of iNO prolong bleeding (43–45). Although there is substantial evidence that low-dose iNO may protect the immature lung through various mechanisms described earlier, RCTs have reported conflicting results on its safety and efficacy. However, interpreting the results of these studies is complicated by design bias (e.g., masked/unmasked), the diverse nature of the study populations, and the timing, dose, and duration of iNO therapy in the various trials. The results of these RCTs are reviewed in the following text.

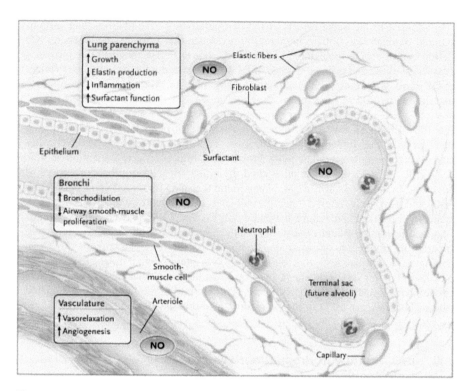

Figure 1 Potential beneficial effects of iNO in the injured premature lung. NO acts in both lung parenchyma and airways to enhance angiogenesis and new alveolar formation, reduce elastin production and promote appropriate distribution of fibrils, decrease the inflammatory response to hyperoxia and mechanical ventilation, transiently improve surfactant function, dilate bronchi, and reduce abnormal proliferation of airway smooth muscle. Animal models of BPD support the proposed effects on alveolar growth, elastin, and airways. iNO acts as replacement therapy for deficient production of endogenous NO secondary to lung immaturity and injury. *Abbreviations*: iNO, inhaled nitric oxide; BPD, bronchopulmonary dysplasia. *Source:* From Ref. 57.

IV. RCTs of iNO Therapy in Premature Newborns with Respiratory Failure

In a small, unmasked, randomized trial of iNO (20 ppm) and dexamethasone treatment, Subhedar et al. reported no differences in survival, CLD, or ICH between iNO-treated infants and controls (46). In a randomized, masked, multicenter clinical trial of low-dose iNO therapy (5 ppm) in severely ill premature newborns with RDS who had marked hypoxemia despite surfactant therapy (a/A O_2 ratio $\leq$ 0.10), iNO acutely improved PaO_2, but did not reduce the incidence of mortality or BPD (47). Notably, there was no increase in the incidence or severity of ICH in this trial, and the incidence of the most severe ICH (grade 4) was 19% for the iNO group and 29% for the control group. The Franco-Belgium study group reported the results of an acute iNO response study (2-hour oxygenation endpoint); however, the brief duration of therapy and a high rate of crossover before the two-hour trial endpoint compromised the interpretation of late outcome measures (48). Hascoet et al. reported the results of an unmasked, randomized trial of iNO in 145 premature newborns with hypoxemic respiratory failure (49). They found no difference between the iNO and control groups in the primary outcome measure (intact survival at 28 days), and no differences in adverse events. As noted by Finer in an accompanying editorial, interpretation of the findings is limited by a relatively high rate of "open-label" iNO use and the lack of important outcomes such as death before discharge and BPD incidence at 36 weeks (50). However, these investigators also studied the effect of low-dose iNO on serum markers of oxidative stress, and found that iNO treatment apparently reduced signs of oxidative stress in these patients (51). Field et al. described the findings of the UK INNOVO trial. In this unblinded study, 108 premature infants with severe hypoxemic respiratory failure were randomized to receive or not to receive iNO (52). There was no difference between the iNO and control group in the main outcome measure (death or severe disability at 1 year corrected age), and no difference in adverse events. Limitations of the study included an 8% crossover to iNO treatment and treatment with other pulmonary vasodilators in 30% of the control group. Moreover, Field describes a lack of equipoise among investigators demonstrated by the observation that 75 infants eligible for enrollment were treated with iNO outside of the trial, leaving only infants with very severe lung disease enrolled in the study (53).

The largest trials of iNO therapy in premature newborns reported to date include the single center study of Schreiber et al. (54), and the multicenter trials of Van Meurs et al. (55), Ballard et al. (56), and Kinsella et al. (57). All of these studies were randomized, controlled, and masked, but have key differences in patient population, disease severity, dose and duration of therapy, and other factors.

Schreiber et al. randomized 207 infants to treatment with iNO or placebo. The main finding of the trial was a reduction in the incidence of BPD and death by 24% in the iNO group. These benefits appeared to accrue predominantly from the subset of newborns with relatively mild respiratory failure (oxygenation index, OI < 6.94). However, in addition to apparent pulmonary benefit caused by low-dose iNO, these authors also reported a 47% decrease in the incidence of severe ICH and periventricular leukomalacia (PVL). Van Meurs et al. enrolled 420 newborns (401–1500 g birth weight) in a multicenter RCT. Although the focus of this study was on premature newborns and the major outcome measure was BPD, the design of the trial was similar to the previous NINOS trial in which term newborns were enrolled and acute changes in oxygenation determined continued treatment with study gas. That is, an acute dose–response study was performed, and only patients who showed significant improvement in PaO_2 were continued on study gas. In striking contrast with other studies, the average duration of iNO treatment was only 76 hours. Overall, they found no difference in the incidence of death/BPD between the iNO and control groups. However, in post hoc analyses, infants with birth weight greater than 1000 g showed a reduction in death/BPD following treatment with iNO (50% iNO vs. 69% control). But a worrisome outcome was suggested in a post hoc analysis of newborns weighing ≤1000 g. This analysis showed an increased risk of ICH/PVL (43% iNO vs. 33% control). However, as noted in an editorial by Martin and Walsh (36), baseline ultrasound examinations were not performed, and it cannot be determined whether these very severely ill infants had ICH before iNO was initiated. Indeed, the severity of illness of infants in this trial of Van Meurs et al. was also markedly different from the study of Schreiber et al. In the Van Meurs trial, the mean OI at enrollment for the iNO group was 23, compared with the median OI of 7.3 in the Schreiber study. This suggests that the degree of illness based on the severity of respiratory failure may be related to iNO safety and efficacy in this population; however, an increased risk of ICH/PVL was not observed in a previous trial of iNO in premature newborns with severe hypoxemic respiratory failure (OI = 30) (31). Other differences between these two trials may offer insights into the disparate outcomes, including the duration of iNO treatment (3 days vs. 7 days), birth weight (839 g vs. 992 g), and gestational age (26 weeks vs. 27.4 weeks). Thus, Van Meurs et al. enrolled smaller, more immature infants with severe respiratory failure who were treated relatively briefly with iNO, making direct comparisons between these two trials problematic.

The results of the two largest randomized, controlled, and masked trials of iNO treatment in premature newborns were recently reported. Ballard et al. randomized 582 premature newborns with birth weights of 500 to 1250 g who required ventilatory support between 7 and 21 days of age (56). Infants were treated with study gas for a minimum of 24 days, and had an estimated OI of 7. They found that the incidence of survival without BPD was increased in the iNO treatment group (43.9%) compared to controls (36.8%) ($p = 0.042$) (Fig. 2). A major finding of this trial was that the benefit of BPD reduction derived almost entirely from the subset of patients enrolled between 7 and 14 days, suggesting that early treatment is important to prevent BPD. There were no differences between the iNO and control groups in adverse events, including medical or surgical treatment of PDA. There also were no differences between the groups in ICH incidence; however, infants were enrolled after the first week of life. Thus, this trial does not help inform the debate about iNO effects on brain injury in the premature newborn.

In the second trial, 793 premature newborns with birth weights of 500 to 1250 g and requiring mechanical ventilation in the first 48 hour of life were randomized to treatment with 5 ppm iNO or placebo gas and treated for 21 days or until extubated (56).

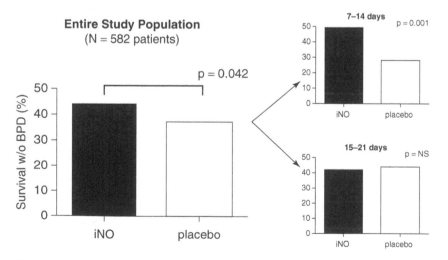

Figure 2 Inhaled NO decreases BPD in mechanically ventilated preterm infants. *Abbreviations*: NO, nitric oxide; BPD, bronchopulmonary dysplasia. *Source:* From Ref. 55.

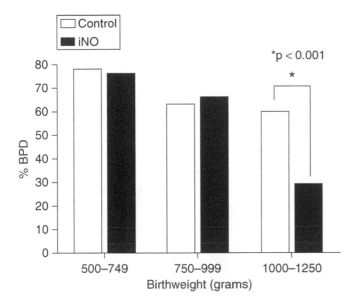

Figure 3 Early inhaled NO treatment of premature newborns with respiratory failure. *Abbreviation*: NO, nitric oxide. *Source:* From Ref. 56.

Overall, there was no difference in the incidence of death or BPD between groups; however, iNO therapy reduced the incidence of BPD for infants with birth weight greater than 1000 g by 50% ($p = 0.001$) (Fig. 3). Low-dose iNO therapy reduced the incidence of PVL ($p = 0.048$), as well as the combined endpoints of ICH, PVL, and ventriculomegaly for the entire study population ($p = 0.032$) (Fig. 4).

INO therapy did not increase the incidence of adverse events including mortality, ICH, PVL, pulmonary hemorrhage, and PDA treatment in any subgroup. In this trial, there was no relationship between OI and brain injury risk, in contrast to the findings of Van Meurs et al. Mechanisms through which iNO therapy might provide neuroprotection in the premature newborn are uncertain and warrant further study. On the basis of laboratory studies, several possibilities exist that include modulation of circulating cells (including neutrophils, monocytes, and platelets) that may occur during NO exposure as they transit the pulmonary circulation. Alternatively, iNO-induced downregulation of lung-derived cytokines may also reduce distant organ injury (58–60). Another possible mechanism may relate to distal delivery of NO or NO-related metabolites through the systemic circulation through red blood cell or protein-mediated pathways (61,62).

V. Effects of iNO on Surfactant Function and Inflammatory Cytokines in Premature Newborns

Previous studies with lung cells in vitro have reported inhibitory effects of iNO on surfactant, including decreased phosphatidylcholine and surfactant proteins (SPs) (63–67). Brief exposure to relatively high concentrations of iNO in several studies of

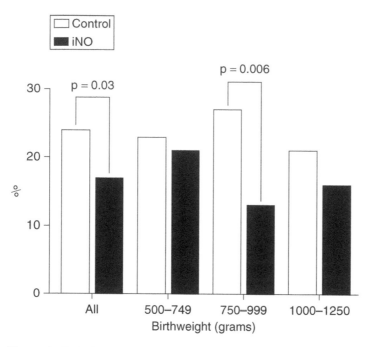

Figure 4 Early inhaled NO treatment of premature newborns with respiratory failure: brain injury. *Abbreviation*: NO, nitric oxide. *Source:* From Ref. 56.

animals caused surfactant dysfunction, decreased SP content, and increased inhibitory proteins in lavage fluid (68,69). By contrast, chronic exposure of infant baboons to a clinically relevant dose of iNO had primarily beneficial effects on surfactant. Although surfactant recovery was slightly reduced, iNO-treated animals had improved phospholipid/protein ratio of surfactant and increased efficiency of SP-B/-C to promote low surface tension (70). As part of the Ballard trial described above, surfactant content, composition, and function were examined in a subpopulation of enrolled infants (71). At baseline, prior to receiving study gas, surfactant function and composition were comparable in the control and treated groups, and there was a positive correlation ($r = 0.43$) between minimum surface tension and severity of lung disease for all infants. Over the first four days of treatment, minimum surface tension increased in placebo infants and decreased in iNO-treated infants ($p = 0.04$ for change from baseline between groups, Fig. 5). There were no significant differences between groups for recovery of large aggregate surfactant and contents of SPs A, B, or C or total protein normalized to phospholipid. On the basis of these findings, iNO treatment of premature infants at risk for BPD does not alter surfactant recovery or protein composition and may transiently improve surfactant function.

NO can have both proinflammatory and anti-inflammatory effects. In the presence of elevated FiO_2, NO is converted to NO_2, peroxynitrite, and other oxides of nitrogen that increase oxidative stress and may initiate or exacerbate pulmonary inflammation. iNO may also modulate the pulmonary inflammatory response by downregulating the

Recovery: Placebo 180±9 µgPL/mg protein (n = 42)
iNO-Treated 178±8 µgPL/mg protein (n = 41, NS)

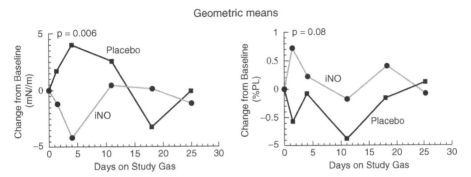

Figure 5 Surfactant recovery, function, and SP-B content in control and treated infants of the NO CLD Trial. iNO treatment did not affect surfactant recovery from tracheal aspirate, transiently improved function (lower minimum surface tension at 4 days), and did not significantly affect content of SP-B. *Abbreviations*: SP-B, surfactant protein B, iNO, inhaled nitric oxide. *Source:* From Ref. 71.

production of inflammatory cytokines (72,73) and by decreasing lung neutrophil accumulation (19,74). Reactive oxygen and nitrogen species increase formation of relatively stable carbonyl adducts of proteins by both direct and indirect oxidation reactions (75). Protein carbonylation can modify protein structure, impair protein function or metabolism, and contribute to disease processes (76). In addition, peroxynitrite modifies proteins (nitration of tyrosine residues), lipids, and DNA and may alter function. Because iNO is coadministered with high FiO_2 into an environment with preexisting inflammation when given to infants at risk for BPD, it is important to consider possible effects of the dose and duration of iNO treatment. As part of the Ballard trial, a subset of 99 infants (52 placebo-treated, 47 iNO-treated), well-matched at baseline, had tracheal aspirate fluid collected at baseline, at 2 to 4 days, then weekly while still intubated during study gas treatment (minimum of 24 days). The fluid was assayed for a panel of inflammatory biomarkers. iNO administration did not result in any time-matched significant change for any of the analytes compared with the placebo-treated group. There also were no significant differences between control and treated infants for concentrations of plasma protein, 3-nitrotyrosine, and carbonylation (Table 1) (77,78).

These laboratory findings indicate that administration of iNO in infants still requiring ventilatory support after the first week of life does not alter tracheal aspirate inflammatory biomarkers or plasma biomarkers of oxidative stress, supporting the safety of this therapy. At present, therefore, iNO therapy to prevent BPD has a high benefit:risk profile. The lack of observed effects of iNO on the various biomarkers, plus the substantial rate of BPD for iNO-treated infants, support future studies of combined therapies to address other components of the pathogenesis of this disease. Potentially, iNO in conjunction with late surfactant treatment or antioxidant or anti-inflammatory agents would further reduce occurrence of BPD.

Table 1 Biomarkers Not Affected by iNO Therapy in the NO CLD Trial

Source	Analyte	Function
Tracheal aspirate	IL-1β	Proinflammatory cytokine
	IL-8	Proinflammatory cytokine
	TGF-β (active)	Anti-inflammatory and profibrotic factor; suppresses surfactant production
	N-acetyl-glucosaminidase	Marker of macrophages
	Hyaluronan	Early inflammatory marker
	α-Epi PGF2	Marker of cell membrane oxidation; mediator of pulmonary hypertension
	Total cells	Inflammatory plus damaged epithelial cells
Plasma		
	Total protein	Indirect indicator of pulmonary edema
	Carbonylation	Protein modification due to oxidative stress
	3-Nitrotyrosine	Protein modification due to oxidative and nitrative stress

Results represent serial determinations during two to three weeks' treatment with iNO or placebo. *Source*: From Refs. 77 and 78.

VI. Follow-up Studies of Premature Newborns Treated with iNO

Long-term outcomes for premature infants treated with iNO are now beginning to be reported. These studies reporting the neurodevelopmental, pulmonary, and health status of iNO-treated premature infants are critical to determining the proper place iNO will have in the treatment of premature infants.

A. Effect of iNO Therapy in Premature Infants on Neurodevelopmental Outcomes

Bennett et al. (79) first reported neurodevelopmental outcomes for the 25 surviving premature infants of a cohort of 42 premature infants treated with iNO in an open, randomized trial of iNO and dexamethasone, initially reported by Subhedar et al. (45). The initial study treated premature infants with iNO for 72 hours, or extubation, and/or dexamethasone. There were no differences at 30 months corrected age in neuro-developmental delay (4/7 vs. 9/14; RR 0.89; 95% CI 0.37–1.75); severe neurodisability (0/7 vs. 5/14, $p = 0.12$) or cerebral palsy (0/7 vs. 2/14, $p = 0.53$) was detected between iNO-treated and control infants.

In contrast, the neurodevelopmental outcomes were significantly better for the 207 premature infants with moderate RDS treated in the Schreiber study (53) as reported by Mestan et al. (80) (Fig. 6). Of the 168 surviving premature infants, 83% were examined at two years corrected age. In the iNO-treated group, 17 of 70 children (24%) had abnormal neurodevelopmental outcomes compared with 31 of 68 children (46%) in the placebo-treated group (RR 0.53; 95% CI 0.33–0.87; $p = 0.01$). Abnormal neuro-developmental outcome was defined as either *disability* (cerebral palsy, bilateral

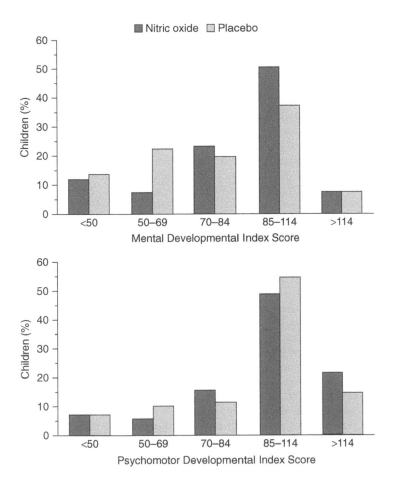

Figure 6 Distribution of scores for the Bayley Scales of Infant Development II. A score of less than 70 on either index indicated impairment. *Source:* From Ref. 80.

blindness, or bilateral hearing loss) or *delay* (no disability, but one score of <70 on the Bayley Scales of Infant Development II). This salutary effect of iNO persisted after simultaneous statistical adjustment for the iNO-induced decrease in BPD and severe intraventricular hemorrhage (IVH)/PVL. Thus, the substantial neuroprotective effect of iNO treatment in this follow-up study appears to be independent of known CNS complications of prematurity.

The improvement in neurodevelopmental outcome in the iNO-treated group in the Schreiber study was primarily due to a 47% decrease in the risk of cognitive impairment [Bayley Mental Developmental Index (MDI) < 70; $p = 0.03$]. In addition to decreasing the number of infants with severe cognitive impairment, there was a nonsignificant trend suggesting that iNO increased the number of patients with scores in the normal range (85–114) compared with infants in the placebo group (Fig. 6). Thus, rather than simply shifting low-functioning infants from the severely impaired group (MDI < 70) to moderately impaired group (MDI 70–84), iNO may have increased the number of children in the normal range. If these findings of improved neurodevelopmental outcomes are corroborated by other studies, iNO will constitute the only postnatal intervention to date that improves neurodevelopmental outcome in preterm infants.

The nonblinded randomized, 34-center trial reported by Field et al. (51) provides little additional data on whether iNO improves neurodevelopmental outcome in premature infants. Premature infants with severe hypoxic respiratory failure (median OI 32) were enrolled only if the attending physician was unsure whether the infant would benefit from iNO (presumably, infants believed by the physician to likely benefit from iNO were treated with open-label NO.) Thus, enrollment in this study was highly skewed toward infants thought likely to die. Unsurprisingly, at one year corrected age, there was no difference in the incidence of death or severe neurological disability (defined as minimal head control or inability to sit or developmental quotient <50) between iNO- and placebo-treated groups.

The follow-up study (81) of the premature infants with similarly severe hypoxic respiratory failure (mean OI 22.5) previously reported by Van Meurs et al. (54) demonstrated similar results to the Field study. At 18 to 22 months corrected age, no difference between groups was detected in the combined rate of death or neurodevelopmental impairment [defined as moderate to severe cerebral palsy, blindness, deafness, or a Bayley Scale (MDI or PDI) < 70]. Of concern, in infants weighing less than 1000 g, the combined incidence of death or cerebral palsy was reported to be higher in the iNO-treated group. However, investigators reported patient outcomes from the time of randomization rather than focusing on only those patients who survived to discharge. Thus, all deaths that occurred during the initial hospitalization were included in the follow-up data set. Evaluation only of children who survived the initial hospitalization, an analysis that can be directly compared with other follow-up studies, demonstrates no significant increase in neurodevelopmental impairment either for the entire study population or in those children who weighed less than 1000 g at birth.

Recently, Tanaka et al. (82) compared the incidence of cerebral palsy in 61 consecutive premature infants (mean gestational age 25.5 weeks; mean birth weight about 820 g) with RDS complicated by persistent pulmonary hypertension over two time periods—1988 to 1993 (pre-iNO) and 1993 to 1999 (iNO era). After 1992, iNO was given to all infants with persistent pulmonary hypertension of the newborn (10–30 ppm). Median duration of iNO treatment was 20 hours. Follow-up exams were performed at three years of age, at which time infants exhibiting abnormal muscle tone in more than one extremity, as well as abnormal movement or posture, were diagnosed with cerebral palsy. In the period after iNO treatment was initiated, the incidence of cerebral palsy was 12.5%, which was significantly lower than the 46.7% observed during the pre-iNO period.

Understanding the true role of iNO in neurodevelopment will require the results of the two largest studies to date, by Kinsella (55) and Ballard (56), as well as those of a currently ongoing multicenter European study. Preliminary results from the Ballard study were recently reported (83). Overall, there were no differences in neurodevelopmental outcomes between the iNO- and placebo-treated groups. It should be noted, however, that the reduction in BPD reported in the initial study was restricted to black and hispanic babies and to those enrolled earlier (i.e., 7–14 days after birth). Such post hoc subgroup analyses have not yet been reported for neurodevelopmental outcomes.

B. Effect of iNO Therapy in Premature Infants on Pulmonary Outcomes

Whether the decreased incidence in BPD reported in some premature infants treated with iNO translates into long-term improved pulmonary status is not yet clear. Hibbs et al. (84) reported on pulmonary outcomes at one year of age for 456 (85%) of the survivors enrolled in the Ballard study. After discharge from the NICU, iNO-treated infants received significantly less bronchodilator treatment (OR 0.53; 95% CI 0.36–0.78), inhaled steroids (OR 0.50; 95% CI 0.32–0.77), systemic steroids (OR 0.56; CI 0.32–0.97), diuretics (OR 0.54; CI 0.34–0.85), and supplemental oxygen (OR 0.65; CI 0.44–0.95) compared with the placebo-treated infants. This report suggests that the improved pulmonary status noted at hospital discharge appears to translate to a decreased requirement for treatments aimed at complications of BPD.

C. Effect of iNO Therapy in Premature Infants on Health Status

At two years corrected age, infants enrolled in the Schreiber study who were treated with iNO had a significantly higher median weight than the placebo group ($p = 0.04$). Furthermore, the iNO-treated infants had significantly higher age- and sex-adjusted z scores for weight ($p = 0.02$). Median height and head circumference were similar between groups. This one kilogram higher median weight persisted through school age, though statistical significance was lost.

To date, no detrimental health outcomes in premature infants treated with iNO have been identified. Hibbs et al. (84) reported no increase in rehospitalizations (OR 0.83; CI 0.57–1.21) at one year post discharge. This was also seen through school age in the Schreiber cohort. Further, Patrianakos-Hoobler et al. (85) recently reported preliminary results for the school-age outcomes of premature infants enrolled in the Schreiber study, and found additional potential iNO-health benefits. They reported a small, but significant, reduction in the number of children with multiple chronic morbidities (e.g., asthma requiring controller medication, failure to thrive requiring nutritional supplements, epilepsy) or technology dependence (e.g., ventriculoperitoneal shunt, gastrostomy tube, tracheostomy).

Thus, the evolving data support the long-term safety of iNO used to treat premature infants with RDS. Whether it will be the pulmonary or neurodevelopmental effects that ultimately serve as the indication for its use remains unclear at this time.

VII. Summary

In order to evaluate whether iNO is a therapy that should result in changing practice in the NICU, one must consider the essential qualities involved in the introduction of a new therapy to clinical practice.

The first consideration is: Is there a significant, untreated clinical problem? Certainly, in spite of therapies that include antenatal corticosteroids; postnatal surfactant replacement; gentler ventilatory methods; and postnatal treatments with steroids, vitamin A, diuretics, and bronchodilators, BPD remains the most severe cause of pulmonary morbidity and mortality in preterm infants. This is particularly true of extremely low birth weight infants less than 1250 g, with 72% of infants less than 750 g having BPD as reported by Vermont Oxford Network data for 2006. BPD is associated with prolonged and expensive ventilatory support and hospitalization, long-term pulmonary complications including asthma, and poor neurodevelopmental outcome. Caffeine has recently been shown to reduce BPD and improve neurodevelopmental outcome; however, the mechanism of this improvement is not understood and most preterm infants already are receiving caffeine as part of their therapeutic regimen. Thus, there is an urgent need for additional therapies for this multifactorial disease.

The second consideration is: Is there evidence for biological plausibility that the proposed therapy will address an aspect of the problem? As discussed above, there is ample evidence from animal models including the baboon, lamb, rat, and piglet that iNO may, in fact, represent replacement therapy in the immature and damaged lung. In addition, treatment may decrease airway resistance, decrease inflammation, improve surfactant function, and improve lung growth and development, and therefore would be expected to be effective in helping to prevent the "New BPD."

The third consideration is: Does therapy make a difference in well-designed, large, clinical trials? The trials as discussed above have demonstrated that (*i*) iNO reduces BPD in infants greater than 1000 g birth weight, (*ii*) in general, less ill infants with a median initial OI of 7.4 or less are the ones who benefit with decreased BPD, (*iii*) treatment within the first two weeks of life—before there has been prolonged exposure to oxidant stress and ventilator volutrauma—appears most effective, (*iv*) treatment of the less ill intubated infants within 48 hours of birth with up to 10 ppm iNO appears to be safe, and in fact, may be neuroprotective. Treatment beginning after 7 days of age beginning with 20 ppm, weaned down to 2 ppm over a 24-day course appears to be safe and prevent BPD in infants between 500 and 1000 g as well as infants greater than 1000 g.

Safety—both short and long term—is the fourth consideration. INO administration appears to be safe in the infants described in the third consideration above. Concern remains about the safety of brief administration of iNO to severely ill infants less than 750 g birth weight, unless the infant has documented pulmonary hypertension. INO has not been associated with any increase in clinical bleeding nor any increase in the common morbidities of prematurity including IVH, PDA, NEC, or ROP. In addition, as described above, in studies on plasma and tracheal aspirates from the NO CLD trial, there has been no evidence of increased inflammation, oxidant stress, or protein modification, and in fact, a transient improvement in endogenous surfactant function in treated infants while they were receiving ≥ 10ppm. Neurodevelopmental outcome through two years of age (discussed above) has also demonstrated the therapy to be safe—and perhaps even beneficial beyond the effects expected with decreased BPD.

A fifth consideration is whether the benefit of treatment is sustained beyond the accepted standard endpoint of survival without BPD at 36 weeks' PMA. In the NO CLD trial, treated infants were more likely to be discharged off pulmonary support at 40 weeks ($p = 0.004$) and significantly less likely to be receiving treatment at one year of age with pulmonary meds including diuretics, bronchodilators, inhaled or systemic steroids, or oxygen therapy.

Finally, evaluation of a new therapy should involve cost-effectiveness considerations. INO is an expensive therapy—however if, as in the NO CLD trial (58), therapy results in significantly fewer days requiring ventilatory support and hospitalization, the therapy (at current US market price) may actually be cost saving (86).

In summary, current evidence supports the use of iNO in infants at high risk of BPD. This includes infants less than 1000 g as well as 1000 to 1500 g who still require ventilatory support at one week of age. Early therapy (with transient exposure up to 10 ppm) of less ill infants (OI < 10) who are intubated in the first 48 hours after birth also appears safe and effective, as well as possibly neuroprotective. We speculate that iNO is a replacement therapy, that is, decreasing airway reactivity and improving lung angiogenesis and alveolarization as in the animal model. Further work is needed to understand the mechanism of potential neuroprotection. INO is appropriate for use in clinical trials in combination with other therapies such as nasal CPAP, superoxide dismutase to reduce oxidant stress, agents to reduce inflammation, and late administration of surfactant to prevent surfactant dysfunction in infants at high risk of BPD. It is reasonable to expect that optimal therapy in a multifactorial disease will require more than a single therapeutic approach and that ideally, by understanding genetic susceptibility of individual infants, therapy may be tailored to the specific infant.

References

1. Kinsella JP, Neish SR, Shaffer E, et al. Low-dose inhalational nitric oxide in persistent pulmonary hypertension of the newborn. Lancet 1992; 340:819–820.
2. Roberts JD, Polaner DM, Lang P, et al. Inhaled nitric oxide in persistent pulmonary hypertension of the newborn. Lancet 1992; 340:818–819.
3. Clark RH, Kueser TJ, Walker MW, et al. Randomized, controlled trial of low-dose inhaled nitric oxide treatment of persistent pulmonary hypertension of the newborn. N Engl J Med 2000; 17:342(7):469–474.
4. Neonatal Inhaled Nitric Oxide Study Group. Inhaled nitric oxide in full-term and nearly full-term infants with hypoxic respiratory failure. N Engl J Med 1997; 336:597–604.
5. Northway WH, Rosan RC, Porter DY. Pulmonary disease following respirator therapy of hyaline-membrane disease. Bronchopulmonary dysplasia. N Engl J Med 1967; 276:357–368.
6. Ricciardolo FL, Sterk PJ, Gaston B, et al. Nitric oxide in health and disease of the respiratory system. Physiol Rev 2004; 84:731–765.
7. Kawai N, Bloch DB, Filippov G, et al. Constitutive endothelial nitric oxide synthase gene expression is regulated during lung development. Am J Physiol 1995; 268:L589–L595.
8. North AJ, Star RA, Brannon TS, et al. Nitric oxide synthase type I and type III gene expression are developmentally regulated in rat lung. Am J Physiol 1994; 266:L635–L641.
9. Shaul PW, Afshar S, Gibson LL, et al. Developmental changes in nitric oxide synthase isoform expression and nitric oxide production in fetal baboon lung. Am J Physiol Lung Cell Mol Physiol 2002; 283:L1192–L1199.
10. Belik J, Shehnaz D, Pan J, et al. Developmental changes in arginase expression and activity in the lung. Am J Physiol Lung Cell Mol Physiol 2008; 294:L498–L504.
11. Afshar S, Gibson LL, Yuhanna IS, et al. Pulmonary NO synthase expression is attenuated in a fetal baboon model of chronic lung disease. Am J Physiol Lung Cell Mol Physiol 2003; 284:L749–L758.

12. Leuwerke SM, Kaza AK, Tribble CG, et al. Inhibition of compensatory lung growth in endothelial nitric oxide synthase-deficient mice. Am J Physiol Lung Cell Mol Physiol 2002; 282:L1272–L1278.

13. Balasubramaniam V, Maxey AM, Morgan DB, et al. Inhaled NO restores lung structure in eNOS-deficient mice recovering from neonatal hypoxia. Am J Physiol Lung Cell Mol Physiol 2006; 291:L119–L127.

14. Kinsella JP, McQueston J, Rosenberg AA, et al. Hemodynamic effects of exogenous nitric oxide in ovine transitional pulmonary circulation. Am J Physiol 1992; 262:H875.

15. Roberts JD, Chen TY, Kawai N, et al. Inhaled nitric oxide reverses pulmonary vaso-constriction in the hypoxic and acidotic newborn lamb. Circ Res 1993; 72(2):246–254.

16. Kinsella JP, Ivy DD, Abman SH. Ontogeny of NO activity and response to inhaled NO in the developing ovine pulmonary circulation. Am J Physiol 1994; 267:H1955–H1961.

17. Kinsella JP, Ivy DD, Abman SH. Inhaled nitric oxide lowers pulmonary vascular resistance and improves gas exchange in severe experimental hyaline membrane disease. Pediatr Res 1994; 36:402–408.

18. Kanwar S, Kubes P. Nitric oxide is an antiadhesive molecule for leukocytes. New Horiz 1995; 3:93–104.

19. Kinsella JP, Parker TA, Galan H, et al. Effects of inhaled nitric oxide on pulmonary edema and lung neutrophil accumulation in severe experimental hyaline membrane disease. Pediatr Res 1997; 41:457–463.

20. Merritt TA, Cochrane CG, Holcomb K, et al. Elastase and α-1-proteinase inhibitor activity in tracheal aspirates during respiratory distress syndrome. J Clin Invest 1983; 72:656–666.

21. Ogden BE, Murphy S, Saunders GC, et al. Lung lavage of newborns with respiratory distress syndrome: prolonged neutrophil influx is associated with bronchopulmonary dysplasia. Chest 1983; 83:31–33.

22. Speer CP, Ruess D, Harms K, et al. Neutrophil elastase and acute pulmonary damage in neonates with severe respiratory distress syndrome. Pediatrics 1993; 91:794–799.

23. Brus F, Van Oeveren W, Heikamp A, et al. Leakage of protein into lungs of preterm ventilated rabbits is correlated with activation of clotting, complement, and poly-morphonuclear leukocytes in plasma. Pediatr Res 1996; 39:958–965.

24. Storme L, Zerimech F, Riou Y, et al. Inhaled nitric oxide neither alters oxidative stress parameters nor induces lung inflammation in premature lambs with moderate hyaline membrane disease. Biol Neonate 1998; 73:172–181.

25. Nelin LD, Welty SE, Morrisey JF, et al. Nitric oxide increases the survival of rats with a high oxygen exposure. Pediatr Res 1998; 43:727–732.

26. Gutierrez HH, Nieves B, Chumley P, et al. Nitric oxide regulation of superoxide-dependent lung injury: oxidant-protective actions of endogenously produced and exogenously admin-istered nitric oxide. Free Radic Biol Med 1996; 21:43–52.

27. Issa A, Lappalainen U, Kleinman M, et al. Inhaled nitric oxide decreases hyperoxia-induced surfactant abnormality in preterm rabbits. Pediatr Res 1999; 45:247–254.

28. MacRitchie AN, Albertine KH, Sun J, et al. Reduced endothelial nitric oxide synthase in lungs of chronically ventilated preterm lambs. Am J Physiol Lung Cell Mol Physiol 2001; 281:L1011–L1020.

29. Afshar S, Gibson LL, Yuhanna IS, et al. Pulmonary NO synthase expression is attenuated in a fetal baboon model of chronic lung disease. Am J Physiol Lung Cell Mol Physiol 2003; 284:L749–L758.

30. Han RN, Babaei S, Robb M, et al. Defective lung vascular development and fatal respiratory distress in eNOS deficient mice: a model of alveolar capillary dysplasia? Circ Res 2004; 94:1115–1123.

31. Balasubramaniam V, Tang JR, Maxey A, et al. Mild hypoxia impairs alveolarization in the endothelial nitric oxide synthase-deficient mouse. Am J Physiol Lung Cell Mol Physiol 2003; 284:L964–L971.
32. Tang JR, Markham NE, Lin YJ, et al. Inhaled nitric oxide attenuates pulmonary hypertension and improves lung growth in infant rats after neonatal treatment with a VEGF receptor inhibitor. Am J Physiol Lung Cell Mol Physiol 2004; 287:L344–L351.
33. Lin YJ, Markham NE, Balasubramaniam V, et al. Inhaled nitric oxide enhances distal lung growth after exposure to hyperoxia in neonatal rats. Pediatr Res 2005; 58:22–29.
34. Mccurnin DC, Pierce RA, Chang LY, et al. Inhaled NO improves early pulmonary function and modifies lung growth and elastin deposition in a baboon model of neonatal chronic lung disease. Am J Physiol Lung Cell Mol Physiol 2005; 288:450–459.
35. Bland RD, Albertine KH, Carlton DP, et al. Inhaled nitric oxide effects on lung structure and function in chronically ventilated preterm lambs. Am J Respir Crit Care Med 2005; 172:899–906.
36. Martin RJ, Walsh MC. Inhaled nitric oxide for preterm infants—Who benefits? N Engl J Med 2005; 353:82–84.
37. Kinsella JP, Neish SR, Shaffer E, et al. Low-dose inhalational nitric oxide in persistent pulmonary hypertension of the newborn. Lancet 1992; 340:819–820.
38. Roberts JD, Polaner DM, Lang P, et al. Inhaled nitric oxide in persistent pulmonary hypertension of the newborn. Lancet 1992; 340:818–819.
39. Abman SH, Kinsella JP, Schaffer MS, et al. Inhaled nitric oxide in the management of a premature newborn with severe respiratory distress and pulmonary hypertension. Pediatrics 1993; 92:606–609.
40. Peliowski A, Finer NN, Etches PC, et al. Inhaled nitric oxide for premature infants after prolonged rupture of the membranes. J Pediatr 1995; 126:450–453.
41. Meurs KP, Rhine WD, Asselin JM, et al. Response of premature infants with severe respiratory failure to inhaled nitric oxide. Preemie NO Collaborative Group. Pediatr Pulmonol 1997; 24:319–323.
42. Abman SH. Bronchopulmonary dysplasia: a "vascular hypothesis." Am J Respir Crit Care Med 2001; 164:1755–1756.
43. Hogman M, Frostell C, Arnberg H, et al. Bleeding time prolongation and NO inhalation. Lancet 1993; 341:1664–1665.
44. Simon DI, Stamler JS, Jaraki O, et al. Antiplatelet properties of protein S-nitrosothiols derived from nitric oxide and endothelium-derived relaxing factor. Arterioscler Thromb 1993; 13:791–799.
45. George TN, Johnson KJ, Bates JN, et al. The effect of inhaled nitric oxide therapy on bleeding time and platelet aggregation in neonates. J Pediatr 1998; 132:731–734.
46. Subhedar NV, Ryan SW, Shaw NJ. Open randomised controlled trial of inhaled nitric oxide and early dexamethasone in high risk preterm infants. Arch Dis Child 1997; 77:F185–F190.
47. Kinsella JP, Walsh WF, Bose CL, et al. Inhaled nitric oxide in premature neonates with severe hypoxaemic respiratory failure: a randomised controlled trial. Lancet 1999; 354:1061–1065.
48. Early compared with delayed inhaled nitric oxide in moderately hypoxaemic neonates with respiratory failure: a randomised controlled trial. The Franco-Belgium Collaborative NO Trial Group. Lancet 1999; 354:1066–1071.
49. Hascoet JM, Fresson J, Claris O, et al. The safety and efficacy of nitric oxide therapy in premature infants. J Pediatr 2005; 146:318–323.
50. Finer NN. Inhaled nitric oxide for preterm infants: a therapy in search of an indication? The search continues. J Pediatr 2005; 146:301–302.
51. Hamon I, Fresson J, Nicolas MB, et al. Early inhaled nitric oxide improves oxidative balance in very preterm infants. Pediatr Res 2005; 57:637–643.

52. Field D, Elbourne D, Truesdale A, et al. Neonatal ventilation with inhaled nitric oxide versus ventilatory support without inhaled nitric oxide for preterm infants with severe respiratory failure: The INNOVO multicentre randomized controlled trial. Pediatrics 2005; 115:926–936.

53. Field DJ. Nitric oxide – still no consensus. Early Hum Dev 2005; 81:1–4.

54. Schreiber MD, Gin-Mestan K, Marks JD, et al. Inhaled nitric oxide in premature infants with the respiratory distress syndrome. N Engl J Med 2003; 349:2099–2107.

55. Van Meurs KP, Wright LL, Ehrenkranz RA, et al. Inhaled nitric oxide for premature infants with severe respiratory failure. N Engl J Med 2005; 353:13–22.

56. Ballard RA, Truog WE, Cnaan A, et al. Inhaled nitric oxide in preterm infants undergoing mechanical ventilation. N Engl J Med 2006; 205:343–353.

57. Kinsella JP, Cutter GR, Walsh WF, et al. Early inhaled nitric oxide therapy in premature newborns with respiratory failure. N Engl J Med 2006; 205:354–364.

58. Viscardi RM, Muhumuza CK, Rodriquez A, et al. Inflammatory markers in intrauterine and fetal blood and cerebrospinal fluid compartments are associated with adverse pulmonary and neurologic outcomes in preterm infants. Pediatr Res 2004; 55:1009–1017.

59. Haynes RL, Baud O, Li J, et al. Oxidative and nitrative injury in periventricular leukomalacia. Brain Pathol 2005; 15:225–233.

60. Aaltonen M, Soukka H, Halkola R, et al. Inhaled nitric oxide treatment inhibits neuronal injury after meconium aspiration in piglets. Early Hum Dev 2007; 83(2):77–85.

61. Palowski JR, Hess DT, Stamler JS. Export by red blood cells of nitric oxide bioactivity. Nature 2001; 409:622–626.

62. Sugiura M, McCulloch PR, Wren S, et al. Ventilator pattern influences neutrophil influx and activation in atelectasis-prone rabbit lung. J Appl Physiol 1994; 77:1355–1365.

63. Bhandari V, Johnson L, Smith-Kirwin S, et al. Hyperoxia and nitric oxide reduce surfactant components (DSPC and SPs) and increase apoptosis in adult and fetal rat type II pneumocytes. Lung 2002; 180:301–317.

64. Haddad IY, Zhu S, Crow J, et al. Inhibition of alveolar type II cell ATP and surfactant synthesis by nitric oxide. Am J Physiol 1996; 270:L898–L906.

65. Lee JW, Gonzalez RF, Chapin CJ, et al. Nitric oxide decreases surfactant protein gene expression in primary cultures of type II pneumocytes. Am J Physiol Lung Cell Mol Physiol 2005; 288:L950–L957.

66. Matalon S, DeMarco V, Haddad IY, et al. Inhaled nitric oxide injures the pulmonary surfactant system of lambs in vivo. Am J Physiol 1996; 270:L273–L280.

67. Salinas D, Sparkman L, Berhane K, et al. Nitric oxide inhibits surfactant protein B gene expression in lung epithelial cells. Am J Physiol Lung Cell Mol Physiol 2003; 285:L1153–L1165.

68. Hallman M, Waffarn F, Bry K, et al. Surfactant dysfunction after inhalation of nitric oxide. J Appl Physiol 1996; 80:2026–2034.

69. Valino F, Casals C, Guerrero R, et al. Inhaled nitric oxide affects endogenous surfactant in experimental lung transplantation. Transplantation 2004; 77:812–818.

70. Ballard PL, Gonzales LW, Godinez RI, et al. Surfactant composition and function in a primate model of infant chronic lung disease: effects of inhaled nitric oxide. Pediatr Res 2006; 59:157–162.

71. Ballard PL, Merrill JD, Truog WE, et al. Surfactant function and composition in premature infants treated with inhaled nitric oxide. Pediatrics 2007; 120:346–353.

72. Kuo HP, Hwang KH, Lin HC, et al. Effect of endogenous nitric oxide on tumour necrosis factor-alpha-induced leukosequestration and IL-8 release in guinea-pigs airways in vivo. Br J Pharmacol 1997; 122.

73. Thomassen MJ, Buhrow LT, Connors MJ, et al. Nitric oxide inhibits inflammatory cytokine production by human alveolar macrophages. Am J Respir Cell Mol Biol 1997; 17:279–283.

74. Chollet-Martin S, Gatecel C, Kermarrec N, et al. Alveolar neutrophils functions and cytokine levels in patients with the adult respiratory distress syndrome during nitric oxide inhalation. Am J Respir Cell Mol Biol 1996; 153:985–990.
75. Stadtman ER. Protein oxidation and aging. Science 1992; 257:1220–1224.
76. Ellis EM. Reactive carbonyls and oxidative stress: potential for therapeutic intervention. Pharmacol Ther 2007; 115:13–24.
77. Ballard PL, Truog WE, Merrill JD, et al. Plasma biomarkers of oxidative stress: relationship to lung disease and inhaled nitric oxide therapy in premature infants. Pediatrics 2008; 121:555–561.
78. Truog WE, Ballard PL, Norberg M, et al. Inflammatory markers and mediators in tracheal fluid of premature infants treated with inhaled nitric oxide. Pediatrics 2007; 19:670–678.
79. Bennett AJ, Shaw NJ, Gregg JE, et al. Neurodevelopmental outcome in high-risk preterm infants treated with inhaled nitric oxide. Acta Paediatr 2001; 90(5):573–576.
80. Mestan KK, Marks JD, Hecox K, et al. Neurodevelopmental outcomes of premature infants treated with inhaled nitric oxide. N Engl J Med 2005; 353(1):23–32.
81. Hintz SR, Van Meurs KP, Perritt R, et al. Neurodevelopmental outcomes of premature infants with severe respiratory failure enrolled in a randomized controlled trial of inhaled nitric oxide. J Pediatr 2007; 151(1):16–22, 22 e11-13.
82. Tanaka Y, Hayashi T, Kitajima H, et al. Inhaled nitric oxide therapy decreases the risk of cerebral palsy in preterm infants with persistent pulmonary hypertension of the newborn. Pediatrics 2007; 119(6):1159–1164.
83. Walsh M, Hibbs AM, Martin R, et al. Neurodevelopmental Outcomes at 24 Months for Extremely Low Birth Weight Neonates in the NO CLD Trial of Inhaled Nitric Oxide To Prevent Bronchopulmonary Dysplasia. Paper presented at: Pediatric Academic Societies, 2008.
84. Hibbs AM, Walsh MC, Martin RJ, et al. One-year respiratory outcomes of preterm infants enrolled in the nitric oxide (to prevent) chronic lung disease trial. J Pediatr 2008; 153(4):525–529.
85. Patrianakos-Hoobler AI, Msall ME, Marks JD, et al. The Effect of Inhaled Nitric Oxide on Medical and Functional Outcomes of Premature Infants at Early School-Age. Paper presented at: Pediatric Academic Societies, 2008.
86. Zupancic JAF, Hibbs AM, Palermo L, et al. Economic evaluation of inhaled nitric oxide in preterm infants undergoing mechanical ventilation. Pediatrics 2009, in press.

25

Vitamin A in the Prevention of Bronchopulmonary Dysplasia

NAMASIVAYAM AMBALAVANAN and WALDEMAR CARLO

University of Alabama at Birmingham, Birmingham, Alabama, U.S.A.

I. Introduction

The term "vitamin A" is the generic term for a group of fat-soluble compounds with the biological activity of retinol and commonly refers to retinol, retinaldehyde, and retinoic acid (RA). The relationship between vitamin A and the lung has been known since the early 20th century. Soon after the discovery of vitamin A in 1913 by McCollum and Davis who observed that the ether extract of egg or butter had a fat-soluble organic substance essential to nutrition in rats (1), McCollum (2) observed in 1917 that animals deficient in "fat-soluble factor A" quite "frequently suffered from prevalent bronchitis." Bloch (3) observed that infants suffering from xerophthalmia frequently had respiratory infections and a higher risk of death and that the provision of milk, cream, and butter could reduce eye disease, promote growth and development, and reduce infectious disease in children. Mori (4) observed histological changes in the larynx and trachea and a high incidence of bronchopulmonary inflammatory lesions in retinol-deficient rats. In 1925, Wolbach and Howe observed squamous metaplasia of the normal mucus-secreting epithelium and occlusion of bronchi with desquamated cells in retinol-deficient rats (5). Research over the past few decades has defined some of the underlying mechanisms for these observations and clarified the critical role of vitamin A in lung development, maturation, inflammation, and repair from injury.

Vitamin A is absorbed from the gut and bound to its transport protein retinol-binding protein (RBP) in the liver, and the retinol-RBP complex is transported in blood in combination with transthyretin (TTR, formerly called prealbumin). Then, retinol is taken up into tissues by a specific membrane receptor and oxidized to its active metabolite RA, and in the retina it is metabolized to retinaldehyde, another active metabolite that helps generate the visual pigment rhodopsin (6). Most (90%) of the body's vitamin A is stored in the liver as retinyl esters. Other major storage sites are the lung and the eye (6).

This chapter will concentrate primarily on the effects of vitamin A in the premature infant and the current research of the key role of retinoids in lung development and in the development of lung pathology. However, preterm infants are not the only neonates who may benefit from vitamin A supplementation. In developed countries, term infants normally have sufficient vitamin A stores and get a sufficient intake of vitamin A either from human milk or from commercial formula. In the developing world, vitamin A deficiency is common in infancy, and vitamin A supplementation has been shown to reduce infant mortality, xerophthalmia, respiratory infection, and gastrointestinal morbidity (7,8). A community-based randomized trial in southern India which infants were given 24,000 IU of oral vitamin A or placebo on days 1 and 2 after delivery showed a 22% reduction in total mortality by six months of age in the infants who received vitamin A (9). The survival curves began to diverge at around two weeks of age and continued to separate until three months of age (9). The impact of vitamin A on survival was limited to infants who were treated before 14 days and to infants of low birth weight (9), suggesting that the effects of vitamin A supplementation would be mostly seen in infants with reduced vitamin A stores at birth. Similar improvements in infant survival with newborn vitamin A supplementation have also been noted in a study in Bangladesh (10).

II. Clinical Research

Benefits of vitamin A supplementation have been demonstrated in preterm infants, and this will be the focus of this section. The fetus accumulates vitamin A in the third trimester, and therefore infants born premature have reduced vitamin A stores (11,12). Preterm infants have lower plasma concentrations of retinol as well as RBP compared with term infants (13,14), which may be secondary to these reduced hepatic vitamin A stores (15). However, there is no direct correlation between serum retinol and gestational age (13) or between liver vitamin A and serum concentrations of vitamin A or RBP (15).

The serum concentrations of vitamin A that indicate adequate "nondeficient" states in preterm infants are not certain but it is usually considered that plasma retinol <0.35 µmol/L (10 µg/dL, 100 µg/L) is associated with reduced hepatic stores and signs of deficiency, while a plasma retinol >0.7 µmol/L (20 µg/dL, 200 µg/L) indicates vitamin A sufficiency (6). It has been suggested that the plasma RBP response (16) and the relative rise in serum retinol concentrations labeled as the relative dose response (RDR) test (17) may be useful in functional assessment of vitamin A stores and may possibly be more closely related to the outcome of BPD than serum retinol (16,17). In a cohort of extremely low birth weight infants who did not receive supplemental intramuscular vitamin A, the serum retinol was 16.2 + 6.2 µg/dL (mean + SD) at 24 to 96 hours after birth and 17.8 µg/dL (7.4 to 63.1; 5th to 95th centiles) 28 days later with 54% having a serum retinol <0.7 µmol/L (20 µg/dL) and 65% with an RDR suggestive of vitamin A deficiency (>10% increase in serum retinol in response to 2000 IU/kg of vitamin A given intramuscularly) (18).

The topic of vitamin A supplementation to prevent mortality and short- and long-term morbidity in very low birth weight infants has been subject to an excellent Cochrane systematic review by Darlow and Graham (12). In this review, randomized or quasi-randomized studies of the effect of vitamin A supplementation on survival, BPD, and vitamin A concentrations in very low birth weight infants were evaluated. Fifteen potentially relevant trials were identified of which eight met eligibility criteria and were included in this systematic review (12). The eight included studies reported outcomes on 653 infants treated with vitamin A and 638 controls. Overall, there was no significant reduction in neonatal death [relative risk (RR) 0.86 (95% CI 0.66–1.11); risk difference (RD) –0.02 (95% CI –0.06, 0.02)] or death before 36 weeks' postmenstrual age (12).

The combined outcome of death or oxygen use at 36 weeks' postmenstrual age using pooled data showed a reduction that reached statistical significance [RR 0.91 (0.82–1.00), RD –0.06 (–0.12, 0.00), number needed to treat (NNT) 17 (8, 1000+)]. Trends were also noted for a reduction in retinopathy of prematurity [RR 0.85 (0.68–1.06), RD –0.10 (–0.24 to 0.03)] and sepsis [RR 0.89 (0.76–1.05), RD –0.05 (–0.11 to 0.02)] (12). The largest randomized trial included in the Cochrane review (12) was the study by Tyson et al. (18) from the NICHD Neonatal Research Network, which will be described further.

Tyson et al. (18) performed a multicenter, blinded, randomized trial to assess the effectiveness and safety of this regimen as compared with sham treatment in 807 extremely low birth weight infants (ELBW; 401–1000 g) in need of respiratory support 24 hours after birth. Infants were enrolled 24 to 96 hours after birth. The mean birth weight was 770 g in the vitamin A group and 769 g in the control group, and the respective gestational ages were 26.8 and 26.7 weeks. Vitamin A was given intramuscularly in view of its poor enteral absorption and unreliable delivery in crystalloid solutions. A dose of 5000 IU (0.1 mL) was given on Monday, Wednesdays, and Fridays for four weeks. The primary outcome of death or chronic lung disease at 36 weeks' postmenstrual age occurred in fewer infants in the vitamin A group than in the control group (55% vs. 62%; RR 0.89; 95% CI 0.80–0.99) for an NNT of 1 additional infant who survived without chronic lung disease for every 14 to 15 infants who received vitamin A supplementation. The mortality rates were similar in the two groups, and the difference in the primary outcome was due to fewer infants with chronic lung disease in the vitamin A group (47% vs. 56%, RR 0.85; 95% CI 0.73–0.98) (18). In addition, nonsignificant trends were noted toward reduced risks of sepsis (RR 0.91; 95% CI 0.77–1.07, $p = 0.25$), intracranial hemorrhage (RR 0.93; 95% CI 0.80–1.09, $p = 0.39$), and periventricular leukomalacia (RR 0.74; 95% CI 0.44–1.25, $p = 0.26$), providing reassurance for possible additional benefit rather than harm. There was no evidence of vitamin A toxicity due to this regimen in this study (18). Serum vitamin A was measured at baseline and at 28 days in the first 300 infants. On study day 28, RDR was evaluated by first collecting a blood sample, administration of a dose of 2000 IU/kg body weight, and obtaining a second blood sample three hours later. Fewer infants in the vitamin A group than in the control group had low retinol concentrations (below 20 µg/dL or 0.70 µmol/ L) on day 28 (25% vs. 54%, $p < 0.001$). An RDR >10%, suggesting low vitamin A status, was found in 22% of infants in the vitamin A group and 45% of infants in the control group ($p < 0.001$).

An evaluation of the neurodevelopmental outcome at 18 to 22 months of age of the infants enrolled in the study of Tyson et al. (18) was reported by Ambalavanan et al. (19). Five-hundred seventy-nine (88%) of the 658 surviving infants were followed up. The primary outcome of neurodevelopmental impairment (NDI) or death could be determined for 687 of 807 randomized infants (85%). Baseline characteristics and predischarge and postdischarge mortality were comparable in both study groups. NDI or death by 18 to 22 months occurred in 190 of 345 (55%) infants in the vitamin A group and in 204 of 342 (60%) of the control group (RR: 0.94; 95% CI 0.80–1.07). RRs for low MDI, low PDI, and CP were also <1.0. Although the change in NDI or death did not reach statistical significance, it should be noted that the study by Tyson et al. (18) was not powered to evaluate small magnitudes of change in long-term outcome.

Despite the data from many studies that have documented a reduction in vitamin A stores and concentrations in extremely preterm infants and the benefit that may be obtained with supplementation, many centers do not currently routinely supplement vitamin A (20). A survey of all ($n = 102$) neonatal-perinatal training program directors (TPD) and 105 randomly selected directors of level III neonatal intensive care units (nontraining program directors, NTPD) was done to evaluate the attitudes and practices among level III NICUs in the United States regarding vitamin A supplementation for ELBW infants (20). Ninety-nine percent of TPD and 94% of NTPD responded. In a minority of programs (20% TPD, 13% NTPD), >90% of eligible extremely low birth weight neonates were supplemented with vitamin A, whereas in most programs (69% TPD, 82% NTPD), routine supplementation was not practiced. Infants in most centers (91% TPD, 81% NTPD) were supplemented vitamin A using a dose of 5000 IU intramuscularly three times per week for four weeks as used by Tyson et al. (18). The most common reason that TPD gave for not supplementing vitamin A is the perceived small benefit, whereas the most common reason for NTPD was that they considered the intervention unproven. These findings indicate inconsistency in practicing evidence-based medicine in neonatal practice, in which therapies are often administered on the basis of weaker evidence of safety and benefit than supports vitamin A supplementation. For example, prevention of one case of early onset group B streptococcal sepsis would need exposure of 250 infants to antibiotics in the intrapartum period and prevention of hemorrhagic disease of the newborn in one infant requires exposure of at least 2000 infants to vitamin K (18). Educational interventions may be required to endorse the benefits and safety of vitamin A supplementation.

It is of interest that 25% of infants in the vitamin A group in the study by Tyson et al. (18) had biochemical evidence of vitamin A deficiency at 28 days despite supplementation. Therefore, it was considered possible that higher doses would reduce the incidence of vitamin A deficiency. In addition, as vitamin A is stored in the liver, it was thought that once-a-week administration may lead to similar serum vitamin A concentrations and magnitude of storage and reduce the need for intramuscular injections three times a week. It was hypothesized that compared with the standard regimen of 5000 IU three times per week for four weeks, (1) a higher dose (10,000 IU 3 × per week) would increase serum retinol and RBP and lower RDRs, and (2) once-per-week dosing (15,000 IU once per week) would lead to equivalent levels, RBP, and RDR. To test these hypotheses, a randomized trial was performed in which extremely low birth weight neonates ($n = 120$) receiving O_2/mechanical ventilation at 24 hours were randomly assigned to (1) standard, (2) higher-dose, or (3) once-per-week regimens (21). Measures of vitamin A deficiency were serum retinol <20 µg/dL, RBP <2.5 mg/dL, and/or RDR >10% on day 28. BPD was defined as O_2/mechanical ventilation at 36 weeks' postmenstrual age. Groups were similar at enrollment (median gestational age, 25 weeks; birth weight, 689 g). Possible toxicity was seen in <5%. The higher dose regimen did not increase retinol or RBP, decrease RDR, or improve outcomes. Infants in the once-per-week regimen had lower retinol levels and higher RDR without an effect on outcomes. Therefore, compared with the standard regimen of 5000 IU three times a week for four weeks, once-per-week dosing worsened and higher doses did not reduce vitamin A deficiency (21).

Vitamin A deficiency reduces RBP but not transthyretin (TTR), while inflammation reduces both RBP and TTR and increases C-reactive protein (CRP), an acute phase reactant. In the trial described earlier in which different vitamin A regimens were evaluated (21), serum RBP, TTR, and CRP were measured in 79 ELBW infants at 28 days (22). The area under the curve (AUC) of the receiver operating characteristic curve analysis evaluated the predictive value of TTR, the RBP/TTR ratio, and CRP for death/ BPD at 36 weeks. It was observed that TTR correlated inversely with CRP ($r = -0.45$, $p < 0.0001$), consistent with TTR being a negative acute phase reactant, and that a higher RBP/TTR ratio predicted death/BPD (AUC 0.68 (CI 0.57–0.78)). The lower TTR and maintained RBP/TTR ratios suggest inflammation rather than vitamin A deficiency as the cause for lower serum vitamin A levels in ELBW infants (22). It is possible that these lower serum vitamin A concentrations in turn accentuate lung injury and predispose to further inflammation and a vicious cycle of additional lowering of vitamin A transport proteins and available vitamin A leading to greater inflammation. Further research is required into the relationship between biochemical vitamin A status, mediators of inflammation, and clinical status.

Most studies have evaluated the use of intramuscular vitamin A but some have also evaluated enteral administration, although vitamin A absorption is possibly less efficient using the enteral route. Rush et al. (23) compared the same dose of vitamin A given intramuscularly as given enterally and found higher mean plasma vitamin A concentrations in those given intramuscular vitamin A. Landman et al. (24) found that a dose of 5000 IU given daily enterally with the early introduction of feeds was comparable to 2000 IU given intramuscularly on alternate days. However, one limitation of enteral supplementation is that many clinicians may be reluctant to provide enteral vitamin A supplementation starting soon after birth, especially if the ELBW infants are not being fed. There is some preliminary evidence that vitamin A can be administered mixed with intravenous lipid emulsions (25,26), and it is possible that one may reduce the need for intramuscular vitamin A supplementation by initially supplementing vitamin A with parenteral nutrition by admixture with the intravenous lipid emulsions, and subsequently supplementing vitamin A with enteral feeds (at a higher dose than with the intramuscular route) when enteral feeds are tolerated. However, randomized trials are required to evaluate this approach and compare its results with standard intramuscular supplementation.

III. Basic Research

Vitamin A (retinol) and its metabolite (RA) play important roles in the development and maturation of the lung as well as for the maintenance of lung alveoli (27). Vitamin A is necessary for the regulation of the proliferation and differentiation of many cell types and in maintaining the integrity of epithelial surfaces. Vitamin A is also necessary for the formation of retinal pigments and in maintenance of immunocompetence.

Vitamin A or its precursor (β-carotene) are obtained from the diet or in the form of supplementation (usually intramuscular) given to preterm infants. Retinol circulates in the blood bound to RBP, and when transferred to cells, is bound to a cytoplasmic protein cellular retinol–binding protein (CRBP-I and CRBP-II) that facilitates its conversion to retinal and then to RA (27). RA is then bound to cellular retinoic acid–binding protein (CRABP-I and CRABP-II). RA enters the nucleus and then binds to nuclear transcription factors to change gene activity. The cellular effects of RA are mediated through the action of two classes of nuclear receptors, the retinoic acid receptors (RARs; activated by all-*trans*-RA and 9-*cis*-RA) and the retinoid X receptors (RXRs; activated by 9-*cis*-RA only) (28,29). RARs are of three major subtypes, α, β, and γ, of which there are numerous isoforms created by alternative splicing and differential promoter usage (28,30). RARs form heterodimers with RXRs and act as ligand-activated transcription factors to regulate downstream gene expression. RXRs can act as homodimers or heterodimers with a variety of orphan receptors such as peroxisome proliferator–activated receptor (28,29). Therefore, complexity in the retinoid signaling system arises from a combination of several forms of RA, multiple cytoplasmic binding proteins and nuclear receptors, and the existence of polymorphic RA response elements (30). Additional diversity occurs by heterodimeric interactions between the RAR and RXR receptors and between nuclear RA receptors and other members of the nuclear receptor superfamily (30).

A. Retinoids in Normal Lung Development

Lung development in humans occurs through a series of developmental stages from the embryonic phase (3–7 weeks), followed by the pseudoglandular phase (7–16 or 17 weeks), the canalicular phase (16 or 17–24 or 27 weeks), the saccular phase (24 or 27–36 weeks), and finally, the alveolar phase (36 weeks onward). The age of change from one stage to another may vary between individuals. The same stages are seen in other mammals although their durations vary. Rodents such as rats and mice have alveolar development that is entirely postnatal (31), which make them good animal models to study lung development. In general, lung development of rodents from birth through the first two weeks of life corresponds to human lung development in the third trimester through the second year of life, the period of greatest interest in research on BPD.

Retinoids are critical mediators of lung development. Morphological analysis of vitamin A–deficient rat fetuses and of retinoic acid receptor (RAR and RXR) mutant mice have demonstrated that RA is essential for lung development (32). Mollard et al. investigated the effects of RA and of a pan-RAR antagonist in cultures of whole embryos and lung explants and noted that retinoid signaling is essential for the formation of primary lung buds and the esophagotracheal septum from the primitive foregut (32). At the pseudoglandular stage, RA signaling through RXR-β, but not RAR-γ, inhibited distal bud formation thereby promoting the formation of conducting airways. In addition, it was seen that the level of CRBP-I in the pseudoglandular lung participated in the control of branching morphogenesis (32). Both RBPs and RAR isoforms are temporally regulated and found within the alveolar septal regions during alveologenesis (28). Alveoli form primarily by septation of saccules, and therefore, it is necessary to consider the factors regulating the formation of alveolar septae. The role of retinoids in the generation and repair of alveoli has been reviewed by McGowan (33). A more general review of control mechanisms of alveolar development and disorders of these control mechanisms in BPD has been performed by Bourbon et al. (34). The septae are composed of alveolar epithelial and endothelial cells, fibroblasts, and a few other (e.g., neuroendocrine, immune) cells (33). Vaccaro and Brody studied the ultrastructural features of postnatal alveolar septal formation in rats from birth to 28 days of age (35). At birth, the rat lung consists of large thick-walled saccules and a cellular interstitium. Interstitial cells have large oval nuclei with scant cytoplasm containing few organelles and scattered lipid droplets. New alveolar septae form between 5 and 15 days of age with thinning of saccular walls. Two types of interstitial fibroblasts are present: one noted at the tips of newly formed septa with myofibroblast characteristics and elastin deposits; the other fibroblast at the base of new septa, filled with lipid and few other cytoplasmic organelles (35). After 15 days of age, alveolar walls become thinner, few new septa form, and interstitial fibroblasts begin to resemble the dormant type of fibroblasts seen at birth. Thus, the process of postnatal alveolarization of lung parenchyma involves differentiation of the interstitial fibroblast and elastogenesis (35). During the second postnatal week, the lipid-laden interstitial fibroblast (LIF) subpopulation may comprise up to 25% of alveolar cells (33). These lipids are primarily neutral lipids and also include retinyl esters. Retinyl esters are most abundant at late gestation and reduce in amount during the phase of alveolarization, accompanied by an increase in the retinol and RA content of the cells (33,36). The utilization of vitamin A stores in the developing lung appears to be independent of the liver stores of vitamin A (36).

Retinoid supplementation increases elastin production by cultured LIF and lung explants (33). McGowan et al. studied mice bearing specific RAR and RXR gene deletions to evaluate the relationships between retinoids and elastin. RAR-β and RAR- γ increase at birth, when the LIF RA content is maximal. The changes in RAR-γ parallel the change in RA, suggesting that RA may signal through RAR-γ. RAR-γ null mice demonstrate reduced alveolar numbers and surface area, increased static compliance, and decreased carbon monoxide diffusion compared with wild-type mice. RAR-γ null mice, which are heterozygote for the RXR-α deletion (RAR-$\gamma^{-/-}$, RXR-$\alpha^{+/-}$), show a reduced elastin gene expression in the LIF as well as decreased lung elastin in alveolar septae (not in airway or vascular walls) with even fewer alveoli and alveolar surface area than RAR-γ null mice (33,37). Therefore, it appears that elastin is one of the key genes in alveolar development and that it is regulated by retinoids. Other key genes that may be involved in lung development and regulated by retinoids are those of the growth factors such as vascular endothelial growth factor (VEGF), platelet derived growth factor (PDGF), and transforming growth factor-beta (TGF-β). It has been shown that prenatal administration of vitamin A increases VEGF in the mouse model (38), and there is some evidence that RA may increase VEGF gene transcription through Sp1 and Sp3 sites in some lung cell lines (39). PDGF is also known to have RA-responsive elements (RARE) (40), and RA upregulates PDGF ligand and receptor expression in neonatal lung fibroblasts (41). RA may stimulate lung development through increasing the expression levels of PDGF-A mRNA and protein (42). RA is known to inhibit TGF-β effects in the lung, ranging from the initial formation of the lung bud (43) to the production of collagen by fibroblasts (44). The balance between TGF-β and RA mediated effects may regulate alveolar septation.

B. Retinoids in Lung Inflammation, Injury, and Repair

Hyperoxia-induced inhibition of alveolarization in newborn mice or rats is often used as an experimental model of BPD. Veness-Meehan et al. (45) showed in a newborn rat hyperoxia model that RA did not initially improve septal formation or decrease airspace size in animals exposed to hyperoxia alone or to hyperoxia plus dexamethasone. However, a late improvement in alveolar septal formation was noted without any effects on elastin expression (46). There was a trend toward increased survival in hyperoxia in animals treated with RA to the extent that combined therapy with RA and dexamethasone resulted in the greatest improvement in animal survival (45). In support of this observation, Garber et al. (47) observed that combined treatment with RA and dexamethasone improved gas exchange and alveolar septation. The exact mechanism by which RA mediates effects during hyperoxia and other models of lung inflammation remain under investigation, and possible mechanisms include cytochrome P450 enzyme regulation (48), modulation of RA pathways such as reduction of CRABP-I and RAR-γ2 by inflammation-induced cytokines such as IL-1β (49). Cho et al. (50) showed that in newborn mice treated with an angiogenesis inhibitor (SU1498), which attenuates alveolar development, RA supplementation maintained mean alveolar volume, alveolar surface area, and endothelial cell volume density. RA also increased the proliferation of human fetal lung capillary endothelial precursor cells in vitro. These results suggest that RA supports the maintenance or growth of the endothelial cell population of the distal lung, permitting postnatal alveolar cell development (50). Pierce et al. evaluated the effects of retinoid supplementation on alveolar elastin expression and deposition and angiogenesis-related signaling in a primate model of BPD (51). It was observed that vitamin A supplementation increased lung elastin expression specifically in alveolar myofibroblasts within alveolar walls but failed to alter morphology or the reduction in angiogenesis genes [VEGF-A, fms-related tyrosine kinase 1 (Flt-1), and tyrosine kinase with immunoglobulin-like and EGF-like domains 1 (TIE-1)] secondary to premature delivery and mechanical ventilation (51). These results suggest that the benefit observed among premature infants receiving retinoid supplementation may not be mediated through enhanced alveolar development but through other mechanisms. However, as previously noted in the section on clinical research, it is possible that part of the insufficient response to vitamin A in this model may be due to inflammation reducing vitamin A transport to the lung, resulting in a state of relative deficiency of vitamin A in the lung despite supplementation. A recent observation is that the combination of vitamin A and RA is able to increase retinol uptake and lung retinyl ester in a synergistic manner in neonatal rats (52) even during concurrent dexamethasone therapy (53). Current studies are under way to determine if this synergistic increase in lung retinyl ester content has functional effects on the reduction of lung injury in newborn animal models. In the preterm sheep model, Bland et al. (54) have shown that preterm lambs that were mechanically ventilated for three weeks demonstrated better alveolar development and capillary development with retinol supplementation as well as a reduction in excessive elastin deposition and an increase in VEGF and its receptor (flk-1). Differences between the primate and sheep models may be due to interspecies differences in alveolar development as well as other differences in methods.

It is possible that the developing alveolus is "plastic" in the sense that degradation of elastin and perhaps other extracellular matrix proteins in the developing alveolar septum by inflammatory stimuli or excessive stretch may lead to a lowering of the height or loss of the alveolar septum, and thereby indicate a reduction in the number of alveoli as the "alveolar ring" at the mouth of the alveolus drops back into the interstitium (as opposed to emphysema, where there is breakdown of preexisting septae). Retinoids may inhibit this breakdown of matrix proteins in the alveolar ring and thereby preserve alveolar structure during stress. That such a mechanism may be present is suggested by studies indicating that RA attenuates cytokine-driven fibroblast degradation of extracellular matrix (55) and can inhibit elastase-induced injury in human epithelial cell lines (56).

There is some evidence that RA may be able to reverse elastase-induced pulmonary emphysema in rats (57), with some improvement in lung function and density measurement on high-resolution computed CT scanning (58). However, benefits of RA in other rat models (59) and in adult mouse models of elastase-induced emphysema have not been noted (60), indicating that model characteristics, strain differences, and species may possibly be important. Provocative research indicating that RA supplementation may induce alveolar regeneration in the adult mouse lung (61) suggests that induction of alveolar regeneration with RA may be a possible therapeutic approach. Before clinical trials of RA for alveolar regeneration are attempted in preterm infants, preliminary safety and tolerability will have to be established as RA also controls the development and maturation of other organ systems such as the central nervous system. Any clinical trials that are performed will need careful monitoring of long-term outcomes that will indicate the safety and benefit of RA supplementation.

IV. Summary and Future Directions

In summary, vitamin A is a critical regulator of lung development, maturation, inflammation, and repair. Preterm infants are deficient in vitamin A and term infants may be only marginally sufficient. Vitamin A deficiency may accentuate lung injury and attenuate normal alveolar development, thereby increasing the risk of BPD. Supplementation of vitamin A has been shown to significantly reduce BPD or death in extremely low birth weight infants but many infants demonstrate biochemical vitamin A deficiency despite supplementation, perhaps due to inadequate vitamin A transport. A better understanding of how vitamin A regulates alveolar development and lung inflammation, and evaluation of methods to improve vitamin A transport to the lungs may help optimize vitamin A prophylaxis and therapy for the reduction of BPD. Research is required into the safety and efficacy of RA supplementation for the maintenance, induction of repair, or regeneration of alveoli in the setting of respiratory distress syndrome and BPD.

References

1. McCollum EV, Davis M. The necessity of certain lipins in the diet during growth. J Biol Chem 1913; 15(1):167–175.
2. McCollum EV. The supplementary dietary relationship among our natural foodstuffs. J Am Med Assoc 1917; 68:1379–1386.
3. Bloch CE. Blindness and other diseases in children arising from deficient nutrition (lack of fat soluble A factor). Am J Dis Child 1924; 27:139–148.
4. Mori S. The changes in the para-ocular glands which follow the administration of diets low in fat-soluble vitamin A; with notes of the effect of the same diets on salivary glands and the mucosa of the larynx and trachea. J Hopkins Hosp Bull 1922; 33:357–359.
5. Wolbach SB, Howe PR. Tissue changes following deprivation of fat-soluble A vitamin. J Exp Med 1925; 42(6):753–777.
6. Mactier H, Weaver LT. Vitamin A and preterm infants: what we know, what we don't know, and what we need to know. Arch Dis Child Fetal Neonatal Ed 2005; 90(2):F103–F108.
7. Humphrey JH, Agoestina T, Wu L, et al. Impact of neonatal vitamin A supplementation on infant morbidity and mortality. J Pediatr 1996; 128(4):489–496.

8. Haidar J, Tsegaye D, Mariam DH, et al. Vitamin A supplementation on child morbidity. East Afr Med J 2003; 80(1):17–21.
9. Rahmathullah L, Tielsch JM, Thulasiraj RD, et al. Impact of supplementing newborn infants with vitamin A on early infant mortality: community based randomised trial in southern India. BMJ 2003; 327(7409):254.
10. Klemm RD, Labrique AB, Christian P, et al. Newborn vitamin a supplementation reduced infant mortality in rural Bangladesh. Pediatrics 2008; 122(1):e242–e250.
11. Malone JI. Vitamin passage across the placenta. Clin Perinatol 1975; 2(2):295–307.
12. Darlow BA, Graham PJ. Vitamin A supplementation to prevent mortality and short-term morbidity in very low birthweight infants. Cochrane Database Syst Rev 2007; (4):CD000501.
13. Brandt RB, Mueller DG, Schroeder JR, et al. Serum vitamin A in premature and term neonates. J Pediatr 1978; 92(1):101–104.
14. Shenai JP, Chytil F, Jhaveri A, et al. Plasma vitamin A and retinol-binding protein in premature and term neonates. J Pediatr 1981; 99(2):302–305.
15. Shenai JP, Chytil F, Stahlman MT. Liver vitamin A reserves of very low birth weight neonates. Pediatr Res 1985; 19(9):892–893.
16. Shenai JP, Rush MG, Stahlman MT, et al. Plasma retinol-binding protein response to vitamin A administration in infants susceptible to bronchopulmonary dysplasia. J Pediatr 1990; 116(4):607–614.
17. Zachman RD, Samuels DP, Brand JM, et al. Use of the intramuscular relative-dose-response test to predict bronchopulmonary dysplasia in premature infants. Am J Clin Nutr 1996; 63(1): 123–129.
18. Tyson JE, Wright LL, Oh W, et al. Vitamin A supplementation for extremely-low-birth-weight infants. National Institute of Child Health and Human Development Neonatal Research Network. N Engl J Med 1999; 340(25):1962–1968.
19. Ambalavanan N, Tyson JE, Kennedy KA, et al. National Institute of Child Health and Human Development Neonatal Research Network. Vitamin A supplementation for extremely low birth weight infants: outcome at 18 to 22 months. Pediatrics 2005; 115(3):e249–e254.
20. Ambalavanan N, Kennedy K, Tyson J, et al. Survey of vitamin A supplementation for extremely-low-birth-weight infants: is clinical practice consistent with the evidence? J Pediatr 2004; 145(3):304–307.
21. Ambalavanan N, Wu TJ, Tyson JE, et al. A comparison of three vitamin A dosing regimens in extremely-low-birth-weight infants. J Pediatr 2003; 142(6):656–661.
22. Ambalavanan N, Ross AC, Carlo WA. Retinol-binding protein, transthyretin, and C-reactive protein in extremely low birth weight (ELBW) infants. J Perinatol 2005; 25(11):714–719.
23. Rush MG, Shenai JP, Parker RA, et al. Intramuscular versus enteral vitamin A supplementation in very low birth weight neonates. J Pediatr 1994; 125(3):458–462.
24. Landman J, Sive A, Heese HD, et al. Comparison of enteral and intramuscular vitamin A supplementation in preterm infants. Early Hum Dev 1992; 30(2):163–170.
25. Porcelli PJ, Greene H, Adcock E. A modified vitamin regimen for vitamin B2, A, and E administration in very-low-birth-weight infants. J Pediatr Gastroenterol Nutr 2004; 38(4):392–400.
26. Greene HL, Smith R, Pollack P, et al. Intravenous vitamins for very-low-birth-weight infants. J Am Coll Nutr 1991; 10(4):281–288.
27. Maden M, Hind M. Retinoic acid in alveolar development, maintenance and regeneration. Philos Trans R Soc Lond B Biol Sci 2004; 359(1445):799–808.
28. Hind M, Corcoran J, Maden M. Temporal/spatial expression of retinoid binding proteins and RAR isoforms in the postnatal lung. Am J Physiol Lung Cell Mol Physiol 2002; 282(3): L468–L476.

29. Kliewer SA, Umesono K, Evans RM, et al. The retinoid X receptors: modulators of multiple hormone signaling pathways. Vitamin A in health and disease. New York: Marcel Dekker, 1994:239–255.

30. Leid M, Kastner P, Chambon P. Multiplicity generates diversity in the retinoic acid signalling pathways. Trends Biochem Sci 1992; 17(10):427–433.

31. Burri PH. The postnatal growth of the rat lung. 3. Morphology. Anat Rec 1974; 180(1): 77–98.

32. Mollard R, Ghyselinck NB, Wendling O, et al. Stage-dependent responses of the developing lung to retinoic acid signaling. Int J Dev Biol 2000; 44(5):457–462.

33. McGowan SE. Contributions of retinoids to the generation and repair of the pulmonary alveolus. Chest 2002; 121 (5 suppl):206S–208S.

34. Bourbon J, Boucherat O, Chailley-Heu B, et al. Control mechanisms of lung alveolar development and their disorders in bronchopulmonary dysplasia. Pediatr Res 2005; 57(5 pt 2):38R–46R.

35. Vaccaro C, Brody JS. Ultrastructure of developing alveoli. I. The role of the interstitial fibroblast. Anat Rec 1978; 192(4):467–479.

36. Shenai JP, Chytil F. Vitamin A storage in lungs during perinatal development in the rat. Biol Neonate 1990; 57(2):126–132.

37. McGowan S, Jackson SK, Jenkins-Moore M, et al. Mice bearing deletions of retinoic acid receptors demonstrate reduced lung elastin and alveolar numbers. Am J Respir Cell Mol Biol 2000; 23(2):162–167.

38. Pinto Mde L, Rodrigues P, Coelho AC, et al. Prenatal administration of vitamin A alters pulmonary and plasma levels of vascular endothelial growth factor in the developing mouse. Int J Exp Pathol 2007; 88(6):393–401.

39. Maeno T, Tanaka T, Sando Y, et al. Stimulation of vascular endothelial growth factor gene transcription by all trans retinoic acid through Sp1 and Sp3 sites in human bronchioloalveolar carcinoma cells. Am J Respir Cell Mol Biol 2002; 26(2):246–253.

40. Pedigo NG, Zhang H, Mishra A, et al. Retinoic acid inducibility of the human PDGF-a gene is mediated by 5′-distal DNA motifs that overlap with basal enhancer and vitamin D response elements. Gene Expr 2007; 14(1):1–12.

41. Liebeskind A, Srinivasan S, Kaetzel D, et al. Retinoic acid stimulates immature lung fibroblast growth via a PDGF-mediated autocrine mechanism. Am J Physiol Lung Cell Mol Physiol 2000; 279(1):L81–L90.

42. Chen H, Chang L, Liu H, et al. Effect of retinoic acid on platelet-derived growth factor and lung development in newborn rats. J Huazhong Univ Sci Technolog Med Sci 2004; 24(3): 226–228.

43. Chen F, Desai TJ, Qian J, et al. Inhibition of Tgf beta signaling by endogenous retinoic acid is essential for primary lung bud induction. Development 2007; 134(16):2969–2979.

44. Redlich CA, Delisser HM, Elias JA. Retinoic acid inhibition of transforming growth factor-beta-induced collagen production by human lung fibroblasts. Am J Respir Cell Mol Biol 1995; 12(3):287–295.

45. Veness-Meehan KA, Bottone FG Jr., Stiles AD. Effects of retinoic acid on airspace development and lung collagen in hyperoxia-exposed newborn rats. Pediatr Res 2000; 48(4): 434–444.

46. Veness-Meehan KA, Pierce RA, Moats-Staats BM, et al. Retinoic acid attenuates O2-induced inhibition of lung septation. Am J Physiol Lung Cell Mol Physiol 2002; 283(5):L971–L980.

47. Garber SJ, Zhang H, Foley JP, et al. Hormonal regulation of alveolarization: structure-function correlation. Respir Res 2006; 7:47.

48. Couroucli XI, Liang YW, Jiang W, et al. Attenuation of oxygen-induced abnormal lung maturation in rats by retinoic acid: possible role of cytochrome P4501A enzymes. J Pharmacol Exp Ther 2006; 317(3):946–954.

49. Bry K, Lappalainen U. Pathogenesis of bronchopulmonary dysplasia: the role of interleukin 1beta in the regulation of inflammation-mediated pulmonary retinoic acid pathways in transgenic mice. Semin Perinatol 2006; 30(3):121–128.

50. Cho SJ, George CL, Snyder JM, et al. Retinoic acid and erythropoietin maintain alveolar development in mice treated with an angiogenesis inhibitor. Am J Respir Cell Mol Biol 2005; 33(6):622–628.

51. Pierce RA, Joyce B, Officer S, et al. Retinoids increase lung elastin expression but fail to alter morphology or angiogenesis genes in premature ventilated baboons. Pediatr Res 2007; 61(6):703–709.

52. Ross AC, Ambalavanan N, Zolfaghari R, et al. Vitamin A combined with retinoic acid increases retinol uptake and lung retinyl ester formation in a synergistic manner in neonatal rats. J Lipid Res 2006; 47(8):1844–1851.

53. Ross AC, Ambalavanan N. Retinoic acid combined with vitamin A synergizes to increase retinyl ester storage in the lungs of newborn and dexamethasone-treated neonatal rats. Neonatology 2007; 92(1):26–32.

54. Bland RD, Albertine KH, Pierce RA, et al. Impaired alveolar development and abnormal lung elastin in preterm lambs with chronic lung injury: potential benefits of retinol treatment. Biol Neonate 2003; 84(1):101–102.

55. Zhu YK, Liu X, Ertl RF, et al. Retinoic acid attenuates cytokine-driven fibroblast degradation of extracellular matrix in three-dimensional culture. Am J Respir Cell Mol Biol 2001; 25(5): 620–627.

56. Nakajoh M, Fukushima T, Suzuki T, et al. Retinoic acid inhibits elastase-induced injury in human lung epithelial cell lines. Am J Respir Cell Mol Biol 2003; 28(3):296–304.

57. Massaro GD, Massaro D. Retinoic acid treatment abrogates elastase-induced pulmonary emphysema in rats. Nat Med 1997; 3(6):675–677.

58. Tepper J, Pfeiffer J, Aldrich M, et al. Can retinoic acid ameliorate the physiologic and morphologic effects of elastase instillation in the rat? Chest 2000; 117 (5 suppl 1):242S–244S.

59. March TH, Cossey PY, Esparza DC, et al. Inhalation administration of all-trans-retinoic acid for treatment of elastase-induced pulmonary emphysema in Fischer 344 rats. Exp Lung Res 2004; 30(5):383–404.

60. Fujita M, Ye Q, Ouchi H, et al. Retinoic acid fails to reverse emphysema in adult mouse models. Thorax 2004; 59(3):224–230.

61. Hind M, Maden M. Retinoic acid induces alveolar regeneration in the adult mouse lung. Eur Respir J 2004; 23(1):20–27.

26

The Use of Antioxidants to Prevent or Ameliorate Bronchopulmonary Dysplasia

JONATHAN M. DAVIS
Tufts University School of Medicine, Boston, Massachusetts, U.S.A.

RICHARD PARAD
Harvard Medical School, Boston, Massachusetts, U.S.A.

I. Introduction

The pathogenesis of bronchopulmonary dysplasia (BPD) is complex and may depend on the nature of the injury, mechanisms of response, or the infant's inability to respond appropriately to the injury process. Although the etiology is multifactorial in nature, prolonged exposure of the lung to supraphysiologic oxygen concentrations does appear to be critically important (1). Under normal conditions, a delicate balance exists between the production of reactive oxygen species (ROS) and the antioxidant defenses that protect cells in vivo. Increased generation of ROS can occur secondary to hyperoxia, reperfusion, or inflammation (2). Alternatively, ROS can increase because of an inability to quench production because of inadequate antioxidant defenses.

The premature neonate may be more susceptible to ROS-induced injury because adequate concentrations of antioxidants may be absent at birth. Frank and Groseclose documented the development of the antioxidant enzymes superoxide dismutase (SOD), catalase, and glutathione peroxidase (GPx) in the lungs of rabbits during late gestation (3). The 150% increase in these enzymes during the last 15% of gestation parallels the maturation pattern of pulmonary surfactant. These developmental changes in the fetal lung allow proper ventilation by reducing surface tension and provide for the transition from the relative hypoxia of intrauterine development to the oxygen-rich extrauterine environment. Premature birth can occur before the normal upregulation of these antioxidant systems and other ROS scavengers (e.g., vitamin E, ascorbic acid, glutathione, ceruloplasmin) and may result in an imbalance between oxidants and antioxidants and an increased risk for the development of BPD.

Many cell, animal, and human studies have suggested that acute and chronic lung injury secondary to prolonged hyperoxia may be ameliorated by administration of antioxidant enzymes, with SOD having significant protective effects (4–7). Three forms of SOD have been identified in mammalian cells; Cu/ZnSOD is present primarily in the cytoplasm, MnSOD in the mitochondria, and extracellular (EC)-SOD (a Cu/Zn containing protein) located in extracellular spaces in adults. However, EC-SOD is primarily intracellular (cytoplasmic) in newborns (4). The only known function of SOD is to convert extremely toxic superoxide (O_2^-) radicals to hydrogen peroxide (H_2O_2) and water. Catalase, GPx, and glutathione reductase then detoxify the H_2O_2 that is produced by SOD, with significant quantities of catalase present in red blood cells. This chapter will review various therapeutic interventions using antioxidants to reduce ROS-induced injury in cell culture experiments, animal models of lung injury, and human trials in preterm infants. Although the use of supplemental antioxidants represents a logical strategy to prevent or ameliorate lung injury from excess generation of ROS, caution must be exercised due to increasing evidence that ROS are critically important second messengers in various cell signaling pathways that control normal cellular functions. In addition, since intracellular generation of ROS is important in bacterial killing by alveolar macrophages and neutrophils, antioxidants may interfere with this process and actually contribute to worsening lung injury.

II. Cell Culture Experiments

A. Lung Epithelial Cells

To determine whether overexpression of antioxidant enzymes in lung epithelial cells could prevent damage from oxidant injury, Ilizarov and colleagues generated stable cell lines overexpressing MnSOD and/or catalase (1.5- to 2-fold increase in activity; Fig. 1) (8). Cells were then exposed to 95% O_2 for 10 days, with 44% to 57% of cells overexpressing both MnSOD and catalase and 37% to 47% of cells overexpressing MnSOD alone being viable compared with 7% to 12% of cells overexpressing catalase alone or

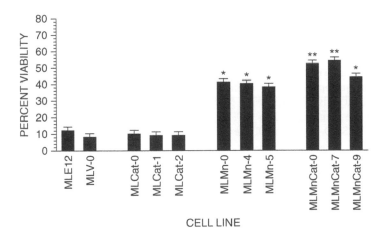

Figure 1 Stable cell lines created in mouse lung epithelial (MLE12) cells. Each bar represents a separate clone. Control cells (MLE), vector alone (MLV), cells overexpressing catalase alone (MLCat, one- to twofold increases), cells overexpressing MnSOD alone (MLMn; one- to twofold), and cells overexpressing both MnSOD and catalase (MLMnCat) were exposed to 95% O_2 for 7 to 10 days. While no improvement in survival was seen in control cells or cells overexpressing catalase alone, cells overexpressing MnSOD had significantly increased survival ($p < 0.05$). Dual overexpression of both MnSOD and catalase resulted in a further small but significant increase in cell survival. *Source*: From Ref. 8.

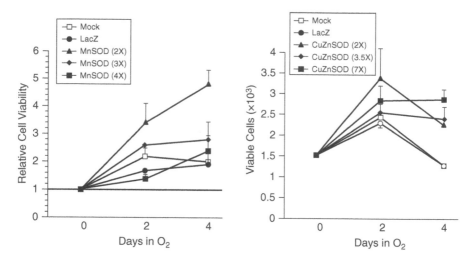

Figure 2 A549 cells (transformed human alveolar epithelial cells) were transduced with recombinant adenovirus–containing gene constructs for LacZ (control), CuZnSOD, or MnSOD. The number of viral particles was progressively increased to reach desired intracellular SOD activity. A two- to threefold increase in activity was found to optimally reduce the growth inhibitory effects of hyperoxia and preserve cell survival. *Source*: From Ref. 9.

control cells ($p < 0.05$). Clonogenic potential of cells overexpressing MnSOD (either alone or combined with catalase) was significantly better than controls. This study demonstrates that overexpression of MnSOD protects cells from hyperoxic injury with catalase offering additional protection only when coexpressed with MnSOD.

It was then important to determine which antioxidant enzymes and level of activity could optimally protect lung epithelial cells against oxidant stress (9). Koo and associates created alveolar epithelial cells overexpressing MnSOD, CuZnSOD, or GPx (alone or in combination). Cells were then exposed to 95% O_2 for up to four days (Fig. 2). Over-expression of either MnSOD or CuZnSOD reversed the growth inhibitory effects of hyperoxia within the first 48 hours of exposure, resulting in a significant increase in cell viability. Optimal protection from hyperoxic injury occurred in cells coexpressing MnSOD and GPx (1.5- to 3-fold increases in activity), with prevention of mitochondrial oxidation appearing to be a critical factor. Other investigators have hypothesized that the generation of ROS activate pro-death signaling pathways within the cell such as c-Jun N-terminal kinase (JNK) and Bax (10,11). In primary rat alveolar epithelial cells, administration of the combined SOD/catalase mimetic EUK-134 reduced activation of Bax at the mitochondrial membrane, cytochrome c release, and cell death. These data indicate that exposure to hyperoxia results in Bax activation at the mitochondrial membrane and subsequent cytochrome c release and cell death, processes that can be reversed by the administration of antioxidant enzymes and antioxidant mimetics.

Next, Arita and associates determined if targeting antioxidants to specific locations within the cell would enhance protection against oxidant stress (12). Cells over-expressing catalase in either the cytosol or mitochondria were exposed to H_2O_2, and cell

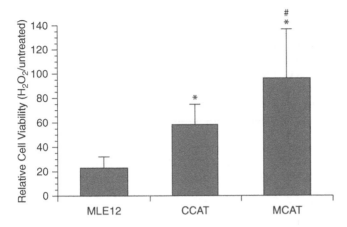

Figure 3 The mitochondrial targeting gene sequence was removed from MnSOD and placed on the human catalase gene. A549 cells were then transduced with LacZ (control), catalase, or mitochondrial targeted catalase. Cells were allowed to recover and were then exposed to 1 mM H_2O_2 for four hours and cell survival determined. Mitochondrial and cytoplasmic catalase activity was determined. Cells overexpressing catalase primarily in the mitochondria had the best survival, despite having lower overall catalase activity than cells with catalase located primarily in the cytoplasm. *Source*: From Ref. 12.

survival, mitochondrial function, and cytochrome *c* release were analyzed. Although all cells had approximately a twofold increase in catalase activity, markers of mitochondrial function and cell survival correlated directly with extent of mitochondrial localization and not overall catalase activity (Fig. 3). The improved protection was observed in both primary and transformed lung epithelial cells. These data indicate that targeting of antioxidants directly to the mitochondria may be more effective in protecting lung epithelial cells against ROS-induced injury.

Since bacterial infection appears to be an important contributory factor in the pathogenesis of BPD, the effects of hyperoxia on bacterial adherence and IL-8 production (an important inflammatory mediator) were examined by Arita and colleagues using lung epithelial cells (13). A 24-hour exposure to 95% O_2 significantly increased *Pseudomonas aeruginosa* adherence by 57% in alveolar and 115% in airway epithelial cells, as well as IL-8 expression. Overexpression of MnSOD significantly reduced bacterial adherence and IL-8 production in response to hyperoxia. These data demonstrate that supplementation with SOD may not only prevent hyperoxic injury but also associated bacterial infection, which would be expected to have a significant impact on BPD.

B. Endothelial Cells

Since disruption in vascular development in the lung is believed to be important in BPD, targeted delivery of drugs to the vascular endothelium may be more specific and effective in reducing ROS-induced endothelial cell injury in the lung. The therapeutic effect of drug targeting to PECAM (platelet/endothelial cell adhesion molecule 1) was evaluated in vivo in the context of pulmonary oxidative stress (14). Catalase was con-jugated to PECAM antibodies and tested in cell culture and mice. Anti-PECAM/catalase (not IgG/catalase) augmented H_2O_2-degrading capacity in cells and prevented H_2O_2 toxicity. Anti-PECAM/catalase (not IgG/catalase) rapidly accumulated in the pulmonary endothelium after intravenous injection in mice and prevented ROS-induced injury and death induced by glucose oxidase coupled with thrombomodulin antibody (anti-TM/GOX; increasing H_2O_2 production). These data validate vascular immunotargeting as a prospective strategy to enhance antioxidant defense in the pulmonary endothelium to prevent acute and chronic lung injury caused by excess ROS.

Using murine lung endothelial cells, Wang and associates demonstrated that hyperoxia caused cell death by a variety of pathways, including an NADPH oxidase–induced production of ROS (15). This process was attenuated by chemical inhibition as well as by genetic deletion of the p47(phox) subunit of the oxidase. Overexpression of heme oxygenase-1 (HO-1) and low concentrations of carbon monoxide prevented hyperoxia-induced caspase activation, cytochrome *c* release, and cell death. Carbon monoxide also attenuated production of ROS and activation of proapoptotic pathways while promoting an interaction of HO-1 with Bax. These results define novel mecha-nisms underlying the protective effects of carbon monoxide during hyperoxic stress.

C. Macrophages/Mononuclear Cells

The effects of hyperoxia and antioxidant enzymes on inflammation and bacterial clearance were studied in mononuclear cells. These cells are known to generate sig-nificant amounts of ROS when exposed to hyperoxia. Mouse macrophages were exposed to either room air or 95% O_2 for 24 hours and then incubated with *Pseudomonas aeruginosa* (16). After one hour, bacterial adherence, phagocytosis, and macrophage inflammatory protein 1α (MIP-1α) production were analyzed. Bacterial adherence increased 5.8-fold ($p < 0.0001$), phagocytosis decreased 60% ($p < 0.05$), and MIP-1α production increased 49% ($p < 0.05$) in response to hyperoxia. Overexpression of MnSOD or catalase significantly decreased bacterial adherence by 30.5%, but only MnSOD significantly improved bacterial phagocytosis and attenuated MIP-1α produc-tion. This suggests that hyperoxia increases bacterial adherence while impairing mon-onuclear cell function, an effect that is significantly blunted by MnSOD. Interventions with SOD could potentially minimize the development of ROS-induced lung injury as well as reducing nosocomial infections that are known to increase the risk for BPD.

As previously mentioned, scavenging of superoxide by SOD may compromise bacterial killing by phagocytes. Walti and colleagues investigated the interaction of exogenous surfactant and recombinant human CuZnSOD (rhSOD) with the antibacterial activity of human blood monocytes (17). Monocytes were preincubated in the presence or absence of (*i*) 1 mg/mL modified natural surfactant; (*ii*) rhSOD (2500 U/mL, Biotec-hnology General Corp., Iselin, New Jersey, U.S.); and (*iii*) bovine catalase (25,000 U/mL). Bacteria (*Legionella pneumophila* or *Escherichia coli*) were then added and incubated for six hours. The antibacterial capacity of monocytes was not impaired by the presence of rhSOD $\pm$ Curosurf and in some instances even potentiated by the addition of rhSOD. Exposure of monocytes to catalase interfered with bacterial killing, suggesting that H_2O_2 production was more important than the generation of superoxide in the process of bac-terial killing. This study demonstrates that rhSOD potentiates the killing of bacteria by human monocytes through the generation of superoxide, which in turn is converted to H_2O_2 in the presence of rhSOD.

III. Animal Models of BPD

Initial studies using rhSOD were performed by Davis and associates on 26 newborn piglets (6). Ten piglets were hyperventilated (arterial PCO_2 15–20 Torr) with 100% O_2 for 48 hours; a second group received identical treatment but was given 5 mg/kg of rhSOD intratracheally at baseline and six piglets were normally ventilated (arterial PCO_2 40–45 Torr) for 48 hours with 21% O_2. In piglets treated with hyperoxia and hyperventilation, lung compliance decreased 42%, and tracheal aspirates showed an increase in neutrophil chemotactic activity (32%), total cell counts (135%), elastase activity (93%), and albumin concentration (339%) over 48 hours (all $p < 0.05$). All variables were significantly lower in rhSOD-treated piglets and comparable to normoxic control values. Immunohistochemistry demonstrated that at 48 hours significant rhSOD was distributed relatively homogeneously in terminal airways. Adding rhSOD to tracheal aspirates of hyperoxic, hyperventilated piglets did not alter neutrophil chemotaxis, suggesting that rhSOD protected the lung by reducing the production of chemotactic mediators. This indicates that acute lung injury caused by 48 hours of hyperoxia and hyperventilation can be significantly ameliorated by prophylactic IT administration of rhSOD.

Other data demonstrating the efficacy of SOD in preventing hyperoxia-induced lung injury come from studies of genetically engineered mice. Transgenic mice lacking MnSOD die within the first 10 days of life in room air, while mice deficient in CuZn or EC-SOD have reduced survival and more lung injury in response to ROS, but a normal life span (18–20). In addition, transgenic mice overexpressing MnSOD in alveolar type II cells are able to survive longer with significantly less lung injury in hyperoxia compared with wild-type controls (21). Furthermore, administration of rAd-CuZnSOD and catalase has been shown to be effective in prolonging survival in rats exposed to hyperoxia for 62 hours (22). The effects of genetic inactivation of MnSOD (SOD2) on O_2 tolerance in knockout mice have not been thoroughly investigated. Homozygous $(-/-)$ and heterozygous $(+/-)$ SOD2 mutant mice were compared with wild-type controls following 48-hour exposure to either room air or hyperoxia (23). Mortality of transgenic mice without any SOD2 activity increased from 0% in room air to 18 and 83% in 50 and 80% O_2, respectively. The administration of N-acetylcysteine (NAC) did not alter mortality of $SOD2^{-/-}$ mice, even though Nagata and colleagues have demonstrated that NAC administration was associated with significant increases in MnSOD activity in addition to glutathione levels in the lung (24). Histopathological analysis revealed abnormalities in saccules of $SOD2^{-/-}$ mice exposed either to room air or to 50% O_2 suggestive of delayed postnatal lung development. In 50% O_2, activities of glutamate-cysteine ligase (GCL) and GPx increased in $SOD2^{-/-}$ (35% and 70%, respectively) and $SOD2^{+/-}$ (12% and 70%, respectively) mice, but glutathione levels remained unchanged. Data suggest that MnSOD is required for normal O_2 tolerance and that in the absence of MnSOD there is a compensatory increase in pulmonary gluta-thione–dependent antioxidant defenses in response to hyperoxia. Although administration of NAC increases glutathione concentrations in cells, it does not appear to prevent ROS-induced injury in the absence of SOD.

Overexpression of SOD could also preserve alveolar development in hyperoxia-exposed newborn mice (4). Newborn EC-SOD transgenic and wild-type mice were exposed to 95% O_2 or air for seven days and bronchoalveolar lavage cell counts, lung EC-SOD activity, oxidized and reduced glutathione, and myeloperoxidase were measured. Total EC-SOD activity in transgenic mice was approximately 2.5×higher than wild-type controls, with hyperoxia-exposed transgenic mice having less pulmonary neutrophil influx and oxidized glutathione than wild type at seven days. In addition, hyperoxia-exposed transgenic EC-SOD mice had significant preservation of alveolar surface and volume density compared with wild-type littermates. Data indicate that SOD is critically important in preventing hyperoxia-induced lung injury and preserving normal alveolar development, supporting the use of this particular class of proteins in therapeutic trials.

Since HO-1 confers protection against a variety of ROS-induced injury, exogenous administration of HO-1 by gene transfer has been examined (25). Intratracheal (IT) administration of Ad5-HO-1 increased the expression of HO-1 mRNA and protein in rat lungs, improved survival, and markedly reduced inflammatory changes and lung injury in response to hyperoxia. Expression of other antioxidant enzymes (MnSOD, CuZnSOD, ferritin) was not affected by Ad5-HO-1 administration. These data suggest the feasibility of high-level HO-1 expression in the rat lung by gene delivery and associated protection against hyperoxia-induced lung injury in an in vivo model.

A catalytic antioxidant (metalloporphyrin AEOL 10113) has been tested in hyperoxia-induced lung injury using a fetal baboon model of BPD (26). Fetal baboons delivered at 140 days of gestation (term = 185 days) and given 100% O_2 for 10 days had increased alveolar tissue volume and septal thickness and decreased alveolar surface area compared with animals given oxygen as needed. Treatment with a continuous intravenous infusion of this antioxidant partially reversed these changes, suggesting that this may represent a novel approach to reduce the risk of pulmonary oxygen toxicity in prematurely born infants.

Peroxiredoxin 6 (Prdx6) is an antioxidant with both GPx and phospholipase A2 activities and is expressed in all major organs, particularly in the lung. Prdx6 uses glutathione as an electron donor to reduce H_2O_2 and other hydroperoxides. Wang and associates have demonstrated that Prdx6-null mice are more sensitive to the effects of oxidants, while mice overexpressing Prdx6 have reduced evidence of oxidation and lung injury in response to prolonged hyperoxia (27,28). It is thought that this unique antioxidant functions mainly by facilitating repair of damaged cell membranes via reduction of peroxidized phospholipids. Other investigators have studied thioredoxin-1 (TRX-1), a small ubiquitous protein that acts as an important ROS scavenger (29). Mice exposed to 98% O_2 were compared with transgenic mice overexpressing human TRX-1 (hTRX-1), with hTRX-1 decreasing alveolar damage, apoptosis, and cytochrome c in the lung. Of interest is that IL-6 (which can have pro- or anti-inflammatory effects) was significantly higher in hTRX-1 transgenic mice than in wild-type mice after exposure to hyperoxia. These studies suggest that overexpression of these unique antioxidants protects against hyperoxia-induced apoptosis in the lung and may be efficacious in the prevention of hyperoxia-induced lung injury.

Pentoxifylline is a phosphodiesterase inhibitor that has been studied in a preterm rat model of hyperoxic lung injury (30). Preterm rat pups were exposed to 100% O_2 for 10 days and injected subcutaneously with saline or 75 mg/kg pentoxifylline twice a day.

Pentoxifylline treatment significantly increased mean survival by three days and reduced fibrin deposition by 66% and total protein concentrations by 33% in the lung compared with untreated hyperoxia-exposed controls. It is unclear whether this agent is effective in preventing ROS-induced lung injury purely by inhibiting phosphodiesterase activity or whether the compound possesses any unique antioxidant properties. Further studies are definitely needed.

The antioxidant vitamins ascorbic acid (vitamin C) and α-tocopherol (vitamin E) are known to inhibit ROS-induced lipid peroxidation. Using a premature baboon model of hyperoxia-induced BPD, Berger and colleagues studied four animals who received high doses of antioxidant vitamins and one animal that received standard dosing and compared them with 21 historical controls who had received standard dose antioxidant vitamin supplementation (31). Although high-dose antioxidant vitamin supplementation significantly raised vitamin C and E concentrations in plasma and the lung, no protective effects could be demonstrated in any physiologic or histologic parameter. These studies question whether raising antioxidant vitamin concentrations alone will be effective in preventing BPD in high-risk preterm infants.

IV. Human Trials of Antioxidants in Preventing BPD

Preterm delivery results in (*i*) insufficient time for placental transfer of essential nutrients; (*ii*) dependence on parenteral nutrition for prolonged periods of time; and (*iii*) an inability to upregulate key antioxidant enzymes. All of these factors may lead to a disruption in a preterm infant's oxidant/antioxidant balance. For instance, trace elements such as copper, zinc, and selenium are essential for normal antioxidant enzyme function. Huston and colleagues measured these elements in a cohort of preterm infants with BPD and noted falling serum levels of zinc and selenium in infants receiving parenteral nutrition as well as a failure to increase serum antioxidant enzymes to predicted levels (32). Since low plasma levels of selenium, α-tocopherol, vitamin A, and other antioxidants within the first three days of life appear to be associated with the development of BPD, many studies have attempted to enhance antioxidant capabilities in preterm infants to improve outcome (1). While several have focused on optimizing parenteral and enteral nutrition by supplementation with key nutritional elements (vitamins A, C, and E, zinc, selenium, copper, manganese, inositol, glutamine, cysteine, and methionine), others have attempted to directly supplement antioxidant status as a strategy to prevent BPD (33). Ironically, when components of parenteral nutrition solution (multivitamin solutions and lipids) are exposed to light, ROS may be generated that increase lipid peroxidation and could worsen outcome in infants developing BPD (34).

Vitamin E (α-tocopherol) scavenges ROS and prevents lipid peroxidation. Preterm infants at risk for BPD are known to be deficient in vitamin E. Randomized controlled trials have consistently failed to demonstrate a statistically significant reduction in the incidence of BPD after intravenous or oral administration of α-tocopherol (35,36). The Cochrane database performed a meta-analysis of 26 separate randomized trials, focusing on 4 studies that included 932 very low birth weight infants, with no demonstrable reduction in the risk of BPD (typical RR 0.89, CI 0.71, 1.13) (37). Of significant concern is the administration of pharmacologic concentrations of vitamin E was associated with an increased risk of sepsis and necrotizing enterocolitis, precluding the routine use of these concentrations in high risk preterm infants (38).

NAC is a source of the essential amino acid L-cysteine and a precursor of the antioxidant glutathione, whose disulfide bond may protect proteins from oxidation. A multicenter, double-blind trial of NAC was conducted in 391 ventilated, extremely low birth weight infants. Infants were randomized by 36 hours of age to receive 16 to 32 mg/kg/day of NAC or placebo intravenously for six days (39). The study failed to show any reduction in survival or the incidence or severity of BPD at 36 weeks corrected age or improved pulmonary function when the infants were studied at term (40). IT NAC has been administered to a small number of ventilated preterm infants with evolving BPD and was not found to improve short-term clinical pulmonary status or pulmonary function (41).

Superoxide dismutase: A randomized trial was performed in which bovine CuZnSOD or placebo was administered by subcutaneous injection every 12 hours to 45 ventilated premature infants with RDS (mean gestational age 28.7 weeks). Plasma SOD levels peaked four hours after dosing. Among the 31 survivors, duration of ventilatory support was shorter, while radiographic scores, days in the hospital, and frequency of clinical symptoms were lower in SOD treated infants (42). When rhSOD became available, pharmacokinetics of IT administration was studied given the short half-life found with intravenous administration. In a cohort of 26 ventilated infants with RDS, a single IT dose (5 mg/kg) resulted in significant increases in SOD activity in serum, tracheal aspirates and urine for two to four days with tracheal aspirate inflammatory markers significantly reduced compared with controls (43). Similar results were observed in 33 preterm infants evaluated for safety and pharmacokinetics of multiple IT rhSOD doses, with dosing every 48 hours over a 14-day period (44). Follow-up (mean 28 months) of these infants suggested that multiple rhSOD doses may reduce the development of asthma and improve neurodevelopmental outcome (45). A multicenter, randomized trial of prophylactic rhSOD was then performed to determine whether IT treatment significantly reduced the incidence of BPD and improved pulmonary outcome at one year corrected gestation age (CGA) (7). Three-hundred two premature infants (600–1200 g at birth) receiving exogenous surfactant at birth for RDS received either IT rhSOD (5 mg/kg) or placebo every 48 hours (as long as intubation was required) up to 1 month of age. There were no differences found in the incidence of death or the development of BPD (at 28 days or 36 weeks CGA). At a median of one year corrected age, 37% of placebo-treated infants had repeated episodes of wheezing or other respiratory illness severe enough to require treatment with asthma medications (e.g., bronchodilators, corticosteroids) compared with 24% of rhSOD-treated infants, a 35% reduction (Fig. 4). In the highest risk infants <27 weeks gestation, 42% treated with placebo-received asthma medications compared with 19% of rhSOD-treated infants, a 55% decrease. Infants <27 weeks gestation who received rhSOD also had a 55% decrease in emergency department visits and a 44% decrease in subsequent hospitalizations. This occurred despite significantly more infants in the placebo group receiving active RSV prophylaxis. This study demonstrates that treatment at birth with rhSOD may reduce ROS-induced pulmonary injury, although this may not be readily apparent when evaluating only early outcomes on the basis of current BPD definitions. But perhaps more importantly, treatment with rhSOD leads to improved clinical status at one year CGA, which as been linked to improvements in pulmonary functions and

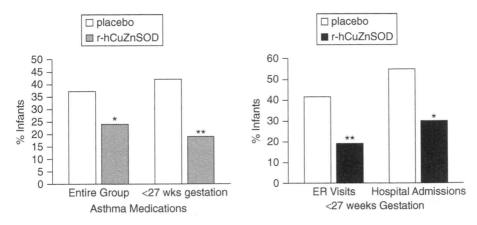

Figure 4 At a median of one year corrected age, the use of asthma medications to treat significant respiratory illness in infants (*left panel*). The entire group is presented as well as a subset of infants <27 weeks gestation at birth. The open bars represent the percentage of placebo controls and the shaded bars the rh CuZnSOD group (*$p = 0.05$; **$p = 0.01$). The right panel shows the number of emergency room visits and hospital admissions (all causes) in a subset of infants <27 weeks' gestation at birth who had received placebo (*open bars*) or rhSOD (*shaded bars*) (*$p = 0.05$; **$p = 0.01$). *Source*: From Ref. 7.

longer-term outcomes (1). Further trials studying the long-term outcome of very preterm infants with rhSOD are currently under way.

Selenium is a trace element necessary for the activity of antioxidant enzymes GPx and thioredoxin reductase. Five-hundred thirty-four infants <1500 g were randomized to receive selenium supplementation (parenteral and then enteral) from week 1 of life until 36 weeks CGA or discharge. No significant differences were seen with respect to short-term outcome defined as oxygen requirement at 28 days of age (46). Unfortunately, longer-term follow-up is not available.

Allopurinol is a structural isomer of hypoxanthine and inhibits the generation of ROS through xanthine oxidase. Boda and colleagues randomized premature infants with RDS to three days of enteral allopurinol (20 mg/kg/day) or placebo and documented decreased serum and urine uric acid levels as well as decreased mortality following active treatment (47). These results were consistent with studies of premature baboons with RDS exposed to hyperoxia, which demonstrated that allopurinol significantly improved respiratory status (48). A trial involving 400 infants 24 to 32 weeks gestation who were randomized to allopurinol (20 mg/kg) or placebo for 7 days found no differences in the incidence of BPD (defined as O_2 requirement at 28 days of life). Infants with higher baseline hypoxanthine levels at birth were at greatest risk for developing BPD (49). Once again, longer-term outcome of treated infants has not been reported.

Ascorbic acid (vitamin C) has both oxidant and antioxidant activities and is thought to contribute to the regeneration of membrane-bound α-tocopherol (31,50). In a trial of 119 preterm infants (mean gestational age 28.4 weeks) randomized to low- or high-dose ascorbic acid supplementation through 28 days of life, no significant differences were seen in the development of BPD between groups (51). Of note, significantly higher baseline serum ascorbic acid levels were detected in six infants who subsequently died, although no direct link could be established.

Inositol is an essential nutrient important in surfactant synthesis and cell growth, which may also function as an antioxidant. In a randomized trial, 230 premature infants (mean gestational age 27.8 weeks) who were randomized to receive at least five days of inositol or placebo, the incidence of BPD was significantly lower in inositol-supplemented infants (52). A meta-analysis of five reports and three randomized trials suggested that the combined outcome of death or BPD was significantly reduced (RR 0.56, 95% CI 0.42, 0.77) in inositol-treated infants (53). Further trials of inositol are currently under way in preterm infants at risk for BPD.

V. Summary

Oxidative injury is well recognized to cause significant cell damage in the lung and appears to be important in the pathogenesis of BPD. A number of therapeutic approaches have been taken to augment endogenous antioxidant activity in preterm infants to significantly reduce the incidence and severity of BPD. While studies in cultured cells and even some animal models have suggested that specific interventions may be efficacious, human trials have met with limited success. Difficulties in interpreting the data from these studies continue to exist, due to varying definitions of BPD used as a primary endpoint. Despite this, the use of rhSOD continues to represent the most promising approach to preventing long-term pulmonary morbidity in high-risk preterm infants.

References

1. Jobe AH, Bancalari E. Bronchopulmonary dysplasia. Am J Respir Crit Care Med 2001; 163:1723–1729.
2. Davis JM, Rosenfeld W. Chronic lung disease. In: Avery G, Fletcher M, MacDonald M, eds. Neonatology. Philadelphia: JB Lippincott Co., 2005:578–599.
3. Frank L, Groseclose EE. Preparation for birth into an O_2-rich environment: the antioxidant enzymes in the developing rabbit lung. Pediatr Res 1984; 18:240–244.
4. Ahmed MN, Suliman HB, Folz RJ, et al. Extracellular superoxide dismutase protects lung development in hyperoxia-exposed newborn mice. Am J Respir Crit Care Med 2003; 167:400–405.
5. Johnson-Varghese L, Brodsky N, Bhandari V. Effect of antioxidants on apoptosis and cytokine release in fetal rat Type II pneumocytes exposed to hyperoxia and nitric oxide. Cytokine 2004; 28:10–16.
6. Davis JM, Rosenfeld WN, Sanders RJ, et al. Prophylactic effects of recombinant human superoxide dismutase in neonatal lung injury. J Appl Physiol 1993; 74:2234–2241.
7. Davis JM, Parad RB, Michele T, et al. Pulmonary outcome at 1 year corrected age in premature infants treated at birth with recombinant human CuZn superoxide dismutase. Pediatrics 2003; 111:469–476.
8. Ilizarov AM, Koo HC, Kazzaz JA, et al. Overexpression of manganese superoxide dismutase protects lung epithelial cells against oxidant injury. Am J Respir Cell Mol Biol 2001; 24:436–441.

9. Koo HC, Davis JM, Li Y, et al. Effects of transgene expression of superoxide dismutase and glutathione peroxidase on pulmonary epithelial cell viability in hyperoxia. Am J Physiol Lung Cell Mol Physiol 2005; 288:L718–L726.

10. Li Y, Arita Y, Koo HC, et al. Inhibition of c-Jun N-terminal kinase pathway improves cell viability in response to oxidant injury. Am J Respir Cell Mol Biol 2003; 29:779–783.

11. Buccellato LJ, Tso M, Akinci OI, et al. Reactive oxygen species are required for hyperoxia-induced Bax active ation and cell death in alveolar epithelial cells. J Biol Chem 2004; 20:279:6753–6760.

12. Arita Y, Harkness SH, Kazzaz JA, et al. Mitochondrial localization of catalase provides optimal protection from H_2O_2-induced cell death in lung epithelial cells. Am J Physiol Lung Cell Mol Physiol 2006; 290:L978–L986.

13. Arita Y, Joseph A, Koo HC, et al. Superoxide dismutase moderates basal and induced bacterial adherence and interleukin-8 expression in airway epithelial cells. Am J Physiol Lung Cell Mol Physiol 2004; 287(6):L1199–L1206.

14. Christofidou-Solomidou M, Scherpereel A, Wiewrodt R, et al. PECAM-directed delivery of catalase to endothelium protects against pulmonary vascular oxidative stress. Am J Physiol Lung Cell Mol Physiol 2003; 285:L283–L292.

15. Wang X, Wang Y, Kim HP, et al. Carbon monoxide protects against hyperoxia-induced endothelial cell apoptosis by inhibiting reactive oxygen species formation. J Biol Chem 2007; 282:1718–1726.

16. Arita Y, Kazzaz JA, Joseph A, et al. Antioxidants improve antibacterial function in hyperoxia-exposed macrophages. Free Radic Biol Med 2007; 15:42:1517–1523.

17. Walti H, Nicolas-Robin A, Assous MV, et al. Effects of exogenous surfactant and recombinant human copper-zinc superoxide dismutase on oxygen-dependent antimicrobial defenses. Biol Neonate 2002; 82:96–102.

18. Melov S, Coskun P, Patel M, et al. Mitochondrial disease in superoxide dismutase 2 mutant mice. Proc Natl Acad Sci U S A 2000; 96:846–851.

19. Carlsson LM, Jonsson J, Edlund T, et al. Mice lacking extracellular superoxide dismutase are more sensitive to hyperoxia. Proc Nat Acad Sci U S A 1995; 92:6264–6268.

20. Reaume AG, Elliott JL, Hoffman EK, et al. Motor neurons in Cu/Zn superoxide dismutase-deficient mice develop normally but exhibit enhanced cell death after axonal injury. Nat Genet 1996; 13:43–47.

21. Wispe JR, Warner BB, Clark JC, et al. Human Mn-superoxide dismutase in pulmonary epithelial cells of transgenic mice confers protection from oxygen injury. J Biol Chem 1992; 267:23937–23941.

22. Danel C, Erzurum SC, Prayssac P, et al. Gene therapy for oxidant injury-related diseases: adenovirus-mediated transfer of superoxide dismutase and catalase cDNAs protects against hyperoxia but not against ischemia-reperfusion lung injury. Hum Gene Ther 1998; 9: 1487–1496.

23. Asikainen TM, Huang TT, Taskinen E, et al. Increased sensitivity of homozygous SOD2 mutant mice to oxygen toxicity. Free Radic Biol Med 2002; 32:175–186.

24. Nagata K, Iwasaki Y, Yamada T, et al. Overexpression of manganese superoxide dismutase by N-acetylcysteine in hyperoxic lung injury. Respir Med 2007; 101:800–807.

25. Otterbein LE, Kolls JK, Mantell LL, et al. Exogenous administration of heme oxygenase-1 by gene transfer provides protection against hyperoxia-induced lung injury. J Clin Invest 1999; 103:1047–1054.

26. Chang LY, Subramaniam M, Yoder BA, et al. A catalytic antioxidant attenuates alveolar structural remodeling in bronchopulmonary dysplasia. Am J Respir Crit Care Med 2003; 167:57–64.

27. Wang Y, Feinstein SI, Manevich Y, et al. Peroxiredoxin 6 gene-targeted mice show increased lung injury with paraquat-induced oxidative stress. Antioxid Redox Signal 2006; 8:229–237.

28. Wang Y, Phelan SA, Manevich Y, et al. Transgenic mice overexpressing peroxiredoxin 6 show increased resistance to lung injury in hyperoxia. Am J Respir Cell Mol Biol 2006; 34: 481–486.

29. Yamada T, Iwasaki Y, Nagata K, et al. Thioredoxin-1 protects against hyperoxia-induced apoptosis in cells of the alveolar walls. Pulm Pharmacol Ther 2007; 20:650–659.

30. ter Horst SA, Wagenaar GT, de Boer E, et al. Pentoxifylline reduces fibrin deposition and prolongs survival in neonatal hyperoxic lung injury. J Appl Physiol 2004; 97:2014–2019.

31. Berger TM, Frei B, Rifai N, et al. Early high dose antioxidant vitamins do not prevent bronchopulmonary dysplasia in premature baboons exposed to prolonged hyperoxia: a pilot study. Pediatr Res 1998; 43:719–726.

32. Huston RK, Shearer TR, Jelen BJ, et al. Relationship of antioxidant enzymes to trace metals in premature infants. J Parenter Enteral Nutr 1987; 11:163–168.

33. Biniwale M, Ehrenkranz R. The role of nutrition in the prevention and management of bronchopulmonary dysplasia. Semin Perinatol 2006; 30:200–208.

34. Brown LA, Gauthier TW. Influence of lung oxidant and antioxidant status on alveolarization: role of light-exposed total parenteral nutrition. Free Radic Biol Med 2008; 45:570–571.

35. Saldanha RL, Cepeda EE, Poland RL. The effect of vitamin E prophylaxis on the incidence and severity of bronchopulmonary dysplasia. J Pediatr 1982; 101:89–93.

36. Watts JL, Milner R, Zipursky A, et al. Failure of supplementation with vitamin E to prevent bronchopulmonary dysplasia in infants less than 1,500 g birth weight. Eur Respir J 1991; 4:188–190.

37. Brion LP, Bell EF, Raghuveer TS. Vitamin E supplementation for prevention of morbidity and mortality in preterm infants. Cochrane Database Syst Rev 2003; 4:CD003665.

38. Johnson L, Bowen FW Jr., Abbasi S, et al. Relationship of prolonged pharmacologic serum levels of vitamin E to incidence of sepsis and necrotizing enterocolitis in infants with birth weight 1,500 grams or less. Pediatrics 1985; 75:619–638.

39. Ahola T, Lapatto R, Raivio KO, et al. N-acetylcysteine does not prevent bronchopulmonary dysplasia in immature infants: a randomized controlled trial. J Pediatr 2003; 143:697–698.

40. Sandberg K, Fellman V, Stigson L, et al. N-acetylcysteine administration during the first week of life does not improve lung function in extremely low birth weight infants. Biol Neonate 2004; 86:275–279.

41. Bibi H, Seifert B, Oullette M, et al. Intratracheal N-acetylcysteine use in infants with chronic lung disease. Acta Paediatr 1992; 81:335–339.

42. Rosenfeld W, Evans H, Concepcion L, et al. Prevention of bronchopulmonary dysplasia by administration of bovine superoxide dismutase in preterm infants with respiratory distress syndrome. J Pediatr 1984; 105:781–785.

43. Rosenfeld WN, Davis JM, Parton L, et al. Safety and pharmacokinetics of recombinant human superoxide dismutase administered intratracheally to premature neonates with respiratory distress syndrome. Pediatrics 1996; 97:811–817.

44. Davis JM, Rosenfeld WN, Richter SE, et al. Safety and pharmacokinetics of multiple doses of human CuZn superoxide dismutase administered intratracheally to premature infants with respiratory distress syndrome. Pediatrics 1997; 100:24–30.

45. Davis JM, Richter SE, Biswas S, et al. Long-term follow-up of premature infants treated with prophylactic, intratracheal recombinant human CuZn superoxide dismutase. J Perinatol 2000; 20(4):213–216.

46. Darlow BA, Winterbourn CC, Inder TE, et al. The effect of selenium supplementation on outcome in very low birth weight infants: a randomized controlled trial. The New Zealand Neonatal Study Group. J Pediatr 2000; 136:473–480.

47. Boda D, Nemeth I, Hencz P, et al. Effect of allopurinol treatment in premature infants with idiopathic respiratory distress syndrome. Dev Pharmacol Ther 1984; 7:357–367.

48. Jenkinson SG, Roberts RJ, DeLemos RA, et al. Allopurinol-induced effects in premature baboons with respiratory distress syndrome. J Appl Physiol 1991; 70:1160–1167.
49. Russell GA, Cooke RW. Randomised controlled trial of allopurinol prophylaxis in very preterm infants. Arch Dis Child Fetal Neonatal Ed. 1995; 73:F27–F31.
50. Berger TM, Frei B. Pro- or antioxidant activity of vitamin C in preterm infants? Arch Dis Child Fetal Neonatal Ed 1995; 72:F211–F212.
51. Turgut M, Başaran O, Cekmen M, et al. Oxidant and antioxidant levels in preterm newborns with idiopathic hyperbilirubinaemia. J Paediatr Child Health 2004; 40:633–637.
52. Hallman M, Pohjavuori M, Bry K. Inositol supplementation in respiratory distress syndrome. Lung 1990; 168(suppl 1):877–882.
53. Howlett A, Ohlsson A. Inositol for respiratory distress syndrome in preterm infants. Cochrane Database Syst Rev 2003; 4:CD000366.

27

Low-Dose Glucocorticoids for Prevention or Treatment of Bronchopulmonary Dysplasia

KRISTI WATTERBERG

University of New Mexico, Albuquerque, New Mexico, U.S.A.

I. Introduction

The inclusion of low-dose glucocorticoid treatment as an emerging therapy for bron-chopulmonary dysplasia (BPD) signals a new chapter in the chronicle of glucocorticoids and BPD. That this new chapter is entitled "low-dose" glucocorticoid treatment is also ironic, signaling as it does that instead of the usual approach to new drug testing—starting with a low dose and escalating after evaluation of efficacy and safety—glucocorticoid therapy for BPD began with very high doses of the powerful synthetic glucocorticoid dexamethasone. Only after documentation of myriad adverse effects, including growth failure and long-term neurodevelopmental compromise, did the pen-dulum swing away from widespread use of high-dose dexamethasone to a very restricted use of any glucocorticoid for BPD. Careful reevaluation of these therapeutic agents in lower doses and alternate preparations may ultimately lead to the emergence of a more nuanced approach to glucocorticoid therapy for this challenging disease, resulting in net benefit. This chapter first briefly reviews the history of glucocorticoid therapy for BPD, then presents the rationale for lower dose therapy, examines differences in glucocorti-coid preparations, reviews current data regarding lower dose therapy, and finally, dis-cusses future directions for research.

II. History: Dexamethasone and BPD

Anecdotal reports of glucocorticoid use for treatment of established BPD began to appear around 1980, as inflammation became recognized as an early and important hallmark of the disease (1–5). The first clinical trials were published in the 1980s, reporting impressive short-term pulmonary benefits in small numbers of patients with established BPD (6–8). All these trials used dexamethasone, at starting doses of 0.5 mg/kg/day, for "its nearly complete glucocorticoid activity and its long half-life, and because there is reasonable experience with its use in neonates and infants" (6). These investigators recommended caution in its use pending assessment of long-term outcomes (6,7), although one study reassuringly reported improved neurological outcome at 15 months in 9 infants treated with 42 days of dexamethasone, compared with those treated with an 18-day treatment course or a placebo (8). This study also reported sustained pulmonary benefit from the longer, 42-day course compared with other groups (8). Widespread clinical enthusiasm and numerous additional studies followed in the 1990s, including studies of very early postnatal treatment designed to prevent BPD, rather than treat the established disease (9). These studies employed different dosing schedules and duration of therapy, but all used dexamethasone at doses ranging from 0.5 to 1.0 mg/kg/day. At the height of enthusiasm for this therapy (1996–1998), three large neonatal networks reported that approximately 25% of *all* very low birth weight (VLBW) infants received glucocorticoid therapy for BPD, probably dexamethasone, though this was not specifically reported (10).

Studies generally supported the utility of dexamethasone in facilitating extubation and improving other short-term pulmonary outcomes; however, they also documented that these high doses of dexamethasone could result in a broad array of short-term adverse effects and, as more long-term outcomes were reported, long-term growth failure, cerebral palsy, and adverse neurodevelopmental outcomes (9,11–13). The enthusiasm for dexamethasone use waned as these adverse neurological effects were documented; by 2003, the large neonatal networks reported that only 3% to 10% of VLBW infants had received postnatal corticosteroid therapy (10).

The close of this era was demarcated by the publication in 2002 of a joint statement by the American Academy of Pediatrics (AAP) and the Canadian Paediatric Society (CPS) which reviewed the literature and concluded that outside of randomized clinical trials (RCTs), "the use of corticosteroids should be limited to exceptional clinical circumstances (e.g., an infant on maximal ventilatory and oxygen support)" (14).

Publication of the alarming long-term adverse outcomes seen following dexamethasone therapy led to a reluctance to use any glucocorticoid for BPD, and to some unintended consequences. For example, the DART study (*D*examethasone: *A Randomized Trial*), which had a primary outcome measure of survival without long-term neurodevelopmental impairments, as recommended by the AAP/CPS statement, was forced to close prematurely in 2002 due to slow patient enrollment (15). With a planned sample size of 814, this RCT enrolled 70 infants born at <28 weeks' gestation or <1000 g birth weight who remained on mechanical ventilation after one week of postnatal age, and treated them with a 10-day lower-dose dexamethasone course (0.15–0.02 mg/kg taper, 0.89 mg/kg total dose). The investigators found that at the end of the treatment period, significantly more infants receiving dexamethasone were successfully extubated (60% vs. 12%), with no increase in death or major disability at two years corrected age (46% vs. 43%) (15,16). Although this study, together with a meta-analysis suggesting that infants at highest risk of BPD may derive neurodevelopmental benefit from dexamethasone therapy (17), may revive interest in studying this drug, at the time of this writing, the website clinicaltrials.gov had no active registered trials of dexamethasone for BPD treatment.

III. Rationale for "Low-Dose" Glucocorticoid Therapy

The basis for using high- or moderately high-dose dexamethasone for BPD was its powerful anti-inflammatory activity in a disease historically characterized by airway inflammation (1,2). Although BPD in the extremely preterm infant is characterized less by lung inflammation and more by arrest of alveolar development (18), mechanically ventilated extremely low birth weight (ELBW) infants continue to have a broad increase in markers of airway inflammation, correlating with the subsequent development of BPD (19–21). Mechanical ventilation results in numerous sources of continuing inflammatory stimuli, such as bacterial colonization of the lower respiratory tract, irritation from the foreign body of the endotracheal tube, microaspiration through the unprotected airway, suctioning procedures and intermittent infections, as well as positive distending pressure. Therefore, anti-inflammatory therapy for BPD continues to make theoretical sense, and efficacy may be achieved at much lower doses, with fewer side effects.

The second reason to consider low-dose glucocorticoid therapy is the emerging concept of a "relative adrenal insufficiency" or "critical illness-related corticosteroid insufficiency," that is, adrenal function that may produce adequate cortisol for normal homeostasis, but be insufficient to respond appropriately to critical illness (22,23). Described first in adults (22,23), the existence of relative adrenal insufficiency would not be surprising in extremely preterm infants, given the immature stage of development of their hypothalamic-pituitary-adrenal axis at that time in gestation (24). Endogenous cortisol modulates the inflammatory response; insufficient cortisol in both animal models and human disease results in significant amplification of inflammation (25–27). Inadequate cortisol response to critical illness or inflammatory stress would therefore place patients at high risk for exuberant inflammatory responses and injury (28).

Several findings support the presence of a relative adrenal insufficiency in extremely preterm infants. First, sicker infants and those receiving vasopressor support have been shown to have decreased cortisol concentrations, rather than the increased concentrations that would be expected under stress (29–31). Additionally, infants subsequently developing BPD have been documented to have decreased cortisol concentrations and/or response to ACTH stimulation during the first week of life compared with infants who recover without BPD (30,32–34). This decreased response may continue for several weeks (35,36). Lower cortisol concentrations have also been linked to elevated markers of airway inflammation in such infants (20). Thus, both because mechanically ventilated preterm infants are exposed to continuing inflammatory stimuli and because they may have inadequate response to these stimuli, low-dose glucocorticoid therapy may have a role to play in the prevention or treatment of evolving BPD.

IV. Glucocorticoid Considerations

A. Different Therapeutic Agents

Although dexamethasone has been the primary glucocorticoid used for treatment of BPD, it is of course far from the only glucocorticoid available. The numerous steroid preparations vary widely in potency, effective biological half-life, glucocorticoid versus mineralocorticoid activity, genomic versus nongenomic effects, and side effect profiles. Although estimates of relative potencies can be found in textbooks (37), it is unclear how accurate these estimates are, both because the effective potency is amplified by the longer serum and biological half-life of synthetic molecules such as prednisone, dexamethasone, and betamethasone, and because the relative potency of different agents varies for different effects over the broad spectrum of glucocorticoid actions. One study comparing the potency and duration of action of dexamethasone to hydrocortisone in suppressing pituitary-adrenal function in adults estimated dexamethasone to be 17 times as powerful as hydrocortisone at time zero; however, because of its longer half-life, its relative effect was amplified to 52 times that of hydrocortisone at 8 hours and 154 times hydrocortisone at 14 hours (38). The prolonged serum half-life of dexamethasone in the preterm infant may therefore further amplify its effect (39,40).

The variability of different glucocorticoid agents for different effects has been demonstrated in other studies. For example, although dexamethasone was found to be almost 50 times more powerful than hydrocortisone in suppressing pituitary-adrenal function or increasing circulating neutrophils, it was only 5 to 17 times more potent in suppressing T-cell populations (41). This variability is particularly evident in the non-genomic effects of different synthetic glucocorticoids. Whereas the classic genomic actions of glucocorticoids occur slowly and require nuclear translocation, transcription, and new protein synthesis, their nongenomic effects occur rapidly (within minutes) and involve numerous interactions with biological membranes, both specific and nonspecific (41,42). When the classical genomic effects of dexamethasone and betamethasone are compared, the drugs appear equally potent; however, their nongenomic effects are quite different. For example, dexamethasone was found to be five times more powerful than betamethasone in suppressing cellular respiration of thymocytes and monocytes (42). These and many other differences in drug profiles make it clear that one steroid molecule cannot be substituted for another with a simple change of dose.

Dexamethasone may also have been an unfortunate choice of therapeutic agent with regard to its actions on the central nervous system (CNS). A large cohort study comparing prenatal betamethasone to dexamethasone found that dexamethasone was associated with a trend for increased risk of Psychomotor Development Index of <70, increased risk of hearing impairment, and decreased likelihood of unimpaired status (43). Another cohort study of antenatal steroids found that betamethasone, but not dex-amethasone, was associated with a decreased risk of cystic periventricular leukomalacia (PVL) (44), whereas a small cohort study comparing postnatal methylprednisolone to dexamethasone treatment for BPD found less cystic PVL in infants treated with methylprednisolone (45). Animal study has suggested that the sulfite preservative in the dexamethasone preparation may play a part (46); however, the reasons for these different effects on human infants remain unclear, although the widely varying potencies of these drugs for different glucocorticoid effects may account for different effects in vivo.

B. Chemical Adrenalectomy

In addition to adverse effects directly attributable to high steroid dosage, exogenous glucocorticoids also may adversely affect the brain by suppressing endogenous cortisol production, resulting in a "chemical adrenalectomy" (47). This effect may be of critical importance in understanding the pathophysiology of the adverse effects of dex-amethasone on neurodevelopmental outcomes. In animal models, investigators have described an "inverted U" pattern for the effects of endogenous cortisol or corticosterone on the CNS, such that both very low and very high concentrations are associated with adverse CNS effects (47–49). Thus, sustained excessive cortisol concentrations produce detrimental effects, particularly in the hippocampus, but the absence of cortisol also adversely affects structure and function (49). Cortisol occupies both mineralocorticoid and glucocorticoid receptors in the brain, binding preferentially to mineralocorticoid receptors at usual physiological concentrations (47,48). Because dexamethasone or other glucocorticoid without mineralocorticoid activity binds only to glucocorticoid receptors and also suppresses cortisol production, it results in a lack of steroid binding to mineralocorticoid receptors in the brain, potentially producing the same CNS effect as adrenalectomy. Consistent with this hypothesis, investigators found that administration of corticosterone to adrenalectomized adult rats protected the hippocampus against the apoptotic effects of dexamethasone (50). In view of the above findings, perhaps future studies of postnatal steroids for BPD should evaluate glucocorticoid agents with some mineralocorticoid activity, or should include low doses of hydrocortisone as an adjunct to therapy.

C. What Is "Low-Dose"?

As the discussion above indicates, it may be difficult to define "low-dose" glucocorticoid therapy. Even if equivalent doses can be determined for the desired respiratory effect, other effects may have different and far-reaching consequences. By any criteria, the doses of dexamethasone historically used to treat or prevent BPD have been very high. Basal endogenous cortisol production in preterm infants is estimated to be about 4 to 7 mg/m^2/day during the first month of life, or about 0.4 to 0.7 mg/day in a 1 kg infant (51). If the potency of dexamethasone is estimated to be 25 to 50 times that of hydrocortisone, a dose of 0.5 mg/kg/day of dexamethasone would be roughly equivalent to 12.5 to 25 mg/kg/day hydrocortisone, or from about 15 to more than 60 times the basal cortisol production rate. Equivalent doses administered to fetal and neonatal animals consistently result in global growth failure and reduced organ weights, as well as decreased brain volume, DNA synthesis, and hippocampal granule cell genesis (52–54). The "low-dose" dexamethasone of 0.1 to 0.15 mg/kg/day studied by several groups of investigators is still equivalent to at least 2.5 and perhaps more than 7.5 mg/kg/day of hydrocortisone, or up to 10 times estimated endogenous production rates (51). Whatever dose of dexamethasone may be chosen, the possible adverse effects of dexamethasone on suppression of endogenous cortisol production are still of concern. Several glucocorticoid preparations do include some mineralocorticoid effect; however, as described above, the effects of any synthetic agent may vary greatly in unpredictable ways. Therefore, the agent least likely to result in unanticipated glucocorticoid effects is hydrocortisone, which, when hydrolyzed, is biologically indistinguishable from native cortisol (37). Although many hydrocortisone preparations contain preservative, unpreserved forms are available and should be used for newborns.

To specifically consider, then, the question of what would constitute "low-dose" hydrocortisone therapy, it seems reasonable to first consider the expected physiological cortisol production rate. Basal cortisol production in humans appears to be somewhat lower than estimated with previous techniques, and to be similar in preterm infants, children, and adults, at about 4.0 to 7.0 mg/m^2/day (51,55,56). Cortisol production should increase in response to stress or illness; however, the calculation of an appropriate hydrocortisone dose for premature infants is difficult. Preliminary pharmacokinetic data indicate that exogenous hydrocortisone has a prolonged and variable serum half-life in this population in the first postnatal week, compared with other patient populations (57,58). While postnatal maturation is likely to shorten the serum half-life, at the time of this writing, no data are available regarding hydrocortisone pharmacokinetics after the first week of life; therefore, assessment of serum cortisol values may be a reasonable method to determine the appropriate dose for an individual patient.

A large randomized trial in ELBW infants during the first week of life found that a hydrocortisone dose of 1 mg/kg/day divided q 12 hours resulted in an average increase in serum cortisol concentration of 5 µg/dL compared with placebo at the end of the first week of life (18.4 vs. 13.0 µg/dL) (59). This is consistent with another study showing that a continuous IV infusion of 1 mg/kg/day of hydrocortisone in preterm infants less than 30 weeks' gestation resulted in an average increase of 14 µg/dL in cortisol concentrations at 24 hours, which decreased to a difference of 7.7 µg/dL by 48 hours and 4.1 µg/dL by 72 hours (22.5 vs. 18.4 µg/dL) (60). These data suggest that three times the estimated basal production rate, or 1 to 2 mg/kg/day in a 1 kg infant, may provide a good starting point for dosing in the first week of life. With maturation of metabolic pathways and renal function after the first week of life, a higher dose may be needed; however, no data are available to answer this question.

V. Evidence Regarding Effects of Low-Dose Glucocorticoids

A. Cohort Studies

One reason for the current reluctance to use glucocorticoid therapy for BPD has been the publication of cohort studies linking *any* postnatal dexamethasone exposure to adverse long-term neurodevelopmental outcomes, both functional and structural. The NICHD Neonatal Research Network, for example, correlated postnatal glucocorticoid treatment for BPD (almost universally dexamethasone) with neurodevelopmental impairment at 18 to 22 months corrected age (61), and a small MRI study correlated typical high-dose dexamethasone treatment with decreased cortical gray matter and cerebral tissue volumes (62). In addition, a study of MRIs performed at term-equivalent age in infants treated with lower-dose dexamethasone (a mean total dose of 2.8 mg/kg) found that even at these lower doses dexamethasone correlated with reductions in total cerebral tissue, subcortical gray matter, and cerebellar volume (63), suggesting that there is no "safe dose" for dexamethasone in the preterm infant.

Although this conclusion may well be valid, it cannot be proven by cohort studies. Cohort studies of postnatal glucocorticoids, as for any therapeutic intervention, are likely to be fatally confounded by unknown variables. Unlike diagnoses, which can be objectively measured and consistently applied within a cohort, the clinical decision to administer a therapy may incorporate numerous factors unlikely to be effectively captured on data forms. Thus, cohort studies of therapeutic interventions cannot be considered evidence of effect, only evidence of the clinician's overall assessment of illness. One cannot be surprised that the infants receiving dexamethasone for BPD—particularly after publication of adverse neurodevelopmental outcomes and the joint statement from the AAP and CPS in 2002 (13,14) —are the sickest infants, as perceived by the clinical care team, and therefore most likely to have worse overall outcomes. Similarly, a very large cohort study found that VLBW infants who received postnatal steroids, primarily hydrocortisone, for hypotension had a significantly higher incidence of intraventricular hemorrhage, PVL, and death than those not treated (64). The authors conclude that these outcomes are likely related to the underlying hypotension, but recommend caution in the use of hydrocortisone for hypotension (64). The question of whether glucocorticoid therapy contributes to those adverse outcomes cannot be answered by such studies, but only by RCTs.

Because, as described above, uncontrolled cohort studies often find an association between a therapeutic intervention and adverse outcomes, a treatment cohort that does as well as its less ill control group is noteworthy. A group of investigators retrospectively compared a cohort of infants at one hospital who were treated with hydrocortisone starting about two weeks of age for BPD (5–1 mg/kg taper over 22 days) and a separate cohort at a different hospital treated with dexamethasone (0.5–0.1 mg/kg taper over 21 days), each to a separate control group at their respective hospitals. They found that hydrocortisone and dexamethasone were equally effective in reducing oxygen dependence (65). At 5 to 7 years of age, however, the children treated with hydrocortisone were similar to their control group in neurological outcome and school performance, whereas those treated with dex-amethasone had an increased incidence of abnormal neurological outcome and need for special education services (65). In an extended study from the same institution, inves-tigators compared neurodevelopmental outcome and MRI findings at school age in 62 infants treated with hydrocortisone with 164 larger, more mature preterm infants, and found no long-term effects on either neurodevelopment or MRI lesions (66).

B. Randomized Trials of Low-Dose Hydrocortisone for BPD

Randomized trials of low-dose hydrocortisone for BPD remain quite limited and include three small studies of 40, 50, and 51 infants and one larger multicenter trial which enrolled 360 patients (59,67–69). The last three studies were halted because of a sig-nificant increase in spontaneous gastrointestinal perforation in hydrocortisone-treated infants in the larger multicenter trial (59). The increase in incidence of this adverse event was seen in those infants who also received indomethacin or ibuprofen shortly after birth—although this finding must be interpreted cautiously, as these therapies were not randomized—and to occur primarily in infants who had significantly higher cortisol concentrations before study randomization (59,69). The association with indomethacin is consistent with a very large clinical dataset, in which early postnatal indomethacin was independently associated with the development of spontaneous ileal perforation (70). Animal studies of the effects of indomethacin and dexamethasone in newborn mice suggest that the apparent synergism of indomethacin and glucocorticoid for spontaneous ileal perforation may be due to simultaneous inhibition of several isoforms of nitric oxide synthase (NOS). Indomethacin was found to inhibit endothelial NOS, whereas dexamethasone inhibited inducible and neuronal NOS (71). This combination of drugs should be avoided if possible, particularly in the first postnatal days.

The first RCT was a pilot study comparing hydrocortisone, started at less than 48 hours postnatal age and continued for 12 days (0.5 mg/kg q 12 hours for 9 days, then half that dose for 3 days), to placebo in 40 intubated ELBW infants at two centers (67). The hydrocortisone-treated group showed a significant improvement in the primary outcome of survival without BPD at 36 weeks' gestation (60% vs. 35% placebo). This study addi-tionally reported that histological chorioamnionitis was a significant risk factor for adverse outcome, and that hydrocortisone treatment appeared to particularly benefit chorioamnio-nitis-exposed infants (67). Two other small RCTs were planned as larger studies, but stopped early for concern of spontaneous gastrointestinal perforation reported in the larger multicenter trial. One employed the same dosing regimen as the first study, randomized 50 patients and reported similar results for the primary outcome, a significant increase in survival without supplemental oxygen at 36 weeks (64% vs. 32%) (68). The other enrolled

51 infants between 501 and 1250 g birth weight, mechanically ventilated at <24 hours of age, and administered a 10-day course of hydrocortisone (2–0.75 mg/kg/day taper) or placebo (69). These investigators also found a trend toward decreased BPD in the hydrocortisone-treated group (28% vs. 42% in the placebo group), and reported that infants with low serum cortisol concentrations appeared to derive more benefit from the therapy.

The multicenter RCT enrolled 360 infants at 9 centers, treating for 15 days (1 mg/kg/day for 12 days and 0.5 mg/kg/day for 3 days). This trial had two primary endpoints: (*i*) survival without BPD at 36 weeks' gestational age and (*ii*) neurodevelopmental outcome at 18 to 22 months corrected age, specifically cerebral palsy, since the incidence of CP may be increased following dexamethasone therapy (13). No difference was found in survival without BPD at 36 weeks' gestational age between study groups; however, in those infants exposed to histological chorioamnionitis, defined as a priori group of interest and diagnosed by central readers, hydrocortisone treatment significantly decreased mortality and improved survival without BPD. With the exception of the increase in spontaneous gastrointestinal perforation discussed above, no short-term adverse effects were found (59).

Neurodevelopmental outcomes were assessed at 18 to 22 months corrected age in 87% of survivors (72). Diagnosis of cerebral palsy was similar between groups (13% treated vs. 14% placebo). Fewer hydrocortisone-treated infants had a Mental Development Index (MDI) more than two standard deviations below the mean (<70) as assessed by the Bayley Scales of Infant Development-II, and more of the hydrocortisone-treated infants showed evidence of awareness of object permanence, an early indicator of prefrontal cortex development (73). Incidence of neurodevelopmental impairment, defined as cerebral palsy, MDI <70, Psychomotor Developmental Index <70, functional blindness, or functional deafness was similar between groups (39% vs. 44% placebo).

One additional RCT used hydrocortisone in conjunction with thyroid hormone, for possible synergy (60). In this study, 253 infants were randomized to placebo or to T3 (6 µg/kg/day) and hydrocortisone (1 mg/kg/day continuous IV infusion) for the first seven postnatal days, with the doses being halved after five days. The authors found no effect of this treatment on death or pulmonary outcomes, including BPD defined as receiving supplemental oxygen at 36 weeks' gestation. From previous work regarding cortisol concentrations over time in infants developing BPD, this course of therapy may have been too short (32,35,36). Of interest, these authors reported a bimodal association between cortisol concentration and outcome, such that infants in the highest or lowest quintile had an increase in death or mechanical ventilation at one week of life (60). This finding is consistent with the observations of others that preterm infants with very low cortisol values had an increased mortality (74), and that those with very high cortisol values had an increase in mortality, severe intraventricular hemorrhage, and other adverse outcomes (33,75).

VI. Current Status and Future Directions

Outcomes from these randomized trials suggest that early low-dose hydrocortisone may decrease BPD in infants at very high risk, particularly for those exposed to prenatal inflammation. Cohort studies also suggest that later somewhat higher dose therapy may facilitate extubation and earlier weaning from oxygen without adverse neuro-developmental effects, a finding that has yet to be confirmed in a randomized trial. These studies found no evidence of adverse neurodevelopmental effects from hydro-cortisone therapy given either during the first postnatal week or later in life. This evidence is limited, and not definitive. Further randomized trials of both early therapy for prevention of BPD and later treatment to facilitate extubation are clearly needed to confirm or refute the short- and long-term benefits reported. As the authors of the first reported clinical trial of dexamethasone said in 1983, "the treatment cannot be recommended without further study of patient selection, dosage schedules, short and long-term side effects, and the mechanisms of its action" (6).

Pending the results of such trials, if the clinician is considering glucocorticoid therapy to facilitate extubation in a patient on high ventilator settings, the evidence presented in this chapter would suggest using hydrocortisone, rather than dexamethasone at any dose. The one previously reported starting dose of 5 mg/kg/day, equivalent to perhaps 0.1 to 0.2 mg/kg/day of dexamethasone, may be reasonable (65). However, considering our limited knowledge of outcomes and the wish to avoid suppression of the hypothalamic-pituitary-adrenal axis, therapy should be limited to as short a course as possible. For example, a dosing schedule similar to the DART study would begin with 5 mg/kg/day hydrocortisone divided q 12 hours for two to three days (15). Extubation can then be attempted; if successful, the dose could be halved for 2 days (2.5 mg/kg/day q 12 hours), halved again for 2 days (1.25/mg/kg/day divided q 12 hours), then given as a once daily dose of 0.5 mg/kg for 2 to 3 days, stopping within 10 days and observing closely for signs of adrenal insufficiency. If extubation is not successful, hydrocortisone can be discontinued after reintubation.

Considering the history of dexamethasone and BPD, the question could be asked, "Should we continue to consider glucocorticoids at all for this disease?" BPD continues to be a leading morbidity of preterm infants, and is a major risk factor for adverse outcomes (10,61,76). The disease has proven remarkably resistant to all therapeutic interventions, and the incidence has not decreased over the last decade (10,76). Indeed, one preliminary report from a database including almost 100,000 infants found that the decrease in use of postnatal dexamethasone for BPD from 1997 to 2006 coincided with an increase in the incidence of severe BPD (defined as positive pressure at 36 weeks' gestational age) in infants <30 weeks' gestation (77). There is good theoretical basis and evidence of efficacy for glucocorticoid therapy for the prevention or treatment of BPD, as outlined in this chapter, whereas other anti-inflammatory medications, such as indomethacin, have shown no utility in this regard (78).

Thus, continued study of glucocorticoids for BPD appears to be warranted. Reviewing the CNS effects of synthetic glucocorticoids versus hydrocortisone, future studies should employ either a less-powerful synthetic agent with some mineralocorticoid activity or, probably more appropriately, hydrocortisone. Which patients to treat, with what dose, and for how long is still not clear, as is the question of how to appropriately monitor dosing. All these questions should be answered within the framework of RCTs that include assessment of long-term outcomes, learning from rather than repeating the experience of high-dose dexamethasone therapy.

References

1. Merritt TA, Cochrane CG, Holcomb K, et al. Elastase and alpha 1-proteinase inhibitor activity in tracheal aspirates during respiratory distress syndrome. Role of inflammation in the pathogenesis of bronchopulmonary dysplasia. J Clin Invest 1983; 72:656–666.
2. Ogden BE, Murphy SA, Saunders GC, et al. Neonatal lung neutrophils and elastase/proteinase inhibitor imbalance. Am Rev Respir Dis 1984; 130:817–821.
3. Kramer LI, Hultzen C. The role of steroids in early bronchopulmonary dysplasia (abstract). Pediatr Res 1978; 12:564A.
4. Pomerance JJ, Puri AR. Treatment of neonatal bronchopulmonary dysplasia with steroids (abstract). Pediatr Res 1980; 14:649A.
5. Hearne AB. Bronchopulmonary dysplasia: treatment success with dexamethasone. J Natl Med Assoc 1982; 74:795–800.
6. Mammel MC, Johnson DE, Green TP, et al. Controlled trial of dexamethasone therapy in infants with bronchopulmonary dysplasia. Lancet 1983; 1(8338):1356–1358.
7. Avery GB, Fletcher AB, Kaplan M, et al. Controlled trial of dexamethasone in respirator-dependent infants with bronchopulmonary dysplasia. Pediatrics 1985; 75:106–111.
8. Cummings JJ, D'Eugenio DB, Gross SJ. A controlled trial of dexamethasone in preterm infants at high risk for bronchopulmonary dysplasia. N Engl J Med 1989; 320:1505–1510.
9. Halliday HL, Ehrenkranz RA, Doyle LW. Early postnatal (<96 hours) corticosteroids for preventing chronic lung disease in preterm infants. Cochrane Database Syst Rev 2003; (1): CD001146.
10. Walsh MC, Yao Q, Horbar JD, et al. Changes in the use of postnatal steroids for bronchopulmonary dysplasia in 3 large neonatal networks. Pediatrics 2006; 118:e1328–e1335.
11. Halliday HL, Ehrenkranz RA, Doyle LW. Moderately early (7–14 days) postnatal corticosteroids for preventing chronic lung disease in preterm infants. Cochrane Database Syst Rev 2003; (1):CD001144.
12. Halliday HL, Ehrenkranz RA, Doyle LW. Delayed (>3 weeks) postnatal corticosteroids for chronic lung disease in preterm infants. Cochrane Database Syst Rev 2003; (1):CD001145.
13. Barrington KJ. The adverse neuro-developmental effects of postnatal steroids in the preterm infant: a systematic review of RCTs. BMC Pediatr 2001; 1:1 [Epub 2001, Feb 27].
14. American Academy of Pediatrics Committee on Fetus and Newborn, Canadian Paediatric Society Fetus and Newborn Committee. Postnatal corticosteroids to treat or prevent chronic lung disease in preterm infants. Pediatrics 2002; 109:330–338.
15. Doyle LW, Davis PG, Morley CJ, et al., DART Study Investigators. Low-dose dexamethasone facilitates extubation among chronically ventilator-dependent infants: a multicenter, international, randomized, controlled trial. Pediatrics 2006; 117:75–83.
16. Doyle LW, Davis PG, Morley CJ, et al., DART Study Investigators. Outcome at 2 years of age of infants from the DART study: a multicenter, international, randomized, controlled trial of low-dose dexamethasone. Pediatrics 2007; 119:716–721.
17. Doyle LW, Halliday HL, Ehrenkranz RA, et al. Impact of postnatal systemic corticosteroids on mortality and cerebral palsy in preterm infants: effect modification by risk for chronic lung disease. Pediatrics 2005; 115:655–661.
18. Coalson JJ. Pathology of bronchopulmonary dysplasia. Semin Perinatol 2006; 30:179–184.
19. Watterberg KL, Demers LM, Scott SM, et al. Chorioamnionitis and early lung inflammation in infants in whom bronchopulmonary dysplasia develops. Pediatrics 1996; 97:210–215.
20. Watterberg KL, Scott SM, Backstrom C, et al. Links between early adrenal function and respiratory outcome in preterm infants: airway inflammation and patent ductus arteriosus. Pediatrics 2000; 105:320–324.
21. Kunzmann S, Speer CP, Jobe AH, et al. Antenatal inflammation induced TGF-beta1 but suppressed CTGF in preterm lungs. Am J Physiol Lung Cell Mol Physiol 2007; 292:L223–L231.

22. Cooper MS, Stewart PM. Adrenal insufficiency in critical illness. J Intensive Care Med 2007; 22:348–362.
23. Marik PE, Pastores SM, Annane D, et al., American College of Critical Care Medicine. Recommendations for the diagnosis and management of corticosteroid insufficiency in critically ill adult patients: consensus statements from an international task force by the American College of Critical Care Medicine. Crit Care Med 2008; 36:1937–1949.
24. Mesiano S, Jaffe RB. Developmental and functional biology of the primate fetal adrenal cortex. Endocr Rev 1997; 18:378–403.
25. Flower RJ, Parente L, Persico P, et al. A comparison of the acute inflammatory response in adrenalectomised and sham-operated rats. Br J Pharmacol 1986; 87:57–62.
26. Nadeau S, Rivest S. Glucocorticoids play a fundamental role in protecting the brain during innate immune response. J Neurosci 2003; 23:5536–5544.
27. Papanicolaou DA, Tsigos C, Oldfield EH, et al. Acute glucocorticoid deficiency is associated with plasma elevations of interleukin-6: does the latter participate in the symptomatology of the steroid withdrawal syndrome and adrenal insufficiency? J Clin Endocrinol Metab 1996; 81:2303–2306.
28. Keh D, Boehnke T, Weber-Cartens S, et al. Immunologic and hemodynamic effects of "low-dose" hydrocortisone in septic shock: a double-blind, randomized, placebo-controlled, crossover study. Am J Respir Crit Care Med 2003; 167:512–520.
29. Scott SM, Watterberg KL. Effect of gestational age, postnatal age, and illness on plasma cortisol concentrations in premature infants. Pediatr Res 1995; 37:112–116.
30. Huysman MW, Hokken-Koelega AC, De Ridder MA, et al. Adrenal function in sick very preterm infants. Pediatr Res 2000; 48:629–633.
31. Ng PC, Lee CH, Lam CW, et al. Transient adrenocortical insufficiency of prematurity and systemic hypotension in very low birth weight infants. Arch Dis Child Fetal Neonatal Ed 2004; 89:F119–F126.
32. Watterberg KL, Scott SM. Evidence of early adrenal insufficiency in babies who develop bronchopulmonary dysplasia. Pediatrics 1995; 95:120–125.
33. Korte C, Styne D, Merritt TA, et al. Adrenocortical function in the very low birth weight infant: improved testing sensitivity and association with neonatal outcome. J Pediatr 1996; 128:257–263.
34. Banks BA, Stouffer N, Cnaan A, et al., North American Thyrotropin-Releasing Hormone Trial Collaborators. Association of plasma cortisol and chronic lung disease in preterm infants. Pediatrics 2001; 107:494–498.
35. Watterberg KL, Gerdes JS, Cook KL. Impaired glucocorticoid synthesis in premature infants developing chronic lung disease. Pediatr Res 2001; 50:190–195.
36. Watterberg KL, Shaffer ML, Garland JS, et al. Effect of dose on response to adrenocorticotropin in extremely low birth weight infants. J Clin Endocrinol Metab 2005; 90:6380–6385.
37. Schimmer BP, Parker KL. Adrenocorticotropic hormone; adrenocortical steroids and their synthetic analogs; inhibitors of the synthesis and actions of adrenocortical hormones. In: Hardman JG, Limbird LE, Goodman Gilman A, eds. Goodman and Gilman's the Pharmacological Basis of Therapeutics. 10th ed. New York: McGraw-Hill, 2001:1649–1677.
38. Meikle AW, Tyler FH. Potency and duration of action of glucocorticoids: effects of hydrocortisone, prednisone and dexamethasone on human pituitary-adrenal function. Am J Med 1977; 63:200–207.
39. Charles B, Schild P, Steer P, et al. Pharmacokinetics of dexamethasone following single-dose intravenous administration to extremely low birth weight infants. Dev Pharmacol Ther 1993; 20:205–210.
40. Lugo RA, Hahata MC, Menke JA, et al. Pharmacokinetics of dexamethasone in premature neonates. Eur J Clin Pharmacol 1996; 49:477–483.

41. Czock D, Keller F, Rasche FM, et al. Pharmacokinetics and pharmacodynamics of systemically administered glucocorticoids. Clin Pharmacokinet 2005; 44:61–98.
42. Buttgereit F, Brand MD, Burmester GR. Equivalent doses and relative drug potencies for non-genomic glucocorticoid effects: a novel glucocorticoid hierarchy. Biochem Pharmacol 1999; 15(58):363–368.
43. Lee BH, Stoll BJ, McDonald SA, et al., National Institute of Child Health and Human Development Neonatal Research Network. Neurodevelopmental outcomes of extremely low birth weight infants exposed prenatally to dexamethasone versus betamethasone. Pediatrics 2008; 121:289–296.
44. Baud O, Foix-L'Helias L, Kaminski M, et al. Antenatal glucocorticoid treatment and cystic periventricular leukomalacia in very premature infants. N Engl J Med 1999; 341:1190–1196.
45. André P, Thébaud B, Odièvre MH, et al. Methylprednisolone, an alternative to dexamethasone in very premature infants at risk of chronic lung disease. Intensive Care Med 2000; 26:1496–1500.
46. Baud O, Laudenbach V, Evrard P, et al. Neurotoxic effects of fluorinated glucocorticoid preparations on the developing mouse brain: role of preservatives. Pediatr Res 2001; 50: 706–711.
47. De Kloet RE, Vreugdenhil E, Oitzl MS, et al. Brain corticosteroid receptor balance in health and disease. Endocrine Rev 1998; 19:269–301.
48. McEwen BS. The brain is an important target of adrenal steroid actions: a comparison of synthetic and natural steroids. Ann N Y Acad Sci 1997; 823:201–213.
49. Sloviter RS, Sollas AL, Neubort S. Hippocampal dentate granule cell degeneration after adrenalectomy in the rat is not reversed by dexamethasone. Brain Res 1995; 682:227–230.
50. Hassan AHS, von Rosenstiel P, Patchev VK, et al. Exacerbation of apoptosis in the dentate gyrus of the aged rat by dexamethasone and the protective role of corticosterone. Exp Neurol 1996; 140:43–52.
51. Heckmann M, Hartmann MF, Kampschulte B, et al. Cortisol production rates in preterm infants in relation to growth and illness: a noninvasive prospective study using gas chromatography-mass spectrometry. J Clin Endocrinol Metab 2005; 90:5737–5742.
52. Howard E. Reductions in size and total DNA of cerebrum and cerebellum in adult mice after corticosterone treatment in infancy. Exp Neurol 1968; 22:191–208.
53. Howard E, Benjamin JA. DNA, ganglioside and sulfatide in brains of rats given corticosterone in infancy, with an estimate of cell loss during development. Brain Res 1975; 92:73–87.
54. Bohn MC. Granule cell genesis in the hippocampus of rats treated neonatally with hydrocortisone. Neuroscience 1980; 5:2003–2012.
55. Linder BL, Esteban NV, Yergey AL, et al. Cortisol production rate in childhood and adolescence. J Pediatr 1990; 117:892–896.
56. Brandon DD, Isabelle LM, Samuels MH, et al. Cortisol production rate measurement by stable isotope dilution using gas chromatography-negative ion chemical ionization mass spectrometry. Steroids 1999; 64:372–378.
57. Watterberg KL, Cook K, Gifford KL. Pharmacokinetics of hydrocortisone in extremely low birth weight infants in the first week of life (abstract). Pediatr Res 2002; 52:713–719.
58. Watterberg KL, Shaffer MS, the PROPHET study group. Cortisol concentrations and apparent serum half-life during hydrocortisone therapy in extremely low birth weight infants (abstract). E-PAS 2005; 57:1501.
59. Watterberg KL, Gerdes JS, Cole CH, et al. Prophylaxis of early adrenal insufficiency to prevent bronchopulmonary dysplasia: a multicenter trial. Pediatrics 2004; 114:1649–1657.
60. Biswas S, Buffery J, Enoch H, et al. Pulmonary effects of triiodothyronine (T3) and hydrocortisone (HC) supplementation in preterm infants less than 30 weeks gestation: results of the THORN trial—thyroid hormone replacement in neonates. Pediatr Res 2003; 53:48–56.

61. Vohr BR, Wright LL, Poole WK, et al. Neurodevelopmental outcomes of extremely low birth weight infants <32 weeks' gestation between 1993 and 1998. Pediatrics 2005; 116:635–643.
62. Murphy BP, Inder TE, Huppi PS, et al. Impaired cerebral cortical gray matter growth after treatment with dexamethasone for neonatal chronic lung disease. Pediatrics 2001; 107:217–221.
63. Parikh NA, Lasky RE, Kennedy KA, et al. Postnatal dexamethasone therapy and cerebral tissue volumes in extremely low birth weight infants. Pediatrics 2007; 119:265–272.
64. Finer NN, Powers RJ, Ou CH, et al., California Perinatal Quality Care Collaborative Executive Committee. Prospective evaluation of postnatal steroid administration: a 1-year experience from the California Perinatal Quality Care Collaborative. Pediatrics 2006; 117:704–713.
65. van der Heide-Jalving M, Kamphuis PJ, van der Laan MJ, et al. Short- and long-term effects of neonatal glucocorticoid therapy: is hydrocortisone an alternative to dexamethasone? Acta Paediatr 2003; 92:827–835.
66. Rademaker KJ, Uiterwaal CS, Groenendaal F, et al. Neonatal hydrocortisone treatment: neurodevelopmental outcome and MRI at school age in preterm-born children. J Pediatr 2007; 150:351–357.
67. Watterberg KL, Gerdes JS, Gifford KL, et al. Prophylaxis against early adrenal insufficiency to prevent chronic lung disease in premature infants. Pediatrics 1999; 104:1258–1263.
68. Bonsante F, Latorre G, Iacobelli S, et al. Early low-dose hydrocortisone in very preterm infants: a randomized, placebo-controlled trial. Neonatology 2007; 91:217–221.
69. Peltoniemi O, Kari MA, Heinonen K, et al. Pretreatment cortisol values may predict responses to hydrocortisone administration for the prevention of bronchopulmonary dysplasia in high-risk infants. J Pediatr 2005; 146:632–637.
70. Attridge JT, Clark R, Walker MW, et al. New insights into spontaneous intestinal perforation using a national data set: 1. SIP is associated with early indomethacin exposure. J Perinatol 2006; 26:93–99.
71. Gordon PV, Herman AC, Marcinkiewicz M, et al. A neonatal mouse model of intestinal perforation: investigating the harmful synergism between glucocorticoids and indomethacin. J Pediatr Gastroenterol Nutr 2007; 45:509–519.
72. Watterberg KL, Shaffer ML, Mishefske MJ, et al. Growth and neurodevelopmental outcomes after early low-dose hydrocortisone treatment in extremely low birth weight infants. Pediatrics 2007; 120:40–48.
73. Noland JS. The A-not-B task. In: Singer LT, Zeskind PS, eds. Biobehavioral Assessment of the Infant. New York, NY: Guildford Press, 2001:312–322.
74. Scott SM, Cimino DF. Evidence for developmental hypopituitarism in ill preterm infants. J Perinatol 2004; 24:429–434.
75. Aucott SW, Watterberg KL, Shaffer ML, et al., for the PROPHET study group. Do cortisol concentrations predict short term outcomes in extremely low birth weight infants? Pediatrics 2008; 122(4):775–781.
76. Walsh M, Laptook A, Kazzi SN, et al., National Institute of Child Health and Human Development Neonatal Research Network. A cluster-randomized trial of benchmarking and multimodal quality improvement to improve rates of survival free of bronchopulmonary dysplasia for infants with birth weights of less than 1250 grams. Pediatrics 2007; 119: 876–890.
77. Harrison MA, Yoder RH, Clark RH. Time-related changes in steroid use and BPD among infants born at 23–32 weeks gestation (abstract). E-PAS 2008: 634451.10.
78. Schmidt B, Roberts RS, Fanaroff A, et al., TIPP Investigators. Indomethacin prophylaxis, patent ductus arteriosus, and the risk of bronchopulmonary dysplasia: further analyses from the Trial of Indomethacin Prophylaxis in Preterms (TIPP). J Pediatr 2006; 148:730–734.

Index

ACE. *See* Angiotensinconverting enzyme
Acetylated low-density lipoprotein, 169
Acidic fibroblast growth factor, 193
Ac-LDL. *See* Acetylated low-density lipoprotein
Acute pulmonary infections, 217
Acute respiratory distress syndrome (ARDS), 320
Acute vasoreactivity testing (AVT), 354
Adenovirus-mediated VEGF therapy, 157
Adult stem cells, 179
AECI. *See* Type I alveolar epithelial cells
AECII. *See* Type II alveolar epithelial cells
AFGF. *See* Acidic fibroblast growth factor
Airway
  development, 89
    control of, 92
  peristalsis, calcium-driven, 4
  pressure, 70
    extubation, 243
  reactivity, 223
α1-proteinase inhibitor (α1-PI), 137, 372
Alveolar-capillary permeability, 137–138
Alveolar crest formation, 224
Alveolar destruction, 183
Alveolar development
  in air-breathing lung, 70–71
  in sheep fetus, 70
Alveolar hypoplasia
  and airway obstruction, 26
  emphysema due to, 8, 13
  and interstitial fibrosis, 16
  phenotypes, 7
  Shh overexpression and, 18
Alveolarization, 167, 224
  aberrant microvascularization and, 224, 226

[Alveolarization]
  after dexamethasone exposure, 236
  angiogenesis and, 168
  apoptosis during, 8
  areal density of αSMA, 62
  chronic ventilation, 227
  disruption of PDGF-A signaling and, 50
  effects of intra-amniotic endotoxin on, 122
  in elastin fibers, 50
  elastogenesis and alveolar septation, 61–64
  epithelial-endothelial interactions, 68–70
  epithelial sodium channel expression and, 249
  exogenous factors for, 7
  extracellular matrix remodeling in, 66–67
  FGF signaling in, 64–65
  fibroblast proliferation, 61
  gene expression in fibroblasts, 65–66
  hormonal control of, 72–73
  lamb model, 227
  late, 60
  mechanical ventilation and, 217
  mesenchymal-epithelial cell interrelationships, 67–68
  and phenotypic changes Smad3 knockout, 17
  in premature infants, 1
  retardation of postnatal lung, 68
  retinoic acid, in control of, 71–72
  role of mechanical factors in, 70–71
  soluble PDGF-βR and, 192
  steps of, 58
  VEGF signaling for, 69
  vs. alveolar septation, 56–58
Alveolar macrophages, 10, 126, 192, 194

Alveolar oxygen tension (PaO₂), 301,
319–320
Alveolar septation, 61–64
Alveolar stage, 5, 24, 89, 95–96, 147, 152
Aminophylline, 377
Amniotic fluids, 119
Angioblasts, 168
Angiogenesis, 68, 69, 70, 90, 91, 167, 168.
    See also Vasculogenesis
  Ang2 induced during, 150
  EPCs levels and, 173
  failure of, 95
  and lung development, 125
  presence of NO, 94
  regulation by Eph and Ephrins, 92
  transcription factors regulating, 148
  VEGF actions on, 152
Angiopoietin 1 and 2, 66, 92
Angiotensin-converting enzyme, 286
Animal models
  of BPD, 152–154
  BPD-type changes in, 118
  of diaphragmatic hernia, 193
  of fetal lung inflammation, 121–124
  proving EGF ligands, positively
      modulating, 19
  of pulmonary immaturity and, 236
Antenatal corticosteroid effects, 128
Antenatal Uu infection, 139
Antiangiogenic factors, 69–70
Antibiotic treatments, for BPD, 366,
    371, 378
Anti-inflammatory cytokines, 135, 136
Anti-inflammatory effects, 249
Antimacrophage chemokine (anti-MCP-1),
    374
Antioxidant enzymes (AOEs), 105, 293
  expression in lung endothelial cells,
      461–462
  expression in lung epithelial cells,
      459–461
  expression in macrophages and
      mononuclear cells, 462–463
  human clinical trials
    allopurinol, 467
    ascorbic acid (vitamin C), 467–468
    inositol, 468

[Antioxidant enzymes (AOEs)
    human clinical trials]
  NAC, 466
  selenium, 467
  superoxide dismutase, 466–467
  vitamin E, 465–466
Antioxidants, 293
  therapy, 371–372
Aortic endothelial cells, 172
Apoptosis
  control, 66
  of inflammatory neutrophils, 134
  of lung cells, 61
Aquaporin 5, 10
Arterial oxygen saturation, 301–302
Arteriogenesis, 168
Artificial ventilation, 314
Asymptomatic bacterial vaginosis, 366

Bacterial endotoxin, 106
BAL. *See* Bronchoalveolar lavage
Barotrauma
  airway pressure induced, 70, 232
  BPD and, 7, 232
  as determinant of lung injury, 139,
      215, 230
Basic fibroblast growth factor, 193
Bayley scale, 437, 438, 479
β-Amino propionitrile, 63
β-Chemokines, 134
β-Galactoside-binding protein, 66
β-Glucoronidase, 137
BFGF. *See* Basic fibroblast growth factor
Bilateral hearing loss, 242
Birth-associated oxidative stress, 302–305
Blood vessels of developing lung, 5
BM-derived MSCs, 184
BM-derived stem cells
  adult lung injury models, 181
    bleomycin-induced lung fibrosis, 182
    elastase-/smoke-induced emphysema,
        182
    LPS-induced lung injury, 182
    MSCs, gene delivery, 183
  lung, engraftment of, 181
  therapeutic potential, 180

BMP-4. *See* Bone morphogenetic protein 4
BMP signaling, 63
Bombesin-like peptide, 136
Bone marrow-derived cells, 179
Bone marrow stromal cells, 180
Bone morphogenetic protein 4, 11, 42, 43
BPD. *See* Bronchopulmonary dysplasia
BPD therapies, 156–157
Branching morphogenesis
  bottlebrush array, 4
  of bronchi in early mouse embryo lung, 2
  EGF ligands role in, 19
  epithelial-mesenchymal interactions role
    in, 12, 40
  fibronectin role in, 24
  IGF role in, 46
  LN variant for, 23
  in lung explants, 151
  RA signaling downregulation, 25
  regulation by FGF, 14–16, 64
  Spry2 levels and, 43
  TGF-βs inhibitory effects on, 16–17
  VEGF role in, 21
Breathsavers quality, 233
Bronchial circulation, develpoment, 98–99
Bronchial submucosal glands, 9
Bronchoalveolar duct junction, 11
Bronchoalveolar lavage, 285
Bronchodilators, 377
Bronchopulmonary dysplasia (BPD), 1,
    188, 201. *See also* Mechanical
    ventilation
  adhesion molecules
    dystroglycan, 282–283
    L-Selectin, 283
  alveolar collapse during expiration, 297
  animal models, 463–465
  antioxidant systems
    glutathione-*S*-transferases, 283
    microsomal epoxide hydrolases, 283
  and arterial oxygen saturation, 301–302
  baboon model, 225, 226, 243
  benchmarking to reduce, 275–277
  caffeine and, 246–247
  candidate genes, 282, 283, 286, 287, 288
  cellular changes, 192
  chest CT images, 229

[Bronchopulmonary dysplasia (BPD)]
  chest radiographic characteristics of
    infants, 333–335
  chronic lung disease, 267
    premature infants, 178
  clinical associations with, 118–121
  definitions, 229–230, 281, 336
    pulmonary outcomes, 270
  development of, 173, 191
  diagnosis of, 209
  differential diagnosis of, 218
  enzymatic antioxidant defenses and,
    106–107
  epidemiology/pathological
    demographic/perinatal risk factors, 230
    experimental evidence, 231–233
    features of, 223, 224
    neonatal antecedents, 230–231
  evidence-based preventive treatments,
    236
  factors contributing to lung disease, 356
  and fetal lung
    inflammation, 127–128
    postnatal associations, 118
  fetal to neonatal transition, 293–300
  forced flows, 332–333
  genetic susceptibility and environmental
    factors, 281
  high-dose glucocorticoids for, 248
  hyperoxia, 183
  incidence, 226–229, 292
  in infants
    chest radiograph of, 211
    common respiratory disease, 280
    incidence of, 209, 210
  inflammatory mediators
    angiotensin-converting enzyme,
      286–287
    antigen processing 1, 288
    factor VII-323 del/ins promoter
      polymorphism, 287
    human leukocyte antigen-A2, 287–288
    insulin-like growth factor 1, 288
    interferon-γ, 284
    interleukin 4, 284
    interleukin 10, 284
    mannose-binding lectin 2, 284

[Bronchopulmonary dysplasia (BPD)
    inflammatory mediators]
    monocyte chemoattractant protein 1,
        284–285
    surfactant proteins, 285–286
    transforming growth factor β, 285
    tumor necrosis factor, 285
    urokinase, 288
inflammatory processes, 297–298
Jobe's hypothesis, 233
lipid nitration products and, 112
long-term outcomes
    cardiovascular outcomes, 409
    gastroesophageal reflux, 410–411
    growth failure, 410
    hearing problems, 412
    neurodevelopmental problems, 411–412
    pulmonary effects, 406–409
    renal problems, 410
    visual problems, 413
low-dose glucocorticoids, 247–248
lung
    function in, 328–329
    microvascular development in,
        152–156
    volumes, 331–332
mild form, 215–216
    evolution of, 217
    outcome of, 218
MSC therapy, effects of, 183–184
multiple births, 281–282
neonatal mortality, 228
neonatal rat model of, 192
new
    baboon model of, 224–226
    evolution of, 217
    outcome of, 218
NIH consensus definition, 270
nonenzymatic antioxidant defenses
    and, 107
Northway, definition of, 267–268
    continuous measures, 269–271
    oxygen utilization, 268–269
    physiological definition, 271–272
oxygenation of blood during fetal
    transition, 300–305
oxygen requirement, evolution of, 213

[Bronchopulmonary dysplasia (BPD]
    oxygen supplementation during
        resuscitation or adaptation
        maneuvers, 303–305
    oxygen therapy and, 108–109
    pathogenesis of, 280–281, 337
    pathogenic factors, 209
    perinatal/postnatal risk factors, 217
    physiological definition, impact of, 272,
        273
    plethysmographic methods, 331
    postnatal contributions, 233
    prediction, 218–219
        clinical scores, 273–274
        risk scores, 274
    prenatal infection and lung inflammation,
        364–365
    prevention, 233–236
        high-frequency ventilation, 246
        inhaled nitric oxide, 236–242
        nasal continuous positive airway
            pressure, 243–244
        nasal intermittent positive pressure
            ventilation, 245
        permissive hypercapnia, 245
    prevention strategies. *See also* Antibiotic
        treatments, for BPD; Antioxidant
        enzymes (AOEs); Glucocorticoids;
        Inhaled nitric oxide (iNO) therapy;
        Vitamin A treatment
        drug therapies, 366–367
        postnatal interventions, 367–374
        prenatal interventions, 365–367
    preventive treatments
        antioxidants, 249
        antiproteinases, 249
        indomethacin, 249–250
    protein nitration targets and, 111
    protein nitrosation/nitrosylation targets
        and, 111–112
    radiographic development, 211
    raised volume rapid thoracic compression
        (RVRTC) method, 331
    rehospitalization of infants, 405
    relevance for, 60–61
    resistance and compliance of respiratory
        system, 329–330

[Bronchopulmonary dysplasia (BPD)]
respiratory failure, 214
severe form of, 210–212
evolution of, 213–214
outcome of, 214–215
stem cell depletion, 183
structure function measurements in, 336
therapeutic efforts, 210
therapies targeting vascular development,
156–157
treatment, 375–379
vulnerability to ROS/RNS and, 106

Caffeine, 371
Calcitonin gene-related peptide, 9
Canalicular stage, 94–95
Cardiovascular outcomes, in BPD, 409
Cartilage oligomeric protein, 66
Catalase, 107
Cathepsin, 137
Caucasians, 212
Cauterization, 4
CCSP-expressing cells, 11
CD31, markers for endothelium, 91
CD11b expression, 134
CD34-expressing cells, 169
CD68-positive macrophages, 134
CDH. *See* Congenital diaphragmatic hernia
Cell
growth lung distension, influence of,
190–191
types, in lung, 9–10
Cell-cell interactions, 72
Cell-matrix interactions, 72
Cellular and endothelial interaction, 134
CFTR. *See* Cystic fibrosis transmembrane
conductance regulator
CFTR gene. *See* Cystic fibrosis transmem-
brane conductance regulator gene
Cftr gene, 9
CFU-Hill assay, 171
CFU-Hill cells, 173
CFU-Hill colonies, 171
CGMP-specific phosphodiesterase
inhibitor, 378
Chemical adrenalectomy, 475–476

Chemoattractants, 26
Chemokinetic factors, 134
Chemotactic factors, 134
Chorioamnionitis, 119, 232, 371. *See also*
Pulmonary inflammation
fetal inflammation from, 127–128
fetal sheep models of, 125
intra-amniotic endotoxin-induced, 124
and lung inflammation in newborn, 121
as postnatal risk factors, 135
with preterm lung, 120
Chromogranin, 9
Chronic airway injury, 9
Chronic airway obstruction, 1
Chronic lung damage, 208
Chronic lung disease (CLD), 267, 314–315
Chronic obstructive pulmonary disease
(COPD)-like phenotype, 269,
388, 399
Circulating angiogenic cells, 171
Circulating neutrophils, 133
Clara cell protein (CC-10), 136
Clara cells, 10, 11
secretory protein, 374
Clara cell–specific protein, 10
CLD. *See* Chronic lung disease (CLD)
CMV. *See* Conventional mechanical
ventilation
Cochrane systematic reviews, 234–235
Congenital diaphragmatic hernia, 63
Connective tissue growth factor, 125, 195
Continuous positive airway pressure
(CPAP), 271, 298–300
Conventional mechanical ventilation, 246
Corticosteroids, 127
Cortisol deficiency, 247
CPAP. *See* Continuous positive airway
pressure (CPAP)
"CPAP or Intubation" (COIN) study, 244
CTGF. *See* Connective tissue growth factor
Cyclin-dependent kinase inhibitor, 189
Cyotokines, 26
Cysteine-rich 61 gene (cyr61/CCN1),
297–298
Cystic fibrosis, 378
transmembrane conductance regulator
gene, 4, 183

Cytochrome P450 monooxygenase
    system, 108
Cytochrome P450 reductase, 10
Cytomegalovirus, 216

Detoxification, 10
Diuretics, 376–377
Dizygotic twins, 282
DNA dye Hoechst 33342, 183
DNA synthesis, 189, 197
Dual oxidases *(DUOX 1, 2),* 109
Dysmorphic microvascular network, 280
Dysplasia, 1
DZ twins. *See* Dizygotic twins

Early blood vessel development, control,
    92–94
Early lung development, 2
  airway peristalsis, 4
  coupling of endothelia with, 4–5
  distal airway branching, complexities of,
    2–4
  genes controlling induction, 2
  hydraulic pressure, impact of, 4
EC. *See* Endothelial cells; Epithelial cells
ECM. *See* Extracellular matrix
EGF. *See* Epidermal growth factor
EGFR. *See* Epidermal growth factor receptor
Elastic fibers, 60
  in developing lung parenchyma, 62
  formation, 62–63
Elastogenesis, 61–64
Electrocardiograms (ECG), 352
EMAP II. *See* Endothelial monocyte-
    activating polypeptide II
Embryonic lung development, 4
Embryonic stem cells, 179
Emphysema-like alveolar destruction, 1
Endogenous NO formation, 110
Endothelial cells, 146
  blood vessels, 167
  characteristics of, 167–168
  mesodermal precursors, 167
Endothelial colony-forming cells, 172
Endothelial monocyte-activating
    polypeptide II, 69, 95, 151

Endothelial nitric oxide synthase, 45, 94,
    96, 99, 110, 152, 156
Endothelial precursor cells, 167
  and BPD, 173
  capillary tubules, 168
  culture of, 170–172
  lung injury, 173
  plating MNCs, 171
  source of, 172
Endothelial progenitor cells, 169–170
Endothelial-specific proteins, 170
Endothelin (ET-1), 100
Endothelium signals, 4
Endotoxin, 126, 374
Endotoxin-induced chorioamnionitis model,
    127
Engrafted marrow cells, 180
ENOS. *See* Endothelial nitric oxide
    synthase
ENOS-deficient mice, 237
Enzymatic antioxidant activity, in
    premature infants, 295
EPCs. *See* Endothelial precursor cells
Epidermal growth factor, 49, 188, 191–192
  receptor, 9, 191
Epithelial cells
  apoptosis, 18, 152, 156, 194
  phenotype of, 180
Epithelial overexpression, of IL-1β, 123
Epithelium and mesenchyme, interaction in
    developing lung, 41
Epoprostenol, 359
Erythromycin treatment, 371
Erythropoietin, 301
Escherichia coli, 118
Esophageal manometry, 391
Exogenous NO, 112
  signaling, 113
Exogenous surfactant, 212
  therapy, 210
Extracellular matrix, 11
  and lung development, 21, 23–24
Extrauterine life, adaptation to, 99–100
Extremely low birth weight (ELBW)
    infants. *See also* Premature infants
  lung mechanics, 297
  respiratory adaptation, 296–297

[Extremely low birth weight (ELBW) infants]
  survival, 292
  use of CPAP, 298–300, 302, 317
Extremely low gestational age (ELGA)
  neonates, survival, 292

Fetal blood, oxygen affinity of, 301
Fetal hemoglobin (HbF), 301
Fetal hypoxia, 301
Fetal lung
  inflammation, 127–128
  monocytes, 127
  surfactant maturation, 25–26
Fetal oximetry (FSpO$_2$), 300
FGF-7, growth factor, 40–41
FGF10, expression as growth factor, 11
FGF-7 binding endogenous receptor, 193
Fgf10-expressing progenitor cells, 11
FGF10-FGFR2b-sprouty signaling, 4
FGF-7 protein, 194
FGFR3 and FGFR4, expression, 64
FGFR-2B receptor, 42
Fgfr2IIIb gene, 65
FGFs. *See* Fibroblast growth factors
FGF-10 signaling, 42, 43
Fibroblast
  apoptosis, 59
  growth factors, 40–42, 193
  proliferation, 61
FISH. *See* Fluorescent in situ hybridization
Flk-1 positive cells, 92, 96
Fluid therapy, 1
Fluorescent in situ hybridization, 181
Fos/Jun heterodimer, DNA-binding of,
  189
Foxa2, transcription factor, 2
FRC. *See* Functional residual capacity
Functional residual capacity (FRC), 231,
  296, 330
  measurements, 331

Galectin 1, 66
Gas
  diffusion surface, 1
  exchange function, 1

Gastrin-releasing peptide, 9
Gastroesophageal reflux, in BPD,
  410–411
GATA-6, for activation of lung
  developmental, 2
GATA DNA sequence, 2
Gelatin-coated plates, 171
Genetic predisposition, 233
Gestation, 268
GH. *See* Growth hormone
Glandular hyperplasia, 213
Glucocorticoids, 366–367
  adverse effects, 475–476
  dexamethasone, 472–473
  early, 368–370
  early inhales postnatal, 370
  late inhaled, 376
  late systemic postnatal, 375–376
  low-dose therapy, 473–474, 476–477
    cohort studies, 477–478
    future prospects, 479–480
    randomized trials, 478–479
    risk-benefit ratio, 248
  vs mineralocorticoid activity, 474–475
Glucocorticosteroids
  hormones, 72–73
Glutathione (GSH), reduced, synthesis of,
  293–294
Glutathione (GSH) peroxidases, 107
Glutathione (GSSG), oxidized, 293
Glutathione-*S*-transferases, 283
Glutathione substrate, 249
GM-CSF. *See* Granulocyte macrophage
  colony-stimulating factor
Goblet cell hyperplasia, 9
G polymorphism, 285
Granulocyte macrophage colony-
  stimulating factor (GM-CSF), 126
Group B streptococcus, 118
Growth factors, 138
  expression pattern and receptors, mouse
    lung, 47
  inhibitors of apoptosis, 197
  repair mechanisms and, 138
Growth failure, in BPD, 410
Growth hormone, 73
GSTs. *See* Glutathione-*S*-transferases

Hearing problems, in BPD, 412
Helium (He) dilution technique, 389
Hematopoietic stem cells, 179
Hemoglobin, 301
Hemoglobin (HbA), adult, 301
Heparin-binding growth factor, 196
Heparin sulfate proteoglycan, 49
Hepatocyte growth factor, 68, 69, 141, 193
  expression of, 194
Hepatocyte nuclear factor, 2
HFJV. *See* High-frequency jet ventilation
HFOV. *See* High-frequency oscillatory
  ventilation
HGF. *See* Hepatocyte growth factor
HIF. *See* Hypoxia-inducible factor
High-frequency jet ventilation (HFJV), 246,
  321
High-frequency oscillatory ventilation
  (HFOV), 321
High-proliferative potential EPCs, 172
High-resolution computed tomography
  (HRCT), 334–335
HLA. *See* Human leukocyte antigen
*Hnf-3/Foxa2*b, survival factor for endo-
  derm, 2
Honeycomb-like structure, 1
HOXA5, homeobox transcription factor, 64
HPP-EPCs. *See* High-proliferative potential
  EPCs
HSCs. *See* Hematopoietic stem cells
HSPG. *See* Heparin sulfate proteoglycan
Human angiopoietin (Ang) family, 150
Human BPD, 154–156
Human fetal lung
  electron microscopy, 168
  vascular casting, 168
Human gestation, 224
Human glutathione peroxidase gene, 189
Human leukocyte antigen, 287
Human lung morphogenesis, 3
Human neonatal lung, 1
Human umbilical vein endothelial cells, 171
HUVECs. *See* Human umbilical vein en-
  dothelial cells
Hyaline membrane disease, 1
Hydraulic pressure, 4
Hydrogen peroxide, 107

Hydrogen peroxide–dependent processes,
  105, 110
Hydroxyl radical (HO•), 108
Hyperoxia, 67, 112, 135, 137, 293
Hypoxia, 98
Hypoxia-inducible factor, 21, 93

IGF-1. *See* Insulin-like growth factor 1
IGF-binding proteins, 46
IGFBPs. *See* IGF-binding proteins
IGFs. *See* Insulin-like growth factors
IGF signaling, 46
IL-1 receptor antagonist, 136
Immune modulation, 126–127
Indomethacin, 370
Infants
  birth weight, 245, 280
  BPD incidence in, 209–210
  chest radiograph of BPD in, 211, 216
  common respiratory disease, 280
  dexamethasone-treated, 248
  preterm birth, 224
Inflammation-induced lung maturation, 123
Inflammation-induced tissue injury, 138
Inflammatory cells, 133
Inflammatory cytokines, 106
Inhaled nitric oxide (iNO), 373–374
Inhaled nitric oxide (iNO) for BPD
    prevention, 112
  clinical trials of, 237–242
  lamb model, 237
  in preterm infants, 242
Inhaled nitric oxide (iNO) therapy, 348, 357
  effects on surfactant and cytokine
    functions, 433–436
  follow-up studies, 436–439
  in premature newborns with respiratory
    failure, 429–430
    randomized trials, 430–433
  rationale for use, 427–429
INO. *See* Inhaled nitric oxide
Inositol, 367–368
Insulin-like growth factor 1, 288
Insulin-like growth factors, 46, 192
Interleukin-6 (IL-6), 119
Interstitial lung disease, 1

Intra-amniotic endotoxin, 128
Intraluminal pressure, 4
Intrapulmonary airway branching, 2
Intravenous prostacyclin (PGI₂), 359

Keap-1. *See* Kelch-like ACH-associating protein 1
Kelch-like ACH-associating protein 1, 112
Keratinocyte growth factor, 42, 193
KGF. *See* Keratinocyte growth factor
Kulchitsky cells, 9

Late alveolarization, 59–60
Late-gestation lung 1 *(Lgl1)*, 67
Lefty-1⁻/⁻ mice, 2
Leptin, 68
LGL1 protein, 67
Lipid nitration products, 112
Lipopolysaccharide, 135, 139, 140
  mouse models of, 181
Lipopolysaccharide-binding protein, 126
Low birth weight, 280
Lower respiratory tract infections, 218
Low inspiratory fractions of oxygen (FiO₂),
    297, 299, 301, 304, 305, 317, 349,
    357, 434, 435
LOX activity, 63, 65
LPS. *See* Lipopolysaccharide
Lung
  cell growth, 190
  growth factors in
    connective tissue growth factor, 195
    epidermal growth factor, 191–192
    fibroblast growth factor, 193
    hepatocyte growth factor, 193–194
    insulin-like growth factor, 192
    placental growth factor, concentration
      of, 196
    platelet-derived growth factors, 192–193
    transforming growth factor, 194–195
    transforming growth factor α, 191–192
    vascular endothelial growth factor,
      195–196
  hypoplasia, 212
  injury, 26

[Lung]
  liquid absorption, 25–26
  maturation, 121–123
  microvascular development, 152
  tissue images, 237
Lung development, 1
  formation of secondary septa, 59
  histological stages in, 5
    alveolar septum formation, 8–9
    alveolar stage, 7–8
    canalicular stage, 5–6
    pseudoglandular stage, 5
    terminal sac stage, 7
  molecular mechanisms of, 11–12
    ECM, 21–27
    peptide growth factors, 14–21
    transcription factors, 12–14
  stages of, 225
    and chronology in human species, 57
  vitamin A role in, 236
Lung endothelium, heterogeneity of,
    172–173
Lung function abnormalities, in BPD
  forced expiratory maneuvers, 393–396
  long-term functions, 396–400
  respiratory mechanics, 391–393
  static lung functions, 389–391
Lung vascular development, 146, 168–169
  angiogenesis as sole mechanism of, 147
  hypothesis of, 147
  regulation of, 148–149
    angiopoietin family, 150
    distal epithelial development and,
      150–151
    VEGF, 149–150
  stages of, 147
Lymphatic hypoplasia, 5

Mammalian bombesin, 196
Mannose-binding lectin, 284
Matrix GLA protein, 151
Matrix metalloproteinases, 23, 66, 137
MBL. *See* Mannose-binding lectin
MCP-1. *See* Monocyte chemoattractant
    protein 1
M3E3/C3 cells, 11

Mechanical ventilation, 336–341
  cochrane meta-analyses, 322
  maldistribution of ventilation, 340
  need for, 315–318
  strategies for limiting, 318–319
  techniques, 319–321
Meconium aspiration, 212
Medicare database, 277
Mesenchymal stem cells, 178, 179–180
  adult human, 180
  characteristics of, 180
  gene delivery, 183
  lung diseases, 180
  paracrine effect of, 182
  therapeutic efficacy of, 183
Mesenchyme cell apoptosis, 15, 21
Metalloprotease-9 activity, 137
Metalloproteinases, 137
Methemoglobinemia, 112, 357
Methylxanthines, 377–378
MGP. *See* Matrix GLA protein
Microfibrils, 297
Microsomal enzymes, 283
Microvascular growth
  immature sheep, 226
  and remodeling, 58–59
MIG. *See* Monokine induced by interferon-γ
Mild hypercapnia, 217
Mitochondrial SOD, 106
MMP14 expression, 67
MMP2 expression and activation, 150
Mmp2-null mice, 67
MMPs. *See* Matrix metalloproteinases
MNCs. *See* Mononuclear cells
Monocyte chemoattractant protein 1, 284, 285
Monocyte/macrophage cells, 170
Monokine induced by interferon-γ, 125
Mononuclear cells, 169
Mononuclear phagocyte system, 10
Monozygotic (MZ) twins, 282
Morphogenetic signaling, 4
MSCs. *See* Mesenchymal stem cells
Mucolytic agents, 378
Mucous (goblet) cells, 9
Multiple occlusion technique (MOT), 392
Mycoplasma, 119

Myeloperoxidase, 137
Myofibroblast apoptosis, 194
MZ. *See* Monozygotic (MZ) twins

NADPH oxidase, 109
Na$^+$ ion transporter protein, 9
Na/K ATPase, 26
NAP1. *See* Nucleosome-associated protein-1
Nasal continuous positive airway
  pressure, 243
Nasal intermittent mechanical ventilation
  (NIMV), in preterm infants, 318
Nasal intermittent positive pressure
  ventilation, 245
NCPAP. *See* Nasal continuous positive
  airway pressure
Neoalveolarization, 59–60
Neonatal lung injury, 192
Neonatal mouse hyperoxia model, 183
Neonatal rabbits, hyperoxia protocol, 191
Neonatal rat pups, FGF-7 mRNA content
  of, 194
Neonatal research network, 271
Neonatology, modern, 292
Neurodevelopmental disabilities, 223
Neurodevelopmental health
  outcomes, 242
Neurodevelopmental problems, in BPD,
  411–412
  academic performance, 418–419
  adaptive functioning, 420
  adverse motor outcomes, 419
  brain injury, 421
  cognitive deficits, 418
  impact of environmental stress, 421
  learning disabilities, 418
  medical management, 421–422
  neurosensory outcomes, 417–418
  psychological and socioemotional
    development, 419–420
  speech, language, and communication
    deficits, 419
Neutrophil apoptosis, suppression
  of, 134
Neutrophil elastase, 372
Neutrophil influx, 133

Newborn intensive care units, 223, 274
Newborn lung mechanics, 297
NF-kB. *See* Nuclear factor kappa B
NICHD neonatal network, 209, 227
NICUs. *See* Newborn intensive care units
NIPPV. *See* Nasal intermittent positive
   pressure ventilation
Nitration, 110
Nitric oxide (NO), 105, 293
  pathway, 99
Nitric oxide synthases, 108
Nitrolinoleic acid, 112
Nitrosation, 110
Nitrosative stress, 110
Nitrosylation, 110
3-Nitrotyrosine, 112
NO-dependent oxidation of hemoglobin,
   112
NO-driven toxicity, 112
Nonenzymatic antioxidant defenses, 107
Norrie disease protein *(Ndp),* 66
Northway, definition of, 267–268
NOS2 activity, 110
Nose continuous positive airway pressure
   (nCPAP), 298–300
NO synthases, 105, 110
NOX 4 in epithelial cells, 109
Nuclear factor-erythroid 2-related factor
   (Nrf-2), 112
Nuclear factor kappa B
  activation of, 189
  dependent mechanism, 123
  dependent pathways, 111, 135
  effects of NO inactivation of, 110
  signaling, 126
Nucleosome-associated protein-1, 173
Null mutation of VEGR3, 5

Obstruction of fluid outflow, 4
Osteoactivin, 66
Osteopontin, 66
Oxidative damage, 136–137
Oxidative stress, 105, 106, 109
  sources of, 108
Oxygen therapy, 108–109, 269
Oxygen toxicity, 190, 212, 215

PaCO$_2$. *See* Partial pressure of carbon
   dioxide
PAECs. *See* Pulmonary artery endothelial
   cells
Parathyroid hormone-related protein, 68
Partial pressure of carbon dioxide, 190
Patent ductus arteriosus, 209
PCR. *See* Polymerase chain reaction
PDA. *See* Patent ductus arteriosus
PDGF. *See* Platelet-derived growth factor
PDGF-AA-induced migration of lung
   fibroblasts, 64
PECAM-1 immunostaining, 155
Pentoxifylline, 379
Peptide growth factors
  BMP subfamily, 17–18
  EGF family growth factors, 19–20
  FGF family, 14–16
  IGFs, 20–21
  PDGF, 20
  SHH pathway, 18–19
  TGF-β/BMP Family, 16
  TGF-β subfamily, 16–17
  VEGF isoforms, 21
  Wnt/β-catenin pathway, 19
Peroxidases, 107
Peroxisome proliferator–activated
   receptors, 112
Peroxynitrite (ONOO⁻), 108
Persistent ductus arteriosus (PDA), 370
Persistent pulmonary hypertension of the
   newborn (PPHN), 319
Phagocytic macrophages, 171
PH development, in BPD. *See* Pulmonary
   vascular disease, in BPD
Phosphodiesterase-5 (PDE-5) inhibitor, 357
PIE. *See* Pulmonary interstitial emphysema
PI3 kinase, 64
Pinch-cock valve function, 4
Pitx2 null mutants, 2
PKC. *See* Protein kinase C
Placental growth factor, 196
Platelet-derived growth factor, 20, 49–50,
   188
  isoforms, 50
Platelet-derived growth factor-A, 7, 20,
   64, 71

Platelet endothelial cell adhesion
      molecule-1, 170
PlGF. *See* Placental growth factor
PMA. *See* Postmenstrual age
PMVECs. *See* Pulmonary microvascular
      endothelial cells
Polymerase chain reaction, 119
Polypeptide growth factors, 197
Positive end-expiratory pressure (PEEP)
      levels, in infants, 390
Post hoc analyses, 276
Postmenstrual age, 226, 281
Postnatal risk factors, 135
Postnatal stem cells. *See* Adult
      stem cells
Potassium channel, 189
PPARs. *See* Peroxisome proliferator–
      activated receptors
Premature infants. *See also* Extremely low
      birth weight (ELBW) infants
   with BPD, 124
   forced expiratory flow studies in,
      394–396
   FRC studies in, 391
   respiratory mechanics studies in,
      392–393
Premature infants, effect of iNO therapy in,
      427–429
   on health status, 439
   on neurodevelopmental outcomes,
      436–439
   on pulmonary outcomes, 439
   with respiratory failure, 429–430
   RCTs of, 430–433
   on surfactant function and inflammatory
      cytokines, 433–435
Primitive larynx, 4
Proinflammatory cytokines, 135
Proinflammatory mediators on the fetal
      lung, 123
Prolyl-hydroxylase domain (PHD)-
      containing protein, 96
Pro213ser polymorphism, 283
Prostacyclin (PGI₂), 99
Prostaglandin synthetase inhibitors,
      370–371
Protective antiproteases, 137

Protein
   nitration targets, 111
   nitrosation/nitrosylation targets, 111–112
Proteinase inhibitors, 230, 372
Protein kinase C, 190
Protein tyrosine kinases, 189
Protein tyrosine phosphatases, 189
Proteolytic damage, 136–137
Pseudostratified ciliated columnar cells, 9
PTHrP. *See* Parathyroid hormone-related
      protein
Pulmonary artery endothelial cells, 172
Pulmonary capillaries, 4
Pulmonary capillary wedge (PCWP), 355
Pulmonary edema, 133, 213
Pulmonary homeostasis, 105
Pulmonary hypertension (PH)
   diagnosis of PH, 350–354
   treatment of PH, 355–359
Pulmonary inflammation, 137, 247
   factors inducing
      chorioamnionitis, 138–139
      hyperoxia, 140
      hypoxia, 140
      infection, 139
      mechanical ventilation, 139–140
   glucocorticoids modulating, 247
   initiation of, 137
   mice lacking TGF-β1 and, 16
   neutrophils and macrophages, role in, 133
   overexpression of *Nkx2.1* and, 13
Pulmonary interstitial emphysema, 210
Pulmonary microvascular endothelial
      cells, 172
Pulmonary neuroendocrine cells, 9
Pulmonary neuroepithelial cells, 189
Pulmonary oxygen toxicity, 190
Pulmonary parenchyma, 232
Pulmonary problems, in BPD, 406–409
Pulmonary vascular disease, in BPD
   abnormalities of the pulmonary
      circulation, 348–349
   cardiac catheterization, 354–355
   diagnosis of PH, 350–354
   treatment of PH, 355–359
Pulmonary vascular resistance, 99, 100
Pulmonary vascular smooth muscle cells, 196

Pulmonary veins, 89
  in developing lung, 5
  development, 92
  from eight weeks' gestation, 98
  having eNOS during fetal life, 99
Pulmonary vessels, origin of, 89–91
Pulse oximetry (SpO$_2$), 301
Putative progenitor endothelial cells, 167
PVR. *See* Pulmonary vascular resistance

RA. *See* Retinoic acid
Radiographic abnormalities, 218
Raised volume RTC technique (RVRTC),
  394
RALDH2. *See* Retinaldehyde
  dehydrogenase 2
Rapid thoracoabdominal compression
  technique (RTC), 393
*RAR*b gene–deleted mice, 72
RA receptors, 44, 71
RARs. *See* RA receptors
R52C mutation, 284
RDS. *See* Respiratory distress syndrome
Reactive nitrogen species (RNS), 105, 109,
  191, 293
Reactive oxygen species (ROS), 105, 109, 293
  intra-/intercellular messengers, 188
Receptor frizzled 1 *(Fzd1)*, 66
Recombinant human copper zinc
  superoxide dismutase, 249
Recombinant human deoxyribonuclease, 378
Redox homeostasis, 189
Reduced glutathione (GSH), 293
Renal problems, in BPD, 410
Resident microvascular endothelial
  progenitor cells, 172
Respiratory distress syndrome (RDS), 1,
  133, 208, 224, 267, 281, 317,
  366, 390
Respiratory failure, 219
Respiratory progenitor cells, 10
Respiratory stem cells, 10
Retinaldehyde dehydrogenase 2, 45
Retinoic acid, 7, 45
  in alveolarization control, 71–72
  downregulation, 196

[Retinoic acid]
  to increase number of alveoli, 8
  and lung morphogenesis, 24–25
  receptors, 44
  signaling, 25
  synthesis and degradation system in
    mammals, 24
Retinoids, 2
Retinoid X receptors
  RXRγ, 66
  subtypes, 44, 71
Reversible protein oxidation, 189
RMEPCs. *See* Resident microvascular
  endothelial progenitor cells
RNS. *See* Reactive nitrogen species
ROS. *See* Reactive oxygen species
RSV-IGIV prophylaxis, 378
RXRs. *See* Retinoid X receptors
Ryan risk score, 274

Saccular stage, 95–96
Sacculi, 296
Salbutamol, 370
Schlafen 4, proliferation regulator, 66
Septal elastogenesis, 61–62
SFPTB. *See* Surfactant protein B
SHH. *See* Sonic hedgehog
SHH-deficient lung explants, 151
Shh signaling, 2
Sildenafil, 348, 357
Single BM-derived stem cell, 180
Single-breath occlusion technique (SOT), 392
SMAD proteins, 48
S-Nitrosothiol, 111
SOD. *See* Superoxide dismutase
Sodium cromoglycate, 370
Sonic hedgehog, 42, 44
SP. *See* Surfactant proteins
SP-C. *See* Surfactant protein-C
Spry family of genes, 42–43
"Squeeze" technique, 332
Stem cells
  definition of, 178–179
  embryonic stem cells *vs.* adult stem cells, 179
  plasticity of, 180
  potency, 179

Superoxide, 105
Superoxide dismutase, 106, 249
Surfactants
    protein B, 41–42
    protein-C
        and CC10-expressing cell lineages, 11
        eGFP donor mice, 181
        lamellar bodies, 184
        SftpC, 10
        proteins, 285
        therapy, 367–368
Systolic PAP, 352
Systolic pulmonary artery pressure
        (sPAP), 352

TAP1. *See* Transporter associated with
        antigen processing 1
T1α protein, 10
Tbx4, for ectopic bud formation, 2
Tei index, 354
TGF-β. *See* Transforming growth factor β
TGF-β1. *See* Transforming growth factor β1
Thioredoxin (TRx), 293
Thrombospondin-1, 70
Thyroid hormone, 73
Thyroid transcription factor-1, 68
Thyrotrophin-releasing hormone (TRH), 367
Tie-2 receptor, 91, 93, 98
TIPP. *See* Trial of indomethacin
        prophylaxis in preterms
Tissue stem cell committee, 180
TLC. *See* Total lung capacity
TNF. *See* Tumor necrosis factor
Toll-like receptor (TLR)-2
    mRNA, 297–298
Toll-like receptor (TLR)-4
    agonist endotoxin, 123
    mRNA, 297–298
Total lung capacity, 231
Transcription factors
    forkhead box transcription factor family,
        12–13
    GLI family of zinc finger transcription
        factors, 14
    Nkx and Hox homeodomain transcription
        factors, 13–14

Transforming growth factor
    α, 191–192
    β, 47–48, 138
    β1, 188
Transition to air breathing,
        25–26
Transmission electron micrographs, 227
Transporter associated with antigen
        processing 1, 288
Trial of indomethacin prophylaxis in
        preterms, 250
Tropoelastin, 61, 62, 297
TSP-1. *See* Thrombospondin-1
Tumor necrosis factor, 284
Type I alveolar epithelial cells, 1
Type I epithelial cells, 10
Type II alveolar epithelial cells, 67
    differentiation, 67, 68, 69
    precursor, 70
    proliferation, 68
Type II pneumocytes, 10, 11

Ulex europeus, 171
Ultrasonographic abnormalities, 242
Ureaplasma urealyticum, 119,
        121, 216
    colonization/infection, 231
    fetal models of, 125
    infection, 371
Urokinase, 288
Uteroglobin, 10

Vascular endothelial growth factor
        (VEGF), 4, 45–46, 91, 124,
        168, 195, 349
    expression of, 195
    induced angiogenesis, 150
    in situ hybridization, 155
    overexpression/ectopic expression
        of, 151
    receptor, 5
    regulators, for expression of, 149
    therapy, 27
Vascular hypothesis, basis of, 196
Vascular injury, 124–125

Vasculogenesis, 12, 45, 146, 167, 168
  distal capillaries develop by, 147
  during early embryonic development,
    168
  in epithelial cells of human fetuses, 93
  initiation of, 21
  pulmonary veins develop by, 92
  pulmonary vessels formation de novo
    by, 91
Vasomotor tone, 167
VEGF. *See* Vascular endothelial growth
    factor
Ventilation, optimal zone of, 231
Ventilator-induced lung injury risk, 190
Ventricular hypertrophy, electrocardiogram
    of, 214
Very low birth weight, 280
Vessel wall, development, 96–98
Visual problems, in BPD, 413
Vitamin A, 9, 25, 44, 71, 107, 236. *See also*
    Retinoic acid

Vitamin A treatment, 371
  clinical evidences, 447–450
  role of retinol and metabolites (RA),
    450–454
Vitamin D3–upregulated protein 1
    (VDUP1), 70
VLBW. *See* Very low birth weight
Volutrauma, 135, 232
Von Willebrand factor, 170

Whole-body plethysmography, 389
Wilson–Mikity syndrome, 218
Wnt signaling, 66

Xanthine oxidoreductase, 108
Xenopus noggin (Xnoggin), 43

Zinc finger proteins, 2